The CD no longer accompanies

this book.

CD files can be found at

www.booksupport.wiley.com

where you enter the ISBN

9780470907573

HANDBOOK OF CLINICAL PSYCHOPHARMACOLOGY FOR PSYCHOLOGISTS

HANDBOOK OF CLINICAL PSYCHOPHARMACOLOGY FOR PSYCHOLOGISTS

EDITED BY
*Mark Muse and
Bret A. Moore*

Illustrations by Gloria Frigola

WILEY

John Wiley & Sons, Inc.

Library of Congress Cataloging-in-Publication Data:

    Handbook of clinical psychopharmacology for psychologists / edited by Mark Muse, Bret A. Moore ;
illustrations by Gloria Frigola.
      p. ; cm.
    Includes bibliographical references and index.
    ISBN 978-0-470-90757-3 (cloth/CD-ROM : alk. paper)
    978-1-118-25965-8 (e-bk.)
    978-1-118-23508-9 (e-bk.)
    978-1-118-22123-5 (e-bk.)
      I. Muse, Mark. II. Moore, Bret A.
      [DNLM: 1.—therapeutic use.   2. Mental Disorders—drug therapy.   3. Psychopharmacology—
methods. QV 77.2]
      615.7'88—dc23   2011044482

Printed in the United States of America

SKY10070896_032524

Writing makes the heart grow fonder.

Let us, then, retire the pen,
and return to family and friend.

MARK MUSE
BRET A. MOORE

Contents

Integrating Care:
A Foreword on Changing Times

Patrick H. DeLeon

Former APA President

Jack G. Wiggins

Former APA President

The enactment of President Obama's landmark Patient Protection and Affordable Care Act [PPACA] (P.L. 111-148; Obama, 2009) represents the most significant change in our nation's commitment for providing high-quality health care to all Americans in our lifetime. As this far-reaching legislation is steadily implemented over the next 5 to 10 years, psychology practitioners will come to appreciate in a very personal and concrete way that the President's plan is fundamentally patient-oriented and definitely not provider-centric. Increasing access to primary health care for all citizens, regardless of where they live and their economic and educational status, is one of the Administration's top priorities. In many ways, this is an exciting time for psychology, with its long-held emphasis upon the psychosocial-economic-cultural gradient of care. Over the years, we have learned that change, however, is unsettling for many of our colleagues (DeLeon & Kazdin, 2010).

In these rapidly changing times, psychology must collectively come to appreciate that our profession today is deemed to be one of the "health care professions," which implies biologically based competencies along with our more traditional psychosociocultural proficiencies. Accordingly, we will soon see that our practitioners will no longer be reasonably able to expect to practice within historically comfortable and isolated "silo" environments. We expect that small individual practices will steadily merge into larger interdisciplinary group practices. Effectively demonstrating that one's clinical services make a real difference in the individual patient's daily life and that they meet objective gold standards will become the expected norm. With the systematic application of telehealth, comparative clinical effectiveness research, and virtual therapeutic realities, licensure mobility will become absolutely necessary. Further, with the dramatically increasing numbers of nonphysician providers being trained by other health disciplines, as well as these disciplines' increasing successes in expanding autonomy and their scopes of practice, psychology simply cannot sit by and remain a passive observer of change. To do so is to steadily and increasingly become obsolete and, ultimately, we would suggest, to be replaced by other more visionary disciplines. In the enactment of PPACA, the states and the Administration have been granted considerable flexibility by the Congress to develop innovative approaches to address this national vision for ensuring high quality health care for all Americans. The times are definitely changing (DeLeon, Kenkel, Oliveira Gray, &

Sammons, in press), and are propitious for courageous innovations such as is found in the prescriptive authority (RxP) movement.

Clinical psychopharmacology is not new to the field of psychology. Psychology has a long history of working with patients who are taking psychotropic medications, as clinicians and as consultants to those who prescribe. In 1998 Wiggins and Cummings (1998) reviewed 1 million mental episodes treated at Biodyne over a 4-year period. They found that upon entering psychotherapy at Biodyne, 68% of patients were already taking prescribed psychotropic medications and, further, that patient reliance upon these medications dramatically decreased to 13% after treatment by one of 8,000 psychologists providing the care. The prescriptive authority movement began philosophically back in 1984, with the suggestion by U.S. Senator Daniel K. Inouye to the Hawaii Psychological Association that obtaining this authority would be in their patients' best interest. Programmatically, the RxP quest began with the enactment of relevant legislation in Indiana (1993), Guam (1998), New Mexico (2002), and Louisiana (2004). Legislatively passed RxP bills were subject to a Governor's veto in Hawaii (2007) and Oregon (2010). Today, in approximately one-third (i.e., 16) of the states, the local psychological association has worked with their state licensing boards to expressly clarify that it is within the scope of their practice for psychologists to consult with clients and/or other practitioners regarding the use of psychotropic medications.[1]

Practitioner scope of practice acts are historically determined by state legislatures. However, the federal health care delivery systems have authorized their practitioners to practice based upon local needs, notwithstanding state imposed limitations (e.g., Medex, Alaskan Native dental extenders, and Department of Defense (DoD) medical corps personnel). Within the Indian Health Service (IHS), Floyd Jennings[2] prescribed with standing orders at the Santa Fe Indian Hospital, New Mexico, during the mid-1980s. Quality assurance reviews of the medical records of his 97 cases were quite positive. Similarly, during this time period, a number of individual psychologists reported to APA that they were prescribing within the then-Veterans Administration (VA).

During the Congressional deliberations on the fiscal year 1989 Appropriations bill for the Department of Defense (DoD), the conferees directed the establishment of a demonstration training project under which military psychologists would be trained and authorized to issue appropriate psychotropic medications. In June 1994 Morgan Sammons and John Sexton became the first two graduates of this program, which ultimately trained 10 psychologists. At its August, 1995, meeting in New York City, the Council of Representatives formally endorsed prescription privileges for appropriately trained psychologists after several years of intensive governance deliberation, thus making it APA policy, and called for the development of model legislation and a model training curriculum (Fox, DeLeon, Newman, Sammons, Dunivin, & Baker, 2009).

By the end of 2008, Glenn Ally[3] estimated that he and his colleagues in Louisiana had written more than 200,000 psychotropic medication orders, including refills,

---

[1]http://rxpsychology.com/State_Opinions_on_Consultation.pdf
[2]Floyd Jennings is a retired psychologist with the Indian Health Service who has documented his historic prescribing experience (Jennings, 2010).
[3]Glenn Ally is current president of APA Division 55, American Society for the Advancement of Pharmacotherapy.

orders in hospitals, patients on multiple medications, and orders to reduce, consolidate, and/or discontinue medications. By October 2010, Jim Quillin[4] estimated that there were 51 medical psychologists practicing in Louisiana and 26 licensed prescribing psychologists in New Mexico. The movement by psychology to obtain independent prescriptive authority has continued to expand and mature, with Bob McGrath[5] estimating that by 2011 there were four major training programs in existence (Alliant International University, Fairleigh Dickinson University, New Mexico State University, and Nova Southeastern University) with approximately 1,500 psychologists having completed their formal training (Cautin, Freedheim, & DeLeon, in press).

Bob McGrath and former DoD prescribing psychologist Morgan Sammons[6] very nicely captured the close relationship between systematically learning more about clinical psychopharmacology in depth and, ultimately, obtaining prescriptive authority. "Prescribing psychology and primary care psychology represent complementary paths to re-engineering the future of professional healthcare practice in psychology. The greatest advantage of primary care psychology over prescribing psychology as a goal is its reliance on the traditional tools of the psychologist as a psychosocial care provider, making it more palatable to key audiences within psychology and medicine. Furthermore, it requires no legislative action. On the other hand, prescriptive authority involves service to the same patient population that is most familiar to psychologists. Although the legislative barriers can be daunting, once overcome, the shift in psychologists' roles is inevitable. There is an existing funding stream for medication management that becomes available to psychologists through third-party payers so that the authorized prescribers can quickly create practice opportunities" (McGrath & Sammons, 2011, p. 117).

As the health care market place evolves under PPACA, we expect that the delivery systems that ultimately surface will closely parallel those of President Nixon's envisioned HMOs or the managed care institutions of President Reagan's era. Experiences with the financing and delivery of mental and behavioral health care during those years would suggest that there will be a concerted effort to integrate this care (and, we would suggest, all other care) within multidisciplinary primary health care delivery systems (i.e., federally qualified community health centers and PPACA's accountable care organizations), rather than returning to a time of specialty "carve-outs." From an organizational frame of reference, the care provided will be integrated and team managed with increasingly fewer individual practice options. Within this health care delivery scenario, those psychologists who have obtained additional specialized training in the physical aspects of care will undoubtedly have a distinct advantage (and market place value), both in their understanding of the basic language of their non-mental health colleagues, as well as their having developed an important clinical appreciation for the intimate relationship between the "mind and body" aspects of patient symptoms.

The Institute of Medicine (IOM) was established in 1970 by the National Academy of Sciences to serve as an advisor to the federal government on policy matters pertaining to the health of the public. Reflecting on the underlying broader policy

[4]James Quillin is past president of the Louisiana Academy of Medical Psychology.
[5]Robert McGrath is past president of APA Division 55, and is director of the RxP training program at Fairleigh Dickinson University.
[6]Morgan Sammons is past president of APA Division 55.

issue of the intimate interrelationship between mind and body, the president of the IOM recently stated, "Improving our nation's general health and the quality problems of our general health care system depends upon equally attending to the quality problems in health care for mental and substance-use conditions. The committee calls on primary care providers, other specialty health care providers, and all components of our general health care system to attend to the mental and substance-use health care needs of those they serve. Dealing equally with health care for mental, substance-use, and general health conditions requires a fundamental change in how we as a society and health care system think about and respond to these problems and illnesses. Mental and substance-use problems and illnesses should not be viewed as separate from, and unrelated to, overall health and general health care. Building on this integrated concept . . . the Institute of Medicine will itself seek to incorporate attention to issues in health care for mental and substance-use problems and illnesses into its program of general health studies" (IOM, 2006, p. x).

In our judgment, there can be no question that over the years psychology's training programs have served the profession very well. Our practitioners are extraordinarily well prepared to meet the mental and behavioral health needs of our citizens. We would even suggest that psychology has more relevant training for serving this subset of our population than any other discipline. And this is especially true for those who have obtained advanced clinical psychopharmacological training, frequently at the postdoctoral master's degree level. From our years of service within the APA governance, as presidents of APA and in many other capacities, we have come to appreciate how diverse the interests are within the family of psychology. As educated professionals, we should appreciate the extent to which clinicians strive for lifelong learning experiences. Given the unprecedented discovery of new knowledge every year, within psychology and each of the related disciplines, it is impossible for any practitioner to systematically keep up-to-date on their own. Although we do not believe that it is necessary for every clinician to seek additional training in the physical and physiological aspects of mental and behavioral health care, we are truly impressed by the growing number of colleagues who have sought to obtain this critical expertise, which undoubtedly will be of direct benefit to a significant subset of their patients. Obtaining advanced expertise in clinical psychopharmacology represents state of the art clinical care and, at the same time, increasingly strengthens the foundation for the profession of psychology, which will inevitably lead to legislative recognition of our discipline's prescriptive authority expertise.

The *Handbook of Clinical Psychopharmacology for Psychologists* is a most timely contribution during this era of health care reform. The editors and authors provide the reader unique psychological perspective on the integration of behavioral treatments with pharmacological approaches. Lamentably, it has become commonplace in physicians' offices to dispense psychotropic medications without an appropriate diagnosis and to do so by providers with little or no training in alternative psychological interventions for behavioral disorders. Using psychotropic medications for a wide assortment of psychological complaints has expanded exponentially since medications have been directly advertised to the public. The bombardment of daily advertising of psychotropic drugs has shifted effective behavioral management away from psychotherapy as the first line of specialty care, to palliative care and symptom relief that in some cases amount to little more than placing a pharmacological Band-Aid over a festering wound. The increased use of drug therapy to replace effective psychological treatments has contributed to the inflationary spiral that the Patient Protection and Affordable Care Act is designed to curtail.

Future federal legislation will undoubtedly have a significant impact on how behavioral health care is delivered as well as how behavioral health specialists are trained to provide this needed care. The critical shortage of behavioral health specialists is pandemic and is well known to makers of public policy. Collaboration among professions is one of the stated goals of the PPACA to improve health care delivery for the benefit of patients. Drs. Muse and Moore, as editors, outline innovative perspective and insights in their chapters dealing with current policy issues and useful up-to-date research findings. The *Handbook of Clinical Psychopharmacology for Psychologists* is designed to present the current state of knowledge of the field of clinical psychopharmacology to practitioners of medical psychology. Practitioners will find detailed information they can incorporate in their services, while the very psychobiosocial model implicit in the *Handbook* may very well become a platform for effecting public policy and training in behavioral health care delivery.

Training for RxP is extensive, as reflected in the content of this book. Psychologists who undergo such training are well versed in the psychobiosocial model, and are proficient enough to write their own training manual. The *Handbook of Clinical Psychopharmacology for Psychologists* is an excellent treatise written for psychologists by psychologists; it is not a book written for physicians—though they may well learn from it—nor should it be. RxP is not a mere replication of the medical curriculum; rather, it fulfills the medical curriculum and surpasses it with its own unique emphasis on the integration of biological components within psychosocial aspects of mental health. It is, in fact, a unique integration and one that we believe is superior to the medical model (McGrath & Muse, 2010). The emphasis is on the psychosocial—for we are, after all, psychosocial scientist-practitioners, yet, our competency has been extended to include the bio, and to put it in its proper place.

In summary, the *Handbook of Clinical Psychopharmacology for Psychologists* is a welcome addition to the growing compendium of psychological literature on the treatment of mental conditions by integrating psychosocial treatments with pharmacotherapeutic options.

REFERENCES

Cautin, R. L., Freedheim, D. K., & DeLeon, P. H. (in press). Psychology as a profession. In D. K. Freedheim (Ed.), *History of psychology. Volume 1 of the handbook of psychology* (2nd ed.), I. B. Weiner (Editor in Chief) (pp. 27–45). Hoboken, NJ: Wiley.

DeLeon, P. H., & Kazdin, A. E. (2010). Public policy: Extending psychology's contributions to national priorities. *Rehabilitation Psychology, 55*(3), 311–319.

DeLeon, P. H., Kenkel, M. B., Oliveira Gray, J. M., & Sammons, M. T. (in press). Emerging policy issues for psychology: A key to the future of the profession. In D. H. Barlow (Ed.), *Handbook of clinical psychology*. New York, NY: Oxford University Press.

Fox, R. E., DeLeon, P. H., Newman, R., Sammons, M. T., Dunivin, D., & Baker, D. C. (2009). Prescriptive authority and psychology: A status report. *American Psychologist, 64*, 257–268.

Institute of Medicine (IOM). (2006). *Improving the quality of health care for mental and substance-use conditions: Quality chasm series*. Washington, DC: The National Academies Press.

Jennings, F. (2010). An introduction to prescription privileges for psychologists: A look back to another time. *Archives of Medical Psychology, 1*, 1–13.

McGrath, R. E. & Muse, M. (2010). Room for a new standard: Response to comments by Heiby. *Journal of Clinical Psychology, 66*, 112–115.

McGrath, R. E., & Sammons, M. T. (2011). Prescribing and primary care psychology: Complementary paths for professional psychology. *Professional Psychology: Research and Practice, 42*, 113–120.

Obama, B. (September 9, 2009). *President Obama's Address to a Joint Session of Congress.* The White House Office of the Press Secretary. The Patient Protection and Affordable Care Act [PPACA] [P.L. 111-148] (HR 3590). (March 23, 2010).

Wiggins, J. G., & Cummings, N. A. (1998). National study of the experience of psychologists with psychotropic medication and psychotherapy. *Professional Psychology: Research and Practice, 29*, 549–552.

About the Editors

Mark Muse, EdD, Ldo (PhD), MP, ABPP, completed his MA and doctorate in clinical research and counseling psychology at Northern Arizona University in 1980 and was subsequently awarded the Licentiate degree in clinical psychology by the Universitat de Barcelona (with PhD cquivalence by the Spanish Ministry of Education) in 1984; he later completed the postdoctorate Master of Science degree in clinical psychopharmacology at Fairleigh Dickinson University in 2008. Dr. Muse holds the Diplomate in counseling psychology from the American Board of Professional Psychology and is licensed as a prescribing medical psychologist by the Louisiana State Board of Medical Examiners, as well as licensed by the Maryland Board of Examiners of Psychologists with competency to consult with patients and providers on psychopharmacotherapy. He served as full professor at the Universitat de Ramon Llull, Barcelona, lecturing in Catalan and Spanish, before returning to the United States in 1998, where he maintains a private practice and provides workshops and consultation to non-mental health physicians on how to integrate psychopharmacology into primary care practice. He is the author of six books in the area of psychology as well as numerous articles that have appeared in professional journals of psychology and medicine. Dr. Muse is publisher/editor of MENSANA Publications.

Bret A. Moore, PsyD, MS, ABPP, completed his doctorate in clinical psychology at the Adler School of Professional Psychology, Chicago, IL, and the postdoctorate Master of Science degree in clinical psychopharmacology from Fairleigh Dickinson University, Teaneck, NJ. He is Assistant Professor of Clinical Psychiatry at the University of Texas Health Science Center at San Antonio and Lecturer in the post doctoral Master of Science program in clinical psychopharmacology at Farleigh Dickinson University. He is licensed as a conditional prescribing psychologist by the New Mexico Board of Psychologist Examiners and board-certified in clinical psychology by the American Board of Professional Psychology. He is the author and editor of four other books, including *Pharmacotherapy for Psychologists: Prescribing and Collaborative Roles*, *The Veterans and Active Duty Military Psychotherapy Treatment Planner, Living and Surviving in Harm's Way*, and *Wheels Down: Adjusting to Life After Deployment*. He is currently preparing, with Stephen Stahl, MD, PhD, *Anxiety Disorders: A Concise Guide and Casebook for Psychopharmacology and Psychotherapy Integration*, to be released by Routledge/Taylor & Francis in 2012. His views and opinions on clinical and military psychology have been quoted in *USA Today*, *New York Times, Boston Globe*, NPR, BBC, and CBC.

About the Contributors

Jonathan M. Borkum holds a PhD from the University of Maine, where he continues as a faculty associate in the psychology department. His book, *Chronic Headaches: Biology, Psychology, and Behavioral Treatment*, published in 2007 by Taylor & Francis, has been cited in headache treatment guidelines issued by the Pain Society of Switzerland and the National Health Service of Scotland. He is on the consulting medical staff of Maine General Medical Center and in full-time private practice with Health Psych Maine, a group psychology practice that draws patients statewide.

William J. Burns, PhD, ABPP, is professor of psychology at the Center for Psychological Studies at Nova Southeastern University (NSU) in Ft. Lauderdale, Florida. He was awarded the Master of Science in clinical psychopharmacology in 2001 from NSU. As clinician, he is board certified by the American Board of Professional Psychology, has been in part-time practice in clinical psychology for 35 years, and supervises diagnostic and treatment practicum students, interns, and fellows in their clinical work. As professor, he teaches neuroscience courses in the neuropsychology concentration for students in the PhD and PsyD programs at NSU. In the NSU master's program in clinical psychopharmacology he is the coordinator of practicum placement and teaches both neuroscience and pathophysiology courses. As researcher, he has conducted studies in pediatric neuropsychology, presents at conferences, and supervises student research and dissertations. He has authored two books, 11 chapters, and over 40 journal articles, and has presented with his students over 200 papers, symposia, and posters at the American Psychological Association (APA), Divisions 55, 40, and 12, National Academy of Neuropsychology (NAN), International Neuropsychology Society (INS), Society for Research in Child Development (SRCD), and the International Conference on Infant Studies (ICIS).

Lisa Cosgrove, PhD, clinical psychologist, is Associate Professor at the University of Massachusetts–Boston, and a Research Lab Fellow at the Edmond J. Safra Center for Ethics at Harvard University. Her current research agenda focuses on two main areas: (1) developing training practices that help mental health professionals think critically about, and try to avoid bias in, psychiatric diagnosis; and (2) addressing ethical dilemmas that arise in the biomedical field because of financial conflicts of interest (e.g., developing more rigorous conflict-of-interest policies when there are collaborations between the pharmaceutical industry and academic institutions; developing patient-centered informed consent guidelines that adequately address the efficacy and safety of psychotropic medications). She is co-editor of *Bias in Psychiatric Diagnosis* and a contributing editor to *Psychiatric Ethics and the Rights of Persons with Mental Disabilities in Institutions and the Community*. Dr. Cosgrove has published over 30 peer-reviewed journal articles and book chapters.

Patrick H. DeLeon, PhD, MPH, JD, received his doctorate in clinical psychology from Purdue University in 1969. His first position was with the University of Hawaii Peace Corps training projects for Fiji and the Philippines and he then worked for the State of Hawaii Division of Mental Health, on both an inpatient and outpatient basis. He began his School of Public Health Internship with U.S. Senator Daniel K. Inouye on the first day of the Watergate hearings, retiring as chief of staff after 38+ years in the Fall of 2011. He has 25+ years of APA governance experience, serving as President in 2000. He was elected as a member of the Institute of Medicine (IOM). He is licensed in Hawaii, a diplomate, and Fellow of APA. Division 55 recently named their student psychopharmacology award after him. He is often referred to as "the grandfather" of psychology's prescriptive authority movement.

Ken Fogel, PsyD, obtained his degree in Clinical Psychology from The Chicago School of Professional Psychology. He holds three bachelor's degrees from McGill University in Canada (physiology, education, and psychology). He is an associate professor at The Chicago School, where he teaches courses in biological bases of behavior, psychopathology, psychological assessment, and clinical psychopharmacology. Dr. Fogel is also the Assistant Chair of Curriculum in the Clinical PsyD department, focusing on student learning and competency development. He currently consults with the Illinois Department of Children and Family Services as part of the Child and Youth Investment Team (CAYIT) program.

George M. Kapalka holds a PhD in clinical psychology and is board-certified in several areas of practice, including clinical psychology, psychopharmacology, child and adolescent psychology, learning disabilities, and forensic psychology. He is a tenured professor (graduate faculty appointment) at Monmouth University, where he currently serves as the Interim Chair of the Department of Psychological Counseling. Dr. Kapalka has been in practice for over 20 years and is licensed to practice psychology in New Jersey, New York, Pennsylvania, and New Mexico. For over a decade, he has been a member of medical staff at Meridian Health, Brick Hospital Division, a primary care hospital. Dr. Kapalka is author of five books and dozens of professional publications and presentations. His latest book, *Pediatricians and Pharmacologically-Trained Psychologists: Practitioner's Guide to Collaborative Care*, was published in 2011 by Springer. He has been interviewed in newspapers, magazines, Internet publications, and on television and radio programs.

Lawrence R. Kotkin, PhD, MS, is a medical and health psychologist who currently focuses on the treatment of chronic illnesses, especially diabetes. He has held board certification in diabetes education, and the Professional Section of the American Diabetes Association placed him in the Who's Who in Diabetes Treatment, Education, and Research. He has been a member of a Diabetes Education Center team, trained at the Einstein College of Medicine's Diabetes Research and Training Center, and served as Supervising Psychologist of the Geriatrics Division at New York's Creedmoor Psychiatric Center. He maintains a private practice and consults with hospitals and schools about the psychological aspects of managing diabetes. He also teaches as an adjunct professor at St. Joseph's College in New York.

Robert E. McGrath received his PhD in clinical psychology from Auburn University in 1984. He is a professor of psychology at Fairleigh Dickinson University, where he currently directs the PhD program in clinical psychology, the postdoctoral

MS program in clinical psychopharmacology, and the certificate program in integrated primary care. He also has an active research program, focusing primarily on the future of professional practice and assessment and measurement, and is the three-time winner of the Martin Mayman Award from the Society for Personality Assessment for his contributions to the theoretical literature in personality assessment. Dr's McGrath's latest book, *Pharmacotherapy for Psychologists: Prescribing and Collaborative Roles,* was published by the American Psychological Association in 2010.

Erin M. McGuinness has worked for several years in the field of Emergency Mental Health, in Chicago, Seattle, and most recently in the U.S.-Mexico border region in El Paso, Texas. Ms. McGuinness holds degrees in psychology and political science from the University of Chicago. She has traveled to communities in 16 countries across five continents observing cultural factors impacting psychological well-being, political decision-making, and public health. Ms. McGuinness is currently attending graduate school at Saint Louis University.

Kevin M. McGuinness, PhD, a clinical psychologist, medical psychologist, and clinical health psychologist, is an active duty commissioned officer of the United States Public Health Service, currently assigned by the Health Resources and Services Administration to a community health center, La Clínica de Familia, in Chaparral, New Mexico. Dr. McGuinness maintains a private practice in Las Cruces, New Mexico, and is a member of the clinical psychopharmacology faculty of New Mexico State University and the Southwest Institute for the Advancement of Psychotherapy. Dr. McGuinness earned his post-doctoral MS in clinical psychopharmacology from Fairleigh Dickinson University and his PhD in clinical psychology from the California School of Professional Psychology. He is a clinical health psychology Diplomate of the American Board of Professional Psychology, a Diplomate of the American College of Forensic Examiners, and a Fellow of the American Psychological Association. Dr. McGuinness is President-Elect of the American Society for the Advancement of Pharmacotherapy and Vice President of the Joshua Foundation, Inc. He has published articles, book chapters, and made numerous presentations addressing topics in chemistry, psychology, and public health.

Jose A. Rey, MS, PharmD, BCPP, is an associate professor of Pharmaceutical Sciences at Nova Southeastern University (NSU), College of Pharmacy, in Ft. Lauderdale, Florida. He is currently the clinical psychopharmacologist for South Florida State Hospital. Dr. Rey's research interests include cosmetic neuropsychopharmacology, geropsychiatry, psychotropic polypharmacy, pain management with antidepressants and anticonvulsants, communication disorders, and clinical and pharmacoeconomic outcomes research with antipsychotics and antidepressants. He has presented his research at national and international meetings. Dr. Rey has published articles, abstracts, and reviews in peer-reviewed journals and has been an invited speaker at state, national, and international meetings. He is currently a member of the American Society of Health-System Pharmacists, the Board of Pharmaceutical Specialties, the College of Psychiatric and Neurologic Pharmacists, and the American Psychological Association. Dr. Rey received his doctorate in pharmacy from the University of Florida, completed an American Society of Health-Systems Pharmacists (ASHP)-accredited specialty residency in psychiatric pharmacy practice at the Gainesville Veterans Administration Medical Center (VAMC) and Shands Hospital in Gainesville, Florida, and is board-certified in psychiatric pharmacy.

Mary (Mimi) Y. Sa, PsyD, MS Psychopharm, has been a conditional prescribing psychologist in New Mexico since 2009. While in New Mexico she worked for the Indian Health Service at both Taos and Mescalero reservations and was recognized by IHS for her services during a teenage suicide epidemic. She has provided clinical services for Native Americans and Latinos for over 10 years in Minnesota and New Mexico and in both rural and urban settings. She serves as the chair of the psychopharmacology division of the Minnesota Psychological Association. Dr. Sa is currently working as a child and adolescent psychologist in central Minnesota at Cambridge Medical Center, with particular emphasis on providing psychotherapy, testing, and psychotropic consultations for pediatricians.

Randall Tackett, PhD, received his MS degree in pharmacology and toxicology from Auburn University in 1977 and his doctorate in pharmacology and toxicology from the University of Georgia in 1979. Following a 2-year postdoctoral fellowship at the Medical University of South Carolina, he returned to the University of Georgia as an assistant professor in the Department of Pharmacology and Toxicology. He is currently Professor of Pharmacology and Toxicology and Graduate Coordinator in the Department of Clinical and Administrative Pharmacy. He also is Director of the Clinical Trials Graduate Certificate Program at the University of Georgia in the Department of Regulatory Affairs. He has developed and teaches in the postgraduate psychopharmacology prescribing program through Alliant University and Fairleigh Dickinson University. For his work in developing the curriculum in these areas, he received the American Psychological Association Presidential Citation in 2000.

Michael R. Tilus received both a PsyD of psychology in marital and family therapy with a concentration in pastoral care and counseling (San Diego) and a postdoctoral MS in clinical psychopharmacology from Alliant International University–California School of Professional Psychology (San Francisco). As a commander on active duty with the United States Public Health Service, an ordained chaplain, and a practicing medical psychologist, he currently serves as the Director of Behavioral Health at Spirit Lake Health Center–Indian Health Service for the Spirit Lake Dakota Reservation at Fort Totten, North Dakota.

Lenore Walker, EdD, is currently a professor at Nova Southeastern University (NSU) in the Center for Psychological Studies where she is Coordinator of the Forensic Psychology Concentration. She earned her doctorate degree in psychology from Rutgers in 1972, with expertise in working with children and their families. She also holds a MS from City College of the City University of New York, and earned a postdoctoral Master's of Science degree in psychopharmacology from NSU in 2006. She is board-certified in clinical psychology and in couples and family psychology by the American Board of Professional Psychology. Dr. Walker has been in private practice for nearly 40 years and, in her work with abused children and their families, has been on national policy-making committees, and has testified numerous times before Congress and in state and federal courts around the United States and other countries; she has also served as advisor to NATO, the ILANUD project of the United Nations, Pan American Health Organization, WHO, and others.

Dr. Walker has authored or co-authored over 15 books and 50+ scientific articles and often travels to conduct training in different countries. In her work at NSU, she trains and supervises doctoral students in forensic psychology who provide psychological evaluations at no charge to families involved with the dependency courts in Broward County, Florida.

Jack G. Wiggins, PhD, completed his graduate studies at Purdue University and subsequently served as APA president; he urged psychologists to seek prescriptive authority in his presidential address in 1993. He has remained active in advocating psychologists' involvement in pharmacotherapy, and he currently serves as editor of the *Archives of Medical Psychology*. His priority at this time is focused on monetizing the value of psychological services by championing reimbursement of psychopharmacologic services provided by licensed psychologists. Dr. Wiggins works to educate leaders in the private and government sectors about the fact that for the past quarter century, pharmacologically trained psychologists have assisted primary care physicians in the prescription of psychotropic medications and have managed treatment outcomes of patients taking these medications; in this vein, he actively promotes reimbursement of specialists within medical psychology who contribute their knowledge and skills in clinical psychopharmacology as an integral component of healthcare.

Massi Wyatt, PhD, has worked as a clinical psychologist in public service for over 10 years since completing his undergraduate degree at Columbia University and his graduate work at Baylor University. He began with the United States Army as an active-duty psychologist for 5 years during the Global War on Terrorism. He served as the psychology consultant at the United States Army Aeromedical Center before leaving active duty service to join the Indian Health Service (IHS) as a civilian. His special interest in multicultural psychology, rural/community psychology, and integrated primary care psychology were well honed during his 4 years as IHS Chief of Behavioral Health at the Ft. Peck Service Unit in northeast Montana. While at Ft. Peck, Dr. Wyatt obtained his MS in clinical psychopharmacology and was instrumental in paving the way for prescribing psychologists obtaining prescription privileges in Indian Health Service. He has continued his work toward prescriptive authority for psychologists (RxP) while returning to work for the Army as the Traumatic Brain Injury (TBI) Program Manager and the Integrated Behavioral Health Champion at Ft. Rucker, Alabama. Dr. Wyatt is also active in education and advocacy activities for RxP by serving as the Membership Chair, Convention Director, and Secretary for APA Division 55—the American Society for the Advancement of Pharmacotherapy.

Robert D. Younger received his PhD in clinical psychology from Auburn University in 1982. He is board-certified in clinical psychology by the American Board of Professional Psychology and completed his postdoctoral master's degree in clinical psychopharmacology from Alliant University, leading to prescriptive authority as a Naval Reserve officer in 1999. He subsequently returned to active duty after September 2001. As a Navy psychologist Dr. Younger deployed three times and prescribed in seven states, on two aircraft carriers, and two foreign countries. He most recently was the director of the Naval Academy Midshipmen Development Center and is currently a Navy captain and prescribing psychologist with the Naval Academy and Naval Health Clinic in Annapolis, Maryland.

List of Illustrations

List of Tables

MEDICAL PSYCHOLOGY
Definitions, Controversies, and New Directions

What's in a name?

—Juliet Capulet

Bret A. Moore

Mark Muse

The field of *medical psychology* includes the specialties of *health psychology*, *rehabilitation psychology*, *pediatric psychology*, *neuropsychology*, and *clinical psychopharmacology,* as well as subspecialties in *pain management, primary care psychology,* and *hospital-based (or medical school-based) psychology*. Yet the term "medical psychology" is an umbrella term: it encompasses the multiple specialties that make up *healthcare psychology,* embracing the *biopsychosocial paradigm* of mental/physical health and extending that paradigm to clinical practice through research and the application of *evidenced-based* diagnostic and treatment procedures.

By adopting the biopsychosocial paradigm, the field of medical psychology has recognized that the Cartesian assumption that the body and mind are separate entities is inadequate, representing as it does an arbitrary dichotomy that works to the detriment of healthcare (Burns, Mueller, & Warren, 2010). The biopsychosocial approach reflects the concept that the psychology of an individual cannot be understood without reference to that individual's social environment (Steele & Price, 2007). For the medical psychologist, the *medical model of disease* cannot in itself explain complex health concerns any more than a strict psychosocial explanation of mental and physical health can in itself be comprehensive (Miller, 2010). Rather, the specialties that constitute medical psychology strive to integrate the major components of an individual's psychological, biological, and social functioning and are designed to contribute to that person's well-being in a way that respects the natural interface among these components.

The biopsychosocial paradigm (Engel, 1977)—or, more aptly, the *psychobiosocial paradigm* (LeVine & Orabona Foster, 2010)—argues not so much for the standard, multidisciplinary division of a person into discrete parts as for the integrated care of the whole person by a professional who is trained to assess and treat all these functional components within his or her specialty area. Indeed, the whole is greater than the sum of its parts when it comes to providing comprehensive and sensible behavioral healthcare.

DEFINITION OF MEDICAL PSYCHOLOGY

The idea that psychologists should be allowed to integrate psychopharmacology and the principles of traditional behavioral science into their clinical practice has been met with considerable controversy. From the perspective of its proponents, progress toward this goal has been slow but steady. Over the past two decades, the debate over whether medication management should be within the purview of psychologists—that is, their right to have *prescriptive authority*—has taken place at professional conferences, in the pages of professional journals (Julien, 2011), before state boards of psychology and medicine, and within academic and legislative halls throughout the country. Although this debate has reflected mainly the opinions of organized psychiatry versus psychologists (Muse & McGrath, 2010a), it has not been exclusively so. One point of contention within professional psychology itself is how the term "medical psychology" should be defined, as well as which areas of applied psychology should have the right to adopt it. For example, Division 38 (Health Psychology) of the American Psychological Association (APA) has taken the stance that the terms "medical psychology" and "medical psychologist" should not be equated with prescriptive authority exclusively (American Psychological Association Division 38, 2010). In a position statement, Division 38 makes the case that the term medical psychology has a long history within the profession and has not been traditionally associated with the right of psychologists to prescribe medication.

In agreement with the concern raised by Division 38 about use of the term medical psychology to mean exclusively the authority to prescribe medication, the *Academy of Medical Psychology* supports an inclusive definition, by which medical psychology is viewed as a specialty within psychology that requires training at the postdoctoral level and utilizes the skills of professionals in clinical psychology, health psychology, behavioral medicine, psychopharmacology, and medical science. This point of view is most consistent with the definition put forth by Division 55 of the APA, the *American Society for the Advancement of Pharmacotherapy,* which states that "[medical psychology] is that branch of psychology that integrates somatic and psychotherapeutic modalities into the management of mental illness, substance-use disorders, and emotional, cognitive, and behavioral disorders" (American Psychological Association Division 55, 2007). This view is also in keeping with the inclusive definition offered 30 years ago by Prokop and Bradley (1981) in the first cogent treatise on the subject entitled "Medical Psychology: Contributions to Behavioral Medicine." Although these authors believed that medical psychology in the 1980s emanated primarily from psychologists housed within schools of medicine, they also foresaw the overlapping of various emerging disciplines, such as health psychology and behavioral medicine.

Much of the concern of Division 38 and other specialties that have traditionally used the term medical psychologist stems from a recent legislative statute in the State of Louisiana in which the term refers specifically to those psychologists licensed by the Louisiana State Board of Medical Examiners to prescribe medications. This statute builds upon the definition issued by the U.S. Drug Enforcement Agency (DEA), which recognizes that the term medical psychologist refers to a *mid-level provider/ practitioner* who has prescriptive authority. The DEA definition notwithstanding, the problem with legislating at a state level the exclusive use of the generic term "medical psychologist" by those psychologists who can prescribe psychotropic medication is that it makes it illegal for other medical psychologists to use the term when referring to themselves within such a jurisdiction. In our opinion, this unfortunate consequence can be avoided by writing future prescriptive authority laws in such a way as to distinguish those medical psychologists who prescribe from those who do not prescribe.

PRESCRIBING MEDICAL PSYCHOLOGY

Since the editors of this volume wish to highlight the integration of clinical psychopharmacology within the psychobiosocial paradigm of medical psychology, we will herein treat the field of *medical psychology* as a generic one, from which springs the discipline of *prescribing medical psychology*, and define it as follows:

> Medical Psychology is a postdoctoral specialty within applied psychology that integrates evidence-based psychological principles with medical science for the purpose of diagnosing and treating emotional, cognitive, behavioral, and psychosomatic disorders. Pharmacologically trained medical psychologists can prescribe, in concert with psychobiosocial interventions, psychotropic medications or advise patients and other professionals about the use of such medication.

Nothing in this definition prevents health, rehabilitation, or pediatric psychologists or neuropsychologists, or any other subspecialty of psychology, such as pain management or primary care psychology, from using the term medical psychology or medical psychologist. The definition does, however, specifically identify a subgroup of medical psychologists who are competent in medication management. Such professionals are referred to here as "prescribing medical psychologists" and are understood to be engaged in the practice of prescribing medical psychology.

In the editors' view, the term prescribing medical psychology most aptly conveys the complexities of this emerging field and captures the rigors of training and clinical practice inherent in integrating psychopharmacology within the psychobiosocial model of health and disease. To refer to individuals who have been trained to be proficient in managing psychotropic medications simply as "prescribing psychologists" does not do justice to their extensive instruction in all aspects of the psychobiosocial model. The individual chapters of this text cover each of the 10 content areas that constitute the subspecialty of prescribing medical psychology and attest to the complex integration of the sciences of psychology and medicine in the preparation of psychologists to prescribe medication.

PRESCRIBING MEDICAL PSYCHOLOGY AND THE PRESCRIPTIVE AUTHORITY MOVEMENT

Because of the broad scope of this subject and space constraints, it would not be prudent to offer a comprehensive review of the history of prescribing medical psychology and the prescriptive authority movement at this juncture.[1] For our purposes

---

[1]The biopsychosocial orientation within psychology has a long and continuous history. The experimental area of psychopharmacology dates back to Emil Kraepelin, a figure pivotal in bridging psychology and psychiatry, who completed studies on the effects of common psychotropic agents such as alcohol in Wilhelm Wundt's psychophysics lab in the 19th century (Müller, Fletcher, & Steinberg, 2006). Early 20th-century psychopharmacologists, such as Harry Hollingsworth (Benjamin, Rogers, & Rosenbaum, 1991), were largely experimental psychologists (Schmied, Steinberg, & Sykes, 2006) who carried out double-blind trials

here, it is more appropriate to highlight the core issues and arguments that propel prescriptive authority within the greater context of medical psychology. These essential arguments illuminate the importance of medical psychology in general and prescribing medical psychology in particular, as well as the reasons why the profession of clinical psychology hinges on the success of this branch of clinical practice.

PROFESSIONAL PSYCHOLOGY IN CRISIS

Professional psychology—that is, the practical application of the science of psychology in the clinical domain—is in danger of becoming obsolete or obviated by other burgeoning professions such as clinical social work and professional counseling. This is due to a multitude of factors, including the shorter preparation time required for the latter groups to pursue their career, preferential contracting by third-party insurance because of the inherently lower costs/reimbursement rates for their services, and effective legislative lobbying by other behavioral health providers to gain competencies that once were reserved for psychologists. Clinical psychology can no longer hold itself out to the public as the sine qua non of psychotherapy. It is, quite literally, being overrun by competitors and ignored by payers. In the eyes of any accountant, this turn of events spells trouble.

Clinical psychology has, indisputably, bona fide differences from other disciplines that offer behavioral health services; traditionally, these differences were founded on this discipline's respect for science and evidence-based approaches, as well as on its development and practice of psychometric-based diagnostic techniques. Still, these differences are largely ignored by third-party payers whose business plan is based on reduced costs rather than on the excellence of a product or outcome. At the same time, large third-party insurers have shifted reimbursement and emphasis from psychotherapy to psychiatric treatment (i.e., psychotropic medication) for an array of conditions that have traditionally been effectively managed with psychotherapy (Olfson & Marcus, 2010).

Medical psychology, on the other hand, not only creates and applies evidence-based diagnostics and interventions, but it does so in an area of practice that is hard to replicate in disciplines with shorter career paths because of the extensive training needed to round out the practitioner in both the psychosocial realm and the biomedical arena. It is the contribution of the medical psychologist in the areas of health, rehabilitation, primary care, and psychopharmacology/substance abuse that sets the profession apart from the typical psychotherapist, who is trained mainly, if not exclusively, in descriptive diagnosis (according to the *Diagnostic and Statistical Manual of Mental Disorders —fourth edition* [*DSM-IV*]) and psychotherapeutic technique. It also

---

involving different psychoactive substances, such as caffeine. Among the 20th-century academicians who contributed significantly during the early stages of prescribing psychopharmacology is the husband-and-wife team of Louis and Ann Marie Pagliaro (Pagliaro & Pagliaro, 1979, 1983, 1986, 1996, 1998a, 1998b, 1999a, 1999b). Clinical involvement of psychology in the practice of prescribing psychopharmacology began in 1986, when the Indian Health Service (IHS) trained a psychologist and granted him prescriptive authority (Jennings, 2010). More recently, pharmacologically trained psychologists have achieved autonomous status as psychobiosocial clinicians with the enactment of various state laws allowing for prescriptive authority and with the simultaneous recognition of prescribing competence for properly trained psychologists by various branches of the federal government, including the Department of Defense (DOD), the IHS, and the Department of Health and Human Services (DHHS) (Dittman, 2003).

sets the prescribing medical psychologist apart from the contemporary psychiatrist (Carlat, 2010a), whose training is based preferentially on the medical model (with its emphasis on "bio") and almost exclusively on the use of a single treatment modality (i.e., medication management). The addition of prescriptive authority to the armamentarium of the medical psychologist will result not only in better-integrated care for his or her clientele, but also in economic viability and solvency, which is the foundation of professional autonomy and sovereignty (Johnson, 2009).

SUPPORT FOR PRESCRIPTIVE AUTHORITY

Filling a Healthcare Gap

Since psychologists began their efforts to incorporate pharmacotherapy into their treatment inventory, the main thrust of their endeavor has been to meet the needs of vulnerable populations. Whether they are treating the underserved (e.g., Native Americans), those in need of targeted and immediate care (e.g., veterans and active-duty military), or those who live in remote areas and are difficult to reach (e.g., residents of rural and frontier communities), psychologists are acutely aware of the millions of people who either go without behavioral healthcare or receive substandard care (Moore, 2010; Moore & McGrath, 2007; Muse & McGrath, 2010b).

Unfortunately, the practice of psychiatry has not adequately met the needs of the most vulnerable and underserved in the population. One need only look at the situation in California to fully appreciate this deficiency. Recent testimony before the California Senate highlighted two alarming facts: approximately 20% of the counties have no practicing psychiatrists, and another 30% are served by five or fewer psychiatrists. As Romney (2007) pointed out, psychiatrists are fleeing remote practice areas in favor of urban and more financially lucrative settings. Although some prescribing medical psychologists may also choose to pursue positions in such settings, most are probably less likely to do so, since the facts show that (a) psychologists already outnumber psychiatrists by about 4 to 1 in rural settings (Hartley, Bird, & Dempsey, 1999) and (b) over half the psychologists who have been trained in pharmacotherapy and are practicing in New Mexico and Louisiana are already serving disadvantaged patients.

Improving Quality and Continuity of Care

Proponents of prescriptive authority for psychologists believe that as the number of psychologists who can effectively integrate pharmacotherapy into psychobiosocial interventions increases, quality of care will also increase. In one respect, this is due to increased access to care in general. Nonetheless, just as important is the fact that those psychologists who choose to add pharmacology training to their knowledge base will emerge as consummate mental health professionals. This is not meant to demean or dismiss the training of psychiatrists, physicians' assistants, psychiatric nurse practitioners, social workers, professional counselors, or psychologists who are not trained in pharmacotherapy. It is, however, meant to highlight the breadth of skills offered by prescribing medical psychologists. Patients who consult a prescribing medical psychologist receive integrated services—that is, diagnostic, consultative, and psychobiosocial care (including pharmacological treatment)—from a single provider rather than fragmented services from multiple providers. Furthermore, the vast majority of prescriptions for psychotropic medications are currently written by non-psychiatric physicians (i.e., family physicians, internists) who have limited training in psychopharmacology and no training in evidence-based psychosocial treatments, so that as the number of prescribing medical psychologists increases, more effective behavioral health services will become inevitable.

RECENT PROFESSIONAL ADVANCES IN PRESCRIBING MEDICAL PSYCHOLOGY

Practice Guidelines

Over the past decade, the specialty that integrates pharmacotherapy with psycho-biosocial interventions has undergone many positive changes. One of the most significant professional developments has been the establishment of *practice guidelines* for pharmacologically trained psychologists. "Practice Guidelines Regarding Psychologists' Involvement in Pharmacological Issues," a document published in 2009 by the APA's Division 55 Task Force on Practice Guidelines (APA, 2011), is the first attempt to address and clarify the professional and ethical issues faced by those psychologists who have incorporated psychopharmacology into their clinical repertoire, whether at the level of (a) actual prescribing of medication, (b) actively collaborating in medication decision making, or (c) providing general information. (See Table 1.1.)

Clarifying a professional practice through the development of guidelines or standards is a necessary part of any applied area of psychology. In formulating the guidelines described above, Division 55 has provided a framework for the integration of pharmacotherapy and psychobiosocial interventions as a distinct specialty instead of relying on professional practice guidelines designed for other disciplines, such as psychiatry, medicine, and nursing.

Expanded Credentialing

As of February 2009, each of three service branches of the U.S. Armed Forces (Army, Navy, and Air Force) had developed its own unique credentialing guidelines for pharmacologically trained psychologists. Although the credentialing section and the commanding general of each military treatment facility must authorize prescription privileges for each prescribing medical psychologist, clear guidance is available to assist them in making informed decisions.

The credentialing of prescribing medical psychologists has also gained momentum in the U.S. Public Health Service, as well as in the Indian Health Service. In 2010, at least three psychologists were credentialed to provide psychopharmacological services to Native Americans at their respective service units, and Earl Sutherland became the first IHS prescribing medical psychologist to be granted a national *DEA prescriber number*, independent of the state-based DEA prescribing numbers issued in New Mexico and Louisiana. According to all estimates, the number of psychologists credentialed to prescribe within the IHS should increase exponentially in the near future.

SPECIALTY CERTIFICATION

Another developmental milestone in the evolution of most areas of applied psychology is specialty certification. The Academy of Medical Psychology allows appropriately trained psychologists to earn the distinction of "Board Certified Medical

Table 1.1 American Psychological Association Practice Guidelines Regarding Psychologists' Involvement in Pharmacological Issues

	Relevant Activities		
	Prescribing	Collaborating	Providing Information
General			
Guideline 1. Psychologists are encouraged to consider objectively the scope of their competence in pharmacotherapy and to seek consultation as appropriate before offering recommendations about psychotropic medications.	X	X	X
Guideline 2. Psychologists are urged to evaluate their own feelings and attitudes about the role of medication in the treatment of psychological disorders, as these feelings and attitudes can potentially affect communications with patients.	X	X	X
Guideline 3. Psychologists involved in prescribing or collaborating are sensitive to the developmental, age and aging, educational, sex and gender, language, health status, and cultural/ethnicity factors that can moderate the interpersonal and biological aspects of pharmacotherapy relevant to the populations they serve.	X	X	
Education			
Guideline 4. Psychologists are urged to identify a level of knowledge concerning pharmacotherapy for the treatment of psychological disorders that is appropriate to the populations they serve and the type of practice they wish to establish, and to engage in educational experiences as appropriate to achieve and maintain that level of knowledge.	X	X	X
Guideline 5. Psychologists strive to be sensitive to the potential for adverse effects associated with the psychotropic medications used by their patients.	X	X	X
Guideline 6. Psychologists involved in prescribing or collaborating are encouraged to familiarize themselves with the technological resources that can enhance decision-making during the course of treatment.	X	X	
Assessment			
Guideline 7. Psychologists with prescriptive authority strive to familiarize themselves with key procedures for monitoring the physical and psychological sequelae of the medications used to treat psychological disorders, including laboratory examinations and overt signs of adverse or unintended effects.	X		
Guideline 8. Psychologists with prescriptive authority regularly strive to monitor the physiological status of the patients they treat with medication, particularly when there is a physical condition that might complicate the response to psychotropic medication or predispose a patient to experience an adverse reaction.	X		

(continued)

Table 1.1   (Continued)

	Relevant Activities		
	Prescribing	Collaborating	Providing Information
Guideline 9. Psychologists are encouraged to explore issues surrounding patient adherence and feelings about medication.	X	X	X
Intervention and Consultation			
Guideline 10. Psychologists are urged to develop a relationship that will allow the populations they serve to feel comfortable exploring issues surrounding medication use.	X	X	X
Guideline 11. To the extent deemed appropriate, psychologists involved in prescribing or collaborating adopt a biopsychosocial approach to case formulation that considers both psychosocial and biological factors.	X	X	
Guideline 12. The psychologist with prescriptive authority is encouraged to use an expanded informed consent process to incorporate additional issues specific to prescribing.	X		
Guideline 13. When making decisions about the use of psychological treatments, pharmacotherapy, or their combination, the psychologist with prescriptive authority considers the best interests of the patient, current research, and, when appropriate, the needs of the community.	X		
Guideline 14. Psychologists involved in prescribing or collaborating strive to be sensitive to the subtle influences of effective marketing on professional behavior and the potential for bias in information in their clinical decisions about the use of medications.	X	X	
Guideline 15. Psychologists with prescriptive authority are encouraged to use interactions with the patient surrounding the act of prescribing to learn more about the patient's characteristic patterns of interpersonal behavior.	X		
Relationships			
Guideline 16. Psychologists with prescriptive authority are sensitive to maintaining appropriate relationships with other providers of psychological services.	X		
Guideline 17. Psychologists are urged to maintain appropriate relationships with providers of biological interventions.	X	X	X

Psychologist" if they are deemed eligible through a peer-review process. In addition, in 2010, a committee of APA's Division 55 applied to the American Board of Professional Psychology to have Clinical Psychopharmacology designated a specialty. The American Psychological Association has also developed a strict procedure for reviewing and awarding official designation to postdoctoral training programs in clinical psychopharmacology (APA, 2009). At this writing, three university-based training progams have achieved APA designation in psychopharmacology: The M.S. Program in Clinical Psychopharmacology at Fairleigh Dickinson University, the Interdisciplinary Master of Arts in Psychopharmacology at Southwestern Institute for the Advancement of Psychotherapy/New Mexico State University (SIAP/NMSU), and the Clinical Psychopharmacology Postdoctoral M.S. Program at the California School of Professional Psychology.

SUPPORT FROM PROMINENT PHYSICIANS

To the consternation of organized psychiatry as well as some members of organized psychology, a number of prominent psychopharmacologists, psychiatrists, and non-psychiatric physicians have openly acknowledged their support of prescriptive authority for prescribing medical psychologists (Carlat, 2010b; Julien, 2011). It remains to be seen how quickly such support will help prescribing medical psychologists become accepted into the mainstream; however, at a minimum, sanction from respected individuals in parallel camps does provide a degree of credibility. Moreover, when critics within psychology who initially—and perhaps reflexively—opposed prescriptive authority (Heiby, 2010) take a less biased look at the training required for prescribing medical psychology and its practice, they will begin to appreciate the rationale for promoting this new and inspiring movement.

FUTURE DIRECTIONS

Prescribing medical psychology is one of the most exciting and professionally relevant areas of psychology today. It has matured considerably over the past few decades and has the potential to shape the future of professional practice, not only with respect to the delivery of services to the traditional mental health population, but also within the medical setting, in which medical psychologists are becoming essential primary care providers (McGrath & Sammons, 2011). Prescribing psychopharmacology has created greater access to care for the most underserved and vulnerable of our society and is responsible for producing some of the most well-rounded health practitioners in the country. It is the editors' hope that these trends will continue. With that in mind, the following three steps need to be taken if prescribing medical psychology is to advance.

Dispense With the "Mid-Level Provider/Practitioner" Mentality

To gain true parity among doctoral-level providers, those psychologists trained in psychopharmacology must dispense with the *"mid-level provider/practitioner"* mentality. For too long psychologists have been relegated to a status within healthcare that does not recognize their skills and abilities. This is compounded 10-fold for prescribing medical psychologists. Accepting lower reimbursement rates from insurance companies and contract agencies, or agreeing to oversight by a physician when the state law doesn't require it, may be the path of least resistance, yet it is a path that will eventually lead to a dead end.

Be Professionally Honest

No doubt some psychologists are interested in gaining prescribing privileges for reasons that are less than altruistic, and to ignore this fact is to risk the sincerity of those who wish to see this specialty develop and succeed. Proponents of prescribing psychopharmacology are concerned about the lack of timely and appropriate psychiatric services to the underserved and vulnerable, believing unequivocally that the power to prescribe is also the power to not prescribe or to unprescribe. Nevertheless, it would be counterproductive to dismiss claims by opponents of prescribing medical psychology that the financial incentive is what makes some psychologists pursue the goal of prescribing. The truth is that at some point prescribing medical psychologists will be remunerated for their investment in training, their competence, and their service to society. Yet, keep in mind that, to date, approximately 1,500 prescribing medical psychologists have undergone training and have received little or no financial reward (Ax, Fagan, & Resnick, 2009). In fact, the first generation of prescribing medical psychologists invested considerable sums of money and many hours of training to pave the way for future psychologists who may, parenthetically, earn more than their contemporary colleagues who have opted for a shorter career path.[2]

There is no need to justify these outcomes, for they are laudable and reflect incentives found in every positive movement within society. The financial incentive for a psychologist to pursue training in prescribing medical psychology is no different from the financial incentive for a researcher to pursue research funding, for a student to choose a specialty track in a medical psychology specialty such as neuropsychology or health psychology, or for a clinical psychologist to enter private practice. Doing something valuable for society and doing something valuable for oneself are not mutually exclusive pursuits (Moore, 2010).

Unify Resources

Although the past decade has witnessed great strides in the area of prescriptive authority, one wonders how much more successful the granting of prescriptive authority would be had there been greater unity among those working to achieve this goal for the betterment of the field. Let us hope that the legendary turf battles between psychiatrists and psychologists do not foreshadow the rise of jealousies among factions of psychologists. If not, perhaps we will end up being "our own worst enemies." It may be inevitable that those who planted the flag—those first intrepid prescribing psychologists—will become the ones who work the hardest to defend the territory gained by limiting mobility of other qualified RxP psychologists. Alternatively, our specialty, which has been honed by the most courageous mental health professionals, might be in a position to address reciprocity for medical psychologists across juridicitions and in a variety

---

[2]According to a recent survey of 17 prescribing medical psychologists in private practice in Louisiana and New Mexico, the "the medium income increase from a prescribing practice is minimally about $20,000 per year" (p. 9). LeVine, E., Wiggins, J., and Masse, E. (2011). Prescribing psychologists in private practice: The dream and the reality of the experience of prescribing psychologists. *Archives of Medical Psychology, 2*, 1–14.

of federal venues, thus circumventing any tendency toward insular jurisdictions. Is it reasonable to limit the scope of practice of one's fellow colleagues when they are fully qualified to exercise their competencies? Can organizations and groups more effectively work together for the common goal of expanding the reach of prescribing medical psychology? Maybe such questions are naïve, but they need to be raised. Let us hope that the answers will lead to a stronger, more committed group of providers.

CHAPTER 1 KEY TERMS

Academy of Medical Psychology: Membership organization that provides board certification, training, and advocacy for medical psychologists.

American Society for the Advancement of Pharmacotherapy: Division 55 of the American Psychological Association (APA), having the primary purpose of enhancing psychological treatments combined with psychopharmacological medications.

Behavioral medicine: A broad, interdisciplinary approach dedicated to understanding physical health and illness through the knowledge and techniques of behavioral science. It seeks to address prevention, treatment, and rehabilitation of illness through incorporating research and practices from psychology, psychiatry, sociology, epidemiology, anthropology, health economics, public health, general medicine, and biostatistics.

Biopsychosocial paradigm: Healthcare approach that stresses the concept that biological, psychological, and social factors all play a significant role in human functioning within the context of disease or illness. (See also *Psychobiosocial paradigm.*)

Clinical psychopharmacology: Science and practice of utilizing pharmacological agents in addressing disorders of mood, sensation, thinking, and behavior.

Drug Enforcement Agency (DEA) prescriber number: A number assigned to a healthcare provider that allows him or her to write prescriptions for controlled substances. This number is used primarily to track patterns of prescribing and to ensure that only appropriate/qualified individuals are involved in prescribing such substances.

Evidence-based practice: Preferential use of mental and behavioral health interventions for which systematic, empirical research has provided evidence of their statistically significant effectiveness as treatments for specific problems.

Health psychology: Area of applied psychology concerned with understanding how biological, psychological, environmental, and cultural factors are involved in physical health and the prevention of illness.

Healthcare psychology: General term used to describe the application of clinical psychological services in the amelioration, elimination, or prevention of psychological, behavioral, and substance-use problems.

Hospital-based psychology: Practice of psychology in a hospital or other medical setting (e.g., medical school).

Medical model of disease: Traditional approach to the diagnosis and treatment of illness as practiced by physicians in the Western world. According to this model, the physician focuses on the defect or dysfunction within the patient, using a cause-and-effect diagnostic orientation and problem-solving therapeutic approach.

Medical psychology: A postdoctoral specialty within applied psychology that integrates evidence-based psychological principles with medical science for the purpose of diagnosing and treating emotional, cognitive, behavioral, and psychosomatic disorders. Pharmacologically trained (prescribing) medical psychologists can prescribe psychotropic medications (in concert with psychobiosocial interventions) or advise patients and other professionals about the use of such medication.

Mid-level provider/practitioner: Healthcare provider who is not a physician but is licensed to diagnose and treat patients, generally under the supervision of a physician. This physician-driven definition is not accurate for medical psychology but is perpetuated by the DEA classification.

Neuropsychology: Discipline within applied psychology that combines neurology, neuroscience, and psychology to study the relationship between the functioning of the brain, cognitive processes, and behavior.

Pain management: Branch of clinical health science that employs an interdisciplinary approach designed to ease the suffering and improve the quality of life of those living with pain. A typical pain-management team includes medical practitioners, clinical psychologists, physiotherapists, occupational therapists, and nurse practitioners.

Pediatric psychology: Discipline within applied psychology concerned with the physical health and illness of children and the relationship of psychological and behavioral factors with health, illness, and disease.

Practice guidelines: Systematically developed statements to assist practitioners and patients in making decisions about appropriate healthcare for specific clinical circumstances.

Prescribing medical psychology: That subspecialty which adds pharmacotherapy to the array of psychobiosocial diagnostic and therapeutic approaches of medical psychology. (See *Medical psychology.*)

Prescriptive authority for psychologists: Political effort to give prescribing rights to pharmacologically trained medical psychologists, enabling them to prescribe psychotropic medications to treat patients who have mental or emotional disorders.

Primary care psychology: Discipline within applied psychology concerned with providing healthcare and mental health services in the primary care setting. It includes the treatment and prevention of disease and the promotion of healthy behaviors in individuals, families, and communities.

Psychobiosocial paradigm: Healthcare approach that is similar to the biopsychosocial model of healthcare delivery but places greater emphasis on the psychological aspect of human functioning within the context of disease or illness, especially mental health.

Rehabilitation psychology: Discipline within applied psychology concerned with assisting a person who has an injury or illness (e.g., chronic, traumatic, and/or congenital) to achieve optimal physical, psychological, and interpersonal functioning.

Chapter 1 Questions

   1. The term "medical psychologist" is a legal/official term for which organization/ state/agency?
      a. New Mexico
      b. Louisiana
      c. Drug Enforcement Agency

    d. Both b and c

    e. None of the above

2. What is the ratio of psychologists to psychiatrists in rural settings?

    a. 1 to 1

    b. 2 to 1

    c. 4 to 1

    d. 10 to 1

    e. 20 to 1

3. Which organizations have specific credentialing guidelines for allowing psychologists to prescribe?

    a. United States Army

    b. United States Navy

    c. United States Air Force

    d. Indian Health Service

    e. All of the above

4. Which of the following is not one of the reasons why some believe that the field of clinical psychology is becoming less relevant in healthcare?

    a. Lower reimbursement rates for providers with master's degree

    b. Expansion of scope of practice by social workers and professional counselors into roles traditionally occupied by psychologists

    c. Decline in training standards in psychology

    d. Resistance to prescriptive authority for psychologists

    Answers: (1) b, (2) c, (3) e, and (4) c.

REFERENCES

American Psychiatric Association. (1994). *Diagnostic and Statistical Manual of Mental Disorders, Fourth Edition* (*DSM-IV*). Washington DC: Author.

American Psychological Association. (2009). *Designation criteria for education and training programs in preparation for prescriptive authority: Approved by APA Council of Representatives.* Washington, DC: Author.

American Psychological Association. (2011). Practice guidelines regarding psychologists' involvement in pharmacological issues. *American Psychologist, 66,* 835–849.

American Psychological Association Division 38. (2010, January 23). Division 38 statement on the use of the term "Medical Psychology." Retrieved from www.healthpsych.org/MedPsych.cfm

American Psychological Association Division 55. (2007, October 18). Minutes of Division 55 board meeting.

Ax, R. K., Fagan, T. J., & Resnick, R. J. (2009). Predoctoral prescriptive authority training: The rationale and a combined model. *Psychological Services, 6,* 85–95.

Benjamin, L., Rogers, A., & Rosenbaum, A. (1991). Coca-Cola, caffeine, and mental deficiency: Harry Hollingsworth and the Chattanooga trial of 1911. *Journal of the History of Behavioral Science, 27,* 42–55.

Burns, D., Mueller, K., & Warren, P. (2010). A review of evidence-based biopsychosocial laws governing the treatment of pain and injury. *Psychological Injury and Law, 3,* 169–181.

Carlat, D. (2010a). *Unhinged: The trouble with psychiatry—A doctor's revelation about a profession in crisis*. New York, NY: Free Press.

Carlat, D. (2010b). Psychologists and prescription privileges: A conversation. *Psychology Today*, March issue.

Dittman, M. (2003). Psychology's first prescribers. *APA Monitor, 34*, 36.

Engel, G. L. (1977). The need for a new medical model: A challenge for biomedicine. *Science, 196*, 129–136.

Hartley, D., Bird, D., & Dempsey, P. (1999). Rural mental health and substance abuse. In T. C. Ricketts (Ed.), *Rural health in the United States* (pp. 159–178). New York, NY: Oxford University Press.

Heiby, E. (2010). Concerns about substandard training for prescription privileges for psychologists. *Journal of Clinical Psychology, 66*, 104–111.

Jennings, F. (2010). An introduction to prescribing privileges for psychologists: A look back in time. *Archives of Medical Psychology, 1*, 1–13.

Johnson, J. (2009). Whether states should create prescription power for psychologists. *Law and Psychology Review, 33*, 167–176.

Julien, R. (2011). Pharmacology training in clinical psychology: A renewed call for action. *Journal of Clinical Psychology, 67*, 1–4.

LeVine, E., & Orabona Foster, E. (2010). Integration of psychotherapy and pharmacotherapy by prescribing-medical psychologists: A psychobiosocial model of care. In R. E. McGrath & B. A. Moore (Eds.), *Pharmacotherapy for psychologists: Prescribing and collaborative roles* (pp. 105–131).Washington, DC: American Psychological Association.

McGrath, R. E., & Sammons, M. (2011). Prescribing and primary care psychology: Complementary paths for professional psychology. *Professional Psychology: Research and Practice, 42*, 113–120.

Miller, G. (2010). Mistreating psychology in the decades of the brain. *Perspectives on Psychological Science, 5*, 716–743.

Moore, B. A. (2010). The future of prescribing psychology. In R. E. McGrath & B. A. Moore (Eds.), *Pharmacotherapy for psychologists: Prescribing and collaborative roles* (pp. 233–239). Washington, DC: American Psychological Association.

Moore, B. A., & McGrath, R. E. (2007). How prescriptive authority for psychologists would help service members in Iraq. *Professional Psychology: Research and Practice, 38,* 191–195.

Müller, U., Fletcher, P. C., & Steinberg, H. (2006). The origin of pharmacopsychology: Emil Kraepelin's experiments in Leipzig, Dorpat and Heidelberg (1882–1892). *Psychopharmacology, 184,* 131–138.

Muse, M., & McGrath, R. (2010a). Training comparison among three professions prescribing psychoactive medications: Psychiatric nurse practitioners, physicians, and pharmacologically-trained psychologists. *Journal of Clinical Psychology, 66*, 1–8.

Muse, M., & McGrath, R. (2010b). Making the case for prescription authority. In R. E. McGrath & B. A. Moore (Eds.), *Pharmacotherapy for psychologists: Prescribing and collaborative roles.* Washington, DC: American Psychological Association.

Olfson, M., & Marcus, S. (2010). National trends in outpatient psychotherapy. *American Journal of Psychiatry, 167*, 1456–1463.

Pagliaro, L., & Pagliaro, A. M. (1979). *Problems in pediatric drug therapy*. Hamilton, IL: Drug Intelligence Publications.

Pagliaro, L., & Pagliaro, A. M. (1983). *Psychopharmacologic aspects of aging.* St. Louis, MO: C. V. Mosby.

Pagliaro, L., & Pagliaro, A. M. (1986). *Drug reference guide to brand names and active ingredients*. St. Louis, MO: C. V. Mosby.

Pagliaro, L., & Pagliaro, A. M. (1996). *Substance use among children and adolescents*. New York, NY: Wiley.

Pagliaro, L., & Pagliaro, A. M. (1998a). *The pharmacologic basis of psychotherapeutics: An introduction for psychologists*. New York, New York: Brunner/Mazel.

Pagliaro, L., & Pagliaro, A. M. (1998b). *Psychologist's psychotropic drug reference*. Philadelphia, PA: Brunner/Mazel.

Pagliaro, L., & Pagliaro, A. M. (1999a). *Clinical psychopharmacotherapeutics for psychologists*. Philadelphia, PA: Brunner/Mazel.

Pagliaro, L., & Pagliaro, A. M. (1999b). *Psychologists' neuropsychotropic drug reference*. Philadelphia, PA: Brunner/Mazel.

Prokop, C., & Bradley, L. (1981). *Medical psychology: Contributions to behavioral medicine*. New York, NY: Academic Press.

Romney, L. (2007, January 6). Prison pay hikes drain staff at state hospitals. *Los Angeles Times*, p. A1.

Schmied, L. A., Steinberg, H., & Sykes, E. (2006). Psychopharmacology's debt to experimental psychology. *History of Psychology, 9*, 144–157.

Steele, S., & Price, J. (2007). *Applied sociology: Terms, topics, tools, and tasks*. Belmont, CA: Wadsworth Publishing.

Chapter 2

INTEGRATING CLINICAL PSYCHOPHARMACOLOGY WITHIN THE PRACTICE OF MEDICAL PSYCHOLOGY

Mark Muse

Bret A. Moore

Integration is the defining characteristic of medical psychology,[1] which purports to integrate the psychobiosocial[2] aspects of human functioning within the diagnosis and treatment of mental health disorders, syndromes, and conditions. One aspect of the practice of medical psychology is *clinical psychopharmacology*, or the management of pharmacokinetics and pharmacodynamics in the treatment of psychological disorders. Clinical psychopharmacology is not engaged in as the sole approach or treatment within medical psychology but is integrated within *multidimensional analyses of behavior* and *multimodal treatment strategies*. Not only are the aspects of human psychology (e.g., behavior, cognition, affect), biology (e.g., genetics, age, sex, race, health/disease), and social context (e.g., family-gender-cultural/ethnic associations, political-economic environment) assessed and weighed for their respective influences on a given individual, they are also integrated within the medical psychologist's orientation and thinking, allowing a holistic approach to understanding and responding to the patient/client.

When engaged in clinical psychopharmacology, the medical psychologist is aware of multiple factors (over and above any particular drug's chemical makeup) that may contribute to a given patient's response. For example, the family history may reveal inherited tendencies in patients with schizophrenia or bipolar disorder (Berrettini, 2000), and if a patient's family member has previously responded positively to a particular medication used to treat the same condition as the patient's, one can predict with some confidence that this same drug can be safely and efficaciously prescribed to the patient (O'Reilly, Bogue, & Singh, 1994).

---

[1]We support integration at the level of the individual practicing professional, as suggested by Daniel Carlat (2011), rather than the fragmented attempt at "integration" among professionals who practice piecemeal specialties. To us, the latter is a multidisciplinary rather than integrated approach.

[2]While medical psychology currently emphasizes the psychobiological aspects of diagnosis and treatment, the social/cultural aspect of clinical analysis and intervention is also acknowledged and may become progressively more important as evidence-based diagnostic and therapeutic strategies are developed in the areas of *clinical anthropology, clinical sociology,* and *social-clinical psychology* (McNally, 2011; Steele & Price, 2004; Rebach & Bruhn, 1991; Rush, 1996, 1999). To the extent that the science and the practice of clinical social interventions are developed, it will become incumbent upon medical psychologists to integrate this type of *psychobiosocial intervention* within their practice (McDaniel, Hepworth, & Doherty, 1992).

Other factors that should be considered in determining the proper role of pharmacotherapy are the patient's belief system (Makela & Griffith, 2003), social support structure, and economic and environmental situation (Roy et al., 2005). For example, the medical psychologist must weigh the benefits of treating a hospitalized patient with the latest, most expensive medication against that patient's ability to afford the prescribed treatment after discharge. A homeless schizophrenic patient who becomes stable while being treated in the hospital with a costly drug that requires strict dose compliance and frequent laboratory monitoring will find it difficult to maintain this regimen upon returning to his or her former indigent lifestyle; a better option would be to initiate treatment in the hospital with a low-cost parenteral preparation that can later be administered and monitored once every 2 to 3 weeks (e.g., haloperidol decanoate, fluphenazine decanoate).

In his writings, Morgan Sammons explicitly describes how medical psychologists can integrate treatment options for an array of emotional disorders by discerning whether it would be better to apply medication or psychotherapy as a *stand-alone treatment* or to combine the two modalities (Sammons & Levant, 1999; Sammons & Schmidt, 2001). Here are just three of his conclusions:

1. In the treatment of obsessive-compulsive disorder (OCD), research indicates that a *single-treatment modality* (behavioral therapy) is more effective than a *combination-treatment modality* (medication-behavioral therapy) when symptoms are primarily compulsive, whereas the reverse is true when symptoms are primarily obsessive.
2. For most other conditions, single-treatment modalities should be attempted before combined treatments are implemented.
3. Not all single-treatment approaches are equal: For example, pharmacotherapy is less effective than psychotherapy as a single-treatment approach when treating a patient who has chronic depression with an Axis II disorder.

Contemporaneous with Sammons' work has been Robert Julien's effort to ferret out differential indications for drug therapy versus talk therapy in his seminal book *A Primer of Drug Action*, now in its 12th edition (Julien, 2005; Julien, Advokat, & Comaty, 2011). Among Julien's conclusions regarding the integration of psychotherapy with pharmacotherapy are the following:

1. In the treatment of phobias (e.g., agoraphobia, simple phobia, and social phobia), cognitive-behavioral therapy (CBT) is more consistent than medications and provides longer-lasting effects;
2. In the treatment of obsessive-compulsive disorder, posttraumatic stress disorder (PTSD), and generalized anxiety, medical and behavioral approaches are equally effective;
3. Psychotherapy (cognitive-behavioral) and medical therapy (selective serotonin-reuptake inhibitors [SSRIs], tricyclic antidepressants, benzodiazepines, and monoamine oxidase inhibitors) are equally effective in the acute treatment of panic disorder, but in this case combining behavioral therapy and medication is superior to either of these monotherapies;
4. In the treatment of major depression, CBT and antidepressant medication are equally effective and display additional efficacy when combined; and
5. In the treatment of eating disorders, CBT is superior to an SSRI.

Prior to the work of both Sammons and Julien, attempts by other investigators to answer the question of when to medicate, when not, and when to combine medication with *psychosocial interventions* drew equivocal results with conflicting conclusions (Weissman, 1981). Fisher and Greenburg (1989) noted what they considered to be an overreliance on drug therapy and concluded that in many of the studies they reviewed the practice of adding medication to psychotherapy yielded no improvement in outcomes. In a later book, Fisher and Greenburg (1997) further argued that pharmacological agents in the treatment of mental disorders are, in general, no more effective than placebo. More recent arguments have been proposed to explain pharmacotherapy's positive clinical results (Moncrieff & Cohen, 2009) by considering psychotropic drugs as nonspecific agents, reminiscent of the *common factors theory* explanation of psychotherapeutic effectiveness (Imel & Wampold, 2008). These agents induce a complex, global response, analogous to the pervasive healing effect of empathy as a nonspecific agent across psychotherapies (Riess, 2010), thus yielding a sense of subjective improvement.

The fact that most psychotherapies are of equal efficacy when compared in meta-analyses—the so-called *Dodo-bird effect* (Wampold et al., 1997)—has led to a search for possible underlying mechanisms, one of which is described in the *Wampold hypothesis* (Sammons, 2010). This view is contrary to the reigning biological paradigm, which assumes that each psychiatric condition has a specific underlying neurological mechanism and that drugs are effective because their respective mechanisms of action differentially address specific imbalances inherent in the disorder being treated. In contrast to this strict biological model, the alternative view suggests that whether one treats depression with norepinephrine or serotonin, cognitive-behavioral or psychodynamic therapy, or pure placebo, it is the interpersonal relationship with a provider and the patient's ensuing expectation for positive change that is largely driving improvement, aided somewhat by the nonspecific *psychobiosocial* effect inherent in all these treatment approaches.

This new line of reasoning complements Stanley Schachter's earlier, experimentally derived *two-factor theory of emotion* (Schachter, 1964; Schachter & Singer, 1962), in which the observer (patient) derives specific meaning from general subjective emotional arousal according to the context in which it occurs. Thus, a specific antidepressant effect might be attributed to SSRIs because it is present when a patient taking these drugs recovers from depression, although a more parsimonious interpretation might be that most therapeutic agents effect positive subjective changes regardless of the specific intervention employed or the condition being treated.

On the other hand, other investigators have proposed differential recommendations for specific disorders.[3] In one of the earliest studies on combining treatment modalities, Hogarty, Goldberg, & Schooler (1974) concluded that a combination of medication and psychosocial interventions prevented relapse in schizophrenic patients. Rush and Hollon (1991) suggested that pharmacotherapy, cognitive therapy, or a combination of both was equally effective in treating nonbipolar and nonpsychotic depression, while pharmacotherapy appeared to be indispensable in

---

[3]Although not a comparison of different biopsychosocial therapies, one meta-analysis of studies of pharmacotherapy in patients with personality disorders may be of interest here. Duggan, Huband, Smailagic, Ferriter, and Adams (2008) acknowledge serious methodological limitations to their study, but after reviewing 35 trials that focused on the use of various drugs to treat a limited sampling of personality disorders, they concluded that anticonvulsants appear to reduce aggressive behaviors while antipsychotics reduce emotional volatility in patients with predominantly borderline personality disorder.

treating bipolar disorder and major depression with psychotic features. With respect to agoraphobia, Mavissakalian (1991), on reviewing six contemporary studies, found that imipramine tended to be as effective as exposure therapy in treating panic, whereas exposure approaches are somewhat more effective in treating phobic behavior; a combination of both approaches appeared to offer some advantage in the treatment of patients who had panic disorder with phobic avoidance. Nevertheless, approximately one fourth of patients who experienced agoraphobia responded equally well to placebo, where about one fourth did not respond to the combination of both pharmacotherapy and exposure psychotherapy. Mavissakalian also indicated that the sequencing of pharmacotherapy—initially for 8 weeks, followed by 16 weeks of imipramine plus exposure therapy—tended to enhance the initial effect achieved with drug treatment alone.

Large-scale studies, as well as expert consensus projects such as the *TMAP* (Kashner et al., 2003), have attempted to shine light on the specific impact of various treatment interventions on particular disorders. Examples of such trials are the *STAR*D* (Fava et al., 2004; Gaynes et al., 2005) and *STEP-BD* (Kogan et al., 2004; Sachs et al., 2003) trials conducted by the National Institute of Mental Health (NIMH); the *TADS*; the *CATIE* (Lieberman et al., 2005); the *CUtLASS* (Jones et al., 2006); and the *MTA* (MTA Cooperative Group, 1999a, 1999b)—all of which are discussed in detail later in this chapter under "Major Studies and Algorithms." Although subtle differences among treatments have been detected, the fact that no substantial, clinically significant differences were found is more impressive.

Although the use of combined therapies has long been assumed to be the gold standard in psychiatric treatment (Conte et al., 1986; Kraly, 2006; Riba & Balon, 2005), Beitman and Blinder (2003) more recently revised such thinking by proposing that combined therapies are not necessarily more effective than their constituent *monotherapies* and should therefore be avoided, unless specific evidence of their comparative effectiveness outweighs the additional cost and potential for an increase in negative side effects (Healy, 2004) of combined treatments. Notwithstanding the undisputed benefits of pharmacotherapy in a subset of disorders, including bipolar disorder, schizophrenia, and major depression with psychotic features, psychotherapy, in addition to its being indicated as a stand-alone approach in an array of other conditions, is generally helpful in supporting the use of medication, since it tends to improve overall compliance (Guo et al., 2010). More to the point, according to Beitman and Blinder (2003), monopsychotherapy has been shown to be effective in patients with major (nonbipolar) depressive disorder, dysthymia, panic disorder, obsessive-compulsive disorder, social phobia, generalized anxiety disorder, bulimia, and primary insomnia; we might suggest that adding medication to the treatment of these conditions is best reserved for those cases in which the potential for side effects is justified by the lack of adequate response to psychotherapy. In mild-to-moderate depression, combined therapy adds little, whereas in severe depression, a combination of medication and psychotherapy appears to increase positive outcomes. In summary, Beitman and Blinder found that the following specific treatments were preferable for particular conditions: family therapy for major depression, CBT for bulimia nervosa, CBT with occasional antidepressant medication for panic disorder, and behavioral exposure for obsessive-compulsive disorder.

Previous research has raised many questions that only recently have yielded answers, with the potential for directing clinical practice. The most recent research (Fournier et al., 2009) indicates that patient variables may influence outcomes within diagnostic categories; for example, if a patient is married, unemployed, or experiencing significant life events, cognitive therapy is likely to result in a better response than anti-depressant medication would be for treating moderate or severe depression. Also, the severity of a given condition such as depression may determine whether there is any advantage at all to medication rather than placebo (Fournier et al., 2010).

Similarly, recent findings point out the subtle interference of medication on the long-term effect of psychotherapy. For example, in the case of sleep disorders, the intermittent use of zolpidem in conjunction with CBT for chronic insomnia (Morin et al., 2009) tends to reduce the effectiveness of CBT, which is more effective singly than when "aided" by as-needed (pro re nata, or PRN) medication. When one attempts to determine the usefulness of combining therapies for the treatment of depression, however, contradictory findings continue to be the theme. March and Vitiello (2009), for example, indicate that the combination of CBT and fluoxetine is superior to the use of either of these agents singly in adolescents with severe to moderate depressive disorders, whereas Kocsis and colleagues (2009) found no advantage to adding psychotherapy to pharmacotherapy for the treatment of chronic depression, and Blier et al. (2009) found that combining fluoxetine with a second antidepressant medication was more effective than fluoxetine alone. Indeed, combining multiple medications has become increasingly common, but there is scant evidence that such *polypharmacy* provides superior results. Mojtabai and Olfson (2010) conclude that these trends "put patients at increased risk of drug–drug interactions with uncertain gains for quality of care and clinical outcomes" (p. 26). Dobson et al. (2008) have pointed out the importance of psychotherapy's effectiveness beyond the treatment stage; in their study, patients who were treated with CBT until remission were only about half as likely to relapse following termination of therapy than patients who were treated with medications until remission.

Studies in attention deficit–hyperactivity disorder (ADHD) tended to confirm the effectiveness of analeptic medication in ameliorating behaviors such as distractedness and hyperactivity, but combination therapy is consistently found to be superior to monopharmacotherapy (Jensen et al., 2005); yet uniformity is lacking with respect to how medication effectiveness is assessed across studies (Faraone et al., 2006), and bias can be ruled out only when variability in study design is more adequately controlled. On the other hand, recent research has indicated that behavioral approaches are unequivocally effective in treating Tourette's syndrome and appear to be as effective as medication (Piacentini et al., 2010).

Apart from clinical research into the differential use of various biopsychosocial interventions in the treatment of emotional distress, psychosocial orientations promulgate theoretical considerations that question the appropriateness of across-the-board medication as *first-line treatment* in the majority of mental health cases (Crystal et al., 2009). Such theoretical stances propose that there are genuine life issues involved in most cases of emotional disturbance and that it is best to treat the disturbance through resolving the issues rather than suppressing symptoms. It is the patient's adjustment to life issues, intrapersonal as well as interpersonal, that defines positive change, and the improvement of symptoms reflects this growth process, which is more likely to occur when the precocious suppression of symptoms by psychotropic drugs has not preempted personal adaptation. A symptom of anxiety does not necessarily imply an anxiety disorder, just as there is a functional side to nearly all emotions (May, 1950), and many symptoms of distress have an adaptive value that can be lost if eliminating symptoms is the only clinical goal in the rush to eradicate a "disorder."

The trend over the last 10 to 15 years has been to increase the role of psychotropics for the suppression of symptoms while reducing the role of psychotherapy

(Olfson & Marcus, 2010). Medical management alone, however, is far more likely to treat symptoms alone without delving into their cause, not only because medications are aimed at symptoms but because they are, by and large, prescribed by clinicians other than mental health professionals (Mark, Levit, & Buck, 2009) who have little or no expertise in evaluating a case beyond the presenting problem (Muse & McGrath, 2010). In contrast to prescribers who are not mental health professionals and to psychiatrists who have specialized in pharmacotherapy to the relative abandonment of psychotherapy (being "motivated by financial incentives and growth in psychopharmacological treatments in recent years" [Mojtabai & Olfson, 2008]), the medical psychologist who can integrate multimodal evaluation and treatment when caring for a patient with an emotional disorder is more likely to concede that a certain amount of "distress" will tend to motivate that patient to make the effort needed for growth. Premature suppression of emotional symptoms runs the risk of delaying or aborting personal adaptation through new learning. When seen in this light, discomfort is a requirement for therapeutic change (Rogers, 1961).

Although we have limited our discussion here to psychotherapy, the larger question concerns the use of *psychosocial interventions* (with psychotherapy being a subset of such interventions) versus *pharmacotherapy* and how these two approaches are best integrated. Another question in the same vein is whether medication can, by its nature, ever be a stand-alone treatment or whether it should be an integral part of psychosocial interventions. Unless a drug is dispensed from a vending machine, with no human contact involved, there is bound to be some form of engagement between the patient and the dispensing professional. Such rapport is the basis of most psychotherapy (Wampold, 2001). How, then, can the true, stand-alone effectiveness of a drug ever be measured when its use is inevitably bound up with the expectations, possible placebo effects, and transference issues inherent in the patient-professional relationship (Busch & Sandberg, 2007; Norcross & Goldfried, 2003)?

A related issue is that of the temporal nature of any research findings, findings which give the impression that even substantiated trends discovered today may be ephemeral, and vanish with time. Case in point is the fact that *placebo effect* is growing within the present mental health treatment zeitgeist (Silberman, 2009), with pharmacological agents acquiring increasing potency as people have come to expect more from them through massive advertisement campaigns that "sell" the product. If the present "biological explanation" of emotional disorders, with its implied need to medicate, were to fall into disrepute or relative disuse (that is, if psychotherapy were to become more popular for whatever reason), some of the research discoveries about the relative effectiveness of one treatment over another may flip, as the placebo effect associated with drugs decreases as a result of generalized skepticism and, perhaps, a parallel re-engendered belief in psychotherapy invests the psychosocial modality with greater placebo.

One approach to circumventing such culturally determined fluctuations in the placebo effect is rooted in the relative immutability of established principles of learning and the application of conditioning for therapeutic effect. Medical psychologists are in a unique position to integrate the effect of conditioned learning that parallels the dispensing of medication so as to reinforce desired therapeutic directions by integrating pharmacotherapy within the behavioral principles of learning. Not only does this create a synergistic therapeutic intervention that enhances the effectiveness of pharmacologic agents, it reduces the acquisition of learned, undesirable secondary effects. Consider these examples of potential applications of behavioral principles in the administration and management of pharmacotherapy:

- In chronic pain syndromes, behavioral therapy (Wolpe, 1969) and behavior modification (Skinner, 1974) can be reinforced by pharmacotherapy within the operant paradigm for motivating patient compliance and efforts toward reha-bilitation (Fordyce, 1976).
- Medication schedules can be managed to avoid positive and negative reinforcement contingencies that promote reliance on and addiction to analgesics (Muse, 1994).
- The medication effect can be used as an unconditioned response for pairing with the conditioned stimulus within the respondent paradigm for countercon-ditioning of phobias (Muse, 2007).
- Aversive substances can be employed as unconditioned stimuli in pairings with the conditioned response of sexual arousal to achieve a *Garcia effect*–like extinction in the treatment of pedophilia (Muse, 1999; Muse & Frigola, 2003).
- A drug-induced, state-dependent learning paradigm can be enlisted to acceler-ate relearning in PTSD (Muse, 1984).
- Drug therapy can be prescribed as an initial mitigator of subjective units of dis-tress (SUDs) attached to hierarchical items in the systematic desensitization of severe vaginismus (Muse, 2010a).
- The placebo effect, thought to account for about 70% of the response to anti-depressant medications (Rief et al., 2009), can act as a booster in stalled stages of psychotherapy to reinforce previous efforts and to facilitate renewed positive expectations in the patient-professional relationship.

SUMMARY

Table 2.1 summarizes what has been covered thus far in our review of past and pres-ent attempts to devise differential interventions in the treatment of psychological conditions to achieve optimal results. This summary is not intended for use by the medical psychologist as a decision tree or algorithm when formulating treatment rec-ommendations; it has been designed merely for heuristic purposes to illuminate trends apparent in the myriad results of research. Clearly, it does not take into account patient variables (e.g., gender, age, race, or ethnicity) or transient contributory factors (e.g., life events), nor does it address the issue of integrating reinforcement contingen-cies of behavioral therapy within pharmacotherapy. In short, Table 2.1 represents all the current limitations inherent in the attempt to force generalized treatment recom-mendations into the dichotomous choice between "drugs" and "therapy."

Major Studies and Algorithms

In order to make heads or tails out of the vast array of treatment options available in the field of mental health, it is incumbent upon the medical psychologist to keep abreast of developments in the science of psychology, as well as to remain current in the field of clinical psychopharmacology. This is not a small task, and for this reason continuing education is far more extensive for medical psychology than for any other subspecialty within applied psychology or perhaps even medicine.

To analyze the studies available, medical psychologists must draw upon their expertise in research and consult primary resource material whenever possible. Each study—whether it be a meta-analysis, a randomized clinical trial, or a case study in the area of psychopharmacology (Muse, 2010b)—has the potential to provide the

Table 2.1   Monotherapy Versus Combined Therapy in Psychobiosocial Treatment of Mental Health Conditions

Research

1. Medication efficacy is hard to calculate, since the greater part of a drug's effect is placebo. This placebo effect also accounts for the greater part of psychotherapy's effect and appears to be culturally bound, thus fluctuating over time as a function of cultural beliefs.
2. Research designs have been inadequate in identifying and separating out effects of medication and psychotherapy on various disorders.
3. Side effects of medication, which are demonstrably greater than with psychotherapy, are not adequately weighed as (negative) outcomes in research that compares this modality with psychotherapy.

Treatment

1. Medication is important (albeit not always effective/efficacious) in:
   a. Treating positive signs of schizophrenia, with clozapine preferred for treatment-resistant symptoms.
   b. Treating mania in bipolar disorder.
   c. Treating depression with psychotic features.
   d. Treating attention deficit–hyperactivity disorder (ADHD), especially the hyperactive type.
2. Medication is of comparable importance to psychotherapy (no better outcome) in:
   a. Treating major depression.
   b. Treating depressive end of bipolar disorder.
   c. Treating panic disorder.
   d. Treating Tourette's syndrome.
3. Medication is of secondary importance to psychotherapy (poorer outcome) in:
   a. Treating negative signs of schizophrenia (second-generation antipsychotics no more effective than first-generation in treating negative symptoms).
   b. Treating depressions other than major depression (adjustment disorder, depression not otherwise specified [NOS]).
   c. Treating obsessive-compulsive disorder.
   d. Treating eating disorders.
4. Medication is generally not indicated (interferes with more effective psychotherapy) in:
   a. Treating simple phobias.
   b. Treating dysthymia.
   c. Treating chronic insomnia.
5. Combining both medication and psychosocial therapy might be indicated for:
   a. Schizophrenia, in which neuroleptics are augmented with systemic, family, or milieu therapy for overcoming the poor social integration involved in negative symptoms and for reducing discontinuation of therapy.
   b. Bipolar disorder with hypomania/mania, in which mood stabilizers are augmented by cognitive-educational approaches intended to help the patient gain insight into the advantage of medication compliance.
   c. Major depression, especially with adolescents, in which medication is augmented by cognitive-behavioral therapy (CBT) approaches in an effort to increase engagement and activity level.
   d. ADHD, in which analeptic medication is paired with CBT approaches aimed at time management, impulse control, and executive functions.
   e. Panic disorder, in which CBT approaches emphasize tolerance of anxiety while selective serotonin-reuptake inhibitors (SSRIs) raise the threshold for manifest panic.
   f. Obsessive-compulsive disorder with a strong obsessive component, in which obsessive symptoms may be adjunctively treated with SSRIs or tricyclic medication while compulsive components are simultaneously treated with behavioral approaches.

Table 2.1   (Continued)

Limitations

1. Current research is dominated by attempts to match diagnosis with treatment modality, paying little attention to subject variables and life event interplay.
2. Little research has been done to optimize the behavioral administration of medications in an effort to integrate medication into behavioral approaches.
3. CBT is overrepresented in controlled studies, leading to the question of how effective are psychosocial interventions in general when only a limited sampling of such interventions is compared to placebo and medication.
4. The medical model has emphasized symptom reduction, reducing the value of emotional distress as a motivator for therapeutic change.

Conclusions

1. Medication is overused in medical practice, given its limited efficacy, its potential for deleterious effects, and the availability of alternative psychosocial treatments of proven value with significantly less side effect profiles.
2. Much more research is needed in the differential effects of medication and psychotherapy on various diagnoses, patient populations, and presenting/underlying life issues before specific, empirically based, authoritative statements can be made with any degree of confidence as to which treatment or combination of treatments might be preferentially recommended.

Table adapted from Muse (2010a).

key to treating a group of patients or, indeed, a particular individual. With an estimated 10,000 randomized, controlled trials being published every year (DeLeon, 2010), the practicing clinician can never commit all relevant studies to memory; therefore, an essential part of the practice of medical psychology is to cultivate the habit of both consulting and revisiting the literature on an ongoing basis, while also relying on certain landmark studies as general points of reference.

Major studies that have been particularly influential in the field of clinical psychopharmacology should be familiar to the medical psychologist and should serve as a general knowledge base. By the same token, certain algorithms may prove useful as guides when one is faced with the complex task of tailoring treatment to specific patients (Fawcett et al., 1999). Several of these major studies and algorithms are summarized in Table 2.2 and are discussed next.[4]

STAR*D Study (Sequenced Treatment Alternatives to Relieve Depression)

This NIMH-funded study was the largest and longest study ever conducted to determine the effectiveness of different treatments for patients with major depression. Over a period of 7 years, the researchers enrolled more than 4,000 outpatients, 18 to 75 years of age, who had not responded to initial therapy with an antidepressant. The study was carried out by psychiatrists and primary care physicians in both private practice and public clinics to reflect the treatments patients typically receive in community settings. This was not a true randomized study with control groups;

[4]One large study worth mentioning, but perhaps not as influential as those cited in Table 2.2, is the SMILE (Standard Medical Intervention and Long-term Exercise) study (Hoffman et al., 2011) in which 202 sedentary adults with major depressive disorder were randomly assigned to either sertraline or aerobic exercise. At the end of this 4-month study, as well as at the 1-year follow-up, antidepressant medication and exercise both proved to be effective but neither was superior to the other.

Table 2.2   Summary of Medication Efficacy in Large Studies and Algorithms

- In the **STAR*D study**, medication efficacy in treating major depressive disorder in adults ranged from about 1/3 to 1/4 to 1/5 for each of three successive attempts; a fourth attempt with treatment-resistant nonresponders yielded a remission rate of less than 10%. With multiple medication switches or augmentation, the cumulative remission rate increased to approximately 60% overall; 40% remained nonresponders, despite up to four successive medication trials. For depressed persons who failed to respond to an antidepressant in the first trial, adding cognitive therapy resulted in the same probability of remission as did switching from one antidepressant medication to another.

- In the **STEP-BD study**, treatment-resistant bipolar patients did not significantly improve when lamotrigine, inositol, risperidone, or antidepressant medication was added to a mood stabilizer, whereas patients who received psychotherapy in addition to medication showed enhanced treatment outcomes for bipolar disorder.

- In the **TADS study**, short-term efficacy in treating depression in children and adolescents was greatest for combined therapy (fluoxetine plus cognitive-behavioral therapy [CBT]) than for either pharmacotherapy or psychotherapy alone. In the long term, combination therapy and CBT monotherapy proved more effective than fluoxetine alone, with CBT somewhat superior to combination therapy on measures of sustained improvement.

- In the **CATIE and CUtLASS studies**, no difference in efficacy was observed between the newer atypical antipsychotic agents and the older neuroleptics, and patients with schizophrenia were relatively noncompliant regardless of which antipsychotic was prescribed. Clozapine was found to be more efficacious than other second-generation antipsychotics in treatment-resistant subjects in the CUtLASS-2.

- In the **TMAP**, some evidence has been presented that treating certain groups of patients according to an algorithm may lead to better recovery results than relying on practitioners' individual decision-making without the structure of consensually developed algorithms.

- In the **MTA study** of children with attention deficit–hyperactivity disorder (ADHD), children placed on medication, either alone or in combination with behavioral approaches, initially showed greater improvement than those treated with behavioral approaches or commuity-based support alone. However, long-term follow-up indicated that medication differences were no longer significant at 3 and 8 years after the initial treatment.

- In the **SOFTABS** on adolescent depression, the great majority of patients recovered from depression within 2 years, yet half of those suffered a relapse within 5 years. Recurrent rates for female adolescents were greater than for male adolescents.

- In the **GLAD-PC Guidelines** for treating adolescent depression in the primary care setting, the expert panel recommended, among other things, that interviews be augmented with standard questionnaires, treatment be based on a collaborative relationship and include evidence-based treatment protocols, and referral be made to mental health professionals as needed, with follow-up reassessment and encouragement to work with these professionals.

indeed, there were no placebo conditions, and patients were allowed to choose among treatment modalities, although the medications within each treatment category were randomly assigned. Four levels of treatment were used, and treatment at each level could continue for up to 14 weeks.

All participants began at Level 1, and were treated with citalopram. Participants who did not become symptom-free or who could not tolerate side effects from citalopram were encouraged to progress to the next level (Level 2), where new treatment choices would be available. Level 2 offered seven different treatments; four of these options "switched" the citalopram participants to either a new medication or talk therapy, and the other three options "augmented" citalopram treatment by adding a new medication or talk therapy to the citalopram they were already receiving. If participants progressed to Level 2, they agreed to have their treatment selected randomly from among the approaches available. Those who joined the "switch" group were randomly assigned to sertraline, bupropion-SR, or venlafaxine-XR, while those who joined the "add-on" group were prescribed either bupropion-SR or buspirone. Participants could also switch to, or add on, cognitive psychotherapy. In Level 3, participants again had the option of either switching to a different medication or adding on to their existing medication. Those who chose to switch their medication were randomly assigned to either mirtazapine or nortriptyline for up to 14 weeks. In the Level 3 add-on group, participants were randomly prescribed either lithium or triiodothyronine (T3) to add to the medication they were already taking. Finally, in Level 4, participants who had not become symptom-free in any of the previous levels were taken off all other medications and randomly switched to one of two treatments: tranylcypromine or the combination of venlafaxine and mirtazapine.

After each level, those participants whose depression did not respond to the treatment were encouraged to go on to the next level of treatment. Participants who fully recovered (reached remission of their depressive symptoms) began the 12-month follow-up process (Gaynes et al., 2005; Rush et al., 2004).

In STAR*D, the outcome measure was "remission" of depressive symptoms (i.e., becoming symptom-free). Perhaps the most significant overall finding was that patients who did not respond to three consecutive trials of antidepressant medication will not be likely to respond when switched to a fourth medication.

In Level 1, about one third of the participants reached remission. In the Level 2 switch group, about 25% of the participants became symptom-free. All three of the switch medications performed about the same and were equally safe and well-tolerated. In the Level 2 add-on group, about one third of the participants became symptom-free. Those who added bupropion experienced less troublesome side effects and a slightly greater reduction in symptoms than those who added buspirone. Level 2 also included cognitive psychotherapy as a switch or add-on treatment; the psychotherapy treatment was equivalent to switching to or adding on of a new psychotropic drug when citalopram was not effective at Level 1 (Thase et al., 2007). In the Level 3 switch group, 12% to 20% of participants became symptom-free, and results with each of the two medications were about equally good, suggesting no clear advantage for either one in terms of remission rates or side effects. In the add-on group, about 20% of the participants became symptom-free, with little difference between the two treatments. In Level 4, 7% to 10% of the participants became symptom-free, with no statistically significant differences between the medications in terms of remission, response rates, or side effects.

In conclusion, about half the participants in the STAR*D study became symptom-free after two treatment levels. Over the course of all four treatment levels, approximately 60% of those who did not withdraw from the study became symptom-free; 40% did not reach remission and, as the level of treatment progressed, treatment-resistant patients were less likely to respond to the interventions.

STEP-BD Study (Systematic Treatment Enhancement Program for Bipolar Disorder)

The STEP-BD study was the largest federally funded study ever conducted for the treatment of bipolar disorder. This long-term study enrolled 4,360 outpatients from 22 sites over a 7-year period (1998–2005). It was designed to find out which treatments, or combinations of treatments, were most effective for treating episodes of depression and mania and for preventing recurrent episodes in people with bipolar disorder.

STEP-BD assessed many of the most established treatments used for bipolar disorder, including mood-stabilizing medications, antidepressants, atypical anti-psychotic medications, and standardized psychosocial interventions that included family-focused treatment, interpersonal/social rhythm therapy, and CBT, all of which were compared with a control treatment that consisted of brief, collaborative patient-professional contact. All psychotherapy treatments were geared toward helping participants and their families better understand the disorder, develop coping strategies, and stick to treatment plans, and they were always given in conjunction with pharmacological therapy. Medications and dosing recommendations were derived from published, evidence-based treatment guidelines (Sachs et al., 2003).

Once enrolled in the STEP-BD program, participants received individualized care that included the best available treatment options. This approach was called the *best practice pathway*. Participants who were 18 years of age or older and whose depression did not improve or who experienced a new depressive episode could enter the randomized clinical trial that examined the effectiveness of different combinations of medication and psychosocial therapy for the depressive phase of bipolar disorder.

The largest randomized trial looked at treatment options for the acute depressive episode and included both medication and psychotherapy. Early results indicated that treatment-resistant bipolar patients did not significantly improve when lamotrigine, inositol, or risperidone was added to their previous treatment regimen (Nierenberg et al., 2006). Subsequent analysis indicated that for depressed people with bipolar disorder who are taking a mood stabilizer, adding an antidepressant medication is no more effective than a placebo (Sachs et al., 2007). Still later findings showed that patients taking medications to treat bipolar disorder are more likely to get well faster and stay well if they receive intensive psychotherapy. There were no significant differences among the three psychotherapies employed (i.e., family-focused therapy, CBT, and interpersonal/social rhythm therapy), but all were superior to a mere collaborative relationship with the provider (Miklowitz et al., 2007). In summary, treatment-resistant patients with bipolar disorder did not significantly improve with the addition of lamotrigine, inositol, risperidone, or an antidepressant medication to a mood stabilizer, whereas patients who received psychotherapy in addition to medication showed enhanced treatment outcomes.

TADS (Treatment of Adolescents With Depression Study)

The TADS was a NIMH-sponsored, multisite clinical research study that examined the short- and long-term effectiveness of antidepressant medication and psychotherapy, as monotherapies as well as in combination with each other, for treating depression in adolescents ages 12 to 17. TADS included 439 participants, ages 12 to 17, from various geographic regions in the United States who were diagnosed with major depression. For the first 12 weeks of the study (Stage 1), participants were randomly assigned to receive one of four treatments: 1. Fluoxetine alone, 2. Placebo alone, CBT alone, or 4. A combination of fluoxetine and CBT. At the end of Stage 1, the participants taking pills were informed whether they were taking placebo or the active medication fluoxetine. Those taking the placebo who were not improved could choose to receive any one of the other three treatments in the study: fluoxetine alone, CBT alone, or combination therapy. Participants who improved while taking placebo were followed for up to 12 weeks and were offered active treatment if their depression worsened during that time. Participants in any of the three active treatment groups (fluoxetine, CBT, or the combination treatment) who improved during the first 12 weeks continued with their assigned treatments for 6 more weeks (Stage 2). Participants who continued to do well in Stage 2 progressed to Stage 3, which lasted another 18 weeks, for a total of 36 weeks of study partici- pation. After the first 12 weeks, 71% of participants who received the combination treatment were much or very much improved. Among those who received fluoxetine alone, 61% improved, and among those who received CBT alone, 44% improved. Among those given a placebo, 35% improved.

Results remained consistent at the end of 18 weeks and at 36 weeks. At 18 weeks, the combination treatment still outpaced the monotherapies with a response rate of 85%, as compared with 69% for fluoxetine alone and 65% for CBT alone. By 36 weeks, the response rate to combination treatment still remained the highest (86%), while the rates for fluoxetine and CBT essentially caught up, at 81% each (TADS Team, 2007). The majority of teens (82%) who reached a sustained positive response by week 12 maintained this level of recovery through week 36. Among those in combination treatment, about 89% maintained improvement for the full 36 weeks. Among those in the fluoxetine-only group, 74% maintained improvement, but among those in the CBT-only group, 97% maintained improvement.

The high long-term success rate of CBT suggests that for teens who initially respond to it, CBT may have a preventive effect that helps to sustain positive improvement and potentially avoid relapse or recurrence. This would be true even if treatment visits become infrequent, as was the case after the first 12 weeks in the TADS study. In addition, the relatively lower sustained success rate for fluoxetine suggests that the effectiveness of fluoxetine therapy may plateau at a certain point for some responders, triggering a need for the addition of psychosocial treatment (Rohde et al., 2008).

By the end of the 36-week trial, 82% of participants had improved and 59% had reached full remission. During the follow-up year, most participants maintained these improvements, and the remission rate climbed to 68%. However, about 30% of the participants who were in remission at week 36 became depressed again during the following year (March & Vitiello, 2009; TADS Team, 2009).

CATIE (Clinical Antipsychotic Trials of Intervention Effectiveness)

This double-blind trial enrolled 1,493 patients with chronic schizophrenia who were randomly assigned to one of the second-generation antipsychotics, including olanzapine, quetiapine, risperidone, or the first-generation drug perphenazine (Lieberman et al., 2005). The results showed poor tolerance for all medications, with 74% of patients discontinuing treatment over 18 months. Olanzapine proved to have the lowest discontinuation rate, but in terms of effectiveness or extrapyramidal side effects, the remaining second-generation drugs did not differ from one another or from the first-generation antipsychotic perphenazine. There was no evidence that second-generation drugs were better than the conventional antipsychotic for alleviat- ing negative symptoms.

For those participants who discontinued the first phase, a second phase was begun that compared clozapine to other second-generation antipsychotics. Ninety-nine sub- jects entered phase 2, and clozapine emerged as significantly better tolerated than other atypical drugs, with more than double the time to discontinuation as compared with the other antipsychotics.

CUtLASS (Cost Utility of the Latest Antipsychotic Drugs in Schizophrenia Study)

CUtLASS was conducted by the National Health Service (NHS) of the United Kingdom (Jones et al. 2006; Lewis et al., 2006) and consisted of several open-label, randomized trials comparing antipsychotic medications according to a standard algorithm for this class of drugs. First-generation and second-generation antipsychotics were compared in one trial, and second-generation antipsychotics were compared with clozapine in the other. Outcomes were determined by judges who were unaware of the treatment assignments. In the first trial, 227 people with schizophrenia were randomly assigned to either a first-generation or a second-generation drug other than clozapine (amisulpride, olanzapine, quetiapine or risperidone). No significant difference could be detected between the first- and second-generation drugs in terms of quality of life or symptoms over the course of 1 year. Moreover, the outcome for the group given the second-generation drugs was no better than that for the group given the first-generation drugs in terms of extrapyramidal side effects. In the second trial, clozapine was compared with five other second-generation drugs (risperidone, olanzapine, amisulpride, zotepine, and quetiapine) in 136 patients who had not responded to at least two previous drugs. On the Positive and Negative Syndrome Scale (PANSS) (Kay, Fishbein, & Opler, 1989), clozapine proved to have a significant advantage over the other drugs in terms of symptom improvements over 1 year.

Algorithms

Algorithms are decision trees that indicate specific therapies for particular phases in the treatment of defined diagnoses, as agreed upon by a panel of experts or a review of the existing literature. Algorithms are expected to be "evidence-based" but are not necessarily put to the test by experimental trials; rather, they tend to stand on their own by virtue of their logic and/or the prestige of those who construct them. David Osser and Robert Patterson (2005) have cited algorithms for depression, bipolar disorder, schizophrenia, panic disorder, PTSD, social anxiety disorder, OCD, generalized anxiety disorder, body dysmorphic disorder, dementia with agitation, personality disorders, ADHD, and a host of other diagnoses, syndromes, and symptoms. The quality of such algorithms varies widely, but the benchmark most referred to as a laudable standard is the Texas Medication Algorithm Project (TMAP), which developed algorithms for treating major depression, bipolar depression, and schizophrenia.

TMAP (Texas Medication Algorithm Project)

The TMAP was started in 1997 with the financial support of several government agencies and private foundation donors, with financial contributions from the pharmaceutical companies whose products were being evaluated. The project proceeded through three phases (Gilbert et al., 1998): The development of expert, consensually agreed upon, evidence-based algorithms; the implementation of the algorithms in public clinics through training programs; and the evaluation of outcomes in terms of effectiveness among a sample of public sector patients treated by algorithm-driven therapy versus treatment-as-usual in public mental health centers. The algorithms went through several revisions as feedback from clinicians was received during the implementation phase, and subsequent evaluation of the applicability of the algorithm for improving care has provided some corroboration of the usefulness of this approach. Suppes et al. (2003), for example, reports that bipolar patients with a history of mania treated according to the algorithm showed significantly more improvement than a comparable group treated without the paradigm of the TMAP algorithm for the treatment of bipolar disorder. As far as the algorithms' current practical value, they are considered by the Behavioral Health Medical Director of the Texas Department of State Health Services to be too out of date to grant copyright permission for their reproduction here (E.A. Becker, personal communication, November 1, 2010).

MTA Study (Multimodal Treatment of Attention Deficit–Hyperactivity Disorder)

The MTA was an NIMH-sponsored study designed to evaluate an algorithm that consisted of the leading treatments for ADHD, including behavioral therapy, medications, and the combination of the two (MTA Cooperative Group, 1999a, 1999b). The study included nearly 600 children, ages 7 to 9, who were randomly assigned to one of four treatment modes:

1. Intensive medication management alone,
2. Intensive behavioral treatment alone,
3. A combination of both, or
4. Routine community care (the control group).

Initial results indicated that combination treatment and medical management alone were both significantly superior to intensive behavioral therapy alone and to routine community care in reducing ADHD symptoms. The study also showed that these benefits lasted for as long as 14 months. In other areas of functioning (e.g., anxiety symptoms, academic performance, parent-child relations, and social skills), combination treatment was consistently superior to routine community care, whereas medication alone and behavioral therapy alone were not. The children in the combination treatment also ended up taking lower doses of medication than the children in the medication-alone group.

Nonetheless, follow-up studies showed that the initial advantages that medication management alone or in combination with behavioral therapy had over purely behavioral therapy or routine community care waned in the years after the controlled treatments ended at 14 months (Jensen et al., 2007; Molina et al., 2009). After 3 years, 45% to 71% of the youth in the original treatment groups were taking medication. However, by the third year, continuing medical treatment was no longer associated with better outcomes. At 8 years, based on reports from parents and teachers as well as self-reports from the children, there were no differences in symptoms or functioning among the youths assigned to the different treatment groups, and children who were no longer taking medication at the 8-year follow-up were generally functioning as well as those who were still on medication.

Other Studies

One final major study and one final algorithm-like study are the *SOFTABS (Survey of Outcomes Following Treatment for Adolescent Depression)* and the *GLAD-PC (Guidelines for Adolescent Depression in Primary Care)*, respectively.

In the SOFTABS, 91.5% of the adolescents studied recovered from depression within 2 years, yet 50% of those who recovered suffered a relapse within 5 years (Curry et al., 2010). Recurrence rates were greater for the female than for the male adolescents (57% vs. 33%, respectively). These results underscore the need for periodic follow-up during the years following remission.

The GLAD-PC was an expert-generated protocol that developed recommendations for the treatment of adolescents within the primary setting (Cheung et al., 2007, 2008; Zuckerbrot et al., 2007). A total of 15 recommendations were generated to cover assessment, treatment and follow-up; the following is an abbreviated summary of some of the recommendations:

- During assessment, personal interviews should be augmented with the use of standard questionnaires.
- Treatment should be based on support and a collaborative relationship with the patient and family and should include evidence-based treatment protocols and referral to mental health professionals as needed.
- Follow-up should include periodic reassessment and active encouragement of referred patients to continue to work with mental health professionals.

Based on desired outcome effectiveness and economic cost-benefit considerations, clinical guidelines for the treatment of alcohol and drug abuse, depression, OCD, PTSD, and generalized anxiety disorder have been developed by the National Institute for Health and Clinical Excellence (NICE), a part of the NHS of the United Kingdom. The guidelines for generalized anxiety disorder and panic disorder (with or without agoraphobia) in adults were based on a review of the literature and expert panel recommendations (National Health Service, 2010). In general, they recommend that generalized anxiety of low intensity be treated within primary care by providing patient education and self-help resources, whereas anxiety of higher intensity or low-intensity anxiety that has not responded to the psychoeducational approach should be treated with CBT, relaxation therapy, or pharmacotherapy. SSRIs should be chosen over benzodiazepines if pharmacotherapy is instituted. If the response to treatment provided within primary care is inadequate, or if the patient poses a threat to himself or herself, a referral to an inpatient or intensive outpatient program is recommended. Guidelines for treating panic disorder follow a parallel course of intervention, with the preference for initial treatment taking place within primary care by professionals trained in psychopharmacotherapy and CBT. If the panic disorder proves resistant to treatment, referral to specialized intensive mental health treatment is recommended.

CONCLUSION

Although evidence-based recommendations in the field of clinical psychopharmacology are tentative at best and premature at worst, attempts to determine "which treatment is suitable for which disorder" have raised hopes that further research will provide more substantiated trends. Such recommendations might emanate from meta-analyses, algorithms, or case studies, but ideally they would be corroborated, whenever possible, through replicable, randomized clinical trials. Recently an effort has been made to assess special populations (Krahn et al., 2006), but greater attention needs to be paid to cofactors such as patient age, gender, and ethnicity, just as diagnoses need to be refined and made more clinically relevant, allowing for spectra of gradation for any fixed term. Treatment modalities have been artificially restricted for convenience in designing comparisons, as medications are tested against a small sampling of existing psychotherapies. There is little evidence to support the notion that one psychotherapeutic approach is universally more effective or more clearly indicated than another, and to date, research has led to the same conclusion for many of the pharmacological agents—that is, there is little evidence to recommend one drug over another.[5] This is not to say that all treatments are equal. Rather, it is an admission of the state of affairs in psychopharmacology and psychotherapy. So little is known, and there is so much to learn. And this admission, we submit, is a powerful reason to promote medical psychologists' involvement, with their solid research training, in the area of clinical psychopharmacology.

CHAPTER 2 KEY TERMS

Algorithms: A problem-solving method that follows a series of steps to arrive at a decision. It is based, with few exceptions, on a mathematical, deterministic model that assumes uniformity in progression from an initial state to a finalized state, following well-defined avenues and options for completing the course. In psychiatry, treatment algorithms have been developed for a host of DSM-IV diagnoses.

Best practice pathway: A term coined in the STEP-BD studies. It was conceived as an alternative to clinical trial studies, and it attempts to recreate the conditions under which various treatment modalities, pharmacologic or psychosocial, are selected in the course of treatment. Subjects are studied within the preexisting relationship with their provider. The patient's/subject's response to treatments is monitored. Although the provider and patient select the treatment modality, the medications or psychosocial interventions within the selected modality are assigned in a random fashion.

CATIE (Clinical Antipsychotic Trials of Intervention Effectiveness): A large, double-blind, randomized clinical trial which revealed no difference between effectiveness of conventional and second generation antipsychotics.

Clinical anthropology: Application of anthropological/cultural concepts within clinical settings.

Clinical psychopharmacology: The practice of psychopharmacology, which, as practiced by medical psychologists, endeavors to critically evaluate research in the area and to integrate evidenced-based pharmacological treatments among proven psychosocial therapies for mental, emotional, behavioral, and somatic disorders.

Clinical sociology: Use of the sociological perspective and/or its tools in the diagnosing and intervention/treatment of social interactions.

Combination-treatment modality: The blending of pharmacotherapy with psychotherapy or with other psychosocial therapies.

Common factors theory: A theory which proposes that different theoretical and evidence-based approaches to psychotherapy and counseling have common components that account for outcome rather than components that are unique to each approach.

---

[5]In the past decade, therapeutic practice in the field of mental health has been decidedly skewed toward pharmacological interventions, hence the substantial increase in the use of psychotropic drugs and the concomitant decline in the practice of psychotherapy (Olfson & Marcus, 2010) even though the rate of compliance with medical regimens is only about 20% (Serna Cruz, Real, Gascó, & Galván, 2011).

CUtLASS (Cost Utility of the Latest Antipsychotic Drugs in Schizophrenia Study): A large, open-label, randomized study based on a treatment algorithm for the pharmacologic treatment of schizophrenia that compared first-generation antipsychotic medications with second-generation antipsychotics, and then compared clozapine with other second-generation antipsychotics. The study found no difference in effectiveness or side effect profiles between conventional and atypical antipsychotics but did find clozapine to be more effective than any other antipsychotic drug for treatment-resistant psychosis.

Dodo-bird effect: Based on psychotherapy outcome studies, this hypothesis states that there is no significant difference between various common psychotherapeutic approaches in terms of client outcome. Also known as the "Dodo-bird hypothesis" (named after the character in *Alice in Wonderland* who, after a footrace, declared that "everyone has won, so all must have prizes").

First-line treatment: A therapy recommended for the initial treatment of a disease. If the disorder does not respond to the first-line treatment, or if there is a reason not to begin first-line treatment (e.g., a dangerous side effect for a given patient), second-line, third-line, and fourth-line therapies may be recommended sequentially.

Garcia effect: Conditioned aversion through strong pairings of a food (conditioned stimulus) to the unconditioned response of nausea after ingesting the toxin-infested food.

GLAD-PC (Guidelines for Adolescent Depression in Primary Care): An expert consensus study that recommended certain guidelines for primary care providers to follow in assessing mental issues among the adolescent population.

Integration: In medical psychology, integration refers to taking psychobiosocial factors into account for an optimal understanding of a person's presenting condition and, ultimately, blending psychobiosocial therapeutic options for maximal treatment effectiveness.

Monotherapies: Sole therapies that are not combined with any other therapy (see also *Stand-alone treatment*).

MTA (Multimodal Treatment Study of ADHD): A large, randomized study that put an algorithm for treating attention deficit–hyperactivity disorder (ADHD) to the test and revealed that medication management of ADHD may be optimally useful only during the first 14 months of treatment.

Multidimensional analyses of behavior: Analyses of the significance of behavior within a holistic perspective. For example, anxiety is not necessarily viewed as a symptom to be medically treated but is understood within the full complexity of the patient's condition. In certain cases, anxiety may be considered functional and/or therapeutic.

Multimodal treatment strategies: The multimodal treatment approach is, arguably, best exemplified by Arnold A. Lazarus (1976), who proposed evaluating and treating the patient on a psychosociobiological spectrum that contained seven measures: behaviors, affective responses, sensory reactions, images, cognitions, interpersonal relationships, and drugs/biological interventions.

Pharmacotherapy: The treatment of disorders through the administration of drugs.

Placebo effect: An effect beyond the result that an active intervention might exert on a subject. In psychopharmacology, a placebo effect is often hypothesized to stem from subject expectation and interpersonal dynamics that are active in the context in which the intervention is delivered. A placebo may exist in combination with an inert substance that is devoid of therapeutic pharmacodynamics or may accompany active ingredients. The placebo effect is not steady; instead, it fluctuates according to the expectation at any given time.

Polypharmacy: The administration of multiple drugs at the same time. Apart from its potential for providing additional benefits derived from multiple agents, polypharmacy implies an increase in interaction among the drugs as well as an increase in exposure to side effects associated with the drugs. Polypharmacy is sometimes used as a pejorative term to indicate overmedication.

Psychobiosocial interventions: Holistic, integrative approaches that assess and treat the client as a multifaceted, yet intimately integrated, functioning entity/organism. The emphasis in medical psychology is on psychology, with profound appreciation for the biosocial aspect of each individual's life and circumstances.

Psychosocial interventions: Mental health therapies, other than biological interventions, that are based on psychological and/or sociological interventions. Examples include individual/group psychotherapy, milieu therapy, family therapy, behavioral engineering, support groups, and a host of other interventions.

Single-treatment modality: See *Monotherapies; Stand-alone treatment*.

SOFTABS (Survey of Outcomes Following Treatment for Adolescent Depression): A large, longitudinal study that found that most adolescents recover from depression within 2 years, but that many relapse. Females were found to relapse more than males.

Social-clinical psychology: Although not a discipline in itself, it represents the interface of social and clinical psychology and is concerned, in part, with the application of research from social psychology toward the alleviation of psychological problems and distress.

Stand-alone treatment: The use of a single-treatment modality, either pharmacotherapy or psychosocial therapy (see also *Monotherapies*).

STAR*D (Sequenced Treatment Alternatives to Relieve Depression): The largest and longest federally funded study to date, STAR*D was conducted to determine the effectiveness of different treatments in people with major depression who have not responded to initial treatment with an antidepressant.

STEP-BD (Systematic Treatment Enhancement Program for Bipolar Disorder): The largest federally funded treatment study ever conducted for bipolar disorder, the STEP-BD ran for over 7 years and was designed to identify which treatments, or combinations of treatments, are most effective for treating episodes of depression and mania and for preventing recurrent episodes in people with bipolar disorder.

TADS (Treatment of Adolescents with Depression Study): A large, federally sponsored clinical research study, the TADS examined the short- and long-term effectiveness of antidepressant medication and psychotherapy both as monotherapies and in combination for treating depression in adolescents.

TMAP (Texas Medication Algorithm Project): An ambitious project that, based on expert consensus, constructed different algorithms for treating several major psychiatric conditions and then tested the accuracy of the algorithms by means of specially designed clinical trials.

Two-factor theory of emotion: This theory postulates that nervous system arousal is interpreted to have significance according to the beliefs and/or the social context in which it is experienced. In a classic experiment (Schachter & Singer, 1962), subjects were given adrenaline, and their behavioral response to this initial physiological arousal was determined by the expectancy that they were led to believe about the effect of the drug.

Wampold hypothesis: A recently coined term to reflect the ideas of Bruce Wampold and his assertion that "at least 70% of the psychotherapeutic effects are general effects (i.e., due to common factors)" and his belief that a significant amount of this effect comes from the interpersonal relationship between therapist and client: "Clearly the person of the therapist is a critical factor in the success of therapy."

Chapter 2 Questions

1. Medical psychologists can contribute to the efficacy and effectiveness of clinical psychopharmacology by
   a. Facilitating nonspecific curative effects of placebo through the therapeutic relationship.
   b. Applying behavioral approaches directly to the management of medications.
   c. Discerning when to use medication or therapy alone or in combination.
   d. All of the above.
2. The fact that most psychotherapies are of equal efficacy when compared in meta-analysis is known as the
   a. Wampold effect.
   b. Dodo-bird effect.
   c. Common factors theory.
   d. Placebo effect.
3. According to Robert Julien, which of the following is *not* correct:
   a. In the treatment of most phobias, cognitive-behavioral therapy (CBT) is more consistent and provides longer-lasting effects than medications.
   b. In the treatment of obsessive-compulsive disorder (OCD), posttraumatic stress disorder (PTSD), and generalized anxiety disorder, medications and behavioral approaches are equally effective.
   c. In the treatment of major depression, CBT and antidepressant medication are equally effective and display additional efficacy when combined.
   d. In the treatment of schizophrenia, atypical antipsychotics are more effective than conventional antipsychotics or psychotherapy.
4. According to Morgan Sammons, which of the following statements is *not* correct:
   a. In the treatment of OCD, a single-treatment modality (behavioral therapy) is more effective than a combination-treatment modality when symptoms are primarily compulsive.
   b. In OCD, a combined-treatment modality (medication-behavioral therapy) is more effective than a single-treatment modality when symptoms are primarily obsessive.
   c. Most single-therapy approaches are equal across all conditions.
   d. Unless there is evidence to the contrary, single-modality treatments should be attempted before combined-modality treatments are implemented.

5. The placebo effect
   a. May be influenced by advertising.
   b. Is a stable factor based on the consumer's expectations regarding a given product.
   c. Is only possible when the agent is inert and devoid of therapeutic value.
   d. Is not a factor in psychotherapy.

6. Beitman and Blinder found which of the following treatments are preferable for which of the following conditions?
   a. Family therapy for major depression.
   b. CBT for bulimia nervosa.
   c. Behavioral exposure for OCD.
   d. All of the above.

7. Learning paradigms, such as classical conditioning, operant conditioning, and social learning (modeling),
   a. Offer little to explain the effects of psychotropic drugs on patients' behavior.
   b. Have indicated that the effects of psychotropic medications are an artifact of placebo.
   c. Offer an additional explanation for the varied effects of psychotropic medications.
   d. Have no clinical application in psychopharmacology.

8. The use of CBT
   a. Is overrepresented in controlled studies.
   b. Is superior to other psychosocial interventions.
   c. Should be considered as an adjunct, not the first choice, in the treatment of mental disease.
   d. Has been overrated.

9. In the STAR*D trials, what percentage of patients remained resistant to anti-depressant medication despite four successive trials with different drugs?
   a. 40%.
   b. 20%.
   c. 10%.
   d. 5%.

10. The STEP-BD study
    a. Proved that adding lamotrigine to a mood stabilizer was superior to a mood stabilizer alone when treating bipolar disorder.
    b. Proved that atypical antipsychotic medication was as effective as mood stabilizers for the treatment of bipolar disorder.
    c. Showed that psychotherapy was of little usefulness as a treatment enhancer in bipolar disorder.
    d. Showed that psychotherapy was an effective adjunct to mood stabilizers in the treatment of resistant bipolar patients.

11. The TADS
    a. Found combination therapy (fluoxetine plus CBT) to be superior to mono-therapy in the short term.

    b. Found combination therapy and CBT monotherapy superior to fluoxetine monotherapy in the long term.

    c. Found CBT superior to combined therapy on measures of sustained improvement.

    d. All of the above.

12. In the CATIE and CUtLASS studies,

    a. Differences were observed between the effectiveness of newer atypical antipsychotic agents over the older neuroleptics.

    b. Patients with schizophrenia were relatively compliant with prescribed medications, regardless of which antipsychotic was prescribed.

    c. Clozapine was found to be no more effective than other second-generation antipsychotics in treatment-resistant subjects.

    d. None of the above.

13. The TMAP

    a. Provided no evidence that treating patients according to the algorithm will improve practitioners' individual decision-making.

    b. Is out of date.

    c. Made no effort to validate its algorithms through clinical studies.

    d. Was a failed attempt to impose the medical model upon clinical decision-making.

14. The MTA study

    a. Showed that adolescents respond well to stimulant medication.

    b. Suggested that medications are more effective in the short-term management of attention deficit–hyperactivity disorder (ADHD) in children.

    c. Found no difference between medication and behavioral management of ADHD in adults.

    d. Found amphetamine to be superior to methylphenidate in the treatment of ADHD.

    Answers: (1) d, (2) b, (3) d, (4) c, (5) a, (6) d, (7) c, (8) a, (9) a, (10) d, (11) d, (12) d, (13) b, and (14) b.

REFERENCES

Beitman, B., & Blinder, B. (2003). *Integrating psychotherapy and psychopharmacology: Dissolving the mind-brain barrier*. New York, NY: W. W. Norton.

Berrettini, W. (2000). Susceptibility loci for bipolar disorder: Overlap with inherited vulnerability to schizophrenia. *Biological Psychiatry, 47*, 245–251.

Blier, P., Ward, H., Tremblay, P., Laberge, L., Herbert, C., & Bergeron, R. (2009). Combination of antidepressant medications from treatment initiation for major depressive disorder: A double-blind randomized study. *American Journal of Psychiatry, 10*, 1176.

Busch, F., & Sandberg, L. (2007). *Psychotherapy and medication: The challenge of integration*. London, UK: The Analytic Press.

Carlat, D. (2011). *Unhinged: The trouble with psychiatry—A doctor's revelations about a profession in crisis*. New York, NY: Simon & Schuster.

Cheung, A. H., Zuckerbrot, R. A., Jensen, P. S., Ghalib, K., Laraque, D., Stein, R. E., & GLAD-PC Steering Group. (2007). Guidelines for Adolescent Depression in Primary Care (GLAD-PC): II. Treatment and ongoing management. *Pediatrics, 120*, 1313–1326.

Cheung, A. H., Zuckerbrot, R. A., Jensen, P. S., Stein, R. E., Laraque, D., & GLAD-PC Steering Committee. (2008). Expert survey for the Management of Adolescent Depression in Primary Care. *Pediatrics, 121*, 101–107.

Conte, H., Plutchik, R., Wild, K., & Karasu, T. (1986). Combined psychotherapy and pharmacotherapy for depression: A systematic analysis of the evidence. *Archives of General Psychiatry, 43*, 471–479.

Crystal, S., Olfson, M., Huang, C., Pincus, H., & Grehard, T. (2009). Broadened use of atypical antipsychotics: Safety, effectiveness, and policy challenges. *Health Affairs, 28*, 770–781.

Curry, J., Silva, S., Rohde, P., Ginsberg, G., Kratochvil, C., Simons, A., . . . & March, J. (2010). Recovery and recurrence following treatment for adolescent major depression. *Archives of General Psychiatry, 150*, 1–8.

DeLeon, P. (2010). A glimpse at an evolving practice environment. *Tablet, 11*(3), 64–67.

Dobson, K., Hollon, S., Dimidjian, S., Schmaling, K., Kohlenburg, R., & Gallop, R. (2008). Randomized trial of behavioral activation, cognitive therapy and antidepressant medication in the prevention of relapse and recurrence in major depression. *Journal of Consulting and Clinical Psychology, 76*, 468–477.

Duggan, C., Huband, N., Smailagic, N., Ferriter, M., & Adams, C. (2008). The use of pharmacological treatments for people with personality disorders: A systematic review of randomized controlled studies. *Personality and Mental Health, 2*, 119–170.

Fawcett, J., Stein, D., & Jobson, K. (1999). *Textbook of treatment algorithms in psychopharmacology*. New York, NY: Wiley.

Faraone, S., Biederman, J., Spencer. T., & Alerdi, M. (2006). Comparing the efficacy of medications for ADHD using meta-analysis. *Medscape General Medicine, 8*, 4.

Fava, M., Alpert, J., Carmin, C., Wisniewski, S., Trivedi, M., Biggs, M., . . . & Rush, A. (2004). Clinical correlates and symptom patterns of anxious depression among patients with major depressive disorder in STAR*D. *Psychological Medicine, 34*, 1299–1308.

Fisher, S., & Greenburg, R. (1989). *The limits of biological treatment of psychological distress: Comparisons with psychotherapy and placebo*. Mahwah, NJ: Erlbaum.

Fisher, S., & Greenburg, R. (1997). *From placebo to panacea: Putting psychiatric drugs to the test*. New York, NY: Wiley.

Fordyce, W. (1976). *Behavioral methods for chronic pain and illness*. St. Louis, MO: C.V. Mosby.

Fournier, J., DeRubeis, R., Hollon, S., Dimidjian, S., Amsterdam, J., Shelton, R., & Fawcett, J. (2010). Antidepressant drug effects and depression severity: A patient-level meta-analysis. *Journal of the American Medical Association, 303*, 47–53.

Fournier, J., DeRubeis, R., Shelton, R., Hollon, S., Amsterdam, J., & Gallop, R. (2009). Prediction of response to medication and cognitive therapy in the treatment of moderate to severe depression. *Journal of Consulting and Clinical Psychology, 77*, 775–787.

Gaynes, B., Rush, A., Trivedi, M., Wisniewski, S., Balasubramani, G., Spencer, D., . . . & Golden, R. (2005). A direct comparison of presenting characteristics of depressed outpatients from primary vs. specialty care settings: Preliminary findings from the STAR*D clinical trial. *General Hospital Psychiatry, 27*, 87–96.

Gilbert, D. A., Altshuler, K. Z., Rango, W. V., Shon, S. P., Crismon, M. L., Toprac, M. G., & Rush, A. J. (1998). Texas Medication Algorithm Project: Definitions, rationale, and methods to develop medication algorithms. *Journal of Clinical Psychiatry, 59*, 345–351.

Guo, X., Zhai, J., Liu, Z., Fang, M., Wang, B., Wang, C., . . . & Zhao, J. (2010). Effect of antipsychotic medication alone vs. combined with psychosocial intervention on outcomes of early-stage schizophrenia. *Archives of General Psychiatry, 67*, 895–904.

Healy, D. (2004). *Let them eat Prozac: The unhealthy relationship between the pharmaceutical industry and depression*. New York, NY: New York University.

Hoffman, B., Babyak, M., & Craighead, W. E., et al. (2011). Exercise and pharmacotherapy in patients with major depression: One-year follow-up of the SMILE study. *Psychosomatic Medicine, 73*, 127–33.

Hogarty, G., Goldberg, S., & Schooler, N. (1974). Drug and sociotherapy in the aftercare of schizophrenic patients. *Archive of General Psychiatry, 31*, 609–618.

Imel, Z. E., & Wampold, B. E. (2008). The importance of treatment and the science of common factors in psychotherapy. In S. D. Brown & R. W. Lent (Eds.), *Handbook of Counseling Psychology* (4th ed). New York, NY: Wiley.

Jensen, P., Arnold, L., Swanson, J., Vitiello, B., Abikoff, H., Greenhill, L., . . . & Hur, K. (2007). Three year follow up on the NIMH MAT study. *Journal of the American Academy of Child and Adolescent Psychiatry, 46*, 989–1002.

Jensen, P., Garcia, J., Glied, S., Crowe, M., Foster, M., Schlander, M., . . . & Wells, K. (2005). Cost-effectiveness of ADHD treatments: Findings from the Multimodal Treatment Study of Children with ADHD. *American Journal of Psychiatry, 162*, 1628–1636.

Jones, P. B., Barnes, T. R., Davies, L., Dunn, G., Lloyd, H., Hayhurst, K. P., . . . & Lewis, S. W. (2006). Randomized controlled trial of effect on quality of life of second- vs. first-generation antipsychotic drugs in schizophrenia: Cost Utility of the Latest Antipsychotic Drugs in Schizophrenia Study (CUtLASS 1). *Archives of General Psychiatry, 63*, 1079–1087.

Julien, R. (2005). *A Primer of drug action: A comprehensive guide to the actions, uses, and side effects of psychoactive drugs*. New York, NY: Worth.

Julien, R., Advokat, C., Comaty, J. (2011). *A primer of drug action: A comprehensive guide to the actions, uses, and side effects of psychoactive drugs* (12th ed.). New York, NY: Worth.

Kashner, T., Carmody, T., Suppes, T., Rush, A., Crismon, M., Miller, A., . . . & Trivedi, M. (2003). Catching up on health outcomes: The Texas Medication Algorithm Project. *Health Services Research, 38*, 311–331.

Kay, S. R., Fishbein, A., & Opler, L. A. (1989). The Positive and Negative Syndrome Scale for Schizophrenia. *Schizophrenia Bulletin, 13*, 261–276.

Kocsis, J., Gelenberg, A., Rothbaum, B., Klein, D., Trivedi, M., Manber, R., . . . & Thase, M. (2009). Cognitive behavioral analysis system of psychotherapy and brief supportive psychotherapy for augmentation of antidepressant nonresponse in chronic depression. *Archives of General Psychiatry, 66*, 1178–1188.

Kogan, J., Otto, M., Bauer, M., Dennehy, E., Miklowitz, D., Zhang, H., . . . & Sachs, G. (2004). Demographic and diagnostic characteristics of the first 1000 patients enrolled in the Systematic Treatment Enhancement Program for Bipolar Disorder (STEP-BD). *Bipolar Disorder, 6*, 460–469.

Krahn, D., Bartels, S., Coakley, E., Oslin, D., Chen, H., McIntyre, J., . . . & Levkoff, S. (2006). PRISM-E (Primary Care Research in Substance Abuse and Mental Health for the Elderly): Comparison of integrated care and enhanced specialty referral models in depression outcomes. *Psychiatric Services, 57*, 946–953.

Kraly, F. S. (2006). *Brain science and psychological disorders: Therapy, psychotropic drugs, and the brain*. New York, NY: W. W. Norton.

Lazarus, A. (1976). *Multimodal Behavior Therapy*. New York, NY: Springer.

Lewis, S. W., Barnes, T., Davies, L., Murray, R. M., Dunn, G., Hayhurst, K. P., . . . & Jones, P. B. (2006). Randomized controlled trial of effect of prescription of clozapine versus other second-generation antipsychotic drugs in resistant schizophrenia. *Schizophrenia Bulletin, 32*, 715–723.

Lieberman, J. A., Stroup, S., McEvoy, J. P., Swartz, M. S., Rosenheck, R. A., Perkins, D. O., . . . & Hsiao, J. K. (2005). Effectiveness of antipsychotic drugs in patients with chronic schizophrenia. *New England Journal of Medicine, 353*, 1209–1223.

Makela, E., & Griffith, R. (2003). Enhancing treatment of bipolar disorder using the patient's belief system. *Annals of Pharmacotherapy, 37*, 543–545.

March, J., & Vitiello, B. (2009). Clinical messages from the Treatment for Adolescents with Depression Study (TADS). *American Journal of Psychiatry, 166*, 1118–1123.

Mark, T., Levit, L., & Buck, J. (2009). Psychotropic drug prescriptions by medical specialty. *Psychiatric Service, 60*, 1167.

Mavissakalian, M. (1991). Agoraphobia. In B. Beitman & G. Klerman (Eds.), *Integrating pharmacotherapy and psychotherapy*. Washington, DC: American Psychiatric Association.

May, R. (1950). *The meaning of anxiety*. New York, NY: Ronald Press.

McDaniel, S., Hepworth, J., & Doherty, W. (1992). *Medical family therapy: A biopsychosocial approach to families with health problems*. New York, NY: Basic Books.

McNally, R. (2011). *What Is Mental Illness?* Boston, MA: Belknap Press.

Miklowitz, D., Otto, M., Frank, E., Reilly-Harrington, N., Wisniewski, S., Kogan, J., . . . & Sachs, G. (2007). Psychosocial treatments for bipolar depression: A 1-year randomized trial from the Systematic Treatment Enhancement Program. *Archives of General Psychiatry, 64*, 419–426.

Mojtabai, R., & Olfson, M. (2008). National trends in psychotherapy by office-based psychiatrists. *Archives of General Psychiatry, 65*, 962–970.

Mojtabai, R., & Olfson, M. (2010). National trends in psychotropic medication: Polypharmacy in office-based psychiatry. *Archives of General Psychiatry, 67*, 26–36.

Molina, B., Hinshaw, S., Swanson, J., Arnold, L., Vitiello, B., Jenson, P., . . . & Houck, P. (2009). The MTA at 8 years: Prospective follow-up of children treated for combination type ADHD in multisite study. *Journal of the American Academy of Child and Adolescent Psychiatry, 40*, 484–500.

Moncrieff, J., & Cohen, D. (2009). How do psychiatric drugs work? *British Medical Journal, 338*, 1535–1537.

Morin, C., Vallieres, A., Guay, B., Invers, H., Savard, J., Merette, C., . . . & Baillargeon, L. (2009). Cognitive behavioral therapy, singly and combined with medication, for persistent insomnia: A randomized controlled trial. *Journal of American Medical Association, 301*, 2005–2015.

MTA Cooperative Group. (1999a). A 14-month randomized clinical trial of treatment strategies for attention-deficit/hyperactivity disorder. *Archives of General Psychiatry, 56*, 1073–1086.

MTA Cooperative Group. (1999b). Moderators and mediators of treatment response for children with attention-deficit/hyperactivity disorder. *Archives of General Psychiatry, 56*, 1088–1096.

Muse, M. (1984). Narcosynthesis in the treatment of posttraumatic chronic pain. *Rehabilitation Psychology, 29*, 155–163.

Muse, M. (1994). The convergence of psychology and psychiatry: The use of behaviorally prescribed medications. *Second International Congress of Eclectic Psychotherapy*: Lyon, France.

Muse, M. (1999). Las parafilias. *Revista de Psicoterapia, 38–39*, 113–121.

Muse, M. (2007). Convergencia de la psicoterapia y la psicofarmacología: El uso de programas para la administración conductual de la medicación. *Revista de Psicoterapia, 69*, 5–10.

Muse, M. (2010a). Combining therapies in medical psychology: When to medicate and when not. *Archives of Medical Psychology, 1*, 19–27.

Muse, M. (2010b). The contribution of case studies to medical psychology research. *Archives of Medical Psychology, 1*, 28–33.

Muse, M., & Frigola, G. (2003). La evaluación y tratamiento de las parafilias. *Revista de Medecina Psicosomática, 65*, 55–72.

Muse, M., & McGrath, R. (2010). Training comparison among three professions prescribing psychoactive medications: Psychiatric nurse practitioners, physicians, and pharmacologically-trained psychologists. *Journal of Clinical Psychology, 66*, 1–8.

National Institute for Health and Clinical Excellence. (2011). Generalized anxiety disorder and panic disorder (with or without agoraphobia) in adults: Management in primary, secondary and community care. NICE Clinical Guideline No. 113. United Kingdom: National Health Service. Retrieved from http://www.nice.org.uk/guidance/CG113

Nierenberg, A., Ostacher, M., Calabrese, J., Ketter, T., Marangell, L., Miklowitz, D., . . . & Sachs, G. (2006). Treatment-resistant bipolar depression: A STEP-BD equipoise random-ized effectiveness trial of antidepressant augmentation with lamotrigine, inositol, or ris-peridone. *American Journal of Psychiatry, 163*, 210–216.

Norcross, J., & Goldfried, M. (2003). *Handbook of psychotherapy integration* (2nd ed.). New York, NY: Oxford University Press.

Olfson, M., & Marcus, S. (2010). National trends in outpatient psychotherapy. *American Journal of Psychiatry, 167*, 1456–1463.

O'Reilly, R. L., Bogue, L., & Singh, S. M. (1994). Pharmacogenetic response to antidepres-sants in a multi-case family with affective disorder. *Biological Psychiatry, 36*, 467–471.

Osser, D., Patterson, R., & Levitt, J. (2005). Guidelines, algorithms, and evidence-based psy-chopharmacology training for psychiatric residents. *Academic Psychiatry, 29*, 180–186.

Piacentini, J., Woods, D., Scahill, L., Wilhelm, S., Peterson, A., Chang, S., . . . & Walkup, J. (2010). Behavior therapy for children with Tourette disorder: A randomized controlled trial. *Journal of the American Medical Association, 303*, 1929–1937.

Rebach, H. M., & Bruhn, J. G. (1991). *Handbook of clinical sociology*. New York, NY: Plenum.

Riess, H. (2010). Empathy in medicine: A neurobiological perspective. *Journal of the American Medical Association, 304*, 1604–1605.

Riba, M., & Balon, R. (2005). *Competency in combining pharmacotherapy and psychotherapy: Integrated and split treatment*. Washington, DC: American Psychiatric Association.

Rief, W., Nstoriuc, Y., Weiss, S., Welzel, E., Barsky, A., & Hofmann, S. (2009). Meta-analysis of the placebo response in antidepressant trials. *Journal of Affective Disorders, 118*, 1–8.

Rogers, C. (1961). *On becoming a person: A therapist's view of psychotherapy*. New York, NY: Houghton Mifflin.

Rohde, P., Silva, S., Tonev, S., Kennard, B., Vitiello, B., Kratochvil, C., . . . & March, J.S. (2008). Achievement and maintenance of sustained improvement during TADS continua-tion and maintenance therapy. *Archives of General Psychiatry, 65*, 447–455.

Roy, R., Jahan, M., Kumari, S., & Chakraborty, P. (2005). Reasons for drug non-compliance of psychiatric patients: A centre-based study. *Journal of the Indian Academy of Applied Psychology, 31*, 24–28.

Rush, A. J., Fava, M., Wisniewski, S. R., Lavori, P. W., Trivedi, M. H., Sackeim, H. A., . . . & Niederehe, G. (2004). STAR*D Investigators Group. Sequenced treatment alternatives to relieve depression (STAR*D): Rationale and design. *Controlled Clinical Trials, 25*, 119–142.

Rush, J. (1996). *Clinical anthropology: An application of anthropological concepts within clinical settings*. Westport, CT: Praeger.

Rush, J. (1999). *Stress and emotional health: Applications of clinical anthropology*. Westport, CT: Auburn House.

Rush, J., & Hollon, S. (1991). Clinical implications of research into specific disorders: Depression. In B. Beitman & G. Klerman (Eds.), *Integrating Pharmacotherapy and Psychotherapy* (pp. 121–142).Washington, DC: American Psychiatric Association.

Sachs, G., Nierenberg, A., Calabrese, J., Marangell, L., Wisniewski, S., Gyulai, L., . . . & Thase, M. (2007). Effectiveness of adjunctive antidepressant treatment for bipolar depression: A double-blind placebo-controlled study. *New England Journal of Medicine, 356*, 1711–1722.

Sachs, G., Thase, M., Otto, M., Bauer, M., Miklowitz, D., Wisniewski, S., . . . & Rosenbaum, J. (2003). Rationale, design, and methods of the Systematic Treatment Enhancement Program for Bipolar Disorder (STEP-BD). *Biological Psychiatry, 53*, 1028–1042.

Sammons, M. (2010). Integrating psychopharmacology into clinical practice: Current trends. ABPP Summer Workshop, Portland, OR.

Sammons, M., & Levant, R. (1999). *Combined psychosocial and pharmacological treatments.* New York, NY: Plenum.

Sammons, M., & Schmidt, N. (2001). *Combined treatment for mental disorders: A guide to psychological and pharmacological interventions.* Washington, DC: American Psychological Association.

Schachter, S. (1964). The interaction of cognitive and physiological determinants of emotional state. In L. Berkowitz (Ed.), *Advances in Experimental Social Psychology.* New York, NY: Academic Press.

Schachter, S., & Singer, J. (1962). Cognitive, social, and physiological determinants of emotional state. *Psychological Review, 69,* 379–399.

Silberman, S. (2009). Placebos are getting more effective: Drugmakers are desperate to know why. *Wired Magazine, 17,* 1–8.

Skinner, B. F. (1974). *About behaviorism.* New York, NY: Knopf.

Serna, C., Cruz, I., Real, J., Gascó, E., & Galván, L. (2011). Duration and adherence of antidepressant treatment (2003–2007) based on prescription data base. *European Psychiatry, 25,* 206–213.

Steele, S. F., & Price, J. (2004). *Applied sociology: Terms, topics, tools, and tasks.* Belmont, CA: Wadsworth.

Suppes, T., Rush, A. J., Dennehy, E. B., Crismon, M. L., Kashner, T. M., Toprac, M. G., . . . & Shon, S. P. (2003). Texas Medication Algorithm Project, Phase 3 (TMAP-3): Clinical results for patients with a history of mania. *Journal of Clinical Psychiatry, 64,* 370–382.

TADS Team. (2007). The Treatment for Adolescents with Depression Study (TADS): Long-term effectiveness and safety outcomes. *Archives of General Psychiatry, 64,* 1132–1143.

TADS Team. (2009). The Treatment for Adolescents with Depression Study (TADS): Outcomes over one year of naturalistic follow-up. *American Journal of Psychiatry, 166,* 1141–1149.

Thase, M., Friedman, E., Biggs, M., Wisniewski, S., Trivedi, M., Luther, J., . . . & Rush, A. J. (2007). Cognitive therapy versus medication in augmentation and switch strategies as second-step treatments: A STAR*D Report. *American Journal of Psychiatry, 164,* 739–752.

Wampold, B. (2001). *Great psychotherapy debate: Models, methods, and findings.* Mahwah, NJ: Erlbaum.

Wampold, B. E., Mondin, G. W., Moody, M., Stich, F., Benson, K., & Ahn, H. (1997). A meta-analysis of outcome studies comparing bona fide psychotherapies: Empirically, "all must have prizes." *Psychological Bulletin, 122,* 203–215.

Weissman, M. (1981). Psychosocial and pharmacological treatments of depression: Evidence for efficacy and research directions. In D. Parron (Ed.), *Combining Psychosocial and Drug Therapy.* Washington, DC: National Academy Press.

Wolpe, J. (1969). *The practice of behavioral therapy.* Elmsford, NY: Pergamon.

Zuckerbrot, R. A., Cheung, A. H., Jensent, P. S., Stein, R. E. K., Laraque, D., & GLAD-PC Steering Group. (2007). Guidelines for Adolescent Depression in Primary Care (GLAD-PC): I. Identification, assessment, and initial management. *Pediatrics, 120,* 1299–1312.

Chapter 3

NEUROSCIENCE

Ken Fogel

George M. Kapalka

Living systems adapt to changes to better survive, but with change there is also the need for stability. Homeostatic balance is the "holy grail" of living things—a state to be sought but never entirely attained. Changes in these systems, whether internal or external, are met by a counterresponse to return the system to its preferred state. In some cases, the range of "play" is very narrow, and the adjustment mechanisms must be sensitive and quick to action.

Psychopharmacological interventions are often designed to tilt the balance in a specific direction, while side effects can be viewed as undesired tilting and the system's response to self-correct. For example, in the modified dopamine model of positive symptoms of schizophrenia, hallucinations are hypothesized to reflect excessive dopaminergic activity in the mesolimbic system. Typical antipsychotic medications, such as dopamine antagonists, are considered to shift the balance toward a normative dopaminergic tone in this pathway. However, over time, the nervous system's response is to return the pathway to its previous level, which might include the *up-regulation* of dopamine receptors, with the potential to cause *tardive dyskinesia*.

At times, the need for homeostasis is pitted against the need for change to adapt to new circumstances. Some circumstances demand that organisms tip away from homeostasis in order to survive, which runs counter to the homeostatic directive. Once the external circumstances have resolved, the directive to return to balance regains primacy. Furthermore, it is highly likely at those times that the balance point for that organism has shifted. In a sense, this process describes evolutionary change.

MODULATION THROUGH CONTROL

Life would not survive without some form of control in an otherwise random or chaotic environment. Maintaining a homeostatic state, which in a sense is investing energy against an increase in *entropy*, typically involves some form of inhibitory action to prevent something from taking place. Conversely, problems often occur when there is a lack of control or overexcitation. Keep in mind that while one cannot drive an automobile without an engine, one would not want to drive an automobile without brakes.

Parallel Processes

In addition to paired excitatory-inhibitory systems (Pavlov, 1927), the delicate balance between homeostasis and change is maintained by duplicate systems that overlap in their function but have inherent differences leading to more fine-tuned control and the capacity to regulate on different levels of functioning (space and time), in some cases providing "back-up" functioning. For example, in response to a stressor, the brain activates both the *sympathetic nervous system* and the *hypothalamic-pituitary-adrenal (HPA) axis*. Both pathways result in the processes and behaviors designed to respond to the stressor, and many of these responses involve mobilization of the same structures and organs. The former response, involving neural pathways, is immediate and relatively quick to resolve, whereas the latter response is hormonal and uses the bloodstream for communication, resulting in a relatively slower and longer-lasting impact.

Topographical Organization

In the service of efficiency and conserving resources, evolution favored optimal adaptive solutions to environmental circumstances. Fitting billions of neurons with trillions of connections into a coconut-sized shell while communicating electrochemical messaging with minimal error, the structures and functions of the nervous system had to be organized logically and topographically. Proximal areas in the environment are represented proximally in the brain, and for the most part, are maintained in this pattern at successive junctions or transfer points. Functions that need a quick response are given a "fast track" and those that play a more crucial role or that operate on a more robust range of stimuli have a larger fraction of "real estate" devoted to them.

Axes of Balance

In the quest for homeostatic balance, living systems have established controls that exist in dynamic opposition, each side in charge of inhibiting the influence of the other. In the nervous system, for example, the sympathetic and parasympathetic branches of the *autonomic nervous system* (ANS) exert opposing influences on many hormonal and visceral body systems in an effort to regulate the body's responsiveness to internal and external environmental forces. An example on a general scale is the glutamatergic and GABAergic neural pathways, which reflect excitatory and inhibitory forces, respectively, at the synaptic level. However, there are many examples in which a neurotransmitter might play both an excitatory and an inhibitory role, as we will see more fully when we discuss *heteroreceptors* and *autoreceptors*. The axis of balance between competing systems is a crucial concept to keep in mind during psychopharmacological interventions, which are essentially designed to "tip the scales" either toward or away from a point on one of these continua or spectra.

THE NEURON

The reason we are capable of ever-growing complexity derives from the established networks of neural pathways. Pathways are, in essence, a chain of individual neurons, each with multiple synapses. Learning, as we understand it, occurs at the level of the synapse. For psychologists who devote a major part of their scienctific study to learning, the capacity to alter pathways of learning in the interest of promoting better adaptability and maintenance of homeostasis is a primary goal. The neuron, which is the building block of the entire nervous system, is a fine place to start in understanding the acquisition of learning. More apropos to our present focus, the purpose of most psychotropic medications is to alter or adjust the function of the synapse. The details of various mechanisms of action notwithstanding, most psychotropic medications can be classified as neurotransmitter *agonists* or *antagonists*, which is another example of how the nervous system, through a series of synapses, achieves balance by having its excitatory and inhibitory structures and functions juxtaposed.

At least one author (LeDoux, 2002) contends that the synapse, being a nonreducible structure, is in fact rightfully regarded as the locus of identity; since that is where learning takes place and forms the basis for memories. Because memories make up the bulk of who we are, the synaptic networks might be where we would expect to "find" our identity. Other authors, among them neuroscientists and neurophysicists, have directed their attention toward the synapse as the potential location of consciousness. In particular, these scientists consider the synapse to be the primary target for the study of neuroquantology, or the application of quantum mechanics and quantum dynamics to neurology (Tarlaci, 2010). Medical psychologists, however, operating from a psychobiosocial orientation, are more likely to view the synapse as the "spark plug" of the nervous system—essential, but not sufficient in itself to bestow identity or explain the myriad systems that work together to contribute to the whole organism.

THE NEURON AS CELL

Neurons are cells, albeit specialized cells.[1] The cell's nucleus holds the genetic code, as embodied in DNA molecules. In neurons, some of the processes of communication and learning involve activating *transcription factors* and other *epigenetic phenomena*. The *endoplasmic reticulum* and *ribosomes* are where key proteins are synthesized according to RNA codes, which in neurons include key enzymes and receptors. The *Golgi apparatus* packages molecules and substances within vesicles, which in neurons will often include neurotransmitters. The cell membrane serves as a boundary and enclosure and, in neurons, represents one of their most distinguishing features.

The *mitochondria* have been characterized as the "power plants" of cells and provide energy to the neuron. Mitochondria also contain rate-limiting enzymes for the processes of *pyrimidine* biosynthesis and *heme* synthesis that are required to make hemoglobin. In the liver, mitochondria are specialized to detoxify ammonia in the urea cycle. Mitochondria are also required for cholesterol metabolism, the synthesis of estrogen and testosterone, neurotransmitter metabolism, and the production and detoxification of *free radicals*. Mitochondria perform all these functions in addition to oxidizing fat, protein, and carbohydrates (Lane, 2005).

Glial Cells

In addition to neurons, various other cells are found within the nervous system. For many years, until relatively recently, glial cells (neuroglia) were labeled "support cells" in the service of neurons. As their name suggests (glia is Greek for "glue"), these cells were believed to hold neurons together. However, the functions of glia have been found to be wide-ranging, as well as crucial for many different functions, including synaptic transmission.

[1]See Chapter 5 for a more detailed description of the human cell.

Astrocytes are the most numerous of the neuroglia and are primarily involved in regulating the chemical environment of the surrounding areas. Such regulation is accomplished in two ways: by absorbing excess potassium during high rates of neuronal firing and by absorbing neurotransmitters (NTs) from synaptic zones. In the 1990s, however, research revealed that some astrocytes released neurotransmitters and manifested some NT receptors on their surface membrane (Cooper, 1995). Thus, in addition to their "classical" roles as support cells, astrocytes are also involved in such processes as communication with neurons and with each other and in modulating communication between neurons.

Microglial cells are the smallest of the neuroglia and are primarily involved in maintaining the physical integrity of the extracellular space by absorbing waste and particles. As part of the *central nervous system* (CNS) immune system, microglia act in a manner similar to that of macrophages in the periphery, proliferating at sites of injury and releasing cytokines.

Oligodendrocytes are myelin-producing cells that wrap around the axons of central neurons. Schwann cells are the *peripheral nervous system* (PNS) equivalents of oligodendrocytes for myelinating peripheral neurons.

Ependymal cells, while not technically glia, are "non-neuron" brain cells. They are located in the internal spaces of the CNS and form the epithelial layer of the *choroid plexus*. Ependymal cells play a role in generating stem cells, as well as controlling exchanges of substances between *cerebral spinal fluid* (CSF) and *interstitial fluid*, but their primary role is in secreting CSF into the ventricles.

Glial cells are more numerous than neurons, at a ratio of 50:1 in some vertebrates. Their rate of growth follows that of typical body cells rather than the limited regrowth of neurons. One implication of this difference in growth rate is that glial cells are far more susceptible to cancer. During instances of brain damage, by either stroke or brain injury, glial cells form a type of scar tissue, the purpose of which is still not entirely clear, but which is partly related to maintaining the integrity of the blood-brain barrier. Astrocyte structure and microglial response combine to hinder axon regeneration in the CNS.

Myelin is composed of layers of membranes, from oligodendrocyte processes and Schwann cells, the primary function of which is to insulate axons. Myelinated axons are not covered uniformly but incorporate gaps of uninsulated membrane along the length of the axon membrane; these gaps are called *nodes of Ranvier*. Myelin is composed primarily of lipids but also includes several types of proteins.

TYPES OF NEURONS

There are numerous ways to categorize neurons, in terms of both structure and function. From a functional point of view, one of the most concrete divisions is based on the direction and purpose of the information relayed by neurons; such a taxonomy distinguishes among sensory neurons, *interneurons*, and motor neurons.

Sensory neurons, or *afferent* neurons, receive information about the environment from sensory receptor cells (not to be confused with synaptic receptors). The function of all sensory receptors is to *transduce* (or "translate") sensory energy into action-potential energy, the common "language" of all neurons. Thus, wavelengths of light, touch pressure, and saltiness are transduced so that the brain can interpret and integrate that information with the rest of the information stored in its networks.

Interneurons are responsible for integration and inter-area processing. They relay information between other neurons, modulating and moderating it as it travels from input to output areas. Interneurons play a crucial role in the process of lateral inhibition, which helps in information processing by boosting the signal-to-noise ratio.

Motor neurons, or *efferent* neurons, convey information to the motor systems for muscles and glands. These effectors carry out the actions and intentions indicated by the integration of sensory information with memories stored from previous experience.

NEURON STRUCTURE

The structures that comprise the neuron are shown in Figure 3.1. Structural features of neural organization can, for the most part, be characterized according to specific functions.

Dendrites and related structures represent the input region and are responsible for collecting information. This information is derived from synapses with other neurons that send NTs across the interneuron gap, called the synaptic cleft. Each dendrite's information status is combined with that of its neighbors to provide an overall message that is further transmitted. In order to increase the surface area for communication across the synapse, dendrites are elaborated into *dendritic spines*. The vast majority of receptor sites are found on dendrites, but receptors also exist on the surface membranes of the axon. Information is initially integrated in the dendritic region, while subsequent integration occurs at the level of the soma.

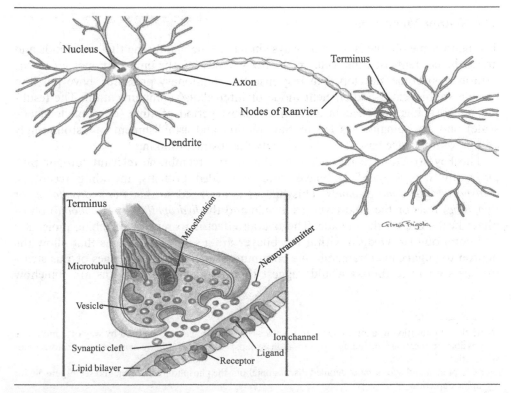

Figure 3.1   The Neuron

Axons receive information via the dendrites[2] and conduct or propagate the information to the end of the neuron. The axon ends at the terminus, as does conduction, but the propagated information does not end with it. The terminal area of the neuron represents the output region. In order to transmit information to the next neuron in the sequence, the terminal ending is structured to send information across the synaptic cleft.

The neuron terminal contains several structures and molecules that have evolved to optimize the transmission of communication between neurons. The gap between neurons, the synapse, is one of the key distinguishing features of the nervous system; yet, recent findings have established that some neurons traverse the synapse and join membranes with adjacent neurons (Biederer, 2002). These neuron-neuron adhesions are produced by the immunoglobulin adhesion molecule SynCAM 1 and presumably occur as a result of repeated stimulation and may represent tangible evidence of learning (Dalva, McClellan, & Kayser, 2007) in a manner similar to the growth of spines on dendritic membranes (Robbins et al., 2010). This is one example of a growing appreciation for *neuroplasticity* through *synaptogenesis* and nerve cell regeneration (Coras et al., 2010).

Although their overall basic structure is common, neurons vary in shape and size, and some of these variations reflect the unique nature of their placement and function in the nervous system. For example, local interneurons manifest short axons in order to communicate quickly and precisely with other proximal neurons. Conversely, neurons in the ascending and descending pathways of the spinal cord have long axons that travel relatively long distances in the body. *Purkinje cell*s in the cerebellum are characterized by an extensive dendritic tree that gathers enormous amounts of input per neuron before sending information downstream.

The Neuron Membrane

The neuron membrane is in many ways similar to the membrane that surrounds and holds the contents of other cells in the body. However, the unique properties of the neuron membrane, developed in response to evolutionary pressures, have put into place a sophisticated and efficient mode of intercellular communication. The resulting network has exploded in a relatively short period of time (on a phylogenetic scale) and, in humans, has led to the creation and establishment of astoundingly complex knowledge bases and the capacity for abstract thinking.

The key structural components of the neuron membrane relevant for our purposes are the *phospholipid* bilayer and embedded proteins, including receptors, *transporters*, and *ion channels*. This bilayer is arranged so that the *hydrophobic* (or *lipophilic*) tails of the lipid layer are inside and the *hydrophilic* (or *lipophobic*) phosphate heads are on the outside. The overall effect is to repel hydrophilic molecules and compounds.[3] Wedged within the bilayer are a series of proteins that allow the neuron to engage in extramembrane communication. The static images of this structure as seen in textbooks would suggest that the embedded proteins are somehow

---

[2]Note that, in addition to axon to dendrite synapses, information can be delivered by way of a multitude of possible connections, including axon-to-axon synapse, axon-to-cell body synapse, and autoreceptor stimulation.

[3]See Chapters 5 and 8 for a more detailed discussion about the phospholipid bilayer, and see Figure 5.6 for a graphic depiction.

anchored or fixed in position; however, the membrane is far more fluid, and the proteins "float" on the surface or form a pore through it. The specific physical and chemical properties of the membrane give it a selectively semipermeable wall—that is, some molecules can pass through, while others cannot. With some exceptions, the smaller, lipophilic molecules can generally pass through, while the larger, ionized lipophobic/hydrophilic molecules cannot. This particular characteristic is central to the entire neural communication process. If the neuron membrane were completely permeable or completely impermeable, the electrochemical-potential energy required for the neuron to function could not be generated.

Inside the neuron, a repository of negatively charged chloride ions and a collection of large, negatively charged protein molecules contribute to the cell's overall negative intracellular charge. The majority of the charge is sustained by macromolecules that cannot pass through the membrane. As a result, the inside of the neuron is slightly negatively charged (approximately -70 millivolts [mV]) relative to the outer, interstitial area. Similarly, smaller *anions* and *cations* (negatively and positively charged ions, respectively) are repelled by the hydrophobic membrane. Other smaller, uncharged particles (e.g., water [H_2O]) and nitric oxide (NO) gas pass freely between the spaces created by the shifting phospholipid chains.

Molecules and compounds move according to electrochemical forces. First, movement occurs along a gradient from an area of higher concentration to lower concentration. Second, opposite charges attract each other, whereas "like" charges repel. The forces combine in one of two ways: Either they are additive, when the electrical force is in the same direction as the concentration gradient, or they cancel each other out, when the concentration gradient opposes the electrical force. The result of these two forces is equilibrium across the membrane, or equilibrium potential, an electrochemical potential equal to voltage. When the equilibrium potential is stable and at baseline, it is called resting membrane potential, or simply resting potential.

Two cross-membrane proteins that are particularly important from the standpoint of neural communication are voltage-gated channels and ion transporters. Both these protein structures allow ions to pass through the membrane that would otherwise be blocked. Each structure, however, responds differentially to specific ions: Voltage-gated channels allow passive access to the interior of the cell, while ion transporters use energy to actively transport ions across the phospholipid membrane. The fact that the channels move ions along the concentration gradient while the active transporters move ions against the gradient also distinguishes between these two types of transportation. Transporters are also crucial for the passage of other substances, such as glucose, and for the reuptake of NTs.

The neuron has voltage-gated channels for potassium (K^+), sodium (Na^+), and calcium (Ca^{2+}) that are sensitive to the electrochemical gradients across the membrane. Thus, the "gate" to the channel opens only when the surrounding membrane reaches a certain voltage threshold. Keep in mind that once a channel opens and ions are allowed to pass, the membrane potential will immediately change as a result. This change may *feed forward* or *feed back*, such that opening the channel will further increase the voltage or return it to a resting state, respectively. Similarly, since channels for specific ions open at different thresholds, the change in voltage due to the opening of one ion channel will influence the change in voltage relative to other ion channels.

Of particular importance to the prescribing medical psychologist is the mechanism whereby voltage-gated channels are targeted by pharmacological agents to influence their functioning. Some drugs affect the channels' propensity for or resistance to opening. For example, some anticonvulsants, which are used as mood-stabilizing medications, have been hypothesized to stabilize membranes (return the neuron to a resting potential) by shifting the threshold of various ion gates—specifically, the sodium, calcium, and potassium gates (Errington, Stöhr, & Lees, 2005).

RESTING POTENTIAL

In order to best remember the "starting point" in the typical neuron, consider that one of the functions of the membrane is to contain structures within it. These structures are proteins and other organic anions, which ionize to a primarily negative charge. As a result, the interior of the neuron is negative. Ions just outside the membrane will be influenced by this electrical force (i.e., cations [positively charged] move inward and anions [negatively charged] move outward). Inasmuch as cells evolved in the context of the oceans (in salt water), organisms have been said to "internalize the ocean," incorporating salt water as extracellular fluid. Thus, sodium chloride (NaCl) is a highly prevalent molecule, ionizing to the elements of Na^+ and Cl^-. A part of the negative resting potential of neurons is derived from the intracellular gradient of Cl^- and the extracellular gradient of Na^+.

Although numerous ions are present in the cell, the primary players in neurotransmission have been narrowed down to a handful. These ions derive from common molecules, and ionization in water provides the electrochemical impetus for neuron communication. In the 1940s and 1950s, Hodgkin and Huxley (1952) measured the ions in a squid giant axon in homeostasis and showed how increasing or decreasing the concentration of any one of the principal ions led to a characteristic change in the membrane potential. In 1943, the *Goldman-Hodgkin-Katz voltage equation,* derived from the *Nernst equation,* accounted for the differential permeability of each ion (McCormick, 2004). Through their observations and experiments, Hodgkin and Huxley established that potassium played a central role in maintaining the membrane potential at its resting level.

The forces on the relevant ions during the resting state are as follows:

- K^+ ions are more numerous inside the neuron and are thus driven out by the concentration gradient, but their positive charge relative to the negatively charged cytoplasm attracts them inward. Overall, there is a constant "potassium leak" out of the neuron, and the K^+ gradient is maintained by the *sodium-potassium (Na-K) pump.*
- Na^+ ions are more numerous outside the neuron and are attracted by the intracellular charge, so the diffusion and electrical forces are additive and create a substantial "pull" toward the inside of the neuron.
- The Na-K pump maintains the concentration gradient by transferring sodium outside and potassium inside. This pump works by an active process that requires energy; it transfers sodium and potassion ions at a ratio of 3 to 2, such that for every three sodium ions it transports out of the cell, it imports two potassium ions into the cell's interior.
- Cl^- flow tends for the most part to be balanced, because the diffusion and electrical forces work in opposite directions. Chloride thus plays a minor role in the determination of the resting potential. Substances that alter the permeability to

Cl⁻ will nonetheless influence the excitability of the membrane and contribute to the communication of information.

- The other key ionic player is Ca^{2+}, although calcium channels are present only at the terminal region of the neuron; thus, Ca^{2+} does not play as much of a role in propagation as it does in transmission.

Maintaining the Potential

The importance of maintaining the resting potential, as noted before, derives from evolutionary principles: This state and process represent the most adaptive options for the survival of the organism and thus for the survival of the species. As such, neurons will adapt to return to the original resting state after momentary changes. In addition to relying on the electrochemical forces described above, the neuron invests energy into maintaining the Na-K pump to keep the potential at around −70 mV. Given the immense number of neurons and frequency of neural firing, the energy cost adds up quickly.

In physics, the concept of "potential" (meaning the potential to do work) characterizes the state of the membrane. The resting potential is a *set point* that results from the initial conditions created by the ions and proteins in the neuron's cytoplasm. The key that "sparks" the change from the resting potential to a dynamic *action potential* is the opening of voltage-gated sodium channels. That is to say, the membrane potential will vary and vacillate with fluctuations in ionic charge on either side of the membrane.[4] When the gate opens, Na^+ ions rush through to reduce the voltage difference between the inside and the outside of the cell. When the voltage reaches a threshold amount, the voltage-gated channels open further and the polarity shifts.

The nature of the initial conditions of the resting potential, and the sudden access to the inside of the neuron provided by the opening of voltage-dependent gates, will result in a sudden inward rush of sodium ions. As more gates open, a cascade follows, and a characteristic pattern of voltage change that lasts about 1 to 3 milliseconds ensues. Keep in mind that the amount of ionic flow is minuscule when compared to the total number of ions present in the vicinity. A typical neuron would be expected to experience an increase of about 0.04% of Na^+ when channels open. When the gate closes, the pump must work to transport ions back out in order to reestablish a transmembrane differential in ion gradient, which results in a return to the resting voltage difference.

Three main categories of changes in membrane potential are relevant for neuron functioning: action potentials, *receptor potentials*, and postsynaptic potentials. These changes in potentials differ based on their location of origin and their properties.

Whereas receptor potentials reflect changes caused by the response of sensory organs to environmental stimuli, action potentials and postsynaptic potentials are the two most important means of transmitting information within the nervous system, in addition to being the most common focus of psychopharmacological interventions. Medications tend to influence action and/or postsynaptic potentials by speeding up, reinforcing, mimicking, dulling, or blocking the sending of signals.

---

[4]In the dendritic segment of the neuron, opening of the sodium channel is usually precipitated by stimulation of a receptor on the postsynaptic membrane from an adjacent firing neuron, while in the axon segment, an internal surge from the action potential triggers the voltage-gated calcium channels.

In neuronal communication, information is transmitted in two phases: First, information flowing within a given neuron, from one end to another, reflects the action potential. Second, information crossing the gap to adjacent neurons reflects neurotransmission. Each of these is discussed in turn.

Behavior of the Neuron

When a neuron is stimulated, local currents are generated by neurochemical activity across the synapse, and they last only a short time and dissipate after a short distance. These currents are temporary because of forces of friction within the neuron; they do not dissipate, however, without leaving an imprint on the cell membrane in the form of a *graded potential*. A graded potential is as strong as the summation of temporary currents impinging upon a local area of the postsynaptic membrane at any given time. Graded potentials increase the leakage of ions across the membrane and affect polarity by increments, creating partial depolarization. If several of these local currents are combined, because of either proximity or simultaneity, the graded potential may shift depolarization sufficiently to cross the threshold for generating an action potential, which is not a graded response but an all-or-none response. Unlike the electric current that characterizes the graded potential, which consists of the flow of electrons, the action potential involves the movement of sodium and potassium ions across the cell membrane.

THE ACTION POTENTIAL (AP)

In trying to understand the mechanisms underlying the AP, bear in mind that there is no true "starting point" and that the process is cyclical. Most texts begin from the "resting state," at −70 mV, when ion movement is presumably in equilibrium. Following this approach, the process begins when the resting potential is depolarized, that is, shifted toward 0 mV by a graded potential. Depolarization refers to movement away from the extreme, or pole. Depolarization occurs as the graded potential creates a leakage of ions across the membrane, usually caused by a partial influx of potassium and sodium ions. If the depolarization is sufficient to reach the threshold of the Na^+ voltage-gated channels (around −50 mV), these channels open, allowing the rapid movement of Na^+ ions inside the cell along both electrostatic and diffusion gradients.

As Na^+ rushes into the neuron, the membrane potential is further depolarized (becoming increasingly positive inside the cell). The extent of the gradients is such that the movement continues past the 0 mV point, and the inside of the neuron becomes positive. As the potential shifts in the positive direction, K^+ voltage-gated channels open, and K^+ ions now move along both gradients toward the interstitial space outside the cell. Recall the relatively higher concentration of K^+ inside, so that diffusion forces these ions outside. In addition, as Na^+ enters and creates an increasingly positive environment, the electrostatic force adds to the diffusion force, accelerating the movement of K^+ ions outward.

Once the membrane potential reaches approximately +30 mV, Na^+ channels close and K^+ channels remain open, so inward Na^+ ion movement stops and outward K^+ ion movement continues. Thus, the inside of the neuron returns to a negative state. In addition, the Na-K pump works to slowly but continuously return these ions to their

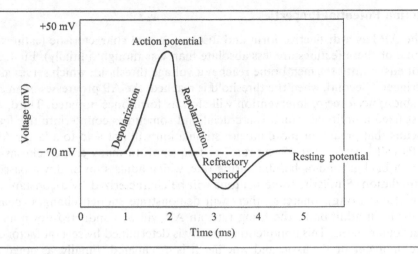

Figure 3.2   Action Potential

resting gradients by ousting sodium while importing potassium to offset the natural leakage of potassium through passive expulsion.[5]

Rather than return to the resting state of −70 mV, the configuration of Na+ and K^+ channels results in a momentary movement beyond the resting state, to a more extreme or hyperpolarized state. This state lasts until the leaked K^+ ions diffuse away from the vicinity of the membrane. At this point, this portion of the membrane is "ready" for the next depolarization. The entire AP sequence can be represented as a characteristic pattern on an oscilloscope graph. (See Figure 3.2.)

Note that the brief period of hyperpolarization makes it more difficult for that patch of membrane to reach the threshold for Na^+ voltage-gated channels to open. This refractory period is crucial for controlling the direction of the AP, since it is more difficult for the potential changes to double back. There are two components to the refractory period: absolute and relative. During the absolute refractory period, the change in voltage inactivates the Na^+ channel, so no further activity is possible, and no AP can occur. During the relative refractory period, the Na^+ channels are active but closed, so the AP is possible but less likely, since the membrane potential is in a hyperpolarized state.

APs propagate along the entire length of the neuron and may be assisted by saltatory conduction, which is the "jumping" of the AP from one node of Ranvier to the next along the myelin sheath that covers the outside of the axon. The term "saltatory" for describing the movement of APs along *myelinated axons* is an unfortunate choice, since it conjures up the image of the electrochemical wave actually "leaping" over the sheaths of myelin. Instead, the electrostatic current flows through the cytoplasm under the sheath until it reaches the next node. The size of the current decreases as it flows owing to friction. However, the membrane at the node of Ranvier is noninsulated and permits an exchange of ions with the interstitial environment, which allows for the propagation of another AP.

---

[5]It should be noted here that there is greater permeability for potassium than for sodium at resting potential and that potassium is passively diffused out of the cell at a greater rate.

Action Potential Properties

The AP has a distinctive form and displays several characteristic features (although some of these features are less absolute than was thought initially). First, an AP will not ensue until the membrane reaches a voltage threshold, which serves as a kind of "trigger." Second, when the threshold is reached, the AP progresses in an all-or-none fashion; no force or intervention will stop its form once initiated. Third, APs manifest fixed amplitude, which is a crucial and sometimes counterintuitive feature. This means that greater or more intense stimulation will not lead to a larger AP. Instead, APs will vary in their "firing rate" or frequency. In many cases, neurons will maintain a background or baseline firing rate, which adjusts up or down based on input stimulation. Similarly, some neurons will be characterized by a constant rate of firing (tonic firing), whereas others will demonstrate sudden changes (phasic firing). Fourth, in addition to the firing rate, an AP will be conducted down an axon at a particular speed. This conduction velocity is determined by several factors, including the diameter of the axon and whether it is myelinated. Finally, as noted above, the nature of the ion channels' activation patterns results in a refractory period, which ensures a specific direction of propagation.

As might be expected, the original model of AP propagation proposed by Hodgkin and Huxley (1952), which was based on the studies of the squid giant axon, were very accurate for describing many cases of neural activity, but this model was limited when it came to understanding central nervous system neurons in the human (Bean, 2007). Some of the key differences reflect the immense variety of ion channels, which results in alterations of the classic AP profile. For example, some central neuron APs manifest wider spikes, longer or shorter refractory periods, and even *after-hyperpolarizations* and *after-depolarizations* (Bean, 2007). In any case, the basic model is correct enough for the purposes of studying general neuronal communication.

The concept of differential velocity is crucial in the functioning of the nervous system, and in this case, faster is not necessarily better. There are four main categories of nerve fiber, based on diameter and myelination. A key example of the need for parallel processes and differential functioning involves the different sizes of nerve fibers in communicating information about pain from the periphery to the CNS. When a painful event occurs, large myelinated fibers carry the information at high speed to the brain and spinal cord, resulting in an immediate reflexive action and subjective response. At the same time, smaller-diameter, nonmyelinated *c fibers* also convey information about the injury, but at a much slower and more prolonged rate. This latter communication stream reflects the ongoing state of the injured tissue, and the experience of pain will be prolonged if the injury is such that it requires attention over a period of weeks.

SYNAPTIC TRANSMISSION

In order for information to be conveyed past the boundaries of a single neuron, it must bridge the gap to the next neuron. The gap, or synapse, is about 20 nanometers (nm) wide. It is literally bridged in some cases and "forded" in others. The type of synapse between the presynaptic and postsynaptic membranes depends on its location. The most common set-up is an axon-to-dendrite connection, or axodendritic synapse. If, instead, the presynaptic axon synapses at the postsynaptic soma or another axon, these are labeled axosomatic or axoaxonic synapses. Other, less common relationships are *axosynaptic, dendrodendritic, axoextracellular,* and *axosecretory.*

In order for a substance to be classified as a neurotransmitter (NT), it must fulfill four criteria (Werman, 1966):

1. It must originate from a neuron, where it is stored and released via depolarization.
2. It must induce effects postsynaptically on a target cell by specific receptors.
3. It must be inactivated or cleared from the synapse through reuptake.
4. It must produce the same effects on nervous tissue in vitro as those produced in vivo.

NTs cross the synapse to bind to receptors on the postsynaptic membrane. The nature of the message is "coded" by the type and amount of NT(s) released. NTs are synthesized in the presynaptic neuron, with the location dependent on the type of NT. Small-molecule NTs are synthesized locally in the terminal, whereas larger, peptide transmitters are synthesized farther upstream and transported along *microtubules* within the axon.

NTs manifest a "life-cycle" from creation to destruction/rebirth that consists of relatively discrete steps. Although some of these steps are facilitated by enzymes, all are potential points for psychopharmacological interventions. The main steps of the life-cycle can be summarized as follows: (a) synthesis of the NT, which then moves into (b) storage within vesicles, which then undergo (c) transport to the terminal button and then await (d) release through *exocytosis* out of fusion pores; once released into the synapse, NTs undergo (e) receptor binding, followed quickly by (f) reuptake or degradation upon release from the receptors.

Although numerous NTs have been identified thus far,[6] the manner in which most of these are synthesized is similar at the core. In essence, substrates must be modified, and enzymes are required to catalyze each reaction or step in the process. The number of steps involved varies according to the NT, as do the enzymes, but the results are the same. The process is governed by the rules of chemistry: The rate of synthesis is only as fast as the slowest step. This rate-limiting step can be due to a limited supply of precursor molecules or to limited enzymatic activity. Conversely, increasing the concentration of precursor or enzyme activity at this step will result in an overall increase in production of the NT.

The NT that is synthesized must be stored until needed for maximum effectiveness. Storage takes place in sacs or vesicles within the terminal, the walls of which are phospholipid-bilayer membranes. Vesicles containing peptides are derived from the Golgi apparatus in the soma. Vesicles that contain small-molecule NTs are also originally produced in the soma but are subsequently re-formed after they release their stored transmitters from endocytotic invaginations of the presynaptic membrane, which result from the release of NT as noted below (Stanford, 2001a). Peptide-containing vesicles

---

[6]Examples of various molecular structures of NTs include amino acids (glutamate, aspartate, γ-aminobutyric acid [GABA], and glycine); monoamines (dopamine, norepinephrine, serotonin, epinephrine, and histamine); and peptides (β-endorphin, substance P). Other structures include gases (nitric oxide), single-atom ions (zinc), and nonamine transmitters (acetylcholine or adenosine). Of the many NTs, glutamate is the most omnipresent in the CNS, accounting for 90% of excitatory synapses. GABA is nearly as widespread, accounting for 90% of inhibitory synapses (Sapolsky, 2005).

must be transported down the axon in order to be released into the synapse, while small-molecule NTs are already close to the membrane where they will be docked. Note that in some areas of the nervous system, NTs are released from varicosities or bulges in the axon rather than from the terminal, but the same process applies.

The release of NT into the synaptic cleft occurs when an AP reaches the membrane of the terminal. Just as the axonal membrane contains voltage-gated Na^+ channels that perpetuate the AP, the terminal membrane contains voltage-gated Ca^{2+} channels. An arriving AP shifts the terminal membrane past the Ca^{2+} gate threshold, opening the channels. At the terminal, the concentration of Ca^{2+} outside the neuron is substantially higher than that inside. Furthermore, the inside of the terminal is still negative. Thus, since the Ca^{2+} has a positive electrical charge, the electrical and chemical gradient forces combine to drive calcium ions immediately into the terminal. In order to return the concentration of Ca^{2+} inside the terminal to its baseline level, a calcium-sodium pump is activated, which requires additional energy.

The increase of Ca^{2+} in the terminal triggers several subsequent processes that ultimately result in the release of NTs. Although the details of the entire process have not been completely mapped out, several components of the process are well known, and many candidate proteins have been identified (Sudhof, 2004). According to one of the more agreed-upon hypotheses, the SNARE (soluble *N*-ethylmaleimide-sensitive fusion protein [NSF] attachment receptor) hypothesis (Sollner & Rothman, 1994), vesicles are docked via proteins (such as *SNAP-25*), and Ca^{2+} activates other proteins (such as *synaptotagmin*) to join the docking complex; this process then leads to the creation of a fusion pore and subsequent release of NT.

Once the NT has been released from the vesicle through the fusion pore, the evacuated vesicle in effect becomes part of the membrane, with the concomitant danger that the terminal membrane will grow to be too large. As part of the recycling process, new vesicles are formed by *endocytosis* of part of the terminal membrane. These new vesicles are coated with proteins (such as clathrin and dynamin), which seem to assist in maintaining the vesicle's structural integrity while being refilled with NT (Zucker, Kullmann, & Schwarz, 2004). The local recycling of vesicle membrane allows for far more rapid processing.

The area at which vesicles dock is called the active zone. The active zone is a disklike structure that contains a hexagonal protein grid. Once filled with NT and docked, vesicles are primed for fusion. At that point, when an AP arrives at the terminal and Ca^{2+} enters the neuron, exocytosis of the NT occurs instantly. The calcium channels are located in close proximity to the docked vesicles to ensure that the process occurs as quickly as possible.

The numerous varieties of synapse in the CNS fall into one of two categories: electrical and chemical. Electrical synapses allow for direct and passive flow of electrical current between neurons through ion channels that are linked together in a *gap junction*. This occurs virtually instantaneously and in either direction. Furthermore, the pore diameter of gap-junction channels is much larger than the voltage-gated ion channels described above. Thus, in addition to ions freely passing through these channels, larger molecules diffuse across the concentration gradient between the two neurons, which is particularly advantageous for hormone-secreting neurons. This last point highlights one of the main purposes of electrical synapses—that is, coordinating between neurons in a linked network. This action is important in, for example, brainstem neurons that generate breathing rhythms, hormone-secreting hypothalamic neurons that release hormones in a large burst into the circulation, and intracellular signaling among glial cells (Kandel & Siegelbaum, 2000).

Chemical synapses are also fast but are much slower relative to electrical synapses. Transmission of neural activity across the synaptic cleft occurs through chemical signaling by NTs. As noted above, the NTs are stored in vesicles in the presynaptic terminal and are released through exocytosis by a process triggered by the influx of Ca^{2+}. Once released, the NTs make the short trip across the synapse and bind to specific receptors on the postsynaptic membrane. The local effect of this NT-receptor binding depends on several factors, including the nature of the NT, the nature of the receptor, the level of excitation of the postsynaptic membrane, and the presence of other substances or molecules in the synapse.

Chemical synapses represent one kind of signaling. Two other types of chemical signaling involve targets that are more distant than a postsynaptic membrane. In paracrine signaling, chemicals are released into the extracellular space to reach a distant target. An example would be the diffusion of the gaseous messenger nitric oxide (NO) through membranes. Endocrine signaling is characteristic of hormones, which are secreted into the bloodstream and lymphatic system and travel to distant targets via the circulatory system.

RECEPTORS

On the other side of the synapse, the postsynaptic membrane often manifests a bustling, crowded area called a postsynaptic density. In anticipation of a deluge of NTs, the postsynaptic receptors are clustered, and many are anchored within the membrane to the cytoskeleton. Furthermore, some proteins within the postsynaptic density bind to the presynaptic membrane, tethering the terminal in an optimal location.

Receptors are very dynamic in structure and process. As proteins in the neural membrane, they float and move laterally and undergo turnover based on circumstances of binding. Two cases are particularly noteworthy, especially in terms of psychopharmacological interventions. In the presence of chronic receptor antagonism, receptors can increase in number, or up-regulate, leading to a situation of increased sensitivity to agonists that come into contact with the postsynaptic membrane. This situation occurs in the case of tardive dyskinesia in response to antipsychotic dopamine antagonists. Conversely, continuous stimulation of receptors, or chronic exposure to agonists, can lead to a decrease in receptor number, or down-regulation. Such desensitization occurs in the case of drug addiction and possibly in medication "poop-out" (e.g., selective serotonin-reuptake inhibitors [SSRIs] are known to sometimes stop working after years of effectiveness).

In general, membrane receptors can be categorized according to their affinity for a particular *ligand*, their selectivity among ligands, their density, their saturability, and their binding reversibility. Families of related receptors can be distinguished by their differential response to specific agonists and antagonists.

- Ionotropic receptors (ligand-gated ion-channel receptors): These types of receptors are a relatively small group of the total number of receptors in the nervous system. Six different NTs are known to fall within this category: glutamate (GLU), gamma-aminobutyric acid (GABA), acetylcholine (ACh), serotonin (5-HT), adenosine triphosphate (ATP), and glycine. The receptor proteins in these cases create the ion channel itself, with transmembrane sections of the protein chain crossing two to four times, forming the pore through which the ions can pass. These receptors are difficult to target in terms of pharmacological intervention because of the speed of action and localized effect.

- Metabotropic receptors (G-protein–coupled receptors): These types of receptors use additional energy as part of their functioning (hence the prefix meaning "metabolism"). They generate a response through the activation of a particular G-protein, a protein that binds guanosine triphosphate (GTP), which transduces the effect of receptor binding to an intracellular response. (The "G" in G-protein stands for guanosine nucleotide-binding protein.) These types of receptors are targets for pharmaceutical development.

Postsynaptic Potentials (PSPs)

At the simplest level, postsynaptic potentials fall into two main categories depending on whether communication is propagated or attenuated. Excitatory PSPs reflect the opening of ion channels that lead to further depolarization and increase the likelihood that an AP will propagate down the postsynaptic neuron's axon. Inhibitory PSPs, in contrast, result from molecular activities that hyperpolarize the membrane or otherwise decrease the likelihood that any further neural communication will ensue. For example, glutamate-activated cationic channels depolarize the membrane and potentially trigger an excitatory postsynaptic potential (EPSP), while GABA-activated anionic (Cl^-) channels hyperpolarize the membrane and trigger an inhibitory postsynaptic potential (IPSP). Note that, for the most part, a single EPSP or IPSP will not exert a significant impact on the membrane but must be "added together" to determine the net effect.

Neural Integration

The summation of postsynaptic potentials, or neural integration, results in a "final value" of membrane potential that may or may not reach threshold for an AP. Clearly, an abundance of EPSPs are likely to do the trick. Conversely, the more IPSPs that enter the equation, the less likely an AP will occur. Integration or summation takes into account both the timing of the PSPs (temporal summation) and their placement (spatial summation). The area of "reckoning" tends to be the axon hillock, the thickened part of the axon just after the soma.

Importance of Inhibition

Although summation occurs all along the membrane from dendrites to soma, the primary "action" occurs at the axon hillock, where the tipping point of an AP "decision" is made. As such, this tends to be the last place for inhibitory influence to prevent propagation of APs. The distribution of axosomatic synapses tends to be such that inhibitory synapses are focused here, acting almost like a failsafe mechanism or "emergency brake" to stop communication.

Second-Messenger Systems

The variety of NT-receptor combinations of ionotropic systems provides a certain level of complexity and flexibility to neuron communication. This complexity of surface communication is increased exponentially with intracellular metabotropic systems that involve coupling with a second messenger (the initial NT being the first messenger). Activation of a metabotropic receptor triggers a chain reaction within the postsynaptic neuron, the layers of which are theoretically infinite. The most common initial step of metabotropic-receptor activity is activation of a G-protein that is coupled to the receptor inside the neural membrane. The variety of G-proteins engage a chain of second-messenger pathways, each of which can trigger a cascade of effects. The activated G-protein tends to trigger an initial effector enzyme, which then activates an internal second-messenger molecule, the identity of which depends on the specific G-protein. (See Figure 3.3.)

The most common second messenger is Ca^{2+}, which acts on a variety of targets, including ion channels. The cyclic nucleotides (cyclic adenosine monophosphate [cAMP] and cyclic guanosine monophosphate [cGMP]) are another category of second messenger, available in abundant supply from ATP and GTP. These cyclic nucleotides either activate *protein kinases* or influence other ligand-gated ion channels. Another category of second messenger derives from the membrane itself, components of which can be converted to inositol triphosphate (IP3) and diacylglycerol (DAG). These second messengers also activate protein kinases, with subsequent downstream effects.

One example of downstream reactions within the neuron stemming from secondary messengers, as set in motion by metabotropic receptors, is the rapid increase in *tyrosine hydroxylase* activity by protein kinase *phosphorylation*. Tyrosine hydroxylase is a key enzyme in the synthesis of catecholamines. Thus, a substance that increases the rate of activity of this enzyme will lead to an increase in the concentration of catecholamines within a particular neuron, with a related impact "downstream." Furthermore, in terms of the relevance of this reaction to psychopharmacology, some theories about its mechanism include effects on second-messenger systems. For example, lithium salts are believed to influence the IP3 system.

As the result of the number of steps and reactions following metabotropic receptor activation, second-messenger systems amplify the size of response, so that a

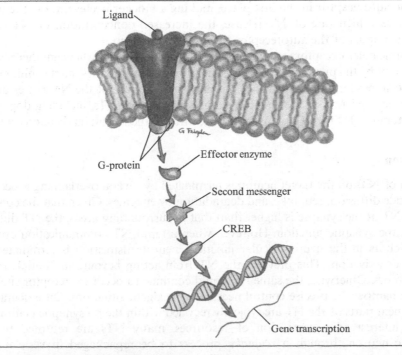

Figure 3.3   G-Protein–Coupled Receptor

single NT-receptor interaction can be multiplied within the neuron and lead to a behavioral response far above that engendered by the initial stimulus.

In addition to the cascade of actions within the postsynaptic cytoplasm, second messengers can also trigger more long-term changes by influencing RNA synthesis of new protein through activating *gene transcription*. The new proteins can, for example, be enzymes, structural elements, channels, or receptors. This is one explanation for the up-regulation of receptors after prolonged synaptic activity. One of the most common transcriptional activators is cAMP response element-binding (CREB) protein. CREB has been identified in the synthesis of *brain-derived neurotrophic factor (BDNF)*, tyrosine hydroxylase, and many neuropeptides, including *enkephalin* and corticotrophin-releasing factor (CRF).

Synaptic Modulation Through Autoreceptors and Heteroreceptors

As noted, inhibition represents a crucial process in life, since chemical reactions must be controlled to exert an impact while not disrupting the processes surrounding the initial action. Two types of receptors provide for additional inhibition and modulation in neuronal firing: autoreceptors and heteroreceptors.

Autoreceptors function as a negative-feedback or thermostat mechanism in which neurons can serve as their own inhibitors. Thus, as the NT is released and exerts an effect on the postsynaptic membrane receptors, it also acts on inhibitory autoreceptors to decrease the release of the NT itself. Some of the neurons that have been found to have autoreceptors are acetylcholine muscarinic (M_2), dopamine (D_2/D_3), gamma-aminobutyric acid ($GABA_B$), serotonin ($5\text{-}HT_{1B}/5\text{-}HT_{1D}$), and histamine ($H_3$). A medication or drug that blocks autoreceptor function would be expected to stop this inhibition and maintain release of the NT. However, this impact is contingent on the amount of NT released. Brief or slight release might be insufficient to activate the autoreceptor in the first place, making a blocker irrelevant. On the other hand, at a very high rate of NT release, the increased concentration of NT could override the impact of the autoreceptor through competition.

Presynaptic heteroreceptors are located at the terminal button, where another neuron controls action by the presynaptic neuron. The proximity of the presynaptic inhibitor to the synapse allows for a fine-tuned level of control over release of the NT. For example, norepinephrine (NE) modulates the release of several other NTs, including dopamine (DA), serotonin (5-HT), and glutamate (GLU), through the NE alpha_2 heteroreceptor.

Termination

The action of NTs on the target neuron is terminated by several overlapping processes, which include diffusion, reuptake, and degradation by enzymes. Given that the concentration of NT at the synapse is higher than that in surrounding areas, the NT diffuses away from the synaptic junction. However, when a rapid NT communication cycle is needed, such as in the neuromuscular junction, neurotransmission is terminated by enzymatic deactivation. This prevents the NT from acting beyond an "initial strike" at the receptors. Otherwise, the same NT could continue to occupy a receptor site and potentially hamper the precise control necessary in exigent situations. Once degraded, the component parts of the NT are typically recycled within the presynaptic neuron.

In the interest of conservation of resources, many NTs are returned to the presynaptic neuron through a *reuptake* process to be repackaged in vesicles and reused. Reuptake can target the whole NT or specific degradation products and is accomplished through active pumps that channel the NT back to the neuron cyto-plasm. The NT is then either *catabolized* through intracellular enzymes, such as *monoamine oxidase (MAO)*, or shunted into vesicles for reuse in the NT cycle. Note that some of the recovered NT is recycled through reuptake, which occurs indi-rectly through glial cells around the synapse. This speeds up the process, as well as isolating the synapse system more completely from surrounding processes.

NEUROTRANSMITTERS

Some texts distinguish transmitters from modulators by the postsynaptic mecha-nism involved—that is, NT receptors are ionotropic channels, while neuromodula-tor (NM) receptors are linked to G-protein and other second-messenger mechanisms. Another distinction is that transmitters are responsible for direct communication of messages across synapses, while modulators indirectly modify postsynaptic messages (von Bohlen und Halbach & Dermietzel, 2006).

One of the advantages of a specific, limited definition for NTs is the expectation of particular targets of intervention, whether for enhancement or for blocking. Neuromodulators, in contrast, play a more varied role. Neuropeptides, for example, are synthesized in neurons and released from terminals, and some bind to postsyn-aptic receptors; however, other peptides are produced in the periphery and bind to receptors within the cell nucleus (Hökfelt et al., 2000).

MAJOR NEUROTRANSMITTER SYSTEMS

Overall, the primary NTs can be divided into two major groups: biogenic amines and small amino acids. Although the amines are more numerous in type, the amino acids are far more prevalent in activity and influence. For the purposes of psychopharma-cology, the following NTs are the most crucial to understand: acetylcholine, dopa-mine, norepinephrine, serotonin, glutamate, and gamma-aminobutyric acid. The three important aspects of each NT system are their (a) location of synthesis, (b) major projection areas, and (c) receptor subtypes. Accounting for these characteristics pro-vides a better sense of the functionality and influence of NTs in the nervous system.

Cholinergic System

Acetylcholine (ACh) plays an important role in both the peripheral and central ner-vous systems. There are three main CNS cholinergic subsystems: spinal cord inter-neurons, striatal interneurons, and projection neurons. ACh is synthesized from acetyl coenzyme A (acetyl CoA) and choline by choline acetyltransferase and is stored in vesicles of cholinergic nerve terminals. After receptor binding, ACh is metabolized by acetylcholine esterase (AChE).

There are two main types of ACh receptors: nicotinic and muscarinic. Nicotinic receptors are composed of five subunits, which create an ion channel.[7] Different com-binations of subunits lead to a wide diversity of nicotinic-receptor subtypes with dis-tinct pharmacological properties, but all lead to depolarization. Although nicotinic

---

[7]See earlier discussion of ionotropic receptors.

ACh receptors are far more common in the periphery, they are present in the hippocampus, cerebral cortex, thalamus, hypothalamus, superior colliculi, and brainstem. Muscarinic receptors are metabotropic and are coupled to G-proteins. The two main classes, M_1 and M_2, are further subdivided into a total of five subtypes. M_1 receptors are located in the cortex, hippocampus, nucleus accumbens, striatum, and amygdalae, while M_2 receptors are found in the thalamus, superior colliculi, olfactory bulb, and brainstem.

Two main projection systems account for the bulk of ACh synthesis in the CNS: the *nucleus basalis of Meynert,* found in the basal forebrain, and the *pedunculopontine tegmental nucleus (PPTN),* found in the brainstem. Through projections to the cortex and hippocampus, the basal forebrain pathways appear to be involved in learning and memory, problem solving, and judgment. The brainstem cholinergic neurons are responsible for the large *pontine-geniculo-occipital (PGO) waves* that characterize the onset of REM sleep. Cholinergic activity is also associated with background cortical excitation.

Dopaminergic System

The dopaminergic system can be roughly categorized by the relative distance between its origins and the target cells. Ultrashort projections, involved primarily in lateral inhibition, include interneurons in the retina and olfactory bulb. Short or intermediate projections include the *tuberoinfundibular pathway* and other pathways that regulate autonomic and endocrine function by connecting hypothalamic nuclei to target cells, as well as dopaminergic neurons in the *periaqueductal gray (PAG)* area.

The most frequently described dopaminergic systems in the context of psychopharmacology are the long pathways originating from the midbrain: the *nigrostriatal, mesolimbic,* and *mesocortical pathways.* (See Figure 3.4.)

Dopamine (DA) is synthesized in a multistep, enzyme-facilitated process with a rate-limiting step from the action of tyrosine hydroxylase. Although this limits the impact of pharmacological intervention from the standpoint of synthesis, some substances, such as the neuropeptide *vasoactive intestinal polypeptide* (VIP), can activate the enzyme. DA must be synthesized within neurons because it cannot cross the *blood-brain barrier (BBB).* The DA neurotransmission process ends with both reuptake and enzymatic deactivation. Reuptake is facilitated by a dopamine transporter (DAT), with different subtypes at the presynaptic and vesicular membranes. DA is deactivated by monoamine oxidase (MAO) and by *catechol-O-methyl transferase (COMT)* both in the synapse and within the terminal.

Five DA receptors have been discovered thus far, which are divided into two main groups: D_1 (D_1, D_5) and D_2 (D_2, D_3, D_4). DA autoreceptors fall within the D_2 group and, as such, are mostly inhibitory; all are metabotropic. D_1 receptors are the most abundant in the forebrain and can be found in the striatum, amygdala, thalamus, midbrain, hypothalamus, and hindbrain; D_2 receptors are also widely distributed, especially in the striatum, midbrain, spinal cord, hypothalamus, and hippocampus; D_3 receptors are found in the basal forebrain, olfactory tubercle, nucleus accumbens, striatum, and substantia nigra; D_4 receptors are found in the frontal cortex, hippocampus, thalamus, striatum, basal *ganglia,* and cerebellum; and D_5 receptors are found exclusively in the thalamus and hippocampus.

DA influences a wide variety of brain functions depending on the specific pathway involved. The mesolimbic and mesocortical systems are involved in goal-directed,

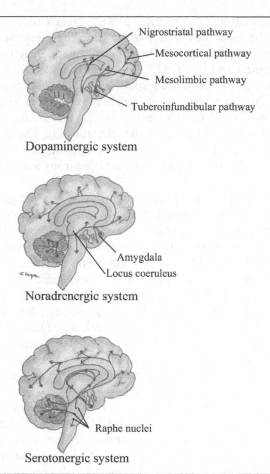

Dopaminergic system

- Nigrostriatal pathway
- Mesocortical pathway
- Mesolimbic pathway
- Tuberoinfundibular pathway

Noradrenergic system

- Amygdala
- Locus coeruleus

Serotonergic system

- Raphe nuclei

Figure 3.4   Neural Pathways

motivation-dependent, and reward-mediated behavior. The nigrostriatal system influences the initiation and maintenance of motor behavior. DA appears to be an essential NT in the hypothalamus, especially in the ventromedial and lateral hypothalamic areas involved in ingestive behaviors, and is also an essential inhibitory transmitter in regulating prolactin.

Noradrenergic System

The primary source of norepinephrine (NE) in the CNS is the *locus coeruleus*, and projections from this area extend throughout the higher- and lower-level systems, most notably the cerebral cortex, hippocampus, and sensory brainstem nuclei (see Figure 3.4). The secondary source for NE is the *lateral tegmental nuclei*, with many of the same projection targets as the locus coeruleus, except for the hypothalamus, which receives most of its adrenergic input from the lateral tegmental nuclei. Although the extent of NE innervation suggests that its impact is diffuse, cortical synapses are highly specialized, and the locus coeruleus exhibits distinct zones with differentiated targets (Stanford, 2001b).

In the periphery, NE is released from postganglionic sympathetic neurons. Norepinephrine derives from enzymatic hydroxylation of dopamine and is a precursor to the formation of epinephrine, which tends to be located primarily in the periphery. For the most part, NE is returned to the presynaptic terminal by nor-epinephrine transporters (NET). As with DA, enzymatic deactivation also occurs by MAO within the neuron and by COMT outside of it.

There are three types of adrenoceptors: (1) alpha-1; (2) alpha-2; and (3) beta. Each of these has three subtypes, all of which are G-protein–coupled: (1) alpha-1A, alpha-1B, and alpha-1D (α1A, α1B, and α1D); (2) alpha-2A, alpha-2B, and alpha-2C (α2A, α2B, and α2C); and (3) beta (β1, β2, and β3). The distribution of receptors in the brain varies, even among layers in the cerebral cortex. Alpha-2A receptors are located on the cell bodies of locus coeruleus neurons and function as inhibitory autoreceptors.

NE-receptor activation can be either inhibitory or excitatory, depending on the brain area where it has occurred. Furthermore, the actions of alpha and beta adrenoceptors are frequently opposed or inverse in their physiological impact. For example, in the periphery, alpha activation results in vasoconstriction, while beta activation leads to vasodilation. Although NE exerts direct NT effects, it also appears to function as a neuromodulator (e.g., on glutamate in the cerebral cortex). Overall, NE activity in the CNS is involved in the regulation of general attention and circadian rhythm, and especially in stress-response. The noradrenergic stress response is mediated in large part by hypothalamic activation of the locus coeruleus. The hypothalamic-pituitary-adrenal (HPA) axis further coordinates the body's reaction to stress by mobilizing cortisol and epinephrine in the adrenal glands.

Two other NE effects with important clinical and pharmacological implications have been characterized. First, noradrenergic activity has been found to influence the emotional impact of a given stimulus, such that the behavioral response can be depicted graphically as an inverted "U"—that is, NE underactivation is ineffective and characterizes a more depressive response, whereas NE overactivation is also ineffective but characterizes a more anxious response. The heightened activity of NE during an extremely stressful situation is blamed in part for the persistence of posttraumatic memories (Nestler, Hyman, & Malenka, 2009). Second, rather than resulting in an overall increase in excitability, NE activity heightens the "signal-to-noise ratio" of incoming information by reducing the underlying level of activity while increasing the response to specific input (Hasselmo et al., 1997). This latter hypothesis provides the basis for one explanation of why stimulants are effective in ADHD.

Serotonergic System

The primary source of serotonin (5-hydroxytryptamine [5-HT]) in the CNS is a cluster of nuclei in the midbrain and brainstem labeled *Raphe nuclei* (see Figure 3.4). Serotonin is synthesized from the precursor amino acid tryptophan, the concentration of which represents the rate-limiting step in the process. This means that conditions that influence the availability of tryptophan will have a profound impact on serotonergic functioning. Since the transport of tryptophan across membranes occurs with other amino acids, the rate of transport will be contingent on those amino acids as well. Serotonergic activity ends with the reuptake of 5-HT into the presynaptic terminal by serotonin transporters (SERT), as well as with MAO deactivation.

Serotonin pathways are interspersed relatively diffusely throughout the brain, with projections to the cerebral cortex, hippocampus, amygdala, basal ganglia, thalamus, hypothalamus, tectum, and ventral horn of the spinal cord. Serotonin receptors are among the most diverse in terms of types and subtypes and numbering between 14 and 16, depending on the source. They consists of two large families of receptors (5-HT$_1$, which has five subtypes, and 5-HT$_2$, which has three subtypes), a ligand-gated receptor (5-HT$_3$), and a miscellaneous group of receptors (with six subtypes). 5-HT$_1$ receptors tend to be inhibitory, with G-proteins that open K$^+$ channels or close Ca^{2+} channels; 5-HT$_{1A}$ and 5-HT$_{1D}$ are autoreceptors; 5-HT$_2$ receptors tend to be excitatory; and the 5-HT$_3$ receptor is excitatory.

Given the widespread projections of serotonergic pathways, it should not be surprising that serotonin modulates several functions in the CNS. Some of the documented areas of functioning include memory and learning, sexual and eating behavior, aggression, sleep, body temperature, and pain perception. Serotonin also plays a role in the activation of the HPA axis, but the mechanism is less well understood.

Glutamatergic System

Glutamate (GLU) is synthesized locally in the cellular Krebs cycle and is stored in vesicles in the terminal of its neuron. Its activity is terminated through reuptake, either directly into the presynaptic neuron or indirectly into nearby astrocytes.

There are four main GLU receptors, three of which are ionotropic and the fourth is metabotropic. Two of the ionotropic receptors, kainate and AMPA (aminohydroxy-methylisoxazole propionate), function in typical fashion, associated with Na$^+$ channels that result in EPSPs. The N-methyl-D-aspartate (NMDA) receptor functions much differently, in that under normal resting conditions the NMDA receptor responds slowly to glutamate, if at all, because of ion-channel inhibition by magnesium ions (Mg^{2+}). If the postsynaptic membrane has been depolarized, however, the Mg^{2+} block is overcome, and the channel can open. At that point, cation influx results in an excitatory response. Additional intracellular processes ensue that result specifically from the entry of Ca^{2+} and lead to long-term potentiation, although they may also result in excitotoxicity.

Eight metabotropic GLU receptor subtypes have been discovered thus far, based on different receptor proteins. Some are presynaptic and some postsynaptic, but for the most part they seem to influence long-term potentiation. Their distribution throughout the CNS varies by subtype.

GLU neurons are very prominent in the cerebral cortex and project to many subcortical structures and areas, including the hippocampus, amygdala, *caudate nucleus,* nucleus accumbens, substantia nigra, and pons. Some specific GLU pathways are (a) cortical-brainstem, which descends from layer-5 pyramidal neurons to neurotransmitter synthesis centers in the midbrain and brainstem; (b) cortico-striatal and cortico-accumbens, which send glutamatergic projections to the striatum and nucleus accumbens, respectively; (c) thalamo-cortical and cortico-thalamic pathways, which comprise ascending and descending GLU fibers, respectively; and (d) cortico-cortical pathways, which allow intracortical communication between pyramidal neurons. Glutamate pathways are also found within the hippocampus, and from the hippocampus to the hypothalamus, nucleus accumbens, and lateral septum.

Glutamate is the primary excitatory NT in the CNS and plays a central role in learning and memory via *long-term potentiation (LTP)*. Other functions include regulating the secretion of pituitary hormones during the reproductive cycle, participating in aspects of neuronal migration during brain development, and integrating environmental stimuli and motor behavior (von Bohlen, Halbach, & Dermietzel, 2006). Given the everpresent danger of excitotoxicity, tight control of glutamate and other excitatory substances is crucial.

GABAergic System

In terms of production, gamma-aminobutyric acid (GABA) is synthesized almost exclusively from glutamate by glutamate decarboxylase, which is present mainly in the cerebellum and pancreas. GABA activity is ended by reuptake through GABA transporters (GAT), followed by enzymatic *transamination* through GABA transaminase (GABA-T). One of the byproducts of this reaction is glutamate. As much as 80% of GABA is returned to the presynaptic terminal through reuptake.

There are three GABA receptors (A, B, and C), all of which increase membrane permeability to Cl^- and thus promote inhibition through hyperpolarization. $GABA_A$ and $GABA_C$ are ionotropic, while $GABA_B$ is coupled to G-protein. $GABA_B$ receptors function as autoreceptors and inhibitory heteroreceptors and appear to be involved in attenuating long-term potentiation. While $GABA_A$ receptors are found throughout the CNS, $GABA_B$ are especially prolific in the cerebral cortex, superior colliculi, cerebellum, and dorsal horn of the spinal cord. $GABA_C$ receptors have been found in the pituitary, and in retinal horizontal and bipolar neurons. In the striatum, nearly 95% of the neurons are GABAergic. There are both GABA interneurons and GABA projection neurons.

GABA is the primary inhibitory NT in the CNS, expressed in 90% of inhibitory synapses and about 30% of all synapses. As a rule, any condition, substance, or alteration that impedes or hinders the GABA system will tend to lead to a state of overexcitation in the CNS, which is potentially dangerous and possibly fatal. Conversely, molecules, substances, and interventions that increase GABAergic tone or activity will result in a reduced level of excitation. The resulting state can be adaptive or maladaptive depending on the extent of the inhibitory process and the context.

Histamine

Most CNS histaminergic neurons originate in the tuberomammillary nucleus of the hypothalamus. These neurons project up through the medial forebrain bundle to the cortex, hippocampus, limbic areas, and hypothalamus. Most histamine neurons also contain other NTs, especially GABA, substance P, and enkephalin (Schwartz et al., 1991). The three histamine receptors discovered thus far—H_1, H_2, and H_3—are all G-protein–coupled. For the most part, histamine inhibits firing in the cerebral cortex via H_1 receptors, although H_1 receptors are excitatory in the hypothalamus. H_2 receptors are also found in the striatum. Less is known about H_3 receptors, but they tend to be autoreceptors. No transporter has been identified; neurotransmission ends with enzymatic deactivation by MAO and *histamine methytransferase*.

Histamine plays a role in mediating arousal and attention, as well as controlling reactivity in the vestibular system. H_1-receptor antagonists (blockers), or antihistamines, cause marked sedation if they cross the BBB. They also prevent motion sickness, likely related to the histaminergic influence on the vestibular system. Some evidence points to histamine's influence on food and water intake and regulation of body temperature (Hough & Green, 1983). Histamine might also influence blood flow in the brain.

Neuropeptides

Since the discovery that some peptides are synthesized in neurons and bind to receptors, the search for substances that act in a similar fashion has yielded a list of more than 50 different, biologically active neuropeptides. Neuropeptides can be grouped into three main categories:

1. Opioid peptides (e.g., enkephalins, endorphins, and dynorphins).
2. Gastrointestinal peptides (e.g., vasoactive intestinal polypeptide [VIP], substance P, neurotensin, neuropeptide Y, and cholecystokinin (CCK]).
3. Pituitary (or hypophysiotrophic) peptides (e.g., vasopressin, oxytocin, somatostatin, thyrotropin-releasing hormone [TRH]).

Neuropeptides differ from the "classical" NTs in many ways. Precursor molecules are large sequences of amino acids that are produced in the nucleus and transported inside vesicles to the terminal, making the process very slow. Precursors are split into smaller fragments until the active peptide is produced. This slow process of synthesis implies that depletion may occur in an active neuron and thus change the pattern of neuronal firing over time. Furthermore, a longer process allows the specific peptide content at any given time to be altered by gene induction and suppression along the way. The rate of release of peptides into the synapse often depends on a higher or more prolonged rate of firing for the larger vesicles to fuse with the membrane and release their contents. In terms of receptor binding, no ionotropic-peptide receptors have been discovered; all are metabotropic, second messenger–coupled. No peptide neurotransmission process ends with reuptake, and no peptide transporters have been found. All peptides are broken down by *peptidases*, which are bound to neuron membranes and which tend to be selective for amino-acid sequences rather than for whole peptides. Furthermore, the peptidases can become saturated if a large amount of peptide has been released. Consequently, excess peptides can diffuse away from the area of the synapse and act on neurons that are distant from the initial site.

Orexin is a highly excitatory neuropeptide hormone, also known as *hypocretin*. It is synthesized in the lateral hypothalamus. The discovery that this key neurotransmitter is deficient in narcoleptic patients provided insights into the sleep-wake cycle, suggesting that orexin plays a role in regulating the sleep-wake transition (Ebrahim et al., 2003). A lack of effective orexin functioning leads narcoleptic patients to experience "sleep attacks," in which the onset of sleep is sudden instead of gradual.

Enkephalins have been identified as endogenous opioids. To date, four opioid receptors have been identified: mu, delta, kappa, and ORL-1. Binding to these G-protein–coupled receptors results in direct inhibition by reducing either the release of NT or membrane excitability. Inhibition can occur pre- or postsynaptically. Kappa-receptor activation closes Ca^{2+} channels, while the other three opioid receptors open K^+ channels. Ascending inhibition of pain messages traveling up the spinal cord results in analgesia, while descending inhibition of the NE and 5-HT pathways reduces the experience of pain. Some indirect excitation can occur through disinhibition in the substantia gelatinosa in the spinal cord and in the hippocampus.

Substance P is a peptide from the *tachykinin* family[8] that has been found to play an important role in pain and inflammation, and possibly in stress, anxiety, depression,

---

[8]Tachykinin peptides are one of the largest families of neuropeptides and are so named because of their ability to rapidly induce contraction of gut tissue.

and reward. High levels are found in the caudate nucleus, nucleus accumbens, colliculi, spinal cord, and olfactory bulb.

Cholecystokinin (CCK) is one of the first gastrointestinal peptides to be discovered in mammal brains. It comprises a family of biologically active fragments, the most neuroactive of which is CCK-8 (octapeptide). CCK-8 neurons and their projections are widespread throughout the CNS. CCK-8 is a frequent cotransmitter with, for example, GABA in the cerebral cortex, DA in the ventral tegmental area (VTA), and enkephalins in the periaqueductal gray (von Bohlen und Halbach & Dermietzel, 2006).

Oxytocin has been called the "love drug" and "cuddle chemical" because of its reported impact on nurturing and social-bonding behaviors. However, recent research suggests that the impact of oxytocin is specific to one's in-group, rather than a general feeling of well-being and affiliation with others (De Dreu et al., 2010, 2011). In any case, such preliminary findings leave many questions about the specificity of neurochemical pathways in invoking particular emotional-behavioral responses, and the extent of modulation by environment (e.g., social context).[9]

Vasopressin inhibits urination, as implied by its other name, antidiuretic hormone (ADH). Its synthetic analog form, DDAVP (l-desamine-8-D-arginine vasopressin), can be used to treat diabetes insipidus and enuresis (Seif et al., 2011). As a neurotransmitter or neuromodulator, vasopressin enhances cognition in learning processes (Ring, 2005). Other actions in the brain include roles in circadian rhythm and blood pressure/temperature regulation, as well as in modifying aggression and social attachment (Young, 2009).

Other Transmitter Substances

Nitric oxide (NO) is a gas, and does not act like other NTs in several ways. It is not stored and can diffuse freely through tissues. Its effect extends beyond the release site, since NO does not act by binding to receptors. This property suggests that NO might be useful for coordinating the activity of a group of neurons within a specific region and mediating learning. NO is produced in many CNS neurons, in addition to peripheral cells. Ca^{2+} plays a key role in the production of NO, particularly in neurons with NMDA receptors. Although its mechanism of action is still unclear, NO tends to act on enzymes that lead to increased neuronal excitability. As such, it should be considered more of a second messenger than a neurotransmitter. NO has been found to result in the release of glutamate and substance P. Overall, NO appears to play a role as a communicator between neurons. Although many studies support the idea of NO as a *retrograde messenger*,[10] especially for NMDA-receptor activation and long-term potentiation, some do not. NO also appears to play a role in excitotoxicity, pain, and possibly epilepsy (Calabrese et al., 2007).

Adenosine, a nucleoside component of ATP, is released during cellular activity as energy is used and ATP is broken down into adenosine diphosphate (ADP) and

[9]See Chapter 2 for Schachter's two-factor theory of emotions.
[10]Retrograde signaling is a phenomenon in which a signal travels from a postsynaptic neuron to a presynaptic one.

cAMP.[11] Adenosine then accumulates in the extracellular space and acts on inhibitory or excitatory A_1, A_2, and A_3 receptors. Adenosine is not a neurotransmitter; it functions as a neuromodulator. Adenosine inhibits pacemaker cells in the heart to slow the heart rate. In the CNS, it inhibits neurons by enhancing the refractory period of the AP. In arousal-system neurons, this inhibition promotes sleep. As an adenosine A_1 antagonist, caffeine acts as a stimulant by inhibiting sleepiness. Adenosine might also serve an anticonvulsant function, since benzodiazepine antiepileptic medications increase adenosine concentration, in addition to their impact on GABA receptors (Dragunow, 1986).

Anandamide is an endogenous cannabinoid, or *endocannabinoid,* that was isolated and elucidated in 1992. Another endocannabinoid is 2-arachidonylglycerol (2-AG). Both these substances derive from membrane lipids, and the mechanism of release is still unclear. They act on two receptor subtypes, the most influential being CB_1. In terms of effect, endocannabinoids appear to regulate synaptic communication through retrograde signaling. In the hippocampus and cerebellum, for example, endocannabinoids inhibit GABA release and thus reduce inhibitory neurotransmission. Other brain areas with CB_1 receptors include the basal ganglia, hypothalamus, and substantia nigra.

Melatonin is an *indole* hormone derived from 5-HT. It is synthesized in the pineal gland, and production is contingent on the rhythm of the suprachiasmatic nucleus (SCN) of the hypothalamus. Peripheral levels of melatonin reflect almost directly the function of the pineal gland and can potentially be used to assess the functioning of the central circadian clock and possible circadian abnormality. Melatonin, while not necessarily a sleep-inducing substance, can promote sleep in recumbent subjects in very dim light. Pharmacotherapy with melatonin has proved to have a positive impact on some circadian-rhythm sleep disorders related to shift work and jet lag (Arendt & Skene, 2005).

Brain-derived neurotrophic factor (BDNF) is an example of a *neurotrophin,* related to nerve growth factor. Neurotrophins can stimulate growth, guide growth to appropriate locations, stimulate gene expression, and promote neuron survival and regeneration after injury. BDNF is believed to hold potential as a neural protector against stress (Huang & Reichardt, 2001).

COTRANSMITTERS

The possibility of multiple NT substances within single neurons increases their complexity and versatility considerably. The combination of individual NTs can result in a compound action that is more effective than the action of either NT alone. Although details are poorly understood, such combinations have been found to play a role in the modulation of sensation and emotion, the perception of pain, and the stress response (Dickenson, 2001). NTs can be combined or coexist in several configurations. Vesicles with classical NTs and neuropeptides can be located within the same axon terminal. Different neuropeptide vesicles can also exist in the same terminal. Some of the more common examples of such combinations

---

[11]See Chapter 5 for a discussion of ATP, ADP, and cAMP.

include ACh + enkephalin, GLU + substance P, 5-HT + substance P, and NE + enkephalin.

DIFFERENTIAL RELEASE OF TRANSMITTERS DUE TO FIRING RATES

Small molecule, "classical" transmitters tend to be stored in vesicles close to, or docked at, the presynaptic membrane. In response to low firing rates, the number of Ca^{2+} channels that open is relatively small, and the concentration of Ca^{2+} tends to open those smaller, docked vesicles. However, when the frequency of stimulation increases, as reflected in more frequent action potentials, the greater amount of entering Ca^{2+} releases neuropeptides stored in larger vesicles that are spread throughout the terminal, in addition to the smaller vesicular release (Hökfelt et al., 2000). Conceptually, this means that a typical rate of firing results in a "standard," immediate, and more localized flow of information. When circumstances increase the firing rate, not only is the "standard" message stronger, as reflected in the release of more NT, but the addition of neuropeptide release extends the range of impact to other neurons, as well as prolonging the action.

NERVOUS SYSTEM: ANATOMY AND STRUCTURAL PHYSIOLOGY

The nervous system can be divided into two broad categories: the central nervous system (CNS) and the peripheral nervous system (PNS). The CNS comprises the brain and spinal cord—no more, no less. All other nervous tissue falls within the category of PNS, which includes sensory neurons and pathways leading to the spinal cord, motor neurons and motor nerves after exiting the spinal cord, cranial nerves that innervate the face and head, and the autonomic nervous system (ANS). The ANS is further subdivided into the sympathetic and *parasympathetic nervous systems*.

THE CENTRAL NERVOUS SYSTEM (CNS)

Brain and Spinal Cord

The brain serves many functions, and its component parts operate to ensure that these functions occur to the best of capacity, within the limits of available resources, within the constraints of the environment (including the size of the skull), and according to the laws of the universe. One way to look at its overarching raison d'être is survival. Viewed from an evolutionary or functionalist perspective,[12] the brain is responsible for maintaining life-support functions. More specifically, at some point beyond its established role as coordinator of nerve impulses and reflexes,

---

[12]The functionalist perspective was well established by William James in his book *Principles of Psychology* (1890).

the brain's development became increasingly predicated on the survival value of learning. The preponderance of its resources were subsequently devoted to using this learning while at the same time continuing to manage life-sustaining functions. Thus, sleep and appetite regulation, as well as a host of other functions, are accompanied by learning and memory creation about these same activities, leading ostensibly to improved adaptation and survival.

The spinal cord, on the other hand, can be considered a vestige of the original impulse/reflex nervous system. Essentially, the spinal cord relays neuronal information between the brain and the rest of the body. Consequently, the spinal cord is composed mainly of tracts and pathways, although some spinal structures play an additional role in mediating or modulating neural activity.

The nervous system has been categorized along several dimensions,[13] most of which are congruent. One of the most rudimentary divisions was derived from the colors of stained brain sections seen on glass slides. White matter reflects the existence of myelin, and thus a preponderance of axons and pathways. Gray matter reflects an absence of myelin, in a sense, and thus reflects "everything else," but primarily neuron cell bodies and other structures.

Another relatively rudimentary division traces evolutionary observations. Cross-species studies have established that many brain areas are common to all organisms with a nervous system, and that "more highly evolved" organisms have developed more specialized areas. An example of categorizing along these lines is Paul MacLean's triune brain concept, or the idea that human brains comprise "three brains in one": low (protoreptilian), middle (paleomammalian, mammal), and high (neomammalian, human) (MacLean, 1970). These rough divisions reflect a hierarchy of functions, such that the most basic functions of life are managed by the lower brain, common to all life forms; midbrain regions represent mammalian evolutionary "achievements" of emotional functioning; and higher regions, which are the most well-developed in humans, reflect higher levels of cognition and complex brain function.

Note that while the triune brain concept is oversimplified and in many ways inaccurate, it can nonetheless serve as a useful metaphor for describing neurological functioning in common-sense terms. For the medical psychologist, such terms translate into a more meaningful way of communicating these concepts to patients. For example, rather than trying to explain to a patient that his or her overwhelming fear is hard to control because of insufficient cortical inhibition of an overactive limbic network, one can cast this situation as "the human brain trying to tame the mammal brain," and so forth.

Another reason for conceptualizing the CNS in developmental terms is that the brain evolved its function along with its structure, and the two become inseparable when viewed from the perspective that *ontogeny recapitulates phylogeny*.[14] Thus, the brainstem "comes online" far ahead of the cerebral cortex and exerts a far more powerful influence on behavior during the first years of life. By the same token,

---

[13]It is customary at this juncture to introduce the idea of localization along axes and planes in order to better describe the position of each structure within the nervous system. However, Dr. Kotkin has provided extensive coverage of such points of orientation in Chapter 5, so we defer to his exposé.

[14]"Ontogeny recapitulates phylogeny," a hypothesis attributed largely to Ernst Heinrich Philipp August Haeckel, states that in developing from embryo to adult, animals go through stages resembling or representing successive stages in the evolution of their remote ancestors.

damage or impairment to lower levels of the brain will have a more profound impact on functioning (e.g., coma) than will damage to higher levels (e.g., memory impairment). Bruce Perry's neurosequential model of development and trauma is an example of effective use of these principles for understanding and treating patients with trauma (Perry, 2006; Perry & Pollard, 1998).

The most common system for categorizing brain divisions follows embryological development. At around one month after fertilization, the zygote's many cells have organized into a tube sandwiched between a plate and crest. The tube's growth and development include the enlargement of three areas that ultimately become the brain's three main divisions: *hindbrain, midbrain,* and *forebrain.* Some researchers further subdivide these segments into four groups: the hindbrain/brainstem, midbrain/diencephalon, limbic brain, and neocortex/forebrain. However, a more commonly used classification includes, in descending order, the *telencephalon* and *diencephalon,* which encompass the forebrain; the *mesencephalon,* or midbrain; and the *metencephalon* and *myelencephalon,* which make up the hindbrain (see Figure 3.5). Although most neuroscientists agree on the end divisions (hindbrain and forebrain), disagreements remain regarding the boundaries of the diencephalon and mesencephalon. Some prefer to obviate that ambiguity by locating the diencephalon in the forebrain and assigning the mesencephalon to the hindbrain structures, thereby removing the midbrain category altogether.

Regardless of the categorization systems that are established based on origin, cell type, and location, virtually all neuroscience texts describe seven main "parts" or areas of the CNS: cerebral hemispheres, diencephalon, midbrain, pons, cerebellum, medulla oblongata, and spinal cord. Of course, each of these "parts" can be subdivided into groups of neurons or "nuclei," but even those groups are described in terms of their "parent" organization. For example, the diencephalic structures (the thalamus and hypothalamus) are made up of many of their own nuclei, each with specific functions within the CNS. Also, the cerebral hemispheres are typically subdivided into the cerebral cortex, basal ganglia, and limbic system.

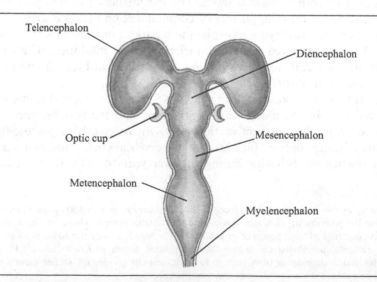

Figure 3.5   CNS Divisions in Early Development

Brain Protection

The most obvious form of physical protection for the brain is the skull. However, the delicate cerebral tissue still needs to be protected inside the skull, just as any fragile item contained within a box. Furthermore, the inside of the skull is not entirely smooth but displays a "stucco" appearance in some areas, which makes it perilous for the brain to hit or graze its casing.

The inner "wrapping" of the brain consists of three layers of tissue, or meninges: The outermost layer, the dura mater, is the thickest and toughest. The innermost layer, the pia mater, is the thinnest and closely envelops the surface of the cortical folds. The middle layer, the arachnoid mater, comprises a weblike network of thin pillars that extend between the dura and pia. The space between the arachnoid and pia mater, or the subarachnoid space, contains the cerebral spinal fluid (CSF).

Within the meninges, the CSF surrounds the CNS, whereas the CSF fills the ventricles, which are spaces within the CNS.[15] As separate spaces, the ventricles are remnants of the developing nervous system, in which the central *neural tube* used to be a continuous pipelike compartment within the enclosed *neural plate*. While the primary purpose of the CSF is to protect the brain structures, circulation of this fluid can serve as a pathway for various substances. For example, melatonin is found at a much higher concentration in the third and lateral ventricles than in the bloodstream. Similarly, metabolic waste material is discharged into the CSF and transported out of the CNS through the blood-brain barrier.

The CSF is similar in composition to blood plasma but contains far less protein. It is produced in large part by the choroid plexus, which is loose connective tissue arranged in *microvilli*. Most of the choroid plexus is found in the lateral ventricles, although it is present in all four. Once CSF is produced, it flows down through the ventricles and the *foramina* and circulates around the spinal column. It then flows into the subarachnoid space, where it circulates through the meningeal system and helps cushion brain tissue against the inside of the skull. The fluid is then absorbed by arachnoid granulations and returned to the venous circulation. Note that the rate of CSF production is such that the entire volume is replenished several times a day.

CSF leaves the CNS through four possible exits: a central canal, the foramen of Magendie, the foramen of Luschka, and the cisterna magna. However, any blockage in the flow can potentially lead to a significant buildup of fluid. If this occurs during early development, *hydrocephalus* ensues. Accumulation of fluid as a result of brain damage can present as a subdural or epidural hematoma, depending on the meningeal depth.

An additional source of protection for the CNS is the blood-brain barrier (BBB), which evolved as a selective filter against many substances. The brain is highly sensitive to the contents of the bloodstream, and the interface between the two must be tightly controlled for proper functioning. The BBB regulates the entrance of circulating blood into brain tissues. In addition to the cell membranes themselves, whose

---

[15]In large part, ventricular size is used as a proxy for the volume of brain matter in the immediate vicinity—that is, the larger the ventricle, the less surrounding brain matter. Thus, an increase in ventricular size, such as that caused by an increase in the volume of CSF, will impinge on the brain matter surrounding it and displace its volume. The assumption has been that this increased size corresponds to decreased brain function. In imaging studies of brains in patients with schizophrenia and dementia, the ventricles appear to be enlarged, with a corresponding reduction in function. However, there have been cases where this relationship does not match the expected theory.

structural properties bar the passage of numerous molecules, the capillary endothelial cells that form the blood vessel walls within the CNS are tightly joined together. Consequently, materials cannot pass through the gaps between cells, whereas they can in the periphery. In addition to these tight junctions, astrocytes extend foot processes around substantial portions of the cerebral capillary system, further regulating the flow of substances in the CNS.

This stands in stark contrast to capillaries in the periphery, where continuous flow in and out of the bloodstream is necessary for tissue exchange. In the CNS, protection far outweighs convenience, because the system cannot easily be repaired. Since substances must pass through the membrane of the cells to access brain tissue, only lipophilic molecules can cross the BBB. For larger, lipophobic molecules that are necessary for survival, such as glucose, other methods are required. Alternative pathways available to substances essential for brain function are transporter proteins, pores, *transcytosis,* and *retrograde neuronal transport* (von Bohlen und Halbach & Dermietzel, 2006).

Brain Nutrition

The brain is a "blood hog," requiring 20% of the body's blood supply to function, even though it represents only 2% of the body's weight. Neurons are more sensitive to oxygen deprivation than are cells in the rest of the body. The supply of oxygen is maintained by two sets of arteries that branch off the dorsal aorta. Vertebral arteries branch off into medullary arteries (which supply the spinal cord) and the basilar artery. (See Figure 3.6.) The internal carotid arteries branch off into the anterior and middle cerebral arteries, which supply the forebrain. The midbrain and hindbrain benefit from both sets of arteries and are supplied by the posterior cerebral, basilar, and vertebral arteries.

One failsafe mechanism that has evolved in the brain's circulation is a "detour" system at the base of the brain that allows for some flow of blood if one of the main arteries should become blocked. This anastomosis, or network of vessels, is called the circle of Willis, named for the researcher who first mapped it out. It comprises joined components of the basilar artery, the internal carotid arteries, the posterior cerebral artery, and the anterior and posterior communicating arteries.

Each of the three cerebral arteries feeds a large cortical region. Loss of blood flow (ischemia) for even a few seconds can be devastating for cellular functioning, since neurons are very sensitive to the chemical environment in which they live. Furthermore, as a result of a potential deteriorating cascade of reactions, a deficiency of oxygen (anoxia) creates a condition that threatens the equilibrium and health of the neurons in the immediate vicinity, leading to brain damage within minutes.

STRUCTURAL AND FUNCTIONAL DIVISIONS OF THE BRAIN

Forebrain

The cerebral cortex, or outer "bark," is the most recognizable and striking feature of the brain. A deep gap down the middle, the longitudinal fissure, separates the cerebral cortex into two symmetrical halves, or cerebral hemispheres. The right and left hemispheres display mainly parallel areas of functioning, such that the similarities far outweigh the differences. However, some of the differences are significant,

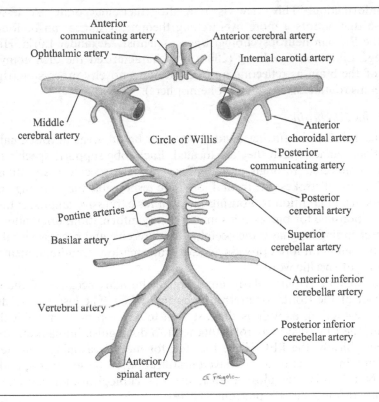

Figure 3.6   Blood Supply to the Brain

especially in terms of communication and information processing, as well as personality and identity. These discrepancies were made particularly cogent by the work of Sperry and Gazzaniga, whose patients underwent operations to treat severe and debilitating seizures. The operations consisted of severing the corpus callosum, which is an interhemispheric bridge of fibers, or *commissure*. The researchers discovered that the two hemispheres would function far more independently were it not for ongoing communication between them via commissures (Sperry, Gazzaniga, & Bogen, 1969).

Hemispheric differences have arguably been exaggerated over the years to the point of ignoring that there are more similarities than differences. Nevertheless, some differences manifest themselves quite clearly, as reflected in stronger tendencies or skills in particular areas of functioning. The most pronounced differences are in language functioning, such that the left hemisphere tends to be dominant for language in most people, in terms of grammar and syntax. On the other hand, the right hemisphere tends to be more highly developed at processing and communicating the underlying meaning in language, or pragmatics, as well as the emotional valence that is crucial in social communication, often reflected in changes in prosody or intonation.

There are few generally accepted theories that can systematically or comprehensively account for the various differences that have been documented over the years, although some come closer than others. The most popularized idea asserts that the left hemisphere is designed for processing linear, logical, syntactic information, whereas the right hemisphere is designed for processing nonlinear, spatial, holistic information. This view is not altogether inaccurate. A lesser-known perspective that adopts a more overarching theoretical stance can be found in the work of the Russian neuropsychologist/neuroscientist Alexander Luria. His student and protégé Elkhonon Goldberg (2002) has characterized the dichotomy between the sides of the brain as reflecting an orientation to novelty processing (right hemisphere) versus routine processing (left hemisphere).

Lobes of the Forebrain

Each hemisphere can be further divided into four broad areas or lobes, named after the skull bones under which they are located. Each lobe supports specific functions, yet all are connected through more diffuse, nonlobe-specific associational areas. Portrayed in broad strokes, the frontal lobes are responsible for planning and engaging movements, in addition to housing the area for expressive language; the parietal lobes are responsible for processing somatosensory information, orientating in space, and comprehending language; the occipital lobes receive and process visual information; and the temporal lobes process auditory information, emotional memories, and the meanings of specific words.

The frontal lobe is particularly important in humans because of the evolution of the "front of the front," or prefrontal cortex (PFC). The last area to develop in our species' evolution, as well as the last area to develop in an individual person's maturation, the PFC plays key roles that tend to distinguish humankind from other animals. Specifically, the PFC is the location for moral reasoning, long-term planning, anticipating consequences, delayed gratification, impulse control, and abstract thinking. Not surprisingly, most forensic neuropsychological inquiries reference the functionality of the accused's prefrontal cortex.

Areas of particular interest within the prefrontal context are outlined in Table 3.1.

Another means of classifying areas of cortex derives from anatomical observations by the neuroscientist Korbinian Brodmann, who developed a system of grouping cortical neurons by differences in cellular organization (cytoarchitecture) and myelin patterns (myeloarchitecture) (Kandel, 2000). He painstakingly mapped out and numbered 47 Brodmann areas on the medial and lateral surfaces of the cortex. Although computerized imaging has since allowed a more accurate three-

---

Table 3.1　Areas of the Prefrontal Cortex

Orbitofrontal cortex (OFC):[1] Moral reasoning, decision making.
Dorsolateral prefrontal cortex (DLPFC):[2] Executive functions, motor planning, organizing responses.
Anterior cingulate cortex (ACC):[3] Motivation, reward-based learning, error detection.
Ventromedial prefrontal cortex (VMPFC):[4] Risk, fear; bridges cognitive and emotional functioning.

---

[1]As a result of the one of the most famous cases in neuroscience, Phineas Gage, OFC was originally earmarked for social and personality functioning (Harlow, 1869). Later, more detailed studies suggested that Gage's brain damage was broader than the OFC.
[2]An important structure in Attention Deficit-Hyperactivity Disorder (Stahl, 2008).
[3]This area is adjacent to the limbic system and appears important in monitoring and verifying cognitive errors and consequent emotional response (Clark et al., 2010).
[4]Although part of the cerebral cortex, and thus "cognitive" in nature, the VMPFC has been shown to attenuate amygdala activity related to fear (Quirk & Mueller, 2008). This area is likely recruited or exercised during treatments that involve exposure for the extinction of phobia.

dimensional representation, Brodmann's system is still referenced for some brain areas more than others.

Cortical Function

White matter, as noted earlier, represents the axon pathways. These fiber systems constitute the primary "information highways" within the CNS. Although the number of different orientations is hypothetically limitless, fibers appear to be organized along three primary axes. More recently, the specific dimensions have been highlighted with the use of diffusion tensor imaging, which has helped demarcate these pathways. The dimensions or axes can be categorized as follows:

Association fibers, which run in the posterior–anterior axis, join the rostral and caudal areas of the CNS. For example, the arcuate fasciculus connects Wernicke's and Broca's areas and plays a significant role in language functioning and expression.

Projection fibers, which run in the inferior–superior axis, join the ventral and dorsal areas. For example, many brainstem areas project "upward" toward the diencephalon and cortex and provide systemic information, while cortical areas project "downward" for inhibitory control and modulation of those areas. The *internal capsule* is a prime example of projection fibers.

Commissures, which run in the medial–lateral axis, join like-cell groups of the left and right hemispheres. As noted above the corpus callosum serves as the primary link between the two hemispheres, and if cut, results in *split-brain phenomena*.

Further Cortical Divisions

Brain areas can also be categorized in terms of functional divisions, which reflect three levels of processing: *Primary cortical areas* are those brain areas that are responsible for processing or organizing information at its most basic. *Secondary cortical areas* process the information further and integrate different variables within the same modality (such as color and line orientation in vision, frequency and location for hearing). Finally, *tertiary cortical areas*, also known as convergence zones, integrate information across modalities.

Research has also established that areas of the cerebral cortex manifest a columnar organization, such that particular aspects of some function or area of the environment are encoded within a "column" of cortex. In some cases, these are considered functional modules, with the most detailed research stemming from studies of the visual system and occipital cortex. In one study in particular, which is considered to support the modular hypothesis, the researchers found that specific visual areas became more active depending on whether the object viewed was a tool or an animal (Martin et al., 1996).

The neurons that make up the cerebral cortex tend to fall into two broad categories: projection neurons and interneurons. Although there are exceptions, projection neurons, which are almost exclusively *pyramidal cells* in the *neocortex*, tend to be excitatory in order to convey information across brain regions. Interneurons, on the other hand, tend to be inhibitory because they are designed to modulate and control the flow of neuronal communications.

All areas of neocortex display the same basic structural organization, with six layers, or laminae, parallel to the surface. This laminar pattern evolved to organize the inputs and outputs of the cerebral cortex more efficiently, given the complexity of the connections involved. Differences across various areas are reflected in variations of laminar thickness, but the number and composition of the layers themselves remain consistent.

Layer 1, sometimes referred to as the "molecular layer," contains few neurons and mostly fibers or axons, some from pyramidal cells in deeper layers. Layers 2 and 4 are granular layers, primarily designed to receive information from sensory areas. These tend to be small, inhibitory interneurons that release GABA. Conversely, layers 3 and 5 are primarily efferent pyramidal neurons that project to motor areas (layer 3 to cortical and layer 5 to subcortical areas). These are descending glutamatergic neurons. Layer 6 is a "multiform layer," primarily encompassing neurons with spindle-shaped bodies that project to the thalamus.

Limbic "System"

The original description of the neurological substrate for emotional functioning as a "system" was based on neuroanatomical observation and appeared to be legitimate for many years. However, as more research blurred the line between emotion and cognition, the concept of a limbic system has become increasingly questionable. Nonetheless, the term has stuck, and for many purposes stands as a useful term for describing emotional functioning at a relatively basic level. Anatomically, the limbic system contains the amygdala, the septum, the hippocampus, the mammillary bodies, and the cingulate gyrus, as well as various other adjacent structures and cortices. (See Figure 3.7.)

Amygdala—The amygdalae, or amygdaloid bodies, are most commonly referred to simply as the amygdala; however, keep in mind that this is not one unitary structure, but rather a set of nuclei, one in each hemisphere. They are typically not visible in a midsagittal section. The amygdala is located in the temporal lobe, at the anterior end of the hippocampal formation.

The amygdala is a highly interconnected set of nuclei, with connections to most other structures in the brain, and to cortical areas in particular (Young et al.,

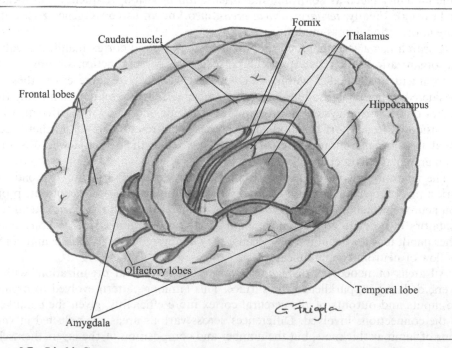

Figure 3.7   Limbic System

1994). As such, it represents an important functional intersection between cognition and emotion. Some functions associated with the amygdala are fear mediation, fear memories, processing of (primarily) negative emotions, and encoding and retrieving emotional memory. The amygdala's central role in the conditioned fear response highlights its related importance in anxiety disorders (LeDoux, 2000; Sah & Westbrook, 2008).

Septum—Several terms are used to refer to the same functional complex, including septal region, septal nuclei, and septal complex. The most important regions for the purposes of mammalian function are the lateral septum and the medial septum. The septal nuclei are involved in circuits between the hypothalamus and hippocampus and are involved in many autonomic behaviors, such as eating, drinking, and sexual behavior. The lateral septum in particular is involved in social memory, parental behavior, and dominant-subordinate relationships. The septum receives substantial excitatory input from the hippocampus and makes many efferent inhibitory connections with the hypothalamus and brainstem. These connections explain in large part the results of early lesion experiments in animals leading to "septal rage," although subsequent studies have been mainly inconsistent. The functions of the medial septum are less clear, especially in humans, but connectivity with the lateral septum and hippocampus suggest a key role in attention and memory, especially in devoting emotional energy to exploration (Numan, 2000). The medial septum is also involved in the circuit that results in the theta-rhythm pacemaker; theta rhythm in the hippocampus is associated with special cognition and memory processing (Wang, 2002).

Hippocampus—Originally included in the Papez circuit as an early conceptualization of the limbic system, the hippocampus represents a clear "crossover" structure between emotion and cognition. It also constitutes what is known as the "paleocortex" or "old cortex," which blurs the distinction between cortical and subcortical structures. The case of Henry Molaison,[16] whose hippocampal formation was bilaterally lesioned, galvanized its role in explicit memory consolidation (Beecher Scoville & Milner, 1957). Specifically, the hippocampus mediates the formation and retrieval of declarative or explicit memories, in contrast to the amygdala's involvement in encoding implicit and emotional memories. In addition, the hippocampus plays a key role in neuroendocrine regulation and stress response. The hippocampus is also central in the ability to locate oneself in space, in large part because of memory for locations.

In some texts, the hippocampus is labeled a "convergence zone" because it connects with association areas from multiple senses and limbic subcortical structures (Damasio & Damasio, 1994; LeDoux, 2002). As a consequence of this convergence of information, hippocampal memories represent complex, conjunctive, multisensory information. The association-cortex connections occur through the *entorhinal area* of the *parahippocampal gyrus*. The "lower" connections, to subcortical regions, occur in large part via the *fornix*.

Several brain areas generate synchronous firing patterns, but the hippocampus has been found to generate three different types of oscillations: theta, sharp waves, and gamma waves. Although the precise function and mechanism of such "pacemaker"

---

[16]Henry Molaison (H.M.) was a research participant for 53 years, first at the Hartford Hospital, then at the Montreal Neurological Institute, and, since 1964, at MIT and the Massachusetts General Hospital. Roughly 100 scientists have interviewed or tested H.M. He died in 2008, at the age of 82.

activities are still unclear, they appear to be linked to integration of neural activities across a distance and other forms of information processing (Frank, 2007).

Mammillary bodies—These hypothalamic nuclei are located medially. They receive information from the hippocampus via the fornix and project to the anterior thalamic nuclei and to the brainstem and spinal cord. They play a role in emotional regulation and learning, and damage to these structures is associated with *Korsakoff's syndrome.*

Anterior cingulate gyrus—The anterior region of the *cingulate cortex* is particularly important in emotional modulation and integration (Vogt, 2009). The cingulate gyrus wraps around the corpus callosum and comprises several cytoarchitectural areas. It can be subdivided into four general regions: anterior cingulate, midcingulate, posterior cingulate, and retrosplenial. Each region has been found to play a role in integrating various functions.

The anterior cingulate cortex (ACC) integrates emotional and autonomic information, and appears to serve as long-term storage for emotional memories. In particular, recent studies have isolated Brodmann area 25 (also known as the subgenual area or subgenual cingulate) as a key player in sad memories and depression. Area 25 also appears to activate behavioral, hormonal, and sympathetic responses to acute stress (Sullivan, 2004). Research involving deep-brain stimulation of this area has been promising in the treatment of resistant depression (Mayberg et al., 2005). Similarly, there is a relatively high concentration of 5-HT_{1A} receptors in the ACC, which might explain the effectiveness of some SSRIs. As would be expected, the ACC receives substantial input from the amygdala and projects to sites that regulate the autonomic nervous system, such as the hypothalamus and periaqueductal gray. The latter projection represents the means by which the ACC mediates the affective component of pain, as well as the opioid placebo effect.

The midcingulate cortex (MCC) appears to represent a decision-making junction or filter in terms of response to rewarding or aversive conditions, especially the former. The MCC has a high density of dopamine inputs and D_1 receptors. It receives reward-based input from the nucleus accumbens and pain-based input from the thalamus. In turn, the MCC projects to the motor system, both cortical and subcortical, and to the periaqueductal gray. More specifically, the MCC appears to contribute to response-selection and approach-avoidance behaviors, and may be involved in OCD and ADHD, both of which partly reflect disorders of response-filtering and decision-making (Bush et al., 2002).

The posterior cingulate (PCC) is associated with integration of visuospatial and self-relevant information, reflected in personal orientation in space, body-orienting behavior, and storage of self-relevant memories. Acetylcholine plays a dominating role as a neuromodulator in the PCC, which highlights the link between decreasing ACh functioning and self-relevant memory loss in Alzheimer's dementia.

The *retrosplenial cortex* has dense reciprocal projections with both the anterior thalamic nuclei and the hippocampus and is implicated in the recall of episodic information. The retrosplenial cortex is one of several brain areas that produce anterograde amnesia when damaged.

Medial temporal lobe—This structure surrounds the amygdala and hippocampus and contains the parahippocampal gyrus, an area of cortex that serves as a transition between the "old" cortex of the hippocampus and the "new" cortex of the temporal lobe. This area of the temporal lobe is involved in integrating multimodal sensory information for storage and retrieval from memory, essentially "attaching" emotional (limbic) meaning to the information. Interactions between the frontal lobes and the medial temporal lobe are important for memory acquisition and retrieval in general. In particular, interactions between the hippocampus and prefrontal cortex are important for memory formation, conscious awareness, and self-awareness. This area has been implicated in several disorders, including bipolar disorder, dissociative disorder, and schizophrenia.

Insula—The insular cortex receives input from the ventromedial thalamus and projects to the orbitofrontal cortex (OFC), amygdala, hypothalamus, and brainstem autonomic nuclei. One line of thought has conceptualized the insula as a "limbic sensory" cortex, in parallel with the "limbic motor" cortex of the anterior cingulate. In particular, the right anterior insula appears to be involved in the experience of *interoception* and emotional awareness (Craig, 2003; Damasio, 1999).

Fornix—Often included in lists of limbic structures, the fornix is a pathway that connects the hippocampus to areas more specifically involved in emotional processing, such as the hypothalamus and basal forebrain.

Stria terminalis—Neurons from the amygdala project to several hypothalamic nuclei, including the preoptic and anterior. This highly myelinated pathway divides the diencephalon from the telencephalon.

The original emotional circuit described by Papez (1937) entailed the following loop: hippocampus to fornix to mammillary body to anterior thalamic nucleus to cingulate gyrus to parahippocampal gyrus back to hippocampus. Subsequently, Paul MacLean (1949) used the term "limbic system" to describe Papez's conceptualization of limbic structures as areas for emotional functioning.

Basal Ganglia

The basal ganglia, while part of the forebrain, are considered subcortical. Their primary role involves integrating motor activity coordination. They also influence movement associated with motivational and emotional functioning, and with reward and expectancy, through connections with limbic structures such as the amygdala. Although voluntary motor commands are derived from the motor cortex, all descending motor track systems connect to the basal ganglia for additional processing of "intent to move." Note that the primary motor cortex, consisting primarily of pyramidal cells, represents the pyramidal motor system. In contrast, the motor pathways derived primarily from the basal ganglia are labeled *extrapyramidal*, and many motor side effects from medications result from their impact on these pathways.

In general, the basal ganglia encompass three subcortical structures: the caudate nucleus, the *putamen*, and the *globus pallidus*. (See Figure 3.8.) However, other areas that play a role in movement coordination and processing include the *substantia nigra*, ventral tegmental area, and *subthalamic nucleus*. The caudate and putamen are often functionally combined as the *striatum*. (One should therefore distinguish between these two structures where they join as constituting the dorsal striatum [anterior caudate nucleus], whereas the nucleus accumbens becomes the ventral striatum and is a part of the putamen.) Unfortunately, adding to the confusion, the putamen and globus pallidus can be grouped together as the lentiform, or *lenticular nucleus*, and part of the globus pallidus extends ventrally to form the ventral pallidum. The reasons for these structural/functional groupings may not be intuitive from the outset, but as one becomes more familiar with them, their linked associations become far more comprehensible.

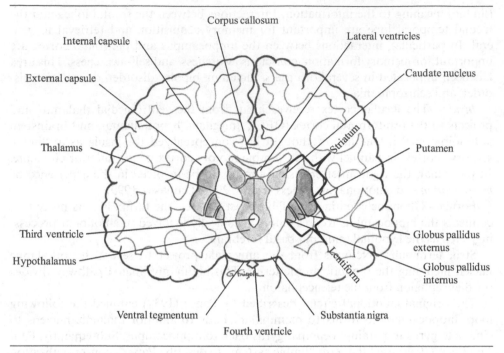

Figure 3.8   Basal Ganglia

These multiple labels and groupings highlight the complexity of connections among the areas in the basal ganglia, which comprise loops and pathways of both excitatory and inhibitory input. This accounts in part for the variety of disorders that arise from damage to the basal ganglia, which could result in under- or overexcitation or under- or overinhibition of motor control.

In terms of functional organization, the basal ganglia can be characterized as input, intrinsic, or output nuclei, depending on where afferent information comes from and where efferent information projects. The input nuclei are the caudate, putamen, and nucleus accumbens. The intrinsic nuclei are the lateral globus pallidus, subthalamic nucleus, substantia nigra (pars compacta), and ventral tegmental area. The output nuclei are the medial globus pallidus, substantia nigra (pars reticularis), and ventral pallidum.

The basal ganglia play a central role in established circuits or loops, four of which exist in parallel and influence motor functions, as well as cognition and emotion. The core circuit comprises a path from cerebral cortex to striatum to globus pallidus to thalamus back to cerebral cortex. Note that, in influencing movement, none of the basal ganglia connect directly to the lower brainstem or spinal cord. The four cortico-striato-pallido-thalamo-cortical circuits of the basal ganglia are motor, association, oculomotor, and limbic.

There are two primary projection neuron types in the striatum: medium spiny neurons and large aspiny neurons. The more numerous neurons are GABAergic and manifest dopamine D_1 and D_2 heteroreceptors. Co-transmitters include substance P and *dynorphin*. Large neurons are cholinergic and excitatory.

Basal Forebrain

This label demarcates structures adjacent to the basal ganglia that interface with their circuits. The nucleus accumbens is a striatum area that interfaces with the limbic and motor systems and is associated with the pleasure/reward center. The accumbens receives strong dopaminergic inputs from the ventral tegmental area of the midbrain, and stimulation of any part of this pathway leads to behavioral reinforcement of that stimulus. Further division between the "core" portion of the accumbens and the "shell" can be made functionally distinct. The shell appears to promote general, unconditioned behaviors that are not necessarily experienced as rewarding. The core, on the other hand, is more involved in establishing reward-based repetition of behaviors (Middleton & Strick, 2001).

The nucleus basalis of Meynert, as noted previously, is one of the key production areas for acetylcholine. It is located in the basal forebrain area but has projections throughout the rest of the brain. These cholinergic neurons are primarily involved in attention, where they enhance processes related to cognition or perception.

Diencephalon

As would be expected for such a complex system, the brain needs a fine-tuned and "well-oiled" system of organization and coordination. Otherwise, the results would be disastrous chaos, and the system could not function in even the simplest ways. The diencephalon encompasses the thalamus and hypothalamus. The *thalamus* is primarily designed for coordination of external stimulation and sensory information and for subsequent organization of motor responses. The *hypothalamus*, by contrast, monitors and regulates internal stimulation and body states and coordination of the subsequent response. Although the distinction is not absolute, one can consider thalamus and hypothalamus as "external affairs" and "internal affairs," respectively.

Thalamus   The thalamus, as a group of nuclei, is charged with imposing order on incoming bursts of information and with beginning to refine "raw stimuli" into more processed signals. This improves the level of sophistication available to subsequent areas, whether interpreting sensory information or communicating "movement orders" to the motor cortex. Many of these thalamocortical pathways are arranged in loops to continually process information and provide feedback.

Thalamic nuclei can be divided and partitioned in various ways. Structurally, a layer of neural fibers, the intralaminar nuclear group, separates a medial group of nuclei from a lateral group, the latter being further divided into ventral and lateral groups. Another group of nuclei, the anterior nuclear group, is the most rostral of the thalamic nuclei.

There are three main functional groups:

1. *Relay nuclei* connect to specific sensory modalities, or subdivisions of the motor or limbic system, forming recursive loops with layer 6 of the specific cortical area that it serves.
2. Association nuclei form similar thalamocortical loops, but link to layer 5 as well as layer 6, so the information has been modulated beyond the relay stage.
3. *Diffuse-projecting nuclei* form connections throughout the cortex and with other thalamic nuclei and influence the overall level of activity and arousal.

As with other brain areas, the nuclei within groups contain both projection neurons and interneurons. Thalamic projections can be specific or nonspecific, depending on whether or not they are characterized by reciprocal connections to specific cortical areas. In large part, thalamic interneurons are GABAergic and can enhance sensory information through lateral inhibition. Thalamic projection neurons tend to be glutamatergic.

Some of the more well-defined connections and functions of thalamic nuclei are as follows: The anterior nuclei are connected to and integrated with the limbic system. They contain the highest density of muscarinic receptors among the thalamic nuclei. Reciprocal connections include the mammillary bodies, hippocampus, cingulate gyrus, and prefrontal cortex. The dorsomedial nucleus is also involved in affective processing, with connections to and from the amygdala, lateral hypothalamus, prefrontal cortex, and orbitofrontal cortex.

The ventral group can be further subdivided into ventral anterior, which links to the globus pallidus, substantia nigra, and premotor cortex; ventral lateral, which bridges cerebral and cerebellar cortex and basal ganglia to cerebral cortex; and ventral posterior (where some researchers include the medial and lateral geniculate nuclei), which receives and integrates somatosensory, auditory, visual, gustatory, and vestibular information into a "body representation," which is then projected to the somatosensory cortex.

The posterior nuclear group (which includes the ventromedial nucleus) comprises input areas for multimodal sensory information, which could reflect a role in the perception of pain and noxious stimuli. Some of these neurons project to somatosensory areas and some to the insula. The lateral nuclear group, which includes the pulvinar, connects to the cingulate gyrus, hippocampus, and septum. The pulvinar projects in large part to the parietal-temporal-occipital (PTO) junction. These nuclei appear to be involved in emotional expression and directed visual attention. The intralaminar nuclei connect widespread areas of cortex, as well as limbic and striatal areas, and receive some cholinergic and monoaminergic projections. These nuclei play a role in cortico-striatal-thalamo-cortical loops, and appear to be involved in sensorimotor integration, general states of awareness and arousal, and/or pain perception.

Hypothalamus   The hypothalamus plays a primary role in coordinating various branches of the nervous and endocrine systems in order to maintain homeostasis. It is seated in a central functional location and monitors links to bodily and mental processes. These nuclei receive inputs from chemical sensory areas (e.g., the status of the gastrointestinal tract, blood pressure, body temperature, and time of day), as well as from limbic emotional and motivational centers. In terms of efferent connections, the hypothalamus targets the pituitary, *autonomic preganglionic neurons*, anterior thalamic nuclei, hippocampus, midbrain reticular nuclei, and higher limbic and cortical structures.

Overall, the hypothalamus receives inputs from almost all areas of the brain and many from the periphery. Some areas in particular are the septal nuclei, orbitofrontal cortex, olfactory bulb, olfactory cortex, retina, amygdala, hippocampus, reticular formation, raphe nuclei, locus coeruleus, and periaqueductal gray. While it is possible to isolate specific nuclei that are afferent targets, there is tremendous processing and integration among hypothalamic nuclei before the shift to efferent connections. Some of the key efferent targets match its afferent connections: orbitofrontal cortex, septum, amygdala, hippocampus, reticular formation, sympathetic nervous system, locus coeruleus, periaqueductal gray, and mediodorsal thalamus.

The following are some relevant hypothalamic nuclei:

- Tuberomammillary nucleus (TMN)—This area produces most of the histamine in the CNS and sends projections throughout the brain. The TMN is involved in the sleep-wake cycle and possibly related to a "switch" in relation to the VLPO (see below).
- Ventrolateral preoptic nucleus (VLPO)—This "sleep center" contains GABA neurons that increase the likelihood of sleep.
- Lateral hypothalamic area (LHA)/posterior hypothalamus (PH)—This is the major production center of orexin/hypocretin, which maintains wakefulness and possibly regulates the "switch" between the VLPO and TMN (Sakurai, 2007). The PH is also involved in temperature regulation.
- Paraventricular nucleus (PVN)—This is the production center for corticotrophin-releasing hormone (CRF); in response to stressors, it activates the HPA axis; also, in concert with the *supraoptic nucleus*, the PVN leads to the production of oxytocin and vasopressin via the posterior pituitary.
- Ventromedial hypothalamus (VMH)—This is a "satiety center," which leads to a decrease in appetite.
- Lateral hypothalamus (LH)—This is a "hunger center," stimulation of which leads to increased appetite.
- Suprachiasmatic nucleus (SCN)—This area responds to light that activates *retinohypothalamic fibers*, resulting in control of the daily activity cycle and biorhythms.
- Mammillary nuclei (part of mammillary bodies)—Connected from the hippocampus via the fornix, these play a role in memory consolidation.

Midbrain (Mesencephalon)

The midbrain is more a location than a structure, as compared with other CNS functional anatomy. Thus, many tracts of higher and lower brain areas pass through the midbrain on their way to their targets. Nevertheless, the midbrain serves as the location of many of its own grouping of neurons that play important roles in the regulation of other functions. Furthermore, these areas are often the targets for psychopharmacological intervention. One way that the midbrain has been subdivided is horizontally, with the dorsal area constituting the tectum and the ventral area the tegmentum. The tectum encompasses the inferior and superior colliculi, which play a role in processing substantial amounts of auditory and visual information, respectively. The colliculi also function in the context of an orienting response to auditory and visual information. The tegmentum, on the other hand, is composed of several groups of nuclei with a variety of functions, although motor functions are strongly represented.

The largest area in the mesencephalon is the substantia nigra. The dorsal, pars compacta segments produce the bulk of the dopamine that projects to the striatum. The ventral, smaller pars reticulata sections are involved in feedback loops to all nuclei of the basal ganglia.

The ventral tegmental area (VTA) incorporates the preponderance of dopaminergic neurons that project to higher-level structures, such as the ventral striatum, amygdala, septum, basal forebrain, and orbitofrontal cortex. As the origin of the mesocorticolimbic system, the projections are primarily dopaminergic, but some of the neurons are GABAergic and glutamatergic.

The periaqueductal gray is not a single unit or nucleus but rather a group of several columns of neurons that run parallel to the cerebral aqueduct. In general, the dorsolateral columns and ventrolateral columns result in related but opposite behaviors in response to situations that demand action. The dorsolateral column results in an orienting and arousal response, increasing heart rate, respiration, and blood pressure, as well as producing (nonopioid) analgesia (Keay & Bandler, 2001). Overall, this reflects a pattern of defensive behavior in response to strong emotional or aversive stimuli. In contrast, the ventrolateral column inhibits movement, lowers blood pressure and heart rate, and produces opioid-dependent analgesia. This overall pattern of behavior resembles the "freezing" response to a threat but more generally a response to pain perception as signaling a need to change behavior. Whether the dorsal or ventral response is chosen in a given situation is not always predictable and more than likely results from descending inputs that take into account situational factors that demand a response from the periaqueductal gray area.

Hindbrain

The reticular formation (RF) is a network of neurons that extends from the top of the spinal cord to the intralaminar nuclei of the thalamus. However, although it crosses several brain areas, it tends to be associated with the hindbrain. Its primary function is influencing the level of overall arousal in the brain or the level of conscious awareness related to physical performance. The RF appears diffuse in structure, but its network, the ascending reticular activating system (ARAS), is highly organized and coordinated to effectively influence motor behaviors. It receives a complex array of sensory stimuli from the spinal cord, as well as blood acidity levels, oxygen concentration of inhaled air, and amount of physical activity from the medulla; and it sends ascending messages via all the main monoaminergic circuits (Brodal, 2010).

The pons and medulla oblongata serve two primary roles each: as a conduit for neural pathways between higher and lower areas, and as a location for nuclei with specific and important life functions. Since the cerebellum is anatomically situated "off to the side" in the lower posterior cranium, it does not share the pathway role. While its primary function is regulating and controlling complex movements, it also plays a role in some aspects of cognition and emotional functioning. The cerebellum is folded like the cerebral cortex but is arranged in three layers rather than six. The top cerebellar layer comprises parallel fibers, the middle layer is marked by large Purkinje cells, and the inner layer is made up of small granule cells.

The pons, as its Latin meaning suggests, serves as a "bridge" from the cerebellum to the rest of the brain. It also houses several important groups of projection neurons. In particular, the locus coeruleus (LC) and raphe nuclei (RN) are located in the dorsal pons (relatively close to the midbrain area). The *pontine nuclei* play an important role in arousal, sleep, and related states of consciousness. The LC sends adrenergic neurons and the RN sends serotonergic neurons throughout the higher levels of the CNS. A large section of the reticular formation passes through the pons.

Finally, located just rostral to the spinal cord is the medulla oblongata, which functions as the "boiler room" of the brain's "corporate offices." This area's structures control vital aspects of functioning, such as breathing, regulating heart rate, maintaining basic muscle tone, swallowing, and vomiting. Damage here usually means coma or death.

Spinal Cord

The spinal cord appears to be a relatively simple and concrete structure, a cable that links the CNS to the rest of the body (i.e., to the peripheral nervous system). Like the brain, it is enveloped by the meninges, which are continuous with the brain and descend the entire length of the CNS.

Examination of a typical cross-section of the spinal cord reveals a pattern that is vaguely shaped like an "H," with limbs designated dorsal horns and ventral horns. (See Figure 3.9.) The relative size and shape of the H varies depending on its location along the length of the cord. As an example of topographical consistency, the dorsal horns relay sensory information toward the CNS, whereas the ventral horns primarily relay motor or other efferent information away from the CNS.

Although the primary distinction entails the inner gray matter surrounded by white matter, further subdivisions are readily apparent. The gray matter, with its fibers oriented in a transverse plane, has been divided into relatively distinct layers or laminae (numbered 1 to 10). The various layers convey different types of information from ascending and descending white matter tracts, or fasciculi. The relative size of the spinal cord decreases as it descends caudally, but the proportion of gray matter to white matter increases at the same time. This results from the change in the number of fibers that share information at successive levels (white matter) and the increased amount of peripheral information that is processed toward the bottom of the spinal cord (Schoenen & Faull, 2004).

The dorsal horns contain groups of neuron bodies called the dorsal root ganglia, which relay primary sensory information of touch, temperature, and pain from the

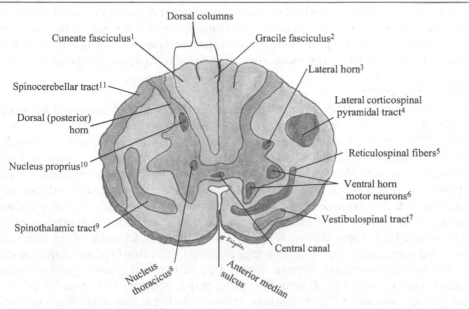

Legend: Dorsal Columns (Ipsilateral sensations) : 1. Upper body discriminate touch, 2. Lower body discriminate touch; 3. Preganglionic sympathetic fibers; 4. Voluntary, skilled movement; 5. Unskilled & involuntary movement; 6. Limb & trunk movement; 7. Trunk & limbs; 8. Proprioception; 9. Touch, pain, temperature; 10. Touch, pain, temperature; 11. Proprioception.

Figure 3.9   Cross-Section of Spinal Cord

trunk and limbs of the body. The somatosensory information that enters the dorsal horn is a *somatotopic* representation of the surface of the skin, a map that is preserved as it reaches the primary somatosensory cortex.

Segments of the spinal cord are named after the vertebrae that house them. Roots pass out of the spine in pairs, with one dorsal pair and one ventral pair for each vertebra. There are 8 cervical, 12 thoracic, 5 lumbar, and 5 sacral roots and 1 coccygeal root. Each spinal nerve's fibers are categorized functionally depending on the direction of flow of information (afferent vs. efferent) and the location of innervation (somatic vs. viscera).

The Peripheral Nervous System (PNS)

Cranial Nerves

The cranial nerves extend out from the brainstem but are considered part of the PNS. These 12, bilaterally symmetrical nerves relay information that is sensory, motor, or both to and from the CNS. The nuclei of these nerves are located in the midbrain, pons, and medulla. Sensory nuclei tend to be located more laterally, whereas motor nuclei are medial. The sensory nerves are the olfactory (I), optic (II), and vestibulocochlear (auditory) (VIII). The motor nerves are the oculomotor (III), trochlear (IV), abducens (VI), spinal accessory (XI), and hypoglossal (XII). The sensory/motor nerves are the trigeminal (V), facial (VII), glossopharyngeal (IX), and vagus (X).[17]

Sensory Components

Sensory receptors take in information from the environment for analysis. Each sensory receptor is designed to respond to a certain modality, and only that modality, according to the law of specific nerve energies. Furthermore, a response occurs only within a restricted range of the variables within the modality. For example, visual receptors in the retina respond only to light energy, and only to the visible range of the electromagnetic spectrum. The receptors' ultimate job is to translate, or transduce, the varieties of information from the environment into neural signals (i.e., action potentials).

Motor Components

Within the somatic PNS, the ventral horn of the spinal cord sends out nerve roots through the intervertebral spaces, which in turn branch into efferent nerves that ultimately terminate in striated muscle. Skeletal muscles are organized into hundreds of motor units, each of which involves a motor neuron that controls discrete bundles of muscle fibers. The neuromuscular junction (NMJ) is the specific type of synapse or junction between the axon terminal of a motor neuron and its muscle-tissue target. The synapse occurs at the motor end plate, a highly excitable region of muscle-fiber plasma membrane responsible for initiating action potentials across the muscle's surface. Acetylcholine is released from the axon terminal of the motor neuron, and subsequent Ca^{2+} release brings about a single, short muscle contraction.

Within the autonomic nervous system (see further on), motor ganglia are associated with innervation of smooth-muscle motor control. The majority of motor ganglia are located in the sympathetic trunks, which are two long chains of ganglia stretching along each side of the vertebral column from the base of the skull to the

---

[17]See Chapter 6 for a more detailed discussion of the function/dysfunction and clinical testing of cranial nerves.

coccyx. Rather than forming typical synapses, autonomic efferent neurons branch substantially near the region of innervation and swell into varicosities, which contain the vesicles of NTs (Brodal, 2010). When released from the varicosities, the NTs diffuse across variable distances, leading to a slower and more prolonged response, in contrast to somatic enervation of skeletal muscle cells.

The visceral motor system is controlled via the enteric nervous system, which is one branch of the autonomic nervous system. More than 20 neurotransmitters and neuromodulators control the function of the smooth muscle of the gastrointestinal system, which contains about as many neurons as the entire spinal cord (Noback et al., 2005). Although it integrates information with the sympathetic and parasympathetic nervous systems, the enteric system operates for the most part independently.

Autonomic Nervous System

Although the *autonomic nervous system (ANS)* technically consists of the sympathetic and parasympathetic branches, their coordination does not exist separately from central, coordinated control by the hypothalamus. Also, although these two branches appear to elicit antagonistic responses (Fig. 3.10), their activities are often parallel and highly coordinated to maintain a stable internal environment (Iversen, Iversen, & Saper, 2000). Nonetheless, target organs will react to one or the other branch in a characteristic fashion. Both sympathetic and parasympathetic systems start with cholinergic neurons that terminate in ganglia in the periphery. Postganglionic neurons then project from these ganglia to the target organs;

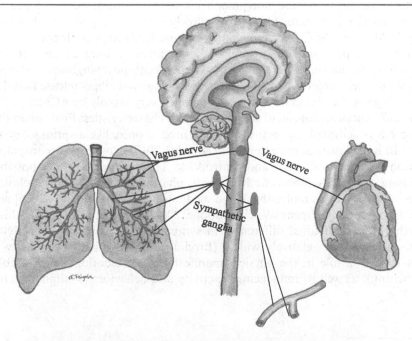

Parasympathetic (vagus) innervation: Slows heart, constricts bronchi.
Sympathetic innervation: Constricts blood vessels, dilates bronchi.

Figure 3.10   Peripheral Innervation of Cardiopulmonary System

sympathetic postganglionic neurons are adrenergic, while parasympathetic postganglionic neurons are cholinergic.

Some implications of the differential functioning of the two branches of the ANS are derived from differences in their composition and organization. The key contrasting facets are their regions of origin from the spinal cord; the NTs in their respective postganglionic fibers; their roles in energy storage, digestion, and overall functioning; and their specificity, which relates to their capacity for regulation and modulation.

The most "famous" aspect of the ANS is the sympathetic nervous system's role in the "fight-or-flight" response.[18] It expends considerable energy and resources toward survival through immediate action. Note, however, that the sympathetic nervous system is not only active during crisis; it also contributes to the daily maintenance of internal balance. Although the parasympathetic system's catch-phrase is less exciting ("rest and digest"), survival remains the overall goal, albeit in the long-term. Some other aspects which distinguish the sympathetic system from the parasympathetic system include the fact that sympathetic activity leads to the production of glucagon, which characterizes the fasting phase of digestion and which results in the release of stored energy from fat and muscle tissue; by contrast, parasympathetic activation of the digestive tract is associated with the secretion of insulin, which characterizes the absorptive phase of digestion, presumably in the presence of food to be metabolized and stored in muscle and fat.

Sympathetic neurons are arranged so that they exit the spinal cord via the thoracic and lumbar segments. They are characterized by short *preganglionic fibers* that then synapse in ganglia that lie parallel to the spinal cord, in the sympathetic trunk or chain. These ganglia then synapse with multiple, long *postganglionic fibers* that fan out over a wide area in innervating their target organs. Furthermore, sympathetic postganglionic fibers release norepinephrine as a neurotransmitter. Since norepinephrine activity is terminated relatively slowly through reuptake or slow degradation by MAO or COMT, the sympathetic response tends to be prolonged.

In contrast, parasympathetic preganglionic fibers, exiting at the cervical and sacral segments, are very long and form synapses with postganglionic fibers in close proximity to their target organs. The short postganglionic fibers release acetylcholine to target organs, the action of which is terminated very rapidly by AChE.

This differential arrangement accounts for two characteristics: First, when the sympathetic NS is activated, the entire system is fired at once, like a sprinkler system set off by a lit match (with some exceptions) (Brodal, 2010). Conversely, parasympathetic activation is far more selective and controllable. There is thus a greater possibility of intervening at a parasympathetic level, both pharmacologically and psychologically (i.e., techniques such as biofeedback and meditation [Takahashi et al., 2005] and possibly chiropractic adjustment [Welch & Boone, 2008] exert their influence at this level).

Furthermore, individual differences in sympathetic nervous system activity have been found to range relatively widely (Brodal, 2010). Sympathetic activity is also known to play a role in the physical manifestation of emotions (such as blushing or blanching), as well as influencing reactivity and behaviors (Maliphant, Hume, &

---

[18]Note that the term "fight or flight" is overly simplified, which is not surprising given how long ago it was coined (Cannon, 1929). For example, other reactions to danger/stress include "freeze" and "fright," and females do not necessarily follow this "rule" (Taylor et al., 2000). Cannon was also one of the first physiologists to introduce the concept of homeostasis and the importance of maintaining an internal balance.

Furnham, 1990; Zahn & Kruesi, 1993). Assessment of autonomic functioning is thus the key to obtaining a complete psychological picture of any given person.

In any case, as noted earlier, the ultimate goal of survival drives the activity of the two nervous systems. Both adjust their contribution to systemic tone based on moment-to-moment body data, with the proximal goal of maintaining homeostasis—which brings the narrative of this chapter full circle.

CHAPTER 3 KEY TERMS

Action potential: A state during which the electrical charge across a membrane rises above the equilibrium set point.

Afferent: Transmitting messages toward the brain (from sensory receptors).

After-depolarization: A period of time, after the action potential, when the neuron remains depolarized rather than entering the refractory period, thus allowing further stimulation and additional action potentials.

After-hyperpolarization: A period of time, after the action potential, when the neuron's polarization falls below the resting potential and initiates the refractory period, during which the neuron is not able to be stimulated to fire.

Agonist: A substance that causes an increase in a reaction (e.g., more release of a neurotransmitter).

Anion: An ion with a negative charge.

Antagonist: A substance that causes a decrease in a reaction (e.g., less release of a neurotransmitter).

Autonomic nervous system: Part of the peripheral nervous system primarily involved in the control of smooth muscles and organs in order to regulate visceral and life-sustaining functions (e.g., digestion, heart rate, respiration).

Autonomic preganglionic neurons: Neuronal cells in the autonomic nervous system that arise from the spinal cord and connect to major ganglia (relay points).

Autoreceptor: A receptor located in the presynaptic neuron that responds to the neurotransmitter released by the same neuron on which it resides.

Axoextracellular: A neuron-to-extracellular space synapse with neurotransmitter release into the interstitial fluid.

Axosecretory: A neuron whose axon terminal synapses with a capillary and releases a neurotransmitter into the circulatory system.

Axosynaptic: A neuron whose axon terminates at another axon at the point where the second axon terminates on a synapse.

Blood-brain barrier: A barrier between the circulatory system and the extracellular fluid in the brain. It is formed along all capillaries by cells that restrict the diffusion of large molecules into the cerebral spinal fluid while allowing small molecules to cross freely. Some molecules (e.g., glucose) traverse the barrier with the aid of specific transport proteins.

Brain-derived neurotrophic factor: A protein found in the nervous system that helps to support the survival of existing neurons and encourage the growth and differentiation of new neurons and synapses.

C fibers: Unmyelinated, afferent neurons found in the somatic nervous system.

Catabolize: To break down complex molecules into simpler molecules or ions.

Catechol-O-methyl transferase (COMT): An enzyme that degrades catecholamine-type neurotransmitters, including dopamine, epinephrine, and norepinephrine.

Cation: An ion with a positive charge.

Caudate nucleus: A C-shaped structure, next to the thalamus, involved in learning, memory, and language functions.

Central nervous system (CNS): All nerve cells within the brain and spinal cord.

Cerebral spinal fluid (CSF): Fluid found around the brain and spinal cord and within the ventricles. Its function is to protect the brain and maintain its chemical stability.

Choroid plexus: A structure in the ventricles of the brain where cerebral spinal fluid is produced.

Cingulate cortex: The portion of the brain immediately inferior to (located underneath) the cerebral cortex and, with other portions of the limbic system, extensively involved in the processing of emotions, memory, and executive functions.

Commissure: A bundle of nerve fibers that join the right and left cerebral hemispheres.

Dendritic spine: Small protrusion from a dendrite that receives input from a single synapse of an axon.

Dendrodendritic synapse: A synapse across which dendrites of adjacent neurons communicate.

Diencephalon: The portion of the brain that includes the thalamus and hypothalamus.

Dynorphin: A family of opioids primarily involved in analgesia that may also play a role in addictive behaviors.

Dyskinesia: A syndrome of repetitive, involuntary movements, often involving the mouth, face, or limbs, that may be caused by some psychotropic medications (e.g., conventional antipsychotics).

Efferent: Transmitting messages away from the brain (toward organs and muscles).

Endocannabinoids: Chemical compounds found in the nervous and immune systems that stimulate cannabinoid receptors.

Endocytosis: A process by which cells absorb molecules by engulfing them.

Endoplasmic reticulum: An organelle with tubules and sacs that are connected to the membrane of the nucleus.

Enkephalin: An endogenous peptide that binds to opioid receptors and is involved in alleviating pain perception.

Entorhinal area: Part of the medial temporal lobe extensively interconnected with the neocortex and primarily involved in memory functions.

Entropy: Lack of order.

Epigenetic phenomena: Changes in phenotype caused by mechanisms other than the underlying DNA.

Exocytosis: Process by which a cell secretes contents into the extracellular space.

Extrapyramidal: The portion of the motor system that lies outside the pyramidal tracts.

Feed-back: The passage of information (e.g., a signal) back to the sending element to affect its reaction (e.g., to change its firing rate).

Feed-forward: The passage of information (e.g., a signal) to the next element in the chain.

Foramina: Openings in the skull bone through which cranial nerves and blood vessels pass.

Forebrain: The largest portion of the brain, including the cortex, thalamus, hypothalamus, basal ganglia, and limbic system.

Fornix: A C-shaped bundle of neuron axons connecting the hippocampus with mammillary bodies and septal nuclei.

Free radical: A molecule with an unpaired electron on an open configuration. Free radicals are implicated in advancing the aging process and underlying many diseases (e.g., cancer).

Ganglia: Groups of cell bodies and dendrites that provide relay points and intermediary connections between various neurological structures (e.g., between the central and peripheral nervous systems).

Gap junction: A connection between cells in which the cytoplasm of adjacent cells connects across the membranes through specialized channels that allow molecules to pass between the two cells.

Gene transcription: The process of copying sections of DNA to form molecules of messenger RNA (mRNA) that bind with other ions or molecules and form proteins, enzymes, etc.

Globus pallidus: The portion of the brain, inferior to (underneath) the cingulate cortex, mostly involved in the planning and control of movements.

Goldman-Hodgkin-Katz voltage equation: An equation used to determine the cell's equilibrium potential, based on the relative charge of all the ions affecting that membrane.

Golgi apparatus: A network of proteins formed from the endoplasmic reticulum into small sacs (vesicles) that break off to deliver products to other structures or to the cell membrane for release outside the cell.

Graded potential: A transient, localized change in cell membrane potential.

Heme: A group of molecules containing an iron atom at the center.

Heteroreceptor: A receptor, usually presynaptic, that responds to several neurotransmitters rather than being coded for one specific neurotransmitter (true for most postsynaptic receptors).

Hindbrain: The portion of the brain closest to the spinal cord that contains the cerebellum, pons, and medulla oblongata and is extensively involved in motor control.

Histamine methyltransferase: An enzyme involved in the metabolism of histamine.

Hydrocephalus: A disorder in which abnormally high amounts of cerebral spinal fluid collect in the brain's ventricles.

Hydrophilic: Attracting water.

Hydrophobic: Repelling water.

Hypocretin: Another name for orexin, a hormone involved in maintaining wakefulness.

Hypothalamic-pituitary-adrenal (HPA) axis: A system of complex influences and feed-back interactions between the hypothalamus and pituitary and adrenal glands involved in mediating stress reactions and many bodily functions.

Indole: A chemical compound that contains benzene and nitrogen.

Insula: The portion of the cerebral cortex involved in the processing of motor, emotion, and cognitive functions.

Internal capsule: The portion of the white matter containing both afferent and efferent axons that run between the cortex and the medulla.

Interneuron: A relay neuron that connects afferent and efferent pathways.

Interoception: Perception of stimuli originating inside the body.

Interstitial fluid: Fluid that surrounds the cells. It is involved in delivering molecules to the cells and removing metabolic waste products.

Korsakoff's syndrome: A type of dementia, usually associated with chronic alcoholism, caused by a deficiency in thiamine and characterized by memory problems, apathy, lack of insight, and poverty of speech.

Lateral tegmental nuclei: An area within the brainstem from which many noradrenergic neurons project into the midbrain.

Lenticular nucleus: The portion of the brain that includes the putamen and the globus pallidus.

Ligand: An ion or molecule that binds to a receptor.

Lipophilic: Attracting lipids (fat cells).

Lipophobic: Repelling lipids (fat cells).

Locus coeruleus: An area within the brainstem from which many noradrenergic neurons originate and project into the midbrain and cortex. It is extensively involved in the processing of anxiety and the fight-or-flight response.

Long-term potentiation: An enhancement in signal transmission between two neurons that results from stimulating them at the same time. It is one of several mechanisms involved in long-term memory.

Mesencephalon: See *Midbrain.*

Mesocortical pathway: A group of dopaminergic neurons projecting from the brainstem to potions of the frontal cortex involved in the processing of motivation and emotion.

Mesolimbic pathway: A group of dopaminergic neurons projecting from the brainstem to portions of the limbic system involved in the processing of emotions, including anxiety and the fight-or-flight response.

Metencephalon: The portion of the hindbrain that includes the pons and cerebellum.

Microtubule: Cylindrical filament that forms the internal skeleton of the neuron and facilitates the movement of vesicles toward the synapse.

Microvilli: Very small membrane protrusions that increase the surface area of the cell membrane.

Midbrain: The portion of the brain between the cortex and the hindbrain involved in the processing of motor, vision, hearing, arousal, sleep, and temperature regulation.

Mitochondria: Membrane-enclosed organelles found mostly in cell body that are involved in the production of energy and maintaining the life-cycle of the cell.

Monoamine oxidase: An enzyme that breaks down monoamine-type neurotransmitters (dopamine, norepinephrine, serotonin, etc.).

Myelencephalon: The portion of the hindbrain that includes the medulla oblongata.

Myelinated axon: An axon enveloped by strands of myelin sheath, increasing the speed with which the axon transmits the action potential along its length.

Neocortex: The outer layer of the cerebral cortex.

Nernst equation: An equation used to determine the equilibrium reduction potential of a membrane.

Neural plate: In a developing embryo, a precursor to the neural tube.

Neural tube: In a developing embryo, a precursor to the central nervous system.

Neuroplasticity: Ability of the brain to change through cortical remapping as a result of one's experience.

Neurotrophin: A group of growth factor proteins involved in the development, survival, and function of neuronal cells.

Nigrostriatal pathway: A group of dopaminergic neurons extending from the brainstem to the striatal region of the basal ganglia involved in motor coordination.

Node of Ranvier: A gap between strands of myelin surrounding the axon of a myelinated cell.

Nucleus basalis of Meynert: A group of acetylcholine-producing neurons in the basal forebrain that has wide projections to the neocortex.

Ontogeny recapitulates phylogeny: A theory proposing that in developing from embryo to adult, individuals go through stages resembling or representing stages in the evolution of our ancestors.

Parahippocampal gyrus: A gray matter area surrounding the hippocampus that is extensively involved in memory encoding and retrieval.

Parasympathetic nervous system: A portion of the autonomic nervous system involved in quieting the fight-or-flight response.

Pedunculopontine tegmental nucleus: A group of acetylcholine-producing neurons in the brainstem with wide projections to various brain areas, especially including the basal ganglia.

Peptidase: An enzyme that breaks down a peptide into its components.

Periaqueductal gray: The portion of the gray matter, in the midbrain, involved in temperature and pain regulation.

Peripheral nervous system (PNS): All nerve cells outside the brain and spinal cord.

Phospholipid: A fat cell that contains a phosphate chemical group.

Phosphorylation: Addition of a phosphate group to a molecule.

Pontine-geniculo-occipital waves: Brain waves that begin from the pons, then move to the thalamus, and end up in the primary visual cortex of the occipital lobe. These waves are most prominent right before rapid eye movement (REM) sleep.

Pontine nuclei: A portion of the pons involved in motor activity.

Postganglionic fibers: Nerve fibers running from the ganglia to other neurological structures (e.g., the peripheral nervous system).

Postsynaptic potential: A change in membrane potential resulting from activation of synaptic input.

Preganglionic fibers: Nerve fibers running from the central nervous system to the ganglia.

Protein kinase: An enzyme that modifies other proteins through phosphorylation.

Purkinje cell: Large neuron located in the cerebellum with unusually elaborate dendrites and dendritic spines.

Putamen: A round structure located at the base of the forebrain involved in learning and motor functions.

Pyramidal cell: A type of neuron, with a characteristic triangular-shaped cell body, present in the neocortex and primarily involved in motor coordination.

Pyrimidine: Heterocyclic compound containing two nitrogen atoms.

Raphe nuclei: Clusters of serotonergic neurons in the brainstem that project into the midbrain and cortex.

Receptor potential: A depolarizing event resulting from inward current flow when a receptor is stimulated, generally moving the cell toward an action potential.

Retinohypothalamic fibers: Projections of neurons that originate in the retinal ganglion cells and project to the suprachiasmatic nucleus.

Retrograde messenger: A molecule that sends messages from postsynaptic to presynaptic neurons.

Retrograde neuronal transport: The process by which molecules are sent back from the neuron's axon to its cell body.

Retrosplenial cortex: A portion of the cingulate cortex primarily involved in the formation of memories.

Reuptake: The process of reabsorption of a neurotransmitter (usually from the synapse) by the same neuron that released it.

Ribosome: Protein synthesized in the nucleus and then released into the cytoplasm, most commonly involved in intracellular protein synthesis.

Set point: A reference level to which relative deviation is compared.

Sodium-potassium (Na-K) pump: An enzyme in the cell membrane that allows three sodium ions to leave the cell for every two potassium ions that enter the cell.

Somatotopic: Maintenance of spatial organization within the central nervous system that reflects the spatial organization of the somatosensory receptors (e.g., areas in the brain that receive information from the sense receptors in the hands are next to areas that receive information from the sense receptors in the arm).

Split-brain phenomena: A term that describes anomalies evident in individuals in whom the corpus callosum has been severed (e.g., the inability to name objects being seen).

Striatum: A portion of the brain that includes the caudate nucleus and the lenticular nucleus.

Substantia nigra: A dopamine-producing brain structure located in the midbrain that is extensively involved in the processing of reward, motivation, learning, and motor control. It is thought to play a major role in addictive behaviors.

Subthalamic nucleus: A portion of the brain, located under the thalamus, involved in impulse control.

Supraoptic nucleus: A portion of the hypothalamus that extensively communicates with the pituitary.

Sympathetic nervous system: A portion of the autonomic nervous system involved in mobilizing the body under stress (fight-or-flight response).

Synaptogenesis: The formation of synapses.

Synaptotagmin: A family of proteins involved in cell membrane fusion.

Tachykinins: A family of peptides found in the gastrointestinal tract that are involved in inducing the contractions of gut tissues.

Tardive: Late in onset (as in tardive dyskinesia).

Telencephalon: The cerebral cortex.

Transamination: A chemical reaction involving the transfer of an amino-acid component from one molecule to another.

Transcription factor: A protein that binds to a portion of DNA and affects how that DNA sequence affects the production of a messenger RNA.

Transcytosis: A process by which molecules within the cell are transported across the interior of a cell.

Transduce: To convert energy from one form to another.

Transporter: A molecule whose primary function is to transport another molecule attached to it (e.g., across the cell membrane).

Tuberoinfundibular pathway: A group of neurons that projects from the hypothalamus to the pituitary.

Tyrosine hydroxylase: An enzyme responsible for the conversion of L-tyrosine to L-DOPA, a precursor for dopamine.

Up-regulation: An increase (e.g., in receptor growth) in response to an opposing action (e.g., a decrease in neurotransmitter).

Vasoactive intestinal polypeptide: A hormone released by many parts of the body (especially portions of the gastrointestinal tract) involved in the regulation of many processes, including digestion and cardiovascular functions.

Chapter 3 Questions

1. Cranial nerve VI is the:
   a. Olfactory nerve.
   b. Trigeminal nerve.

  c. Abducens nerve.

  d. Facial nerve.

2. The locus coeruleus begins projections for pathways primarily innervated by which neurotransmitter?

  a. Dopamine

  b. Norepinephrine

  c. Serotonin

  d. Histamine

3. The pons is most involved in regulating:

  a. Motor activity.

  b. Emotions.

  c. Sleep.

  d. Hormone levels.

4. The enteric nervous system is part of all of the following except:

  a. Central nervous system

  b. Peripheral nervous system

  c. Autonomic nervous system

  d. Visceral motor system

5. Sympathetic neurons are arranged so that they exit the spinal cord via the _____ segments.

  a. Thoracic

  b. Lumbar

  c. Both a and b

  d. Neither a nor b

6. Dorsal root ganglia relay:

  a. Motor control signals.

  b. Enteric system messages.

  c. Touch, temperature, and pain.

  d. Cardiac control signals.

7. The tectum and tegmentum are portions of:

  a. Hindbrain.

  b. Midbrain.

  c. Forebrain.

  d. Cingulate cortex.

8. Mammillary bodies play an important role in:

  a. Activating the fight-or-flight response.

  b. Motor control.

  c. Memory consolidation.

  d. Appetite control.

9. The paraventricular nucleus produces:

  a. Catecholamines.

  b. Thyroid-stimulating hormone.

c. Histamine.

d. Corticotropin-releasing hormone.

10. The nucleus basalis of Meynert is one of the key production areas for:

   a. Acetylcholine.

   b. Cortisol.

   c. Dopamine.

   d. Serotonin.

11. Cerebral spinal fluid is produced in large part by the:

   a. Pituitary.

   b. Choroid plexus.

   c. Fornix.

   d. Microvilli.

12. Melatonin is most closely related to which neurotransmitter?

   a. Dopamine

   b. Histamine

   c. GABA

   d. Serotonin

13. The active effect of neurotransmitters on the target neuron is terminated by:

   a. Diffusion.

   b. Enzymatic degradation.

   c. Reuptake.

   d. All of the above

14. Nitric oxide transmits messages primarily through:

   a. Endocrine signaling.

   b. Chemical signaling.

   c. Paracrine signaling.

   d. Synaptic transmission.

15. At the start of the action potential:

   a. Sodium enters the cell and potassium leaves the cell.

   b. Potassium enters the cell and sodium leaves the cell.

   c. Sodium and potassium leave the cell while chloride enters the cell.

   d. The sodium-potassium pump temporarily ceases operation.

   Answers: (1) c, (2) b, (3) a, (4) a, (5) c, (6) c, (7) b, (8) c, (9) d, (10) a, (11) b, (12) d, (13) d, (14) c, (15) a.

REFERENCES

Arendt, J., & Skene, D. J. (2005). Melatonin as a chronobiotic. *Sleep Medicine Reviews, 9*, 25–39.

Bean, B. P. (2007). The action potential in mammalian central neurons. *Nature Reviews Neuroscience, 8*, 451–465.

Beecher Scoville, W., & Milner, B. (1957). Loss of recent memory after bilateral hippocampal lesions. *Journal of Neurology, Neurosurgery, and Psychiatry, 20*, 11–21.

Biederer, T., Sara, Y., Mozhayeva, M., Atasoy, D., Liu, X., Kavalali, E., & Südhof, T. (2002). SynCAM, a synaptic adhesion molecule that drives synapse assembly. *Science, 30*, 1525–1531.

Brodal, P. (2010). *The central nervous system: Structure and function* (4th ed.). New York, NY: Oxford University Press.

Bush, G., Vogt, B. A., Holmes, J., Dale, A. M., Greve, D., Jenike, M. A., & Rosen, B. R. (2002). Dorsal anterior cingulate cortex: A role in reward-based decision-making. *Proceedings of the National Academy of Sciences USA, 99*, 523–528.

Calabrese, V., Mancuso, C., Calvani, M., Rizzarelli, E., Butterfield, D. A., & Stella, A. M. G. (2007). Nitric oxide in the central nervous system: Neuroprotection versus neurotoxicity. *Nature Reviews Neuroscience, 8*, 766–775.

Cannon, W. B. (1929). *Bodily changes in pain, hunger, fear, and rage.* New York, NY: Appleton-Century-Crofts.

Clark, D., Boutros, N., & Mendez, M. (2010). *The brain and behavior.* Cambridge, UK: Cambridge University Press.

Cooper, M. S. (1995). Intercellular signaling in neuronal–glial networks. *Biosystems, 34*, 65–85.

Coras, R., Siebzehnrubl, F. A., Pauli, E., Huttner, H. B., Njunting, M., Kobow, K., . . . & Blümcke, I. (2010). Low proliferation and differentiation capacities of adult hippocampal stem cells correlate with memory dysfunction in humans. *Brain, 133*, 3359–3372.

Craig, A. D. (2003). Interoception: The sense of the physiological condition of the body. *Current Opinion in Neurobiology, 13*, 500–505.

Dalva, M., McClellan, A., & Kayser, S. (2007). Cell adhesion molecules: Signaling functions at the synapse. *National Review of Neuroscience, 8*, 206–220.

Damasio, A. R. (1999). *The feeling of what happens: Body and emotion in the making of consciousness.* Orlando, FL: Harcourt.

Damasio, A. R., & Damasio, H. (1994). Cortical systems for retrieval of concrete knowledge: The convergence zone framework. In C. Koch & J. L. Davis (Eds.), *Large-scale neuronal theories of the brain* (pp. 61–74). Cambridge, MA: MIT Press.

De Dreu, C., Greer, L., Van Kleef, G., Shalvi, S., & Handgraaf, M. (2011). Oxytocin promotes human ethnocentrism. *Proceedings of the National Academy of Science.* Published ahead of print January 10, 2011.

De Dreu, C., Greer, L., Van Kleef, G., Shalvi, S., Handgraaf, M., Baas, M., ... & Feith, S. (2010). The neuropeptide oxytocin regulates parochial altruism in intergroup conflict among humans. *Science, 11, 328*, 1408–1411.

Dickenson, A. H. (2001). Peptides. In R. A. Webster (Ed.), *Neurotransmitters, drugs and brain function* (pp. 251–264). Chichester, UK: Wiley.

Dragunow, M. (1986). Adenosine: The brain's natural anticonvulsant? *Trends in Pharmacological Sciences, 7*, 128–130.

Ebrahim, I. O., Sharief, M. K., de Lacy, S., Semra, Y. K., Howard, R. S., Kopelman, M. D., & Williams, A. J. (2003). Hypocretin (orexin) deficiency in narcolepsy and primary hypersomnia. *Journal of Neurology, Neurosurgery, and Psychiatry, 74*, 127–130.

Errington, A., Stöhr, T., & Lees, G. (2005). Voltage gated ion channels: Targets for anticonvulsant drugs. *Current Topics in Medicinal Chemistry, 5*, 15–30.

Frank, M. G. (2007). Hippocampal dreams, cortical wishes: A closer look at neuronal replay and the hippocampal-neocortical dialogue during sleep. *Cell Science Reviews, 3*, 161–171.

Goldberg, E. (2002). *The Executive brain: Frontal lobes and the civilized mind.* New York, NY: Oxford University Press.

Harlow, J. (1869). Recovery from the passage of an iron bar through the head. *Boston Medical and Surgical Journal, 3*, 116–117.

Hasselmo, M., Linnster, C., Patil, M., Ma, D., & Cekic, M. (1997). Noradrenergic suppression of synaptic transmission may influence cortical signal-to-noise ratio. *Journal of Neurophysiology, 77*, 3326–3339.

Hodgkin, A. L., & Huxley, A. F. (1952). A quantitative description of membrane current and its application to conduction and excitation in nerve. *Journal of Physiology, 117*, 500–544.

Hökfelt, T., Broberger, C., Zhi-Qing, D. X., Sergeyev, V., Ubink, R., & Diez, M. (2000). Neuropeptides: An overview. *Neuropharmacology, 39*, 1337–1356.

Hough, L. S., & Green, J. P. (1983) Histamine and its receptors in the nervous system. In A. Lajtha (Ed.), *Handbook of neurochemistry* (pp. 187–211). New York, NY: Plenum Press.

Huang, E., & Reichardt, L. (2001). Neurotrophins: Roles in neuronal development and function. *Annual Review of Neuroscience, 24*, 677–736.

Iversen, S., Iversen, L., & Saper, C. B. (2000). The autonomic nervous system and the hypothalamus. In E. R. Kandel, J. H. Schwartz, & T. M. Jessell (Eds.), *Principles of neural science* (4th ed., pp. 960–981), New York, NY: McGraw-Hill.

James, W. (1890). *Principles of psychology: Volume I.* Republished (1950) by Dover Publications.

Kandel, E. R. (2000). The brain and behavior. In E. R. Kandel, J. H. Schwartz, & T. M. Jessell (Eds.), *Principles of neural science* (4th ed., pp. 5–18), New York, NY: McGraw-Hill.

Kandel, E. R., & Siegelbaum, S. A. (2000). Overview of synaptic transmission. In E. R. Kandel, J. H. Schwartz, & T. M. Jessell (Eds.), *Principles of neural science* (4th Ed., pp. 175–186), New York, NY: McGraw-Hill.

Keay, K. A., & Bandler, R. (2001). Parallel circuits mediating distinct emotional coping reactions to different types of stress. *Neuroscience & Biobehavioral Reviews, 25*, 669–678

Lane, N. (2005). *Power, sex, suicide: Mitochondria, and the meaning of life.* New York, NY: Oxford University Press.

LeDoux, J. E. (2000). Emotion circuits in the brain. *Annual Review of Neuroscience, 23*, 155–184.

LeDoux, J. E. (2002). *Synaptic self: How our brains become who we are.* New York, NY: Penguin.

MacLean, P. D. (1949). Psychosomatic disease and the "visceral brain": Recent developments bearing on the Papez theory of emotion. *Psychosomatic Medicine, 11*, 338–353.

MacLean, P. D. (1970). The triune brain, emotion, and scientific bias. In F. O. Schmitt (Ed.), *The neurosciences second study program* (pp. 336–349). New York, NY: Rockefeller University Press.

Maliphant, R., Hume, F., & Furnham, A. (1990). Autonomic nervous system (ANS) activity, personality characteristics and disruptive behaviour in girls. *Journal of Child Psychology and Psychiatry, 31*, 619–628.

Martin, A., Wiggs, C. L., Ungerleider, L. G., & Haxby, J. V. (1996). Neural correlates of category-specific knowledge. *Nature, 379*, 649–652.

Mayberg, H. S., Lozano, A. M, Voon, V., McNeely, H. E., et al. (2005). Deep brain stimulation for treatment-resistant depression. *Neuron, 45*, 651–660.

McCormick, D. A. (2004). Membrane properties and neurotransmitter actions. In G. M. Shepherd (Ed.), *The synaptic organization of the brain* (pp. 39–77). New York, NY: Oxford University Press.

Middleton, F. A., & Strick, P. L. (2001). Revised neuroanatomy of frontal-subcortical circuits. In D. G. Lichter & J. L. Cummings (Eds.), *Frontal-subcortical circuits in psychiatric and neurological disorders* (pp. 44–58). New York, NY: Guilford.

Nestler, E. J., Hyman, S. E., & Malenka, R. C. (2009). *Molecular neuropharmacology: A foundation for clinical neuroscience.* (2nd Ed.), New York, NY: McGraw-Hill Medical.

Noback, C. R., Strominger, N. L., Demarest, R. J., & Ruggiero, D. A. (2005). *The human nervous system: Structure and function.* Totowa, NJ: Humana Press.

Numan, R. (2000). *The behavioral neuroscience of the septal region.* New York, NY: Springer-Verlag.

Papez, J. W. (1937). A proposed mechanism of emotion. *Archives of Neurology & Psychiatry, 38*, 725–743.

Pavlov, I. P. (1927). *Conditioned reflexes.* London: Oxford University Press.

Perry, B. D. (2006). Applying principles of neurodevelopment to clinical work with mal-treated and traumatized children: The Neurosequential Model of Therapeutics. In N. Webb (Ed.), *Working with traumatized youth in child welfare* (pp. 27–52). New York, NY: Guilford Press.

Perry, B. D., & Pollard, R. (1998). Homeostasis, stress, trauma, and adaptation: A neurode-velopmental view of childhood trauma. *Child and Adolescent Psychiatric Clinics of North America, 7*, 33–51.

Quirk, G. J., & Mueller, D. (2008). Neural mechanisms of extinction learning and retrieval. *Neuropsychopharmacology, 33*, 56–72.

Ring, R. H. (2005). The central vasopressogenic system: Examining the opportunities for psy-chiatric drug development. *Current Pharmaceutical Design, 11*, 205–225.

Robbins, E., Krupp, A., Perez de Arce, K., Ghosh, A., Fogel, A., Boucard, A., . . . & Biederer T. (2010). SynCAM 1 adhesion dynamically regulates synapse number and impacts plasticity and learning. *Neuron, 68*, 894–906.

Sah, P., & Westbrook, F. (2008). The circuit of fear. *Nature, 454*, 589–590.

Sakurai, T. (2007). The neural circuit of orexin (hypocretin): Maintaining sleep and wakefulness. *Nature Reviews Neuroscience, 8*, 171–181.

Sapolsky, R. (2005). *Biology and human behavior: The neurological origins of individuality.* Chantilly, VA: The Teaching Company.

Schoenen, J., & Faull, R. L. M. (2004). Spinal cord cyto- and chemoarchitecture. In G. Paxinos & J. K. Mai (Eds.), *The human nervous system* (2nd ed., pp. 190–232), San Diego, CA: Elsevier.

Schwartz, J. C., Arrang, J. M., Garbary, M., Pollard, H., & Ruat, M. (1991). Histaminergic transmission in the mammalian brain. *Physiology Reviews, 71*, 1–51.

Seif, S., Zenser T., et al. (2011). DDAVP (l-Desamino-8-D-arginine-vasopressin) treatment of central diabetes insipidus: Mechanism of prolonged antidiuresis. *Journal of Clinical Endocrinology & Metabolism, 46*, 381–388.

Söllner, T., & Rothman, J. E. (1994). Neurotransmission: Harnessing fusion machinery at the synapse. *Trends in Neurosciences, 17*, 344–348.

Sperry, R. W., Gazzaniga, M. S., & Bogen, J. E. (1969). Interhemispheric relationships: The neocortical commissures, syndromes of hemisphere disconnection. In P. J. Vinken & G. W. Bruyn (Eds.), *Handbook of clinical neurology* (pp. 273–290). Amsterdam, Holland: Elsevier.

Stahl, S. (2008). *Stahl's essential psychopharmacology: Neuroscientific basis and practical appli-cations.* Cambridge, UK: Cambridge University Press.

Stanford, S. C. (2001a). Neurotransmitter release. In R. A. Webster (Ed.), *Neurotransmitters, drugs and brain function* (pp. 81–104). Chichester, UK: Wiley.

Stanford, S. C. (2001b). Noradrenaline. In R. A. Webster (Ed.), *Neurotransmitters, drugs and brain function* (pp. 163–186). Chichester, UK: Wiley.

Sudhof, T. C. (2004). The synaptic vesicle cycle. *Annual Review of Neuroscience, 27*, 509–547.

Sullivan, R. M. (2004). Hemispheric asymmetry in stress processing in rat prefrontal cortex and the role of mesocortical dopamine. *Stress, 7*, 131–143.

Takahashi, T., Murata, T., Hamada, T., Omori, M., Kosaka, H., Kikuchi, M., . . . & Wada, Y. (2005). Changes in EEG and autonomic nervous activity during meditation and their association with personality traits. *International Journal of Psychophysiology, 55*, 199–207.

Tarlaci, S. (2010). A historical view of the relation between quantum mechanics and the brain: A neuroquantologic perspective. *NeuroQuantology, 8*, 120–136.

Taylor, S. E., Klein, L. C., Lewis, B. P., Gruenewald, T. L., Gurung, R. A. R., & Updegraff, J. A. (2000). Biobehavioral responses to stress in females: Tend-and-befriend, not fight-or-flight. *Psychological Review, 107*, 411–429.

Vogt, B. A. (2008). Regions and subregions of cingulate cortex. In B. A. Vogt (Ed.), *Cingulate neurobiology and disease* (pp. 3–31). Oxford, UK: Oxford University Press.

von Bohlen und Halbach, O., & Dermietzel, R. (2006). *Neurotransmitters and neuromodulators: Handbook of receptors and biological effects*. Weinheim, Germany: Wiley.

Wang, X. (2002). Pacemaker neurons for the theta rhythm and their synchronization in the septohippocampal reciprocal loop. *Journal of Neurophysiology, 87*, 889–900.

Webster, R. A. (2001). *Neurotransmitters, drugs and brain function*. Chichester,UK: Wiley.

Welch, A., & Boone, R. (2008). Sympathetic and parasympathetic responses to specific diversified adjustments to chiropractic vertebral subluxations of the cervical and thoracic spine. *Journal of Chiropractic Medicine, 7,* 86–93.

Werman, R. (1966). Criteria for identification of a central nervous transmitter. *Comparative Biochemistry and Physiology, 18*, 745–766.

Young, L. (2009). The neuroendocrinology of the social brain. *Frontiers in Neuroendocrinology 30*, 425–428.

Young, M. P., Scannell, J. W., Burns, G. A. & Blakemore, C. (1994). Analysis of connectivity: Neural systems in the cerebral cortex. *Reviews in the Neurosciences, 5*, 227–250.

Zahn, T. P., & Kruesi, M. (1993). Autonomic activity in boys with disruptive behavior disorders. *Journal of Psychophysiology, 30*, 605–614.

Zucker, R. S., Kullmann, D. M., & Schwarz, T. L. (2004). Release of neurotransmitters. In J. H. Byrne & J. L. Roberts (Eds.), *From molecules to networks: An introduction to cellular and molecular neuroscience* (pp. 197–244). San Diego, CA: Elsevier.

Chapter 4

NERVOUS SYSTEM PATHOLOGY

Mark Muse

Jonathan M. Borkum

Massi Wyatt

Diseases of the nervous system are particularly relevant to the prescribing medical psychologist. When performing a biopsychosocial assessment and determining differential diagnoses and treatment, the medical psychologist must take into account biological determinants in order to understand the neurological basis of certain emotional and behavioral conditions and appreciate the possible biological impact of pharmacological agents on nervous system functioning.

In this chapter, we present nervous system diseases of diverse origin, including genetically acquired, congenitally developed, and environmentally induced. There is usually no clear line, however, dividing conditions according to particular origins, and the majority of disorders have more than one potential etiology, while an interplay of multiple causes is perhaps more the rule than the exception. We review here neurodegenerative/cognitive disorders, such as Alzheimer's disease; neurodevelopmental conditions, such as autism spectrum disorder; mental retardation and genetically linked intellectual disorders, such as Rett's syndrome; neurovascular disorders, such as stroke; seizure disorders; infections; psychological disorders with a neuropathological basis, such as schizophrenia, affective disorders, and attention deficit–hyperactivity disorder (ADHD); movement disorders; extrapyramidal dysfunctions; traumatic brain injury; sleep disorders; and chronic pain. Diagnostic methods for identifying neurobehavioral disorders, such as electroencephalography (EEG) and neuroimaging, are also discussed.

NEURODEGENERATIVE/COGNITIVE DISORDERS

Dementia

Cognitive decline with advancing age is a near universal occurrence. However, when decline is associated with severe impairment, the medical psychologist needs to be aware of various neuropathological processes that may be implicated, as well as available pharmacological and psychosocial remedies. In this section, we provide an overview of the more common neurocognitive disorders associated with advanced age. Although these disorders may appear to be diverse, certain substrates will recur: an abnormal accumulation of proteins, inflammation, oxidative damage, and the consequent destruction of neurons and sometimes glial cells.

Alzheimer's Disease

Alzheimer's disease is the leading cause of dementia, with a current prevalence in the United States of approximately 5 million (Butterfield & Sultana, 2007), accounting for between 50% and 80% of all cases of dementia (Daviglus et al., 2010). With advancing age being the primary risk factor, combined with increases in life expectancy, the prevalence of Alzheimer's is expected to rise sharply in the developed world (Farlow, Miller, & Pejovic, 2008).

Clinically, Alzheimer's disease involves the development of multiple cognitive deficits, including memory and at least one additional area such as *executive functioning*, language, the ability to recognize objects, or the ability to carry out motor activities (American Psychiatric Association, 1994; Daviglus et al., 2010). Pathophysiologically, the hallmarks of Alzheimer's disease are *neurofibrillary tangles* within neurons and, extracellularly, plaques of *amyloid beta (Aβ)* peptide (Butterfield & Sultana, 2007). The latter has given rise to the amyloid hypothesis of Alzheimer's pathophysiology.

The Amyloid Hypothesis

Amyloids, known to pathologists for 150 years, are extracellular deposits of filaments, termed *fibrils* (Haass & Selkoe, 2007). Amyloid beta (Aβ), specifically, is a peptide comprising 40 or 42 amino acids ($Aβ_{40}$, $Aβ_{42}$). These are fragments of a protein, *amyloid precursor protein (APP)*, produced when first beta and then gamma *secretases* cleave the precursor protein. $Aβ_{42}$ is particularly toxic because it is hydrophobic and therefore tends to form aggregates (Haass & Selkoe, 2007; Selkoe, 2004). The *plaques* may be diffuse and relatively benign (or at least in the early stage), or they may be surrounded by dystrophic axons and dendrites, and by *activated microglia* (Selkoe, 2004). The precursor protein itself, *APP*, resembles a cell-surface receptor, although what it is receiving and what effect the reception has are unknown (Selkoe, 2004). That Aβ plays a key role in Alzheimer's is supported by the fact that familial cases (which are very rare, yet instructive) involve mutations encoding the Aβ or nearby regions of APP or encoding gamma secretase. That is, the mutations either increase the production of $Aβ_{42}$ or increase the tendency of the peptide to aggregate into *oligomers*.[1]

How does Aβ cause neural damage? Possibly, the plaques may not be the central problem; their surface area is small and their filaments relatively inert. Rather, it appears that smaller units of 2 to 12, self-aggregated $Aβ_{42}$ peptides dissolved in the extracellular fluid interfere with synaptic signaling.[2] The original plaques, however, do not resolve and may serve as a reservoir from which oligomers may dissolve and reaggregate extracellularly (Haass & Selkoe, 2007). Moreover, mouse models of *Down syndrome*, a condition also characterized by high levels of amyloid precursor protein, suggest that the protein (or a downstream product) interferes with the retrograde transport of nerve growth factor from the hippocampus to the cell bodies of the cholinergic neurons of the basal forebrain (Salehi et al., 2006). Without the nerve growth factor, these neurons become quiescent, reducing excitatory input to the hippocampus and thus its capacity for the long-term synaptic potentiation believed to underlie learning and memory. A third, nonexclusive possibility is that after it coalesces into filaments, Aβ provokes an *inflammatory cascade*. We will return to this last possibility below.

---

[1]Other genes, such as apolipoprotein ε4, function as lower-grade risk factors. For example, apolipoprotein ε4 seems to promote the aggregation of Aβ into filaments (Haass & Selkoe, 2007; Selkoe, 2004).

[2]How this interference takes place is not clear. There might be specific Aβ receptors, Aβ might adhere nonspecifically to the synaptic membrane, or ringlike oligomers might bind to the synapse, forming extraneous, artificial pores (Haass & Selkoe, 2007).

Why does Alzheimer's disease exist at all? Gamma secretase seems to form part of a receptor, called the *notch receptor*, which is crucial for cell-to-cell communication. Thus, one theory holds that cleavage of APP into $A\beta_{42}$ is simply an unintended consequence that has persisted because it does not affect survival until after reproductive age (Selkoe, 2004).

Neurofibrillary tangles. The intracellular *neurofibrillary* tangles are made up of *tau*, a protein normally involved in stabilizing the microtubule scaffolding within neurons (Bellettato & Scarpa, 2010). Tau is usually highly soluble, but the tangles— filaments of two helical protein strands wound around each other and hyperphosphorylated—are not soluble at all (Selkoe, 2004). Under the amyloid hypothesis, the presence of neurofibrillary tangles is thought to be a secondary phenomenon, reactive to the extracellular $A\beta$ deposits (Selkoe, 2004). But tau may yet prove to be central. It can be the sole mutation involved in a class of dementias referred to as *frontotemporal lobular degeneration*, discussed further on (Haass & Selkoe, 2007). And a compound designed to prevent formation of neurofibrillary tangles has performed very well in Phase 2 trials for treating Alzheimer's disease (Opar, 2008).

Lysosomal dysfunction. Proteins and smaller peptides, including tau and $A\beta_{42}$, are a normal part of metabolism. Like other proteins, they are subject to turnover. The old proteins are delivered to *vacuoles* within the cell, where enzymes (proteases) and acid degrade them (Bellettato & Scarpa, 2010). There is some evidence that these vacuoles, termed *lysosomes*, or the machinery that delivers proteins to them become dysfunctional in Alzheimer's disease. The result is a buildup of incompletely digested proteins that disrupt neural functioning by toxicity or simply by clogging intracellular traffic (Pimplikar et al., 2010). That is, the buildup of $A\beta_{42}$ and of hyperphosphorylated tau may be a side effect of the true problem. In a mouse model, a drug that partially restores lysosomal function also improves cognition (Spilman et al., 2010).[3]

Mitochondrial dysfunction. Ineffective lysosomes may be a result of impaired energy production by the mitochondria (Cardoso et al., 2010). Mitochondrial DNA shows an abnormal number of mutations, and key mitochondrial enzymes such as cytochrome c oxidase show decreased function in Alzheimer's disease (Moreira et al., 2006; Swerdlow & Khan, 2004). This might explain why aging is such a strong risk factor for Alzheimer's; in normal aging, mitochondrial mutations accumulate and enzyme function declines (Cardoso et al., 2010). The mitochondrial hypothesis might also suggest a novel role for $A\beta$. In its soluble form, it can damage mitochondria, potentially setting up a vicious cycle. It is possible that the extracellular plaques of $A\beta$ are actually a defense by the neurons, a way of sequestering the excess peptide.

Oxidative stress. Mitochondrial dysfunction can be the cumulative effect of oxidative stress. Conversely, inefficient mitochondria produce an abnormally large amount of reactive oxygen species. Thus, it is possible that oxidative stress is a core problem in Alzheimer's disease.

Neuroinflammation. Although the blood-brain barrier usually protects the central nervous system (CNS) from infiltration by white blood cells from the periphery (see, in contrast, the discussion of multiple sclerosis below), the brain has its own innate immunity, provided by the *microglia* that surround and encase neurons (Milligan & Watkins, 2009). In their resting state, the microglia sample the chemical environment.

---

[3]Parenthetically, the proton-pump inhibitors used to treat gastroesophageal reflux cross the blood-brain barrier and inhibit the enzyme pumps used to acidify lysosomes. This has led to speculation, so far untested, that they may increase the risk of Alzheimer's disease (Fallahzadeh, Borhani Haghighi, & Namazi, 2010).

When activated, they take on the shape of *macrophages*, phagocytizing intruders and secreting proinflammatory *cytokines* such as interleukin-1β (IL-1β) (Frank-Cannon et al., 2009). Since Aβ is a toxin, microglia presumably have a role to play in eliminating this toxin. There is some evidence for this hypothesis. In test-tube experiments, microglia can internalize and clear Aβ. Also, IL-1β, although it increases production of APP, also upregulates tumor necrosis factor-α converting enzyme (TACE), a form of α-secretase, which provides an alternative processing pathway for APP so that it is not transformed into Aβ (Tachida et al., 2008). Furthermore, vaccination against Aβ can prevent or slow the course of Alzheimer's disease (Hock et al., 2003).[4]

It is also likely, however, that this protective process can go awry. Proinflammatory cytokines may block the ability of microglia to phagocytize Aβ (Koenigsknecht-Talboo & Landreth, 2005), leaving them in a state of chronic activation. The resulting chronic inflammation may damage nearby neurons by the excess production of nitric oxide (Block & Hong, 2005; Block, Zecca, & Hong, 2007). Moreover, correlational studies suggest that activated microglia may be responsible for the aggregation of diffuse plaques into the more toxic *neuritic plaques* (plaques surrounded by atrophied dendrites and axons). Thus, the challenge may be not to eliminate inflammation but to shift it from a chronic to the more efficacious acute form.

Altered cell signaling. One final corollary in the genesis and maintenance of Alzheimer's are the types of mutations that give rise to familial Alzheimer's disease; these mutations may also affect the intracellular signaling pathways involved in cell survival, as opposed to *apoptosis*, and in short- and long-term *synaptic plasticity* (Pimplikar et al., 2010).

Treatment of Alzheimer's Disease

Pharmacotherapy. Although currently available treatments for Alzheimer's disease are limited in number and efficacy, they do offer some benefit. Second-generation *cholinesterase inhibitors* have been approved for the treatment of mild-to-moderate Alzheimer's disease (donepezil, galantamine, *rivastigmine*), and donepezil has also been approved for severe disease. They are designed to compensate for the loss of cholinergic transmission by slowing the breakdown of acetylcholine in the synapse (Farlow, Miller, & Pejovic, 2008). They have slightly different mechanisms of action: While all three inhibit acetylcholinesterase, rivastigmine also inhibits butyrylcholinesterase, and galantamine modifies nicotinic acetylcholine receptors (Bhasin et al., 2007).

Clinical improvements are modest but tend to be seen in all domains—cognitive, behavioral, and daily functioning. Although these three medications are roughly equal in efficacy, a lack of response or intolerable side effects with one medication does not predict a similar result in the same patient for another medication within the same class. In other words, someone who has an adverse reaction to donepezil may respond well to rivastigmine. Side effects are mostly gastrointestinal (diarrhea, nausea, abdominal pain), although headaches, muscle cramps, fatigue, syncope, and sleep disturbance have also been reported (Farlow, Miller, & Pejovic, 2008).

Approved for severe Alzheimer's, and showing additive benefit with donepezil, is memantine, an inhibitor of NMDA-type glutamate receptors. The logic behind reducing glutamatergic transmission is to prevent the *excitotoxicity* believed to contribute to the loss of neurons. Memantine, like the cholinesterase inhibitors, shows

---

[4]So far, this has not been clinically useful because of the occasional side effect of severe brain inflammation, or *meningoencephalitis* (Orgogozo et al., 2003).

modest benefits in the realms of cognition, behavior, and daily activities. It has few side effects and is generally better tolerated than the cholinesterase inhibitors. Its utility for mild and moderate Alzheimer's, however, is questionable (Farlow, Miller, & Pejovic, 2008).

All these treatments appear to be symptomatic, partially slowing the clinical decline while having no effect on the underlying disease process. So far, this appears true even for memantine, which is presumed to prevent excitotoxicity. Clearly, pharmacological agents are needed that, based on our current understanding of Alzheimer's pathophysiology, would truly blunt the underlying neurodegeneration. A number of such disease-modifying agents are in preclinical or early clinical development (see Table 4.1).

Lifestyle. Epidemiological studies suggest a rather markedly lower risk of dementia in people who exercise, maintain a healthy weight, are well educated, stay involved in social interaction and cognitively challenging activities, and eat a diet high in fruits, vegetables, vitamin E, and fish (Farlow, Miller, & Pejovic, 2008). In vitro and animal models have shown that the flavonoids found in fruits and vegetables have anti-inflammatory and antioxidant properties (Rezai-Zadeh et al., 2008; Zhao, 2009), increase the activity of *ATPase* (Chen et al., 2008; Song et al., 2009), and prevent the buildup of Aβ (Wang et al., 2009). Although clinical trials are lacking for most of these, they appear to be reasonable steps to achieve a prudent lifestyle.

Cognitive-Behavioral Therapy. Cognitive rehabilitation and "reality orientation" have received empirical support in a meta-analysis (Sitzer, Twamley, & Jeste, 2006) and in a Cochrane Review (Spector et al., 2000), respectively. Reality orientation involves providing environmental cues to help the patient remain oriented. Also, support for the caregiver and environmental modifications for the patient can minimize behavioral disturbances. Psychobiosocial interventions are a significant strategy in the management of Alzheimer's, since atypical antipsychotics, which might otherwise be prescribed for such disturbances, have been shown to increase the risk of cerebrovascular events, falls, and death (Farlow, Miller, & Pejovic, 2008).

Frontotemporal Dementias

The *frontotemporal dementias* are a heterogeneous class of disorders involving profound brain atrophy and gradual deterioration, not of memory as in Alzheimer's disease, but of personality, social functioning, language, and motor skills (Roberson, 2006). Studies from the United Kingdom suggest a prevalence of 0.015% of these types of dementias among middle-aged adults 45 to 64 years of age, placing it behind Alzheimer's among the early-onset dementias (Piguet et al., in press).

Pathophysiology The underlying physical disease is better seen at the level of the individual dementia subtypes, for which the symptoms seem to reflect the predominant areas of brain atrophy (Josephs, 2008; Roberson, 2006) (Table 4.2).

Cortical degeneration is most noticeable in *laminae II and III*, which take on a spongy appearance because of the numerous small vacuoles. These layers are particularly important for connections between different regions of cortex (Josephs, 2008; Roberson, 2006).

In nearly all cases, the frontotemporal dementias share a feature with other neurodegenerative disorders: the abnormal accumulation of proteins. The proteins are found inside neurons and glia. The most common protein, accounting for about 58% of cases, is hyperphosphorylated tau, as in Alzheimer's disease (but usually without the amyloid plaques) (Roberson, 2011). Thus, the genes most frequently associated

Table 4.1 Potential Disease-Modifying Strategies in Alzheimer's Disease

Strategy	Advantages	Disadvantages	Status of Therapy
Inhibit beta secretase	Mouse models suggest few adverse effects	Inhibitors difficult to find	Rosiglitazone—development stopped; Other agents—phase 1 trials completed or ongoing
Partially inhibit gamma secretase	Is key step in Aβ formation	Possible risk of cancer or toxicities in the thymus, spleen, and GI system	Semagacestat—development stopped; Other agents—in phase 1 or 2 trials
Modulate gamma secretase	Shifts site of gamma secretase action, producing $A\beta_{38}$ instead of $A\beta_{42}$		Tarenflurbil—failed in phase 3 trial; CHF 5074—in phase 1 trials
Vaccinate against amyloid beta (Aβ)	Shown to clear Aβ and slows cognitive decline in some people	Vaccines that stimulate T cells have caused meningoencephalitis; elderly patients might not mount an immune response	AN-1972—phase 2 trial discontinued owing to meningoencephalitis; Other agents—in phase 1 or 2 trials
Administer monoclonal antibodies to Aβ	Seems to prevent inflammatory side effects		Several agents are in phase 3 trials
Administer polyclonal intravenous (IV) immune globulin	IV immune globulin already FDA-approved for immune deficiency	Requires repeated IV administration; expensive	IV immune globulin—phase 3 trial ongoing
Prevent binding of Aβ oligomers to neuronal membranes	May reduce neurotoxicity of Aβ		Phase 3 trials ongoing
Prevent plaque formation by interfering with Aβ aggregation	May allow increased clearance of Aβ; may reduce levels of tau		Tramiprosate—no efficacy in phase 3 trial; PBT2—successful in phase 2 trial

Strategy	Rationale	Concerns	Clinical status
Inhibit phosphorylation of tau	Neurofibrillary tangles of hyperphosphorylated tau are the earliest sign of Alzheimer's		Davunetide—successful in phase 2 trial; Nicotinamide (vitamin B_3)—phase 2 trial ongoing
Prevent aggregation of tau protein	Neurofibrillary tangles of hyperphosphorylated tau correlate with severity	Because methylene blue dyes the sclera and urine, a blinded study is unlikely	Methylene blue—successful in phase 2 trial
Preserve mitochondrial function	Latrepirdine has been used previously as an antihistamine in Russia	Depression and dry mouth seen in 14% of participants in a large trial	Latrepirdine—phase 3 trial ongoing
Administer antioxidants	Few side effects; at dietary levels, generally recognized as safe	Limited efficacy in established disease so far; high doses of vitamin E may increase mortality; ginkgo biloba associated with risk of bleeding	Vitamin E—mixed results, ongoing study; Ginkgo biloba—most studies show no effect; Epigallocatechin gallate (EGCG)—phase 2 and 3 trials ongoing; Resveratrol—early trial ongoing
Administer anti-inflammatory drugs	Already FDA-approved for other uses	GI and renal toxicity; might inhibit clearance of Aβ by microglia	Numerous agents have failed in clinical trials

Sources: Duara et al. (2009); Farlow, Miller, & Pejovic (2008); Haass & Selkoe (2007); Mangialasche et al. (2010); Matsuoka et al. (2008); Medina, Caccamo, & Oddo (2011); Neugroschl & Sano (2010); Opar (2008); and Selkoe (2004).

Table 4.2   Frontotemporal Dementia Subtypes

1. *Frontotemporal dementia, behavioral variant*, is a syndrome of marked personality change, loss of executive functioning, and disinhibited and inappropriate behavior for which there is little insight. Neurodegeneration is most apparent in the orbitofrontal and *anterior cingulate cortex*.
2. *Semantic dementia* is characterized as a progressive loss of word meaning and knowledge about objects. At first, superordinate categories may be used in place of the object name (e.g., tool instead of screwdriver) but in time, the knowledge of what a screwdriver is used for may be lost. Here, the atrophy is strongest at the temporal poles, usually moreso on the left.
3. *Progressive nonfluent aphasia* is characterized by slow effortful, telegraphic, and ungrammatical speech; atrophy is found in particular at the left frontal lobe.
4. *Frontotemporal dementia with motor neuron disease* combines the behavioral (although sometimes language) features of frontotemporal dementia with the motor impairment of amyotrophic lateral sclerosis. Degeneration is particularly prominent in the posterior frontal lobe.
5. *Corticobasal syndrome* involves a variety of asymmetrical motor and cognitive deficits implicating the cortex. Motor problems include apraxia, myoclonus, and "alien limb phenomenon," in which the limb is experienced as moving by itself. Atrophy is primarily frontal and parietal.
6. *Supranuclear palsy* involves slowed, jerky movements; spinal rigidity, with backward extension and an upward gaze; and eventually, slurred speech and difficulty swallowing. In this disorder, atrophy is concentrated in the *tegmentum* in the midbrain and the *superior cerebellar peduncle*.

with frontotemporal dementia are those that encode tau or that affect the structure of tau, how much of it is produced, or the ratio between its subforms. In another 33% of cases the protein is *TDP-43*, a protein that normally helps regulate gene transcription and whose aggregation seems to be involved in *amyotrophic lateral sclerosis*. In a few cases, the implicated proteins are *neurofilament* and α-internexin. In some cases, the neurons show *inclusion bodies* suggestive of a proteinopathy, but the constituent protein has not yet been identified (Josephs, 2008; Roberson, 2006).

Treatment is purely supportive, with no empirically validated or disease-modifying therapies yet in place. Hopefully, the recent progress in developing pharmaceutical agents for the neurofibrillary tangles see in Alzheimer's disease will turn out to have benefit for the tau-positive frontotemporal dementias.

Dementia With Lewy Bodies   Dementia with Lewy bodies (DLB) appears late in life as a progressive impairment in cognition and markedly fluctuating alertness and attentiveness, combined with visual hallucinations and such parkinsonian motor impairments as postural instability, gait difficulties, and relative absence of facial expression. (Tremor is seen less often than in Parkinson's disease.) The fluctuations in alertness can take place over minutes, hours, or days (McKeith et al., 2004). Signs of autonomic instability, such as orthostatic hypotension, urinary incontinence, constipation, impotence, and trouble eating and swallowing, are often present as well, as are vivid dreams that the patient may seem to act out (McKeith et al., 2005). Depression, dizziness, and syncope may also be present. In addition to the visual hallucinations there can be systematized delusions and auditory hallucinations (Jellinger, 2007).

DLB is not at all rare, affecting perhaps 0.5% of the nursing-home population over the age of 65, 5.0% of those over age 85, and approximately 10% to 20% of all patients with dementia. This would make it the second most common form of dementia after Alzheimer's disease (McKeith et al., 2004). The average age of onset is 71 years, and men seem to be affected more frequently than women (Kövari, Horvath, & Bouras, 2009). Histologically, there is Alzheimer's-type brain pathology but also the presence of Lewy bodies, which are also found in Alzheimer's but are prototypically characteristic of Parkinson's disease. Despite this overlap in underlying pathophysiology, DLB can be distinguished clinically from Alzheimer's disease and its timecourse differs from that of the dementia accompanying Parkinson's disease (McKeith et al., 2004).

In contrast to Alzheimer's disease, memory is well preserved early in the course, with impairment seen mostly in the realms of executive, visuospatial, and visual-constructive functioning. The hallucinations are well formed and are often of people or animals (Jellinger, 2007).

Pathophysiology. In imaging studies, patients with DLB show some gray matter atrophy, although not nearly as much as in Alzheimer's disease, and their temporal lobe, hippocampus, and amygdala are relatively spared. Rather, in DLB one sees mostly white matter changes and atrophy in the *putamen* and *caudate nucleus. Positron emission tomography (PET)* and *single-photon emission computed tomography (SPECT)* scans show hypometabolism in much of the cortex (Jellinger, 2007). There is also a marked loss of cholinergic neurons, which may account for the visual hallucinations, along with Lewy bodies in the anterior and inferior temporal lobe and amygdala (involved in generating complex visual images) (Kövari, Horvath, & Bouras, 2009; McKeith et al., 2005).

Like Alzheimer's disease, Parkinson's disease, Huntington's disease (*chorea*), and frontotemporal dementia, DLB involves the intraneuronal accumulation of a misfolded protein. In DLB, the protein *alpha-synuclein (AS)* is the same as in Parkinson's (Jellinger, 2007). As with Aβ, we do not yet know whether the key pathology leading to Lewy bodies is the overproduction of AS, its misfolding, or a failure of the normal protein-degrading machinery in the cell (McKeith et al., 2004). What AS should be doing in the cell is not clear. However, its localization to axon terminals suggests that it may play a role in the transport of synaptic vesicles, help regulate neurotransmitter (dopamine) release, or contribute to synaptic plasticity. In vitro studies suggest that when bound to unsaturated lipids in the cell membrane, it may function as an antioxidant. The combined presence of AS and Aβ may be particularly toxic, with Aβ inhibiting the breakdown of AS filaments (Jellinger, 2007).

Lewy bodies probably first appear in the lower medulla and spread over time to the pons, midbrain, *substantia nigra pars compacta*, limbic structures, and finally the prefrontal and association areas of the cortex. Their presence in portions of the limbic system (anterior cingulate and *transentorhinal cortex*) and in the prefrontal cortex is a strong indicator of dementia (Kövari, Horvath, & Bouras, 2009).

Pharmacotherapy. Treatment involves identifying and addressing the most important individual symptoms.

The visual hallucinations and disturbance in rapid-eye-movement *(REM)* sleep are thought to reflect impairment of the cholinergic system. Thus, cholinesterase inhibitors are the treatment of choice. Rivastigmine has the advantage of demonstrated efficacy in a double-blind, placebo-controlled trial (Emre et al., 2004; McKeith et al., 2000). However, comparison with open label data raises the possibility that donepezil has greater efficacy than rivastigmine or galantamine (Bhasin et al., 2007). Presumably because of the prominent cholinergic deficit, cholinesterase inhibitors appear to be more effective for DLB than for Alzheimer's disease (Samuel et al., 2000). Indeed, not just the hallucinations, but sleep disturbance, anxiety, apathy, and cognitive impairments seem to respond to this class of medication (McKeith et al., 2004). The amelioration of visual hallucinations seems to correlate with improvements in cognition and attention, suggesting that poor alertness may play a role in the hallucinations (McKeith et al., 2005).

Depression is generally treated with selective serotonin reuptake inhibitors (SSRIs) or serotonin-norepinephrine reuptake inhibitors (SNRIs), taking care to avoid medications with anticholinergic properties such as amitriptyline or paroxetine (McKeith et al., 2005). Traditional antipsychotics (D_2-receptor blockers) are contraindicated. About half the people with DLB show severe hypersensitivity to neuroleptics, with exacerbation of parkinsonian motor symptoms, impaired consciousness, and a two- to three-fold increase in mortality (McKeith et al., 2005; Tateno, Kobayashi, & Saito, 2009). Atypical antipsychotics are presumed to be safer, but since severe reactions have been reported, they should be used with great care (McKeith et al., 2004, 2005).

The sleep difficulty characteristic of DLB might contribute to the fluctuations in alertness during the day and, through this, to the visual hallucinations (McKeith et al., 2004). Besides cholinesterase inhibitors, treatments for insomnia include clonazepam (0.25 mg qhs), *melatonin* (3 mg qhs), or quetiapine (12.5 mg qhs). The doses may be carefully titrated upward, with monitoring for efficacy and side effects (McKeith et al., 2005). Motor symptoms are generally addressed with levodopa, starting at low doses and titrating slowly so as not to exacerbate the hallucinations and delusions (McKeith et al., 2005).

So far, there are no known disease-modifying treatments for DLB, yet the outlook for neuroprotection does not seem entirely bleak. Despite the marked and progressive neurological impairment, the degree of cortical atrophy in DLB seems to be limited (McKeith et al., 2004).

Nonpharmacological treatment. So far, nonpharmacological strategies have not been studied in DLB. However, because a poor alertness level is thought to contribute to the cognitive impairments and visual hallucinations, a stimulating environment and social interaction may be helpful (McKeith et al., 2005).

Summary of Neurodegenerative Disorders

Amidst all the complexity attending our understanding of the neurodegenerative disorders, a surprising simplicity also emerges: Neurodegenerative diseases that on the surface appear to be very different from one another actually share the common etiology of filaments of misfolded protein. Moreover, when formed into oligomers, these disease-causing amyloid proteins—Aβ, *alpha-synuclein*, huntingtin (in Huntington's chorea), *islet amyloid polypeptide* (in type II diabetes), and the *prion protein*—are so similar to one another in structure that they bind to the same artificial antibody (Haass & Selkoe, 2007). Whether this means that a single intervention will one day effectively treat all these disorders remains in the realm of unfettered possibility.

MENTAL RETARDATION

Mental retardation is highly diverse with respect to its etiology, with only about 25% of cases so far traceable to a known genetic cause and only 50% to 70% traceable to *any* cause. Among those that are genetic, over 1,200 syndromes have been identified (Dierssen & Ramakers, 2006; Gothelf et al., 2005). The more common causes include *Down syndrome*, *fragile X syndrome*, in utero exposure to toxins (including alcohol) or viruses (rubella, herpes simplex, cytomegalovirus), and subsequent exposure to birth trauma, hypoxia, malnutrition, or hypothyroidism (Dierssen & Ramakers, 2006). Here, we focus on two of the more common etiologies.

Down Syndrome

Down syndrome is named after J. Langdon Down, who in the mid-19th century pioneered its recognition as a discrete diagnosis. It is the most common known form of inherited intellectual disability, affecting 1 in 732 live births in the United States (Sherman et al., 2007). About 50% of people with Down syndrome have congenital heart defects (usually involving the septum or heart valves), and 10% have digestive abnormalities, such as a blockage of the upper small intestine (duodenal atresia) or its constriction by a ring of pancreatic tissue (annular pancreas) (Sherman et al., 2007).

Down syndrome results from having a third (extra) copy of chromosome 21 (*trisomy* 21). By far the strongest risk factor is advanced maternal age at conception, presumably because of malfunction of the *meiotic machinery* that separates the two copies of the chromosome. In a small minority of cases, the problem may be that the two copies are joined in such a way that they are particularly difficult to separate (e.g., *telomeric exchange*) (Sherman et al., 2007). Presumably, there are environmental risk factors as well, including maternal exposures before and during pregnancy, but these have not yet been confirmed with any certainty (Sherman et al., 2007). Clinically, the resulting cognitive deficits are a relatively global, mild-to-moderate mental retardation, with *syntax*, *verbal short-term memory*, and declarative memory being particularly affected (Gardiner et al., 2010).

Pathophysiology

Having three copies, rather than two, of chromosome 21 means that most of the proteins encoded by the 500+ genes on the chromosome are overproduced by about 50%. Because these proteins interact with numerous other systems, the underlying physiology of Down syndrome is complex and still poorly understood. In mouse models, however, key features appear to be an alteration in the expression of and responsiveness to *nerve growth factors*, affecting development and neuroplasticity (Gardiner et al., 2010). Macroscopically, there is reduced volume in the human brain, specifically in the cerebellum and the frontal and temporal cortices (Gardiner et al., 2010). Physiologically, again using a mouse model, there is excessive inhibitory input into the hippocampus relative to excitatory input (Hanson et al., 2007).

The gene encoding amyloid precursor protein, which we encounter when discussing Alzheimer's disease, is on chromosome 21. Thus, a consequence of trisomy 21 is an overproduction of this protein, leading to β amyloid deposits as early as age 10, followed by a gradual increase in Alzheimer's-like pathology over the next 20 years (Selkoe, 2004). This is separate from the mental retardation seen from birth in these individuals and raises hope that antiamyloid treatments for Alzheimer's disease will be of benefit in the later stages of Down syndrome as well (Reeves & Garner, 2007).

Pharmacotherapy

An overweighting of inhibitory input to the hippocampus led to the hypothesis that $GABA_A$ antagonists would partially reverse deficits in learning and memory. In fact, very good results have been reported in mice with *pentylenetetrazole* (Fernandez et al., 2007). Intriguingly, the improvement persisted for months after drug administration. Whether similar results can be achieved in humans remains to be seen.

Pentylenetetrazole was used clinically in the 1950s as a circulatory and respiratory stimulant, but FDA approval was withdrawn in 1982 in part due to the risk of seizures with higher doses (Reeves & Garner, 2007).

The reduction in cerebellar volume may be due to diminished responsiveness of its neurons to the growth factor known as *sonic hedgehog*. In mice, a sonic hedgehog agonist restored cerebellar volume (Roper, et al., 2006). Because sonic hedgehog has widespread effects, the risk of unintended consequences is high, and its clinical application will most likely be deferred for many years.

Fragile X Syndrome

The *fragile X syndrome* is relatively common, affecting 1 in 4,500 males and 1 in 9,000 females. Males generally have moderate-to-severe mental retardation, with particular deficits in short-term memory, executive functioning, arithmetic, and visuospatial skills. Females, having an extra, unaffected copy of the X chromosome, may show only mild or even no intellectual disability (Gothelf et al., 2005), depending on the degree to which the mutated versus the normal X chromosome is active (*activation ratio*) (Hagerman, 2006).

Pathophysiology

In this syndrome, a set of three nucleotides on the X chromosome is abnormally repeated and *hypermethylated*, such that a nearby gene, *FRM1*, is silenced (Oostra & Chiurazzi, 2001). This gene encodes a protein that regulates the production of many other proteins in the neuron (Hagerman, 2006). The results may include increased glucocorticoid and decreased $GABA_A$-receptor function, a reduction in AMPA-type glutamate receptors, and enhanced signaling through the metabotropic glutamate receptor type 5 (mGluR5) (Hagerman, 2006). All these effects imply altered synaptic functioning.

The protein encoded by *FMR1* also seems important in developmental axonal path-finding (Oostra & Chiurazzi, 2001). Thus, we might expect disrupted neural circuitry. In fact, imaging studies show an enlarged caudate nucleus in this syndrome, the volume being negatively correlated with IQ, and reduced white matter density in the tracts from the frontal cortex to the head of the caudate (Gothelf et al., 2005). Impaired connections between the frontal cortex and the *basal ganglia* may be a specific effect of the gene silencing. There are also indications of reduced hippocampal volume.

Moreover, dendritic spines in the fragile X syndrome are numerous but of a thin, unstable, immature form rather than the stubby or mushroom-shaped spines typically found in adults and thought to encode memories (Dierssen & Ramakers, 2006). This may suggest a deficit in synaptic pruning (Dierssen & Ramakers, 2006). Alternatively, it may reflect the importance of the metabotropic glutamate receptor type 5 in *long-term synaptic depression*. The enhanced depression may partially counteract the *long-term potentiation* involved in strengthening synapses and lead to weak, poorly developed connections between neurons (Hagerman, 2006).

Pharmacotherapy

In summary, fragile X syndrome involves enhanced functioning of the metabotropic glutamate receptor type 5 and a reduced number of AMPA-type glutamate receptors. This suggests that mGluR5 antagonists and medications to stimulate AMPA receptors would be of use in treating the disorder; both agents are in the early stages of development (Hagerman, 2006). Also, lithium interferes with the production of inositol triphosphate (IP3), part of the downstream signaling cascade of mGlu5, and may turn out to have clinical utility in fragile X (Hagerman, 2006).

Currently, though, treatment focuses on the psychiatric symptoms that often accompany the fragile X syndrome: SSRIs for anxiety, anticonvulsants or atypical antipsychotics (especially aripiprazole) for aggression and mood instability, and stimulant medication for attention deficit–hyperactivity symptoms (Hagerman, 2006).

Rehabilitation

Individuals with the same level of the protein encoded by *FMR1* can differ considerably in level of behavioral and cognitive functioning, with environment probably accounting for much of the difference. Thus, behavioral therapy, occupational and speech therapy, and special education are all important in the treatment of persons with the fragile X syndrome (Hagerman, 2006).

NEURODEVELOPMENTAL DISORDERS

The term *neurodevelopmental disorders* pertains to abnormalities in the growth of the CNS. Convention classifies neurological disorders manifesting in infancy and childhood under this label.

Neurodevelopmental disorders often begin in the earliest stages of embryonic CNS development—that is, growth of the primitive *neural tube*. In humans, the neural tube originates from the outer layer of embryonic cells called the *ectoderm* and rapidly differentiates into sections that evolve into the mature human brain. The primordial rhombencephalon and mesencephalon form the hindbrain and midbrain, respectively. The diencephalon turns into the thalamus and hypothalamus. From the telencephalon area of the neural tube, the cerebral cortex develops.[5] By the end of 18 weeks of gestation, most cortical cells have migrated and differentiated into the gross structure of the human brain. This early embryonic cell stage is often the target of the pathophysiological mechanisms underlying neurodevelopmental disorders. Even minor aberrations can result in clinically severe symptoms in the early stages of neural development. However, the maturation of the brain continues for years in a sensitively timed progression, and both endogenous and exogenous causes of pathology can affect the normal development of the CNS at any stage of growth (Taylor-Flusberg, 1999).

The etiologies of the neurodevelopmental disorders can be broadly separated into two categories: genetic (endogenous) and acquired (exogenous). Genetic disorders can be further delineated into metabolic disorders (e.g., *phenylketonuria*), structural malformations (e.g., microcephaly, tuberous sclerosis), and chromosomal abnormalities (Down syndrome, *Williams' syndrome*). Acquired causes of neurodevelopmental disorders include infectious diseases (e.g., congenital syphilis, encephalitis), injury/trauma/neglect (e.g., premature birth, malnutrition, perinatal asphyxia, shaken-baby syndrome), and *teratogen exposure* (e.g., heavy-metal poisoning).

Neurodevelopmental disorders encompass irregularities across the entire spectrum of neurological function. They may affect only one area, as in sensorimotor disorders (e.g., cerebral palsy, congenital blindness, multiple sclerosis), emotional/behavioral

---

[5]See Figure 3.5.

disorders (e.g., reactive attachment disorders, ADHD), cognitive disorders (e.g., intellectual disability, autism), and seizure disorders, or they may impact multiple domains, depending on the etiology, location, and course of the disorder (e.g., fetal alcohol syndrome, traumatic brain injury).

In the following sections, we review some common and/or well-defined examples of neurodevelopmental disorders that medical psychologists are likely to encounter in clinical practice or in the scientific literature. There are over 100 defined inherited diseases of the central and peripheral nervous systems (Wiedeholt, 2000), so only a few have been selected for this review.

Although very familiar to most readers, *autism spectrum disorder* will be reviewed here in order to address the changes in diagnostic criteria and classifications proposed in the upcoming fifth edition of the *Diagnostic and Statistical Manual of Mental Disorders* by the American Psychiatric Association (*DSM-5*). Motor cortex dysfunction, traumatic brain injury (TBI), and seizures are reviewed elsewhere in more detail in this volume, as is mental retardation. Most readers of this resource are already well-versed in the field of emotional/behavioral disorders of childhood, and for this reason some of the more ubiquitous *DSM* disorders involving psychosocial etiologies (e.g., reactive attachment disorder) or mixed sociobiological etiologies (e.g., ADHD) will not be covered here. Finally, disorders that are currently deemed too inconclusive or controversial to be categorized as neurodevelopmental disorders have been omitted. For example, sensory integration dysfunction (sensory processing disorders) and Pediatric Autoimmune Neuropsychiatric Disease Associated with Streptococcus (*PANDAS*) have not yet been recognized as diagnoses in the *DSM* or the International Classification of Disease, despite being currently diagnosed in clinical settings. Readers are encouraged to continue to follow the developing empirical research and wait for future references for guidance.

Autism Spectrum Disorder

Autistic disorder is an example of a complex disorder with evidence of genetic and acquired pathophysiology that manifests numerous cognitive, sensorimotor, and behavioral symptoms. *Autism spectrum disorder* (ASD) is a term used to describe a series of psychiatric and neurological disorders called *pervasive developmental disorders* that includes autistic disorder. The five forms of ASD previously delineated in the *DSM-IV* were autistic disorder, Asperger's syndrome, Rett's disorder, childhood disintegrative disorder, and pervasive developmental disorder–not otherwise specified (PDD-NOS) (American Psychiatric Association, 2000). However, the *DSM-5* work group of the American Psychiatric Association (American Psychiatric Association, 2011) has proposed subsuming only four of the previous pervasive developmental disorders under the one diagnostic code of autistic disorder—autism spectrum disorder—thus deleting Rett's disorder from this listing in the *DSM-5*.

Epidemiological reviews of autism spectrum disorders are marred by inconsistencies. In the 1990s, the incidence of autism diagnoses increased incongruously, most likely due to changes in definitions, public awareness, and availability of services. With the advent of new diagnostic criteria to be implemented in the *DSM-5*, the data will likely be further complicated. However, current estimates suggest a prevalence of all autism spectrum disorders to be around 6 per 1,000 children in the United States. Estimates of the individual ASD conditions are 1 to 2 per 1,000 for autistic disorder, 0.6 per 1,000 for Asperger's syndrome, 0.02 per 1,000 for childhood disintegrative disorder, and up to 3.7 per 1,000 for PDD-NOS (Newschaffer et al., 2007).

The term *autism spectrum disorder* has often been used interchangeably by the lay public to describe the prototypical diagnosis of autistic disorder. With the proposed changes of the *DSM-5* work group, there will be only one diagnosis remaining. The proposed *DSM-5* guidelines for autism spectrum disorder require the following:

A. Persistent deficits in social communication and social interaction across contexts, not accounted for by general developmental delays, and manifest by all three of the following:
   1. Deficits in social-emotional reciprocity; ranging from abnormal social approach and failure of normal back-and-forth conversation through reduced sharing of interests, emotions, and affect and response to total lack of initiation of social interaction.
   2. Deficits in nonverbal communicative behaviors used for social interaction, ranging from poorly integrated verbal and nonverbal communication through abnormalities in eye contact and body-language or deficits in understanding and use of nonverbal communication to total lack of facial expression or gestures.
   3. Deficits in developing and maintaining relationships appropriate to developmental level (beyond those with caregivers), ranging from difficulties adjusting behavior to suit different social contexts through difficulties in sharing imaginative play and in making friends to an apparent absence of interest in people.
B. Restricted, repetitive patterns of behavior, interests, or activities as manifested by at least two of the following:
   1. Stereotyped or repetitive speech, motor movements, or use of objects (such as simple motor stereotypes, echolalia, repetitive use of objects, or idiosyncratic phrases).
   2. Excessive adherence to routines, ritualized patterns of verbal or nonverbal behavior, or excessive resistance to change (such as motoric rituals, insistence on same route or food, repetitive questioning, or extreme distress at small changes).
   3. Highly restricted, fixated interests that are abnormal in intensity or focus (such as strong attachment to or preoccupation with unusual objects, excessively circumscribed or perseverative interests).
   4. Hyper- or hyporeactivity to sensory input or unusual interest in sensory aspects of environment (such as apparent indifference to pain/heat/cold, adverse response to specific sounds or textures, excessive smelling or touching of objects, fascination with lights or spinning objects).

The proposed criteria conceptualize the previous distinct disorders as points on the spectrum of the single disorder. The clinical presentation that was once termed Asperger's syndrome will now meet the new criteria for autistic disorder because the previous autistic disorder criterion of spoken-language deficits has been removed. Although estimates that as many as 75% of patients currently diagnosed with autistic disorder display IQs in the intellectual disability range, the new criteria do not address cognitive delays or deficits. Patients who meet the criteria for the diagnosis of both autistic disorder and intellectual disability will be diagnosed with both disorders. Those patients previously diagnosed with Asperger's syndrome, who tend to function in the average to superior intellectual range, will still meet the ASD criteria without being diagnosed with intellectual disability. Rett's syndrome (referred to as "Rett's disorder" in the *DSM-IV*) has also been removed from the proposed *DSM-5* but is no longer included in the autism spectrum disorders. Now that a specific genetic marker has been identified as causing Rett's syndrome, it will now be considered an etiological specifier to be added on to the diagnosis of autistic disorder when appropriate (e.g., "autistic disorder associated with a known medical condition of Rett's disorder"). Many genetic disorders are known to have high rates of comorbidity with autistic disorder (e.g., fragile X syndrome, tuberous sclerosis), and Rett's syndrome will now be added to the list.

The comorbidity with genetically linked disorders is evidence of the heritability influence on autistic disorder. Other genetic support includes twin studies that suggest the heritability of 0.7 to 0.9 for ASD; evidence suggests that siblings of autistic children are about 25 times more likely to be diagnosed with autism than the general population (Geschwind, 2009). Despite this robust evidence, a direct genetic link or defect has still not been identified, and other theories continue to be explored. The teratogen theory is supported by some evidence. One study reported an association between maternal exposure to *organochlorine pesticides* in the first trimester of pregnancy and the subsequent development of ASD in the child (Samson, 2007). However, the celebrity-endorsed claims of vaccination-induced ASD have not produced much empirical support.[6]

Brain-imaging studies continue to look for specific pathophysiological mechanisms to explain ASD. For instance, postmortem analysis of the brains of autistic children has suggested reductions for $GABA_B$ in the cingulate cortex and *fusiform gyrus*. The cingulate cortex is associated with the evaluation of social relationships, emotions, and cognition. The fusiform gyrus is associated with evaluating faces and facial expressions (Oblak, Gibbs, & Blatt, 2010). Furthermore, research has consistently demonstrated high levels of platelet serotonin in the bloodstream of autistic children (Cuccaro et al., 1993), and a disruption in the normal brain synthesis of serotonin in autistic children and their family members (Chugani et al., 1999). However, the mechanism of autistic disorder continues to prove complex, and the "smoking gun" has yet to be identified.

There does not seem to be any clear pharmacological treatment that alleviates the primary symptoms of autism. Nonetheless, there is research demonstrating the effective use of medications to manage secondary symptoms. For instance, atypical antipsychotics might help to minimize the self-harm caused by stereotypic movements and may decrease aggression in emotional dysregulation. Antidepressants and stimulants might help increase focus and decrease restricted interests. Finally, antiepileptic medications are used to control seizures that can be comorbid with autistic disorder.

Fetal Alcohol Syndrome

Fetal alcohol syndrome is an example of an acquired neurodevelopmental disorder. According to one study, fetal alcohol syndrome is the leading preventable cause of

---

[6]The British medical journal *Lancet* recently announced that a 1998 study published in that journal by the physician Andrew Wakefield linking autism to vaccination was an elaborate fraud, perpetrated by the author of the article (Wakefield et al., 1998).

intellectual disability in the world (Abel & Sokol, 1987). It is 100% preventable if the mother does not use alcohol during pregnancy. Alcohol can damage the brain at any point during a pregnancy, and no amount of alcohol has been identified as safe to drink. Alcohol crosses the placenta and results in fetal alcohol concentrations comparable to those in the mother, whereas clearance of alcohol from the fetal liver is less than 10% of that in the mother. The Centers for Disease Control and Prevention estimate that approximately 12% of pregnant women reported drinking alcohol within 30 days prior to being surveyed (CDC, 2009).

Statistical analysis is difficult due to inconsistent diagnostic criteria and limited methodological factors. Nevertheless, the incidence of disorders related to fetal alcohol syndrome in the United States is estimated to be 1 to 3 cases per 1,000 live births, and as high as 1 out of 100 live births when evaluated according to expanded criteria for alcohol-related neurodevelopmental disorders (Sampson, Streissguth, & Bookstein, 1997).

The terms *fetal alcohol spectrum disorders* and *alcohol-related neurodevelopmental disorders* are used to describe patients with dysfunctions related to prenatal alcohol that do not display the characteristic facial features required in other diagnostic systems. For example, the Centers for Disease Control and Prevention requires evidence of prenatal exposure to alcohol, significant growth deficits, functional CNS abnormalities, and the presence of three specific structural anomalies in order for fetal alcohol syndrome to be diagnosed. The three facial abnormalities include a smooth *philtrum*, thin vermilion border of the upper lip (appearing as a thin upper lip), and short *palpebral fissures* (appearing as decreased width of the eyes). A smooth philtrum appears as a flattening of the indentation between the nose and upper lip, and this divot (or groove) flattens with increased prenatal alcohol exposure. All three facial signs increase in degree of severity relative to the degree of prenatal exposure.

The structural effects on the brain are also affected by the degree, and timing, of the prenatal exposure to alcohol. Myriad anatomical anomalies are common. These include microcephaly, agenesis of the corpus callosum, and *cerebellar hypoplasia* (Stratton, Howe, & Battaglia, 1996). Other systems of the body are affected as well. Growth deficiency (defined as lower than the 10th percentile for normal height and weight, adjusted for gestational age) is also a characteristic trait of fetal alcohol syndrome patients. Other structural signs common to fetal alcohol syndrome include skeletal defects, cardiac flaws, and renal impairments.

The neurobehavioral symptoms of fetal alcohol syndrome are numerous. Intellectual disabilities and learning disorders are some of the more familiar symptoms. Other related disabilities include hyperactivity and inattention, impulse control problems, deficient fine motor skills, hearing loss, memory impairment, language delays, seizure disorder, and poor interpersonal skills. Owing to the obvious behavioral difficulties facing these children early in development, they are more likely to be diagnosed with disorders such as ADHD, oppositional defiant disorder, mood disorders, and antisocial behavior/conduct disorder. Some of these disorders can develop as secondary disabilities later on. There is also evidence to suggest that children diagnosed with fetal alcohol syndrome are at high risk for developing substance abuse disorders (Streissguth et al., 1996). Although there are numerous treatment modalities that effectively mitigate or manage these secondary disorders, there is no evidence that pharmacological and behavioral interventions are successful in reversing the primary symptoms in patients diagnosed with fetal alcohol syndrome.

GENETICALLY LINKED INTELLECTUAL DISORDERS

Angelman Syndrome/Prader-Willi Syndrome

Angelman syndrome is an example of genetic imprinting in which genes are expressed in a child according to the genotype of the carrier-parent, in classic Mendelian fashion. *Prader-Willi syndrome* was the first intellectual disorder proven to result from genetic imprinting in humans. Both the Angelman and Prader-Willi syndromes result from the absence or inactivation of genes on chromosome 15. However, in Angelman the genetic defect is inherited from the mother and in Prader-Willi it is inherited from the father. Both disorders are characterized by intellectual and developmental delays, severely impaired speech, obesity, seizure disorder, stereotypical movements (especially jerking of the hands that looks like the flapping of wings), excessive laughter or smiling, and an outgoing, happy demeanor and intense desire for social interaction (Ledbetter et al., 1981). Both are extremely rare, yet they display a very recognizable phenotype. Diagnosis is based on developmental delays, characteristic hand-flapping and personality traits, abnormal EEG and seizures, and deletion or inactivity on chromosome 15. There is no cure for either the Angelman or the Prader-Willi syndrome; however, medications can be used to manage seizures.

Rett's Syndrome

Rett's syndrome was formerly classified as a pervasive developmental disorder. However, since the initial publication of the most recent version of the *DSM-IV*, evidence has emerged suggesting that the disorder is caused by mutations in the MECP2 gene, located on the X chromosome. The MECP2 protein is apparently crucial for nervous system development beyond the initial stages (Maezawa et al., 2009). In less than 10% of patients with Rett's syndrome, the mutation is found on the genes for CDKL5 or FOXG1; in rare cases, no gene mutation can be identified. It is thought that 95% of cases involve de novo mutations in the fetus. Virtually all known cases are female. It is believed that male fetuses with the mutated X chromosome do not survive to term because the male fetus has only one defective X chromosome, whereas females have one defective and one normal X chromosome. All males with Rett's syndrome known to have survived have also been diagnosed with Klinefelter's syndrome, in which the male has an extra X chromosome in addition to the Y chromosome and the defective X chromosome (XXY).

The progression of Rett's syndrome begins with seemingly healthy development for 6 to 18 months. After the initial progression, a period of stagnation begins, which is then followed by a period of regression of previously acquired developmental skills regress. Early on, the regression may appear similar to autistic behavior. The child may display stereotypical hand-flailing, loss of oral language and motor skills, general lack of interest in others, and inconsolable fits. The Rett child will also display distinctive breath-holding, sighing, and hyperventilation. Following the regression period, some functioning may return, including social interest; however, the child will rarely regain vocal communication or purposeful use of hands.

Most girls with Rett's syndrome survive to adulthood and into their 50s and 60s, although most continue to have severe disability. Patients diagnosed with this syndrome are prone to seizures, gastrointestinal dysfunction, and scoliosis. Surgeries and lifelong therapy may be necessary, depending on the severity of the disability.

Smith-Magenis Syndrome

The Smith-Magenis syndrome (SMS) is an example of a disorder that is often confused with Down syndrome, yet as development continues toward puberty, the disorder takes on its own characteristics. Like Down syndrome, SMS is not inherited but is still congenital and is caused by genetic aberration of the *gametes* (as in Down syndrome). SMS has been linked to deletions in the gene for retinoic acid–induced 1 (RAI-1) of the short arm (p) of chromosome 17, so another name for this disorder is the 17p– syndrome (Smith et al., 1986). The genetic abnormalities in SMS are thought to occur during formation of the reproductive cells (eggs or sperm) or during early fetal development. Studies have not indicated heritability contributions, and SMS patients are typically the only ones with SMS in their families. The chance of conceiving with an aberrant egg or cell increases with age. However, the disorder is still exceedingly rare, occurring in about 1 in 25,000 individuals.

SMS is often confused with Down syndrome in childhood, but the phenotypical signs become more apparent with age, and a definitive diagnosis can be made with genetic testing. The most characteristic traits in SMS patients are *brachycephaly* (in which the face appears similar to the Down syndrome faces until puberty), mild-to-moderate mental retardation (with an intellectual range similar to that in Down syndrome), a hoarse voice (which becomes distinct from that in Down syndrome with age), and an aggressive/labile personality. SMS patients also tend to display common behavioral problems that might differentiate them from other intellectual disabilities, such as self-soothing by hugging themselves and licking of the fingers, excitable touching of others, and inverted sleep-disorder patterns. Along with its resemblance to Down syndrome, this disorder is often misdiagnosed as other psychiatric disorders, including ADHD, autistic disorder, and obsessive-compulsive disorder (OCD), owing to their characteristic behaviors.

There is no cure for SMS. However, numerous other sites besides the neurobehavioral system are affected by the genetic abnormality and can be treated. For instance, scoliosis, cardiac defects, hearing/vestibular disturbances, vision deficits, and kidney defects are symptoms of SMS that might respond to medical treatment. Likewise, medications can be utilized to manage symptoms such as sleep disturbance, hyperactivity, and emotional lability.

Tuberous Sclerosis and Neurofibromatosis

Tuberous sclerosis is an example of a rare genetic disease that causes structural abnormalities across multiple systems in the body. The genetic disturbance is not directly related to cognitive function; however, when these nonmalignant tumors grow in the brain, neurodevelopmental disorders will result. Symptoms can range from intellectual disability, cognitive disturbance, seizures, and increased intracranial pressure to numerous other neurological dysfunctions. Typically, CNS symptoms may manifest as similar to intellectual disabilities, learning disorders, ADHD, OCD, or autistic disorder. One study claimed that between 25% and 60% of patients with tuberous sclerosis met the behavioral criteria for autistic spectrum disorder (Harrison & Bolton, 1997). The disease is caused by a mutation of either of two genes that encode for the proteins hamartin and tuberin. These two proteins act as tumor-growth suppressors and are thus agents that regulate cell proliferation and differentiation. Without the protein tumor supressors, tumors will affect the entire body. Signs depend upon the location and severity of the disorder and can range from mild skin abnormalities to kidney failure, stroke, and cancer. Treatment depends on the location and severity of the disorder. Treatment with the immunosuppressant drug *rapamycin* was found to be effective at shrinking tumors in animals. Human studies are being conducted to test rapamycin in the treatment of tuberous sclerosis (Tuberous Sclerosis Alliance, 2009).

Although central *neurofibromatosis* and tuberous sclerosis are genetically distinct diseases, both produce *hamartomas* (benign focal malformations) of supporting cells in the CNS, as well as malformation of other tissues. In neurofibromatosis, tumors grow within the nervous system, beginning in the supporting cells that surround the nerves and the myelin sheath. In both these disorders, tumors grow on nerves and lead to other abnormalities, such as skin changes and bone deformities. The major symptom is usually pain, together with tingling and other sensory changes.

Wilson's Disease

Wilson's disease is an example of a disorder that manifests neurological symptoms, including mental deficiency (Das & Ray, 2006), through a genetic mutation that affects the metabolism of copper. This mechanism is absent in early neurodevelopmental stages and does not exhibit neurological dysfunction until relatively later in life (e.g., adolescence and adulthood). The pathophysiology of Wilson's disease involves genes that control the transport of copper out of the bloodstream and into the liver for breakdown and storage. The mutated gene disrupts this normal metabolic mechanism, and excessive amounts of copper are transported to tissues throughout the body. The copper migrates particularly to the kidneys, eyes, and brain. In the brain, copper tends to inordinately affect the basal ganglia, putamen, and globus pallidus, which disturbs coordination of movement, processing of stimuli, and regulation of mood.

Wilson's disease usually becomes manifest between the ages of 10 and 20 years. The disease occurs in 1 to 4 people per 1,000. Around 40% of symptoms pertain to hepatic functioning, 35% are neurological, and 10% are psychiatric (Ala et al., 2007). Symptoms will normally present in childhood as liver dysfunction. However, in young adults, psychiatric and neurological symptoms may appear. These include dysarthria, dysphagia, tremor, dystonia, headache, seizure, emotional lability, and psychosis. Once symptoms become evident, death may ensue within 2 to 3 years if no treatment is begun. Treatment consists primarily of copper-removing medications such as *penicillamine*. Restrictive diets and possible liver transplant are also potential treatments (Wiederholt, 2000).

VASCULAR DISORDERS OF THE NERVOUS SYSTEM

Cerebrovascular disease is defined as a pathological process involving the blood vessels in the brain. The pathophysiological mechanisms underlying this disease include occlusion, rupture, and malformation of the veins, arteries, and capillaries of the brain, but cerebrovascular disease can also result from damage due to excessive pressure and necrosis from bleeding into cerebral cavities.

Cerebrovascular Accident

The most common type of cerebrovascular disease is the *cerebrovascular accident—* more commonly referred to as a stroke. A stroke is a focal, nonconvulsive, neurological deficit caused by a vascular lesion. The lesion results in an adequate supply of oxygen and glucose to the brain. The lack of oxygen is known as *ischemia*. Over time, ischemia can progress to *infarction* (the formation of an area of cell death) in a specific part of the brain. The ensuing neurological dysfunction is related to the site affected by the ischemia or infarction. During a stroke, neurological dysfunction occurs suddenly, but the sequelae may last longer than 24 hours, if the victim survives that long.

Cerebrovascular accident is the third leading cause of death in the United States (about 144,000 annually), and it is the leading cause of serious, long-term disability (AmericanHeart.org, 2010). Each year, about 795,000 people suffer a stroke, and about 185,000 of these strokes represent recurrent attacks. Nearly three-fourths of all strokes occur in people over the age of 65. Each year, about 55,000 more women than men have a stroke. However, the incidence of stroke among men younger than 55 years is greater than that in women. The rate of stroke in African-Americans is higher than that in European Americans across the life span.

Ischemic Strokes

The most common type of stroke is the obstructive ischemic stroke, accounting for 87% of all strokes. Such strokes are called "ischemic" because when a cerebral artery becomes completely blocked, or occluded, a sufficient amount of oxygen cannot be delivered to areas of the brain beyond the occlusion. Brain cells that are not adequately oxygenated begin to die, and eventually infarction occurs.

There are several mechanisms by which the blood vessels become occluded in an ischemic stroke. An event caused by a traveling clot (or *embolus*) is described as a *cerebral embolism*. The "clotting" mass is commonly a vascular fatty plaque that breaks off from the vessel wall and enters the bloodstream. Clots can also consist of coagulated blood, a bundle of foreign material, a clump of bacteria, or even a conglomeration of gas bubbles. Emboli can travel from their point of origin and become obstructive either suddenly or over the course of a few days. Sometimes a small plug of cells will increase in mass like a snowball as it travels, eventually becoming large enough to block the flow of blood through the vessel. At other times the embolus might be traveling from a larger blood vessel into a smaller one, finally becoming lodged within a restrictive space and causing a rapid onset of symptoms.

Another typical kind of occlusion results from *cerebral thrombosis*. This occurs when fatty plaques build up on the arterial walls and narrow the diameter of the blood vessel (the lumen) enough to restrict blood flow. Cerebral thromboses can develop over hours or days and could present clinically as a slow progression of CNS dysfunction.

Occlusion can also develop as a result of *cerebral atherosclerosis* and *cerebral vasculitis*. Cerebral atherosclerosis is caused by the thickening and hardening of the arteries, resulting in restricted blood flow. In cerebral vasculitis, inflammation and spasm of the blood vessel decreases the size of the lumen and disrupts blood flow.

Intracerebral Hemorrhagic Strokes

The second most frequently occurring stroke is the *intracerebral hemorrhage*, accounting for 10% of strokes in the United States. Intracerebral hemorrhage is defined as excessive bleeding inside the brain. The major causes are hypertension, blood disorders, exposure to toxins, and cerebral artery defects. The onset of hemorrhagic strokes is rapid and the prognosis is poor in victims who remain unconscious for longer than 48 hours.

A ruptured *aneurysm*—usually secondary to hypertension—is the most common cause of hemorrhagic stroke. An aneurysm is a balloon-like protrusion of the blood vessel wall that can be the result of hypertension, congenital vascular defects, occlusion, or infection. Rupture of a weakened vascular wall will produce excessive bleeding into the intracerebral space. Furthermore, intracranial hemorrhage can also be caused by congenital *arteriovenous malformations* that are susceptible to vessel leakage.

Subarachnoid hemorrhage, or bleeding into the space between the arachnoid membrane and the pia mater, which cover the brain, occurs in approximately 3% of strokes. This type of hemorrhage can lead to immense pressure on brain tissue and thus cause severe injury. Although subarachnoid hemorrhages can be caused by a traumatic brain injury as well as a stroke, most cases result from rupture of a brain aneurysm. The primary presentation of a subarachnoid hemorrhage is a "thunderclap headache," so severe and sudden that it warrants treatment in the Emergency Department. Subarachnoid hemorrhage is associated with a poor prognosis and a 50% mortality rate.

Distribution of Blood Supply to the Brain

The dysfunction following a cerebrovascular accident depends largely on the site in the brain affected by the injury. Many specific structures in the cerebrovascular system are at greater risk for injury and generate certain predictable presentations owing to their locations. It is important to familiarize oneself with the major pathways of circulation in order to understand the pathophysiology of cerebrovascular disease.

Although the brain represents only 2% of the body by weight, it is supplied with about 20% of the body's total blood supply. Blood flows from the neck into the brain through two branches of major blood vessels—the internal carotid arteries and the vertebral arteries. The two vertebral arteries flow through the cervical spine toward the posterior part of the brain, where they conjoin to form the *basilar artery* at the base of the medulla oblongata. The basilar artery is the primary blood vessel supplying the brainstem. The two internal carotid arteries—one left and one right—flow through the neck to supply the anterior part of the brain. These arteries branch out to form the anterior cerebral arteries and the middle cerebral arteries.

The basilar artery, the two internal carotid arteries, and the two anterior cerebral arteries connect together to form the *circle of Willis* before splitting up into smaller branches to provide the primary blood supply of the brain. (See Figure 4.1.) If one thinks of the cerebrovascular system as a transportation route for shipping blood, the circle of Willis would be the "bypass" or "roundabout" in which the major highways join together before splitting into smaller local roads in "Brain City." The circle of Willis creates multiple routes by which blood can reach its destination. As in a circular bypass in a major city, if there is blocked traffic on one road, the vehicles (blood cells, in this analogy) can change directions and find a detour. This structural design reduces the chances of ischemia in the event of a cerebrovascular occlusion.

The *anterior cerebral arteries* (both left and right) supply blood to the anterior areas of the cerebrum: the orbital frontal lobes, cingulate gyrus, medial surface of the frontal lobe, parietal lobes, anterior portions of the corpus callosum, anterior portions of the basal ganglia, and internal capsule. Motor and sensory functions in the contralateral lower limbs are significantly impacted by injury. Incontinence often occurs with anterior cerebral artery occlusion. However, if the blockage occurs prior to reaching

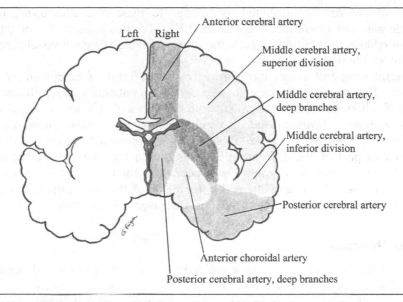

Anterior cerebral artery

Left   Right

Middle cerebral artery, superior division

Middle cerebral artery, deep branches

Middle cerebral artery, inferior division

Posterior cerebral artery

Anterior choroidal artery

Posterior cerebral artery, deep branches

Figure 4.1   Blood Supply to the Brain
Adapted from Blumenfeld, H. (2010). *Neuroanatomy through clinical cases* (2nd ed.). Sunderland, MA: Sinauer Associates.

the anterior communicating artery, which connects the right and left anterior cerebral arteries, functioning is usually well preserved owing to collateral circulation.

The *posterior cerebral arteries* arise out of the basilar artery. As the name indicates, they primarily irrigate the posterior portion of the cerebrum (occipital lobe, visual cortex, and parts of the temporal lobe) but also serve the cerebellum and brainstem. Occlusion of the posterior cerebral arteries causes visual problems, vestibular difficulties, pain and temperature insensitivity, and dysfunction of the cranial nerves (oculomotor, facial, vagus, and hypoglossal nerves).

The *middle cerebral arteries* (both left and right) are not considered part of the circle of Willis; structurally, they are located between the anterior and posterior cerebral arteries. They are the largest cerebral arteries and supply the most extensive area of the cerebral cortex, much of the lateral aspects of the hemispheres, and parts of the lateral cerebrum, anterior temporal lobes, and insular cortices, as well as Broca's and Wernicke's areas. As branches of the internal carotid arteries, the middle cerebral arteries are commonly involved in cerebral thrombosis, since plaques tend to form in these vessels. Several very distinct signs are seen with occlusion of the middle cerebral arteries, such as contralateral loss of sensory-motor control of the face and upper extremities. Injury to the dominant hemisphere (usually left) will usually generate aphasia symptoms, while injury to the nondominant hemisphere might cause neglect syndromes. Midbrain syndrome (*Weber's syndrome*) is also a common reaction. A very reliable sign of damage to the middle cerebral arteries is the *ipsilesional gaze shift*, in which the pupils look toward the side of the body that has been affected by the injury.

Many small blood vessels branch from the middle cerebral arteries and travel deep into the brain to supply the thalamus, basal ganglia, and internal capsule. *Lacunar disease* is caused by rupture or occlusion of these small blood vessels. Almost 25% of ischemic strokes can be attributed to damage to these structures owing to their minuscule diameter (Weinstein & Swanson, 1998). For this reason, 70% of intracerebral hemorrhages in hypertensive patients can be attributed to small-vessel ruptures in this region of the brain.

A careful review of recent medical history and lifestyle is helpful in ruling out cerebrovascular disease as the cause of impairment in patients with significant neurological difficulties. For instance, a patient who presents with a history of hypertension, diabetes, coronary heart disease, hypercholesterolemia, and/or substance abuse (tobacco) is at high risk for stroke. In such cases, cerebrovascular disease should be considered as part of the differential diagnosis when one is exploring the etiology of the patient's neurological symptoms. Especially in the evaluation of patients with dementia, an understanding of the pathophysiology of the symptoms can be used to differentiate vascular dementia from various other types of dementia.

Vascular Dementia

Vascular dementia tends to display a rapid progression of symptoms, depending on the area and mechanism of action of the injury. In contrast, many other neurological disorders—such as Alzheimer's dementia, Lewy body disease, Parkinson's disease, and Huntington's chorea—display a slow and subtle progression in cognitive impairment. Vascular dementia is second only to Alzheimer's as the most frequent type of dementia diagnosed in the United States. The prevalence is 1.5% in most western countries. Around 25% of all stroke victims develop dementia symptoms within 1 year of the cerebrovascualr accident (Knopman, Rocca, & Cha, 2002). The prognosis is poorer for patients diagnosed with vascular dementia, as opposed to Alzheimer's dementia, with 39% of patients dying within 5 years (Brodaty et al., 1993). Vascular dementia can put patients at higher risk for Alzheimer's disease. In fact, symptoms often result from a combination of both neurovascular disease and Alzheimer's disease.

Like any other neurovascular disease, dementia can be caused by hemorrhage, occlusion, vascular disease, or any combination thereof. It can result from injury to a specific area of the brain or from an aggregation of insults to multiple sites, or it can be due to one large stroke or several smaller/briefer infarctions. These brief cerebrovascular accidents are known as *transient ischemic attacks* (TIAs).

Transient Ischemic Attacks

TIAs (mini-strokes) have traditionally been distinguished from stroke because symptoms are temporary, lasting less than 24 hours. The American Heart Association and American Stroke Association have recently adopted a definition that focuses more on the lack of permanent infarction and less on the limited time course. The new criteria describe "a transient episode of neurological dysfunction caused by focal brain, spinal-cord, or retinal ischemia, without acute infarction" (Easton et al., 2009).

Symptoms arising from a TIA are acute and focused and usually resolve within 1 hour. They include temporary numbness or tingling (paresthesia), weakness on one side of the body (hemiparesis), disorientation and difficulty speaking (aphasia), loss of vision in one or both eyes (amaurosis fugax), and sudden severe headache. Loss of consciousness is very uncommon. In the United States, 200,000 to 500,000 people suffer TIAs annually. Mini-strokes are often perceived as being a warning sign for an impending full-blown stroke, but patients who experience a TIA have only a 15% probability of having another within 3 months, although about one third of patients with a TIA will have an acute stroke at some time in the future; still, the risk of sudden death from a heart attack is higher in TIA patients than the risk of death from stroke (Adams et al., 2003).

Treatment of Vascular Dementia

No approved pharmacological treatment exists for vascular dementia, which should be managed in a manner designed to decrease targeted symptoms. For example, psychotropic medications can be used to treat secondary symptoms of vascular dementia, such as anxiety and psychosis. Preventive measures should be considered, and risk factors for cerebrovascular disease (e.g., tobacco dependence) should be treated when present. Cholinesterase inhibitors, which include donepezil, rivastigmine, and galantamine, have proven symptomatic efficacy in Alzheimer's disease and may also have a role in the treatment of vascular dementia (Bowler, 2003).

OTHER CNS DISORDERS

Multiple Sclerosis

Multiple sclerosis (MS) is an autoimmune disease affecting the myelin sheaths of nerves in the brain and spinal cord. Its onset is generally between ages 20 and 50, and it is twice as common in women as in men (Milo & Kahana, 2010). Symptoms can include numbness and paresthesia, localized muscle weakness, lack of coordination, visual disturbances affecting one eye, double vision, dizziness, and vertigo (Milo & Kahana, 2010). Approximately 85% of cases start with intermittent relapses that may resolve partially or completely (relapsing-remitting MS), which typically shifts over 10 to 15 years to a steady, progressive course (secondary progressive MS). For 15% of patients, the disease is steadily progressive from the outset (primary progressive MS) (Milo & Kahana, 2010). Globally, about 1 million people are affected by MS (Martinelli Boneschi et al., 2003).

The hallmark of MS is the presence of localized regions of demyelination, disseminated in space (multiple locations within the CNS) and in time (new lesions appearing in a relapsing or progressive course). The foundation of the diagnosis is the neurological exam, while evidence of white matter lesions on magnetic resonance imaging (MRI) and the presence of abnormal bands of immunoglobulin G on cerebral spinal fluid analysis support the diagnosis and help rule out alternative diseases. A delay in the visual evoked response can indicate the presence of a lesion in the visual pathways (Myhr, 2008).

The lesions of MS can occur in any part of the brain or spinal cord, leading to neurological deficits that vary from person to person and over time in the same person (Lassmann, 2007). However, because they tend to start in the vicinity of small veins, lesions are more common where veins are plentiful: in the optic tracts and nerves, the subcortical white matter, the white matter around the ventricles, the *cerebral peduncles*, and the spinal cord (Lassman, et al., 2011).

Genetics is key in susceptibility to the disease, and the concordance rate for MS in monozygotic twins is 30%. That the rate is well below 100%, however, suggests that the disease also requires an environmental trigger. What this trigger might be is not known, but as a result of epidemiological studies, suspicion has fallen on infections during childhood or adolescence (Lassmann et al., 2011), particularly with the Epstein-Barr virus, a portion of whose nuclear antigen closely resembles a segment of myelin basic protein (Milo & Kahana, 2010). Thus, an immune response to the virus might accidentally target myelin as well. Other factors associated with MS are living in a northern latitude, being of northern European descent, having limited exposure to sunlight, and having inadequate levels of vitamin D (since sunlight and vitamin D modulate the immune system) (Milo & Kahana, 2010).

Pathophysiology

The relapsing-remitting phase of MS, in which plaques form and then burn out or sometimes heal, and the progressive phase, characterized by diffuse and increasing brain atrophy, appear to be two relatively independent processes (Lassmann, 2007).

The plaques form around venules because the acute inflammation that causes their formation is driven by infiltrating *lymphocytes*. These lymphocytes appear to destroy the myelin sheath and sometimes the *oligodendrocytes*. The axons themselves are not targeted and may be spared, or they may sustain collateral damage. Sometimes the demyelination is followed by a later stage of remyelination, depending on how well the glial progenitor cells have held up and on whether the chemical environment of the plaque is conducive to remyelination (Lassmann, 2011).

The chronic, progressive stage of MS seems to involve two processes: One consists of much greater demyelination in the cortex, extending in from the meninges, suggesting the diffusion of an inflammatory or toxic factor, and the other is diffuse atrophy throughout the brain, possibly because of chronic, low-grade inflammation by the microglia (Lassmann, 2007).

Pharmacotherapy

Intravenous and/or oral methylprednisolone is used to shorten the duration of acute relapses. However, it does not seem to increase the amount of recovery or lower the risk of future relapses (Sellenbjerg et al., 2005). To improve long-term prognosis, four therapies have been approved by the FDA to ameliorate the disease course: three are immunomodulatory (interferon-β, glatiramer acetate, and natalizumab), and one is immunosuppressive (mitoxantrone) (Myhr, 2008).

The available immunomodulator medications merely slow the course of relapsing-remitting MS. However, a new drug, GEMSP, so far tested only in animals, appears to inhibit CNS infiltration by white blood cells, prevents CNS damage, and—new for any drug—prevents the development of MS in animals (Mangas, Coveñas, & Geffard, 2010). Lithium also seems to prevent the development of MS in animals, making it a prime candidate for studies in humans (Mangas, Coveñas, & Geffard, 2010). Lithium would have another advantage over currently approved medications in that it can be taken orally rather than by injection or infusion. Other oral medications that are anti-inflammatory, neuroprotective, or immunosuppressive or that prevent the infiltration of white blood cells into the CNS are either under development or being adapted from cancer therapy to MS. Whether any of these will provide the right balance between efficacy and side effects is not yet known (Gasperini & Ruggieri, 2009).

Immunosuppression is, of course, the most logical way to treat an autoimmune disease, but there is a catch: The same processes that allow macrophages to be recruited into an inflamed plaque also allow oligodendrocytes to be recruited and differentiated to form new myelin. Thus, if immunosuppression is too vigorous, it could, in theory, prevent healing (Lassmann, 2007).

HIV Encephalopathy

Dementia usually presents as a late-stage complication of infection with the human immunodeficiency virus (HIV) after systemic immunosuppression has become symptomatic. HIV *encephalopathy* is less common since the advent of the highly active antiretroviral protease inhibitors in the mid-1990s. Nonetheless, HIV dementia continues to occur because of eventual failure of the medications or possibly as a long-term consequence of their toxicity (Koutsilieri et al., 2007). Of note, although HIV can gain access to the brain, antiretroviral drugs cannot. Even in well-treated HIV infection, the CNS can harbor an inaccessible pool of the virus (Koutsilieri et al., 2007).

Pathophysiology

The earliest signs of HIV encephalopathy are psychomotor slowing, apathy, depression, and memory problems, as well as increased sensitivity to dopamine antagonists. Not surprisingly, then, neuroimaging and autopsy studies suggest that deterioration of the basal ganglia is particularly characteristic of this encephalopathy, although diffuse atrophy of gray matter, white matter, or both, manifests later in the course (Koutsilieri et al., 2007).

HIV seems to enter the CNS via macrophages, where it then infects the microglia. Neurons themselves do not have the requisite receptors, so any damage to them is likely secondary. There is some evidence for direct neurotoxicity by *virus coat proteins*, excitotoxicity of neurons, and damage because of altered intracellular signaling pathways. However, the strongest evidence points to inflammatory and oxidative stress as a byproduct of chronic microglial activation (Koutsilieri et al., 2007). Why are the basal ganglia the target of HIV? No putative pathophysiological mechanism has elucidated the region-specific action of HIV infection, yet in vitro evidence suggests that dopamine, which is ubiquitous in the basal ganglia, may activate the virus by increasing oxidative stress and, simultaneously, may increase the vulnerability of cells to damage (Koutsilieri et al., 2007).

Pharmacotherapy

The involvement of the basal ganglia led to the application of selegiline, an antiparkinsonian medication, and initial studies suggested some improvement in cognition. In a simian model, however, consistent with a facilitative role for dopamine in HIV infection, selegiline increased viral load, the expression of *tumor necrosis factor–α* (a proinflammatory cytokine produced by microglia), and neurodegeneration (Koutsilieri et al., 2007).

Other directions currently under study include calcium-channel blockers (e.g., nifedipine) and blockers of NMDA-type glutamate receptors (e.g., memantine) to prevent excitotoxicity (Koutsilieri et al., 2007). Antioxidants and anti-inflammatory agents such as nitric oxide synthase blockers and *interleukin-10* (an anti-inflammatory cytokine) are also being explored.

TRAUMATIC BRAIN INJURY (TBI)

TBIs are typically categorized into three groups, depending on severity. The Department of Defense uses a similar system that presents clear criteria based on the person's level of consciousness and the time period during which the alteration of consciousness lasts. A mild TBI corresponds to a score on the *Glasgow Coma Scale* greater than 13—indicating minimal alteration of consciousness (Teasdale & Jennett, 1974). Any posttraumatic amnesia should be briefer than 24 hours, and loss of consciousness should last no more than 30 minutes. A moderate TBI will lead to a Glasgow Coma Scale rating between 9 and 12, which generally indicates someone with dysfunctional speech, impaired motor reflexes, and/or oculomotor dysfunction. However, persons with moderate TBI may still be able to open their eyes, respond to painful stimuli, and generate comprehensible words. A moderate TBI may result in posttraumatic amnesia for no longer than 1 week and loss of consciousness for less than 1 day. To classify as a severe TBI, the person must be unconscious for longer than 24 hours or have posttraumatic amnesia in excess of 7 days. The Glasgow score will be 8 or lower, generally indicating nonresponsiveness or impaired responsiveness in reaction to painful stimuli.

Concussion (Mild TBI)

According to the American Congress of Rehabilitation Medicine (1993) criteria, a person with a mild TBI will have had a trauma-induced physiological disruption of brain function, as manifested by at least one of the following:

1. Any period of loss of consciousness.
2. Any loss of memory for events before and after the accident.
3. Any alteration in mental state at the time of the accident (e.g., feeling dazed, disoriented, confused).
4. Focal neurological deficits that may or may not be transient.

The term *mild TBI* is used interchangeably with the term *concussion*. An individual suffering from a concussion may remain conscious and experience a brief alteration in consciousness; however, other symptoms may persist in the hours or days following. Symptoms of concussion include memory deficits, headache, confusion, lightheadedness, dizziness, blurred vision, photosensitivity, ringing in the ears, irritability, mood lability, depression, fatigue, and insomnia. When these symptoms follow a concussion and persist for longer than 3 months, the condition is sometimes referred to as *postconcussive syndrome*.

Postconcussive Syndrome

The *DSM-IV, TR* of the American Psychiatric Association (2000) defines postconcussional disorder in the following manner:

1. A history of head trauma that has caused significant cerebral concussion.
2. Evidence from neuropsychological testing or quantified cognitive assessment of difficulty in attention (concentrating, shifting focus of attention, performing simultaneous cognitive tasks), or memory (learning or recalling information).
3. Three (or more) of the following occur shortly after the trauma and last at least 3 months: Becoming fatigued easily, disordered sleep, headache, vertigo or dizziness, irritability or aggression with little or no provocation, anxiety/depression/ affective lability, changes in personality (e.g., social or sexual inappropriateness), and apathy or lack of spontaneity.

4. The symptoms in criteria B and C have their onset following head trauma or else represent a substantial worsening of preexisting symptoms.

5. The disturbance causes significant impairment in social or occupational functioning and represents a significant decline from a previous level of functioning. In school-age children, the impairment may be manifested by a significant worsening in school or academic performance dating from the trauma.

6. The symptoms do not meet criteria for dementia due to head trauma and are not better accounted for by another mental disorder (e.g., amnesic disorder due to head trauma, personality change due to head trauma).

Pathophysiology

The pathophysiology of postconcussive syndrome is thought to be related to diffuse axonal injury. Diffuse axonal injury describes extensive damage to neuronal axons in the white matter tracts in the brain as a result of forceful, rapid acceleration and deceleration. A shearing injury occurs when axons rub against each other with great force, resulting in white matter lesions. The damage caused by diffuse axonal injury is widespread, as opposed to a focal injury that affects one area of the brain. However, most likely to be affected are the frontal and temporal lobes. Diffuse axonal injury is one of the leading causes of death in TBI. It is observed in trauma due to motor vehicle trauma. One preventable form of diffuse axonal injury is the *shaken-baby syndrome*.

It is believed that the lesions on the axons are not necessarily caused by the mechanical forces stretching the neuron. Evidence suggests that a delayed biochemical cascade takes place hours after the initial impact. Chemical processes that involve the Ca^{2+} cation, cell enzymes, and the cytoskeleton are activated when the axon is damaged, and the subsequent changes lead to neuron separation and cell death (Arundine et al., 2004; Cohen et al., 2005).

Despite the numerous potential symptoms experienced by victims of concussion, it is very infrequent for these symptoms to endure longer than 90 days. Estimates are that up to 80% of patients with concussion will recover functioning within 7 days. Over 95% of patients suffering a single, noncomplicated concussion make a complete recovery by 90 days. Some experts believe that the true incidence of postconcussive syndrome could be lower than 1%, depending on how the disorder is measured (McCrea, 2008). Evidence supports the assertion that the persistence of symptoms in postconcussive syndrome is influenced more by psychological or psychosocial factors than by the pathophysiology of a mild TBI. For instance, an analysis of data on Operation Iraqi Freedom veterans demonstrated that mild TBI–related problems became nonsignificant once researchers controlled for symptoms of posttraumatic stress disorder (PTSD) and depression (Hoge et al., 2008). Also, 40% of patients with physical trauma not related to brain injury and 90% of depression patients without physical trauma met the diagnostic criteria for postconcussive syndrome when surveyed (Boake, McCauley, & Levin, 2004; Iverson, Zasler, & Lange, 2006). Furthermore 74% of patients who reported postconcussive symptoms 12 months after the injury were found to be engaged in lawsuits or were suspected of malingering (Rutherford, Merrett, & McDonald, 1979).

Second Impact Syndrome

Although symptoms from a single concussion are likely to resolve, the results of a second injury occurring shortly after the first can be lethal. The condition known as *second impact syndrome* occurs when a person suffers another concussion before the brain has had an opportunity to recover from the first concussion. The incidence is exceedingly rare and the true rates are unknown owing to deficiencies in quality data. Although there is some controversy as to whether this syndrome really exists, most documented cases come from adolescents and young adults who play contact sports; the immaturity of the adolescent brain may be a factor in the pathophysiology. The clinical implication is obvious: Strenuous efforts must be undertaken to avoid secondary injuries after a concussion to prevent this tragedy. Animal studies indicate that mild impacts within 24 hours of a previous impact cause a breakdown of the blood-brain barrier and brain swelling (Lovel & Fazio, 2008). In humans, the symptoms can be abrupt. After an apparent mild blow, the person suddenly passes out. Brainstem compression quickly follows, and the result is coma or death.

Primary and Secondary Brain Injury

As observed in secondary impact syndrome, it is not always the trauma or lesions to the brain tissue that cause the most harm. At times, it is the ensuing complex cascade of biological processes that can cause damage. Brain injury is therefore often categorized as either primary or secondary to distinguish the cause.

Primary brain injury is the destruction to tissue that occurs at the moment of trauma. Tissue is torn, blood vessels are ruptured, and cells are killed instantly upon insult. In contrast, *secondary brain injury* involves a complex set of subsequent cellular processes and a biochemical chain of events that occurs after the initial trauma. Focal damage during primary brain injury causes dysfunction related to the particular area of the brain that is compromised. Nonetheless, secondary brain injuries are often diffuse and can affect a wide range of brain functions, leading to dysfunction of greater scope. The secondary injuries can exacerbate the primary injuries and worsen the impact of the TBI. Secondary injuries are among the leading cause of death in patients with TBIs.

The pathways involved in diffuse axonal injury are an example of how secondary brain injury occurs. The mechanical forces unleash an influx of ions into the neuron, *phospholipidases* and *proteolytic enzymes* are activated, mitochondria cell membranes are damaged, and second-messenger systems are triggered. Eventually, this progression leads to axon separation and cell death (Smith & Meancy, 2000). Other secondary brain injuries include disruption of the blood-brain barrier, exocytosis from changes in neurotransmitter concentrations (e.g., glutamate), ischemia as a result of blood loss or occlusion, lesions resulting in changes to cell integrity, and the release of factors that cause inflammation and increase intracranial pressure. In fact, most of the secondary injuries listed here will lead to several of the other processes, and a chain reaction of brain-injurious events may occur.

Pharmacotherapy After TBI

There is very little empirical evidence that any pharmacological treatment will improve functioning after a TBI. One review found mild support for psychostimulants as treatment for apathy, inattention, and slowness in brain-injured patients (Crownshaw, 2004). Notwithstanding the lack of evidence in the pharmacological treatment of neurological sequelae, many studies support the use of medications to treat the problematic behavioral problems caused by brain damage. Some patients require sedative medications to help control the agitation and poor tolerance of frustration observed following a TBI. There is evidence to argue for the use of anticonvulsants, antidepressants, and high-dose beta blockers in the treatment of agitation and aggression. Nevertheless, there has been discussion in the literature against using heavily sedating drugs in TBI patients because of the cognitive side effects. Crownshaw (2004), for example, warns that lithium and some neuroleptics cause deterioration in patients with TBI. In one of the most robust studies to date, Comper and colleagues (2005) found that psychosocial/psychoeducational approaches have accumulated the greatest empirical validation for effective intervention in patients diagnosed with mild TBI.

SEIZURE DISORDERS

The term *seizure disorder* is widely considered to be interchangeable with epilepsy. However, having seizures is not equivalent to having a diagnosis of epilepsy. For the purposes of this chapter, seizure disorder will refer to the wide spectrum of disorders involving seizures. For instance, seizures caused by structural brain abnormalities, overdose of medications, and TBIs and pseudoseizures can all be categorized under the umbrella term *seizure disorders*. The term *epilepsy* properly refers to the specific subtype of seizure disorder that is diagnosed upon having more than one unprovoked seizure during one's lifetime.

Seizures in general are classified broadly as either partial (i.e., originating in a relatively small focus of the brain) or general (i.e, bilateral and without local onset). An epileptic seizure is defined as a single event, based on clinical or EEG data (Brown & Holmes, 2008) and lacking an identifiable cause, such as trauma or a chemical insult.

Epilepsy

Epilepsy is diagnosed when a patient has at least two seizures that occur at least 24 hours apart over the span of their lifetime and that have no known cause (Mayo Clinic, 2011). Epilepsy is the most common primary brain disorder and the second most common neuropsychiatric cause of disability in the world (Engel & Pedley, 1998). According to statistics presented by the Epilepsy Foundation, epilepsy is chosen as the diagnosis in the majority of persons with seizure disorders, since no cause can be identified in 70% of all new cases. Epilepsy and seizures affect almost 3 million Americans of all ages, at an estimated annual cost of $15.5 billion in direct and indirect costs. Approximately 200,000 Americans are diagnosed with epilepsy for the first time each year. A bimodal distribution shows the highest incidence of epilepsy among persons under age 2 and over age 65. Epidemiological trends suggest that more cases are being diagnosed in the geriatric population and fewer in the pediatric population. By the age of 75, approximately 3% of all Americans will have been diagnosed with epilepsy. The incidence of epilepsy diagnosis is higher among males, African-Americans, and members of lower socioeconomic classes (Epilepsy Foundation, 2011).

Approximately 50 million people are diagnosed with epilepsy worldwide, with around 90% of all cases diagnosed in the developing world (WHO, 2011). While such statistics may reflect the greater reporting of cases in developed nations rather than a difference in the rate of occurrence, further statistics demonstrate that certain subgroups are at higher risk for epilepsy. For example 25.8% of children with mental retardation, 13% of children with cerebral palsy, and 50% of children with both disabilities will be diagnosed with epilepsy. Alzheimer patients and stroke patients are more likely to develop comorbid seizures than the general population. Furthermore, around 33% of all patients who have had an unprovoked seizure are likely to have a recurrence of seizure and be diagnosed with epilepsy. Although 70% of epileptic patients treated with antiepileptic medication can expect to remain free of seizures for 5 years or more, three fourths of patients in the developing world receive inadequate treatment; 10% of U.S. patients with seizure disorders fail to respond to antiepileptic medication (Epilepsy Foundation, 2011).

Other Causes of Seizures/Convulsions

Ten percent of the American population will experience at least one seizure in their lifetime (Epilepsy Foundation, 2011). Over 300,000 Americans per year will suffer their first convulsion. Forty percent of Americans who experience their first seizure will be children under 18 years of age. Around 75,000 to 100,000 first-time seizures are categorized as *febrile seizures* due to fever in children under the age of 5.

Sixty percent of all seizures occurring worldwide have no identifiable cause and are described as idiopathic seizures. On the other hand, the known causes of secondary seizures (also known as symptomatic seizures) include head trauma, infarction, CNS infections, fever, exposure to toxins or drugs, and structural anomalies (e.g., brain tumors). Other factors include hormone fluctuations, stress, sleep patterns, and photosensitivity. According to the Epilepsy Foundation, the most common trigger for unexpected seizures is the failure to take medication as prescribed. Cerebrovascular disease appears to be the most common risk factor for seizures in the elderly. For children, fever, perinatal complications or injury, and congenital/genetic conditions are associated with the onset of seizures.

Specific Types of Seizures

In 1981, the International League Against Epilepsy recommended a nomenclature system for seizures called the International Classification of Epileptic Seizures (ICES) that continues to be used currently (ILAE, 1981). Seizures are grossly categorized as generalized versus partial seizures, and these two broad categories are further broken down into numerous major subtypes.

The terms *generalized seizures* and *partial seizures* describe the location of the seizure—specifically, whether the excessive electrical activity has affected the whole brain or whether the neurological abnormality has been confined and localized to a specific brain region. Generalized seizures occur when electrical abnormalities spread throughout the entire brain across both hemispheres. A partial seizure does not involve the entire brain; instead, the electrical activity remains restricted to a specific region. The limited region of the brain in a partial seizure is called an *epileptic focus*, and this type of seizure is also called a *focal seizure*. The presentation of a partial seizure depends heavily on the location of the seizure activity. For example, excessive firing of the motor cortex might result in stereotypical movements, whereas a seizure focused in the olfactory bulb might result in perceptual abnormalities.

A hybrid form, a partial-generalized seizure, also exists and might best be described as a partial seizure evolving into generalized *tonic-clonic convulsions*, in which a seizure that began as a partial seizure spreads to other parts of the brain and becomes a generalized seizure.

A special category of seizure, because of its intensity and life-threatening risks, is *status epilepticus*. This term is generally applied to convulsions that last more than 30 minutes (Annals of Emergency Medicine, 2004). Most episodes resolve themselves, but mortality among persons in status epilepticus is 20%.

Generalized Seizures   Generalized seizures can be divided into several other subtypes. A *tonic-clonic seizure* (previously called a grand-mal seizure) is typically associated with "convulsive fits" of epilepsy. It consists of two distinct phases: *tonic* and *clonic*. The tonic phase involves the sudden loss of consciousness, followed by muscle rigidity that often leads to collapse. Loud vocalizations are caused by strong exhaling of air from the lungs. The tonic phase of the seizure usually lasts for less than 1 minute. It is followed by the clonic phase, which is typically characterized by the rapid muscle twitches and violent limb-shaking seen in persons with epilepsy. The eyes may roll back, the jaw may contract and damage the tongue, and incontinence may occur. A period of sleep due to physical and emotional exhaustion occurs immediately following the conclusion of the seizure. This is called the *postictal sleep* and usually lasts from 5 to 30 minutes. Finally, upon awakening, the person will be disoriented and experience total amnesia until consciousness gradually returns.

Absence seizures. Absence seizures (previously called *petit-mal seizures*) typically occur between the ages of 5 and 10, and the child is often thought to have childhood absence epilepsy. The presentation includes the altered consciousness seen in generalized, tonic-clonic seizures but without the forceful motor convulsions. The observation of significant motor events, other than mild automatism, will rule out this disorder. In absence seizures, consciousness is interrupted and the person will become unresponsive for a brief period of time. The seizure is brief, lasting just seconds, and may occur hundreds of times throughout the day. Most likely, the child will not remember the seizure after it is over and will resume preseizure activities. Therefore, a child who appears to "space out" at school may be experiencing an absence seizure. This type of seizure can progress to a full tonic-clonic seizure. Treatment is effective in managing the epilepsy in 65% of those affected, while as many as 90% are likely to experience a remission of symptoms by the conclusion of adolescence. In at least one study, almost half the patients who did not received incomplete seizure management went on to develop juvenile *myoclonic epilepsy* (Wirrell et al., 1996).

Myoclonic seizures. A myoclonic seizure involves a very brief (< 0.1 second), involuntary contraction of the muscles of the face, tongue, arms, or legs that appears to be a jerky movement. Myoclonic seizures are most apt to occur when waking after a night's sleep. A myoclonic movement that is repeated at regular intervals every few minutes may be characterized as a clonic seizure. These clonic seizures are characterized by motion in reflex arcs, such as movements of the knee or ankle.

Atonic seizures. In contrast to the motor contractions seen in myoclonic seizures, an *atonic seizure* results in the sudden loss of muscle tone and of consciousness for a brief period (< 15 seconds). In some cases an individual may become briefly paralyzed in a focused part of the body. Atonic seizures typically begin in childhood and may persist into adulthood. Injuries can occur as a result of falling or banging one's head. Atonic seizures are sometimes referred to as "drop attacks." A head bobbing motion is also common, owing to the release of muscle tone in the neck.

Partial Seizures   Partial seizures are divided into two categories according to the degree of consciousness of the victim while the seizure is underway. A complex seizure occurs when the level of consciousness is altered significantly. If consciousness is not affected, then the seizure is classified as a simple seizure.[7]

During a *complex partial seizure*, the individual may lose consciousness or may experience a significant alteration in consciousness. He or she might lose an awareness of time, become disoriented to self and situation, or stare into space and be unresponsive. Despite this alteration of consciousness, the individual may continue to perform simple, nonpurposeful movements such as hand-rubbing, lip-smacking, or walking in circles. The victim's behavior may appear inappropriate to the situation owing this to alteration in awareness, with no memory of previous actions. Yet, because of its subtleness, this behavior might not be recognized as indicating a seizure.

During a *simple partial seizure* (SPS), consciousness and awareness remain intact. Nonetheless, awareness of the seizure and the ensuing psychological, sensory, and motor symptoms might also exacerbate the person's ability to respond appropriately. To observers, the person may appear to have had an alteration in consciousness, while to the patient, the episode may be characterized as an anxiety attack. Awareness of the seizure, with memory retained, is typically referred to as an *aura*. The ICES defines an aura as "that portion of the seizure which occurs before consciousness is lost, and for which memory is retained afterwards." If a patient experiences an aura without progressing to a complex seizure, they may be diagnosed as having had an SPS.

ICES further subdivides the SPS into sections according to the area of the CNS that has been affected[8]—that is, the area of the brain that is most likely responsible for the characteristic presentation of symptoms. An SPS with motor signs involves clonic discharges in the sensorimotor cortex that cause jerky movements, possibly restricted to one area of the body. Discharges from the tonic-supplementary motor area (SMA) and the premotor region produce sustained contractions and unusual limb postures. *Phonatory activation* of the primary or supplementary motor cortex produces vocalizations, speech arrest, or aphasia (Kotagal & Lüders, 1998).

An SPS involving the somatosensory and primary sensory cortex usually elicits positive or negative sensations contralateral to the discharge. Symptoms associated with seizures from the postcentral gyrus include tingling, numbness, pain, heat, cold, agnosia, phantom sensations, and sensations of movement. The visual association cortex is the probable origin of complex visual hallucinations and *photopsias*. Auditory SPS from the auditory cortex typically are perceived as simple sounds, rather than words or music.

Perceived odors from the *orbitofrontal cortex* are usually unpleasant and often have a burning quality. Gustatory seizures are usually of temporal lobe origin and typically produce an unpleasant, often metallic taste. Vestibular seizures include vertigo, tilting sensations, and vague dizziness. Emotional and distorted perceptual symptoms emanating from SPS arise predominantly from the temporal and

---

[7]All generalized seizures involve loss of consciousness and are presumed to fall within the "complex" category. Therefore, generalized seizures do not require any classification on this domain.
[8]Another subtype, *epilepsia partialis continua* (Kojewnikoff syndrome), includes stereotypical periodic to semiperiodic clonic activity that may persist for years and is often refractory to treatment.

limbic regions, including the amygdala, hippocampus, and parahippocampal gyrus. Perceptual hallucinations or illusions associated with SPS are usually complex, visual, auditory, and associated with feelings of déjà vu. Fear and anxiety are the usual emotions, but the seizure can also elicit happiness, sexual arousal, and anger. Cognitive symptoms include feelings of depersonalization, unreality, forced thinking, or feelings that may defy description (Ajmone-Marsan & Goldhammer, 1973).

SPS can also involve the autonomic nervous system. The most common cardiac manifestation of seizure is sinus tachycardia with arrhythmias, with bradycardia occurring infrequently. Seizures from the superior portion of the posterior central gyrus can result in genital sensations, while sexual auras arise more from the limbic or temporal regions. *Ictal orgasms* have been reported, although rarely (Janszkyab et al., 2004). Postictal neurological deficits can occur after an SPS as a negative manifestation of the area of function affected by the seizure (e.g., *Todd paralysis*) (Calleja, Carpizo, & Berciano, 1988; Kaada & Jasper, 1949; Keilson, Hauser, & Magrill, 1989).

Treatment of Seizure Disorders

Most anticonvulsant medication works via three primary mechanisms to decrease transmission of the electrochemical signal by altering the ion flow across the neuron cell membrane. The first mechanism is inactivation of the Na^+ ion channel. By inhibiting Na^+ cations from entering the cell, anticonvulsant drugs decrease the chance that the neuronal impulse will be potentiated. Drugs involved in Na^+ inhibition include phenytoin, carbamazepine, oxcarbazepine, valproic acid, lamotrigine, topiramate, and gabapentin. Another pharmacodynamic mechanism of anticonvulsant medication includes inactivation of Ca^{2+} ion channels. By keeping Ca^{2+} channels closed longer this type of medication also decreases the probability of excess electrical discharge through the neuron and release of neural transmitters from the axon bundle. Phenytoin acts on Ca^{2+} ion channels. Finally, many anticonvulsant medications work by increasing GABA transmission, which in turn hyperpolarizes the neuron cell through the action of the Cl^- anion. Again the transmission of the action potential is decreased, and seizure activity is reduced. All benzodiazepines use this mechanism, and phenytoin, carbamazepine, oxcarbazepine, valproic acid, gabapentin, and topiramate also share this action (Stahl, 2007).

Vagus nerve stimulation (VNS) uses an implanted stimulator that sends electric impulses to the vagus nerve. VNS is not a frontline therapy; instead, it is reserved for patients who have exhausted their medical options. VNS represents an intermediate approach between medications and surgery. The FDA limits the use of VNS to patients older than 12 years of age (Mapstone, 2008). Its mechanism of action is not fully understood, but theories include (a) alteration of norepinephrine release by projections of a solitary tract to the locus coeruleus, (b) elevated levels of inhibitory GABA related to vagal stimulation, and (c) inhibition of aberrant cortical activity by reticular system activation (Ghanem & Early, 2006).

When all other treatment options have been exhausted, the surgical removal of small areas of damaged tissue that are leading to disabling focal seizures can be employed. Patients with partial seizures, focal seizures, or childhood hemiplegia are the best candidates for such surgery. In addition, patients with secondary generalized seizures that start on one side of the brain and progress to both hemispheres can elect to undergo *corpus callosotomy*, in which the tract of neurons that bridge the two hemispheres (the corpus callosum) can be severed, thereby removing the pathway that is needed for the seizure to spread (Brodie & Kwan, 2002).

Seizures and seizure disorders are diagnosed through careful clinical interviews in which symptom presentation and medical history are noted. Often the most common test for ruling in seizures is electroencephalography. The EEG records brain waves that can be detected by wires connected to the cranium. Electrical signals from brain cells are recorded and may display certain patterns during seizures and during the intervals between seizure activity. Imaging methods such as computed tomography (CT) or MRI scans are useful for ruling out any anatomical abnormalities that could be contributing to the seizures. Positron emission tomography (PET) has also been used to identify areas of the brain that are producing seizures. Nevertheless, in at least one study, PET did not prove to be superior to EEG in identifying abnormalities in the general population (Swartz et al., 2002).

BEHAVIORAL/PSYCHOLOGICAL DISORDERS WITH A NEUROPATHOLOGICAL BASIS

Schizophrenia

The symptoms of schizophrenia are represented by three syndromes: a psychomotor syndrome comprising poverty of speech, decreased spontaneous movement, and blunted affect; a disorganization syndrome, involving incongruous affect and disturbances in the structure of thought; and a *reality distortion syndrome*, involving auditory hallucinations, persecutory delusions, and ideas of reference (Liddle, 1987). The psychomotor syndrome constitutes what are often referred to as the negative symptoms of schizophrenia, while the reality distortion syndrome constitutes the positive symptoms (Hanson et al., 2010; Liddle, 1987). Not surprisingly, pathophysiological investigations have focused on motivational systems, systems subserving the integration of information processing across brain regions, and executive functioning.

The prevalence of schizophrenia has remained constant over at least the last century, suggesting that any genes involved in the disorder must, in certain contexts, have enough survival benefit to outweigh the harm to reproductive fitness conferred by schizophrenia itself (Tandon, Keshavan, & Nasrallah, 2008).

Familial aggregation is strong. Identical twins of people with schizophrenia have a 40% to 50% risk of developing the disorder. Heritability (variance due to genes and the gene–environment interaction) is estimated to be 80%. Genes showing a possible association with schizophrenia include those for dopamine receptors D_1 to D_4, the metabotropic glutamate receptor, catechol-O-methyl-transferase (an enzyme that degrades catecholamines), neuroregulin-1 (*NRG1*), and *dysbindin-1* (*DTNBP1*). No specific gene has emerged as having dominant importance, however. Schizophrenia may be due to small contributions from a large number of genes, or it may be a heterogeneous disorder with different genes involved in different patients, or it may not be the genes at all but the pattern in which they are expressed (*epigenetic factors*) (Tandon, Keshavan, & Nasrallah, 2008).

Environmental risk factors are equally important. Those factors with relatively strong effects (a relative risk of 2 to 3) include geographical migration (with the children of immigrants being affected more than the immigrants themselves); living in an urban area (with a dose-response relationship: the more urban, the more risk); infection or malnutrition of the mother during the first or second trimester of pregnancy; marijuana use in adolescence; and complications before, during, or after birth. Smaller effects are seen with paternal age over 35 at the time of conception, male gender, and possibly birth during winter, especially in places with harsh winters. Psychosocial stress has also been linked to schizophrenic episodes, although whether it is a risk for the disease itself or simply explains the timing of acute flare-ups, has not been teased apart (Tandon, Keshavan, & Nasrallah, 2008).

Pathophysiology

The pathophysiology of schizophrenia remains poorly understood—so much so that we may not be dealing with a single disorder at all but rather a collection of disorders with similar clinical presentations. Nonetheless, a number of neurobiological abnormalities appear to be correlated with the diagnosis (Keshavan et al., 2008):

• Decreased volume of the frontal, temporal, and parietal cortices (Honea et al., 2008). This abnormality appears to be specific to the gray matter and possibly to the *pyramidal neurons* of lamina III, which is involved in the corticocortical connections that integrate processing between brain regions (Garey, 2010).

• Decreased volume of the thalamus, even after correcting for smaller brain volume (Byne et al., 2009). The thalamus is a logical focus for studies of schizophrenia because certain fibers that coordinate between brain regions pass through it (i.e., fast, myelinated cortico-thalamo-cortical pathways (Byne et al., 2009).

• Dysfunction of the prefrontal cortex. This abnormality is suggested by mild atrophy evident on *volumetric MRI*; decreased blood flow on *functional MRI* and PET scans, decreases in N-acetyl aspartate (a marker for neuronal, or at least mitochondrial, integrity) and in phosphomonoester (a marker for the integrity of dendrites) on magnetic resonance spectroscopy; and in autopsy studies, a reduction in dendritic spines and axon terminals in the prefrontal cortex.

• Dysfunction of the hippocampus, medial temporal cortex, and primary and secondary auditory cortex, as suggested by findings on volumetric MRI and in auditory event-related potential studies.

• Loss of cerebral asymmetry, as seen globally on volumetric MRI and histological studies of pyramidal cell density (which should be higher in the dominant hemisphere).

• Loss of integration across brain regions, as suggested by decreased volume or integrity of white matter (e.g., in the corpus callosum and tracts connecting the frontal and temporal lobes [Gothelf et al., 2005]) and by loss of EEG power in the gamma range (30 to 80 Hz). Coherence, or synchronization across brain regions in the gamma range, is thought to play a role in the integration of brain activity.

Complementing these are a number of suspected neurotransmitter abnormalities, as follows:

• Dopamine—Perhaps dopamine is hypoactive in mesocortical structures (e.g., medial frontal cortex, involving D_1 receptors) and hyperactive in mesolimbic (D_2) structures. This is suggested by the D_2-receptor antagonism characteristic of all antipsychotic medications, the psychotomimetic properties of amphetamines (which facilitate dopamine release and inhibit its reuptake), imaging studies that suggest higher rates of dopamine synthesis in the *striatum*, and evidence that dopamine-receptor occupancy is increased in the striatum (Laruelle et al., 2005). Striatal dopamine seems to be responsible for the positive symptoms specifically. Of note, for an antipsychotic drug to be maximally effective, it appears that it must reduce striatal dopaminergic tone to below the level found in healthy subjects (Laruelle et al., 2005).

- Glutamate—Decreased glutamatergic signaling through NMDA-type receptors is suggested by postmortem studies and by the ability of NMDA-receptor antagonists (ketamine, phencyclidine) to mimic the positive and negative symptoms of schizophrenia. Moreover, agonists at the NMDA receptor have shown clinical benefit (Keshavan et al., 2008; Laruelle et al., 2005). Because bidirectional negative-feedback loops seem to connect striatal dopamine and prefrontal glutamate systems, excessive dopaminergic and deficient glutamatergic transmission may be two sides of the same coin. That dopaminergic tone must be reduced to below normal levels implies that dopamine may not be the key target. Rather, antipsychotic drugs may be indirectly upregulating glutamatergic transmission in the cortex (Laruelle et al., 2005).
- GABA—Gamma-aminobutyric acid has been found to be underactive in the prefrontal cortex on autopsy studies.
- Acetylcholine—A decrease in muscarinic-type acetylcholine receptors has been found in postmortem studies, with supportive results from genetics and functional neuroimaging.
- Serotonin—Abnormalities in serotonin activity is a possibility, as suggested by the efficacy of atypical antipsychotics which block 5-HT_{2A} receptors .

To date, there is no widely accepted definitive theory to tie all these findings together. We are left with pieces of the puzzle, a collection of tantalizing hints, and hypotheses for future treatment directions. One attempt to synthesize various hypotheses into a cogent paradigm has been offered by Steven Stahl (2009). Stahl proposes that dopamine is involved in both the mesolimbic and the mesocortical pathways to promote positive and negative signs of schizophrenia—that is, hyperactivity in the mesolimbic pathway creates positive signs such as hallucinations and delusions, while hypoactivity in the mesocortical pathway leads to negative signs, such as cognitive impairment, lack of motivation, and anhedonia. Stahl further proposes that dopamine activity is intricately related to serotonin and glutamate activity; in the case of schizophrenia, the interplay among dopamine, serotonin, and glutamate may form a functionally autonomous loop that sustains the imbalance contributing to psychosis. The effectiveness of atypical antipsychotics, which mainly target $5\text{HT-}2_A$ heteroreceptors, is attributed to breaking up this loop.

The pathophysiological correlates of symptom clusters have also been examined, with the goal of advancing treatment. The negative symptoms of schizophrenia (psychomotor syndrome) correlate with reduced functioning of the ventral striatum, suggesting that decreased reactivity to rewards could underlie the lack of motivation (Hanson et al., 2010). Increased activity in the amygdala also correlates with negative symptoms (Hanson et al., 2010).

Pharmacotherapy

First-generation antipsychotics, introduced in the early 1950s, are antagonists at the D_2-dopamine receptor (Seeman & Lee, 1975). They include the oral medications chlorpromazine (Thorazine, Largactil), loxapine (Loxapac), methotrimeprazine (Nozinan, Levoprome), perphenazine (Trilafon), sulpiride (Meresa, Bosnyl), and trifluoperazine (Stelazine); the long-acting injectables fluphenazine (Prolixin) and pipothiazine (Piportil); and, available for either of these delivery routes, flupenthixol (Depixol), haloperidol (Haldol), and zuclopenthixol (Acuphase). Also generally included among the typical antipsychotics is thioridazine (Mellaril). These agents are effective when they occupy between 55% and 70% of striatal D_2-dopamine receptors. The primary side effect—extrapyramidal, or parkinsonian, motor symptoms—emerges when receptor occupancy is above 80%, allowing for a narrow therapeutic window (Laruelle et al., 2005). Traditional antipsychotics may also elevate serum *prolactin* levels (Seeman, 2002).

Long-term antipsychotic use may lead to *tardive dyskinesia* (TD)—repetitive, involuntary, purposeless movements that can involve the lips, jaw, tongue, and face; the arms or legs; and/or the respiratory system (Margolese et al., 2005). Tardive dyskinesia is thought to arise from compensatory upregulation of D_2 receptors (Remington, 2007), although degeneration of striatal cholinergic and GABAergic neurons has also been suspected (Margolese et al., 2005). With typical antipsychotics, the annualized incidence of tardive dyskinesia appears to be 3% to 5% over the first 5 years of treatment (Kane et al., 1982). It is unclear whether the risk levels off or continues to rise with longer-term use (which, of course, is characteristic in the clinical setting). In addition to the use of D_2-receptor antagonists, risk factors for tardive dyskinesia include being elderly and the use of psychotropic agents to treat an affective disorder rather than schizophrenia (Remington, 2007).

Most second-generation antipsychotics are antagonists at dopamine D_2 and serotonin 5-HT$_2$ receptors. In contrast to first-generation antipsychotics, which bind more tightly to D_2 receptors than does dopamine itself, binding by the atypical antipsychotics is looser; the drug occupies the receptor frequently but briefly throughout the day (Seeman, 2002). Medications in this class include amisulpride (Solian), aripiprazole (Abilify), clozapine (Clozaril), olanzapine (Zyprexa), quetiapine (Seroquel), risperidone (Risperdal), sertindole (Serdolect), ziprasidone (Geodon), zotepine (Nipolept), and most recently iloperidone (Fanapt) and asenapine (Saphris) (Leucht et al., 2009a, 2009b; Potkin et al., 2008; Weber & McCormack, 2009). These are oral medications, with risperidone also available as a long-acting injection.

In a study involving 1,432 patients, olanzapine appeared to have greater effectiveness than quetiapine and ziprasidone, although this may in part reflect the fact that more patients in the trial had been taking olanzapine prior to the start of the study (Lieberman et al., 2005). Three head-to-head comparisons have found greater treatment adherence with olanzapine than with other atypical antipsychotics in patients with chronic schizophrenia (Johnsen & Jørgensen, 2008). Clozapine appears to have specific benefit for patients whose schizophrenia has been refractory to treatment with other medications (McEvoy et al., 2006).

It seems that tardive dyskinesia is much less likely to occur with atypical antipsychotics. From the evidence available so far, an annualized incidence of 0.8% has been estimated—not too different from the spontaneous incidence of tardive dyskinesia in schizophrenia (Correll, Leucht, & Kane, 2004; Shirzadi & Ghaemi, 2006). Moreover, with the atypical antipsychotics, preexisting tardive dyskinesia appears to go into remission (Remington, 2007). However, whether these favorable properties will continue with long-term use, polypharmacy, or use for conditions other than schizophrenia is not yet known (Remington, 2007).

The main side effect for second-generation antipsychotics is an increased risk of *metabolic syndrome* and therefore cardiovascular disease: weight gain and increases in fasting blood-glucose levels and cholesterol levels. Among the medications in this class, olanzapine and clozapine are somewhat more likely to cause metabolic changes, while amisulpride, aripiprazole, and especially ziprasidone are less likely to do so. Quetiapine, risperidone, and sertindole fall in an intermediate range (Rummel-Kluge et al., 2010), although quetiapine, like olanzapine, has been associated with increased risk of heart disease (Daumit et al., 2008).

Head-to-head trials in clinical populations vary and suggest no difference in efficacy between first- and second-generation antipsychotics as a class (Lieberman et al., 2005). Lieberman concludes, however, that olanzapine was less likely to be discontinued by patients and physicians than was perphenazine, a first-generation antipsychotic with moderate potency. Surprisingly, at least in studies lasting for 1 year, there may not be a difference in objectively determined motor side effects between first- and second-generation antipsychotics (Foussias & Remington, 2010).

Current antipsychotics of both generations show efficacy specifically for the positive symptoms of schizophrenia. A modest effect on negative symptoms is probably due to a reduction in depression and anxiety rather than a true targeting of negative symptoms (Hanson et al., 2010). Still, there may not be a sharp line between depression and negative symptoms, and SSRIs have been shown to provide benefit as adjunctive treatment (Sepehry et al., 2007). More experimentally, one study showed that N-methylglycine (sarcosine), an agonist at NMDA-type glutamate receptors, reduced both positive and negative symptoms of schizophrenia (Lane et al., 2010).

Prevention

Minocycline, an antibiotic related to tetracycline, has neuroprotective properties and was of benefit in a study of acute psychotic episodes in young patients with schizophrenia (Levkovitz et al., 2010). In individuals at high risk for schizophrenia, a 12-week trial of omega-3 fatty acids reduced the risk of conversion to schizophrenia from 27.5% to 5% over the next 40 weeks (Amminger et al., 2010).

Attention Deficit–Hyperactivity Disorder (ADHD)

ADHD involves persistent and developmentally inappropriate behavior in the realms of overactivity, inattention, and impulsiveness. The disorder can be subdivided into a predominantly inattentive type, a predominantly hyperactive-impulsive type, and a type that combines symptoms from both categories (American Psychiatric Association, 1994). Neuropsychological studies suggest abnormalities in vigilance, working memory, planning, response suppression, and motivation (Nigg, 2005; Willcutt et al., 2005). Except for motivation, all these abnormalities fall within the realm of executive functioning; however, deficits in executive functioning are not necessary or sufficient for a diagnosis of ADHD (Tripp & Wickens, 2009).

The differences in motivation, attentiveness, and perhaps response inhibition seem to derive from a preference for an immediate, albeit small, reward over a greater, delayed reward. There appears to be an impairment in the development of *secondary reinforcers*, that is, *reinforcers* that acquire their rewarding properties because they signal a later, more primary reward. Since positive reinforcement is signaled in the brain by a phasic release of dopamine, the impairment has been described as a "dopamine transfer deficit," or the failure of the dopamine burst to transfer from the primary reinforcer to conditioned cues (Tripp & Wickens, 2009).

The *heritability coefficient* for this disorder is quite high, approximately 0.8, which is probably due to small contributions from many genes. Among these, genes encoding the dopamine D_4 and D_5 receptors and the *transporter proteins* for dopamine and serotonin reuptake are most strongly implicated, but each likely accounts for no more than 4% of the variance in symptoms (Tripp & Wickens, 2009).

Among environmental factors, smoking during pregnancy increases the risk of ADHD in the child by 2.7-fold, in a dose-response relationship. Smoking appears particularly deleterious for individuals harboring a particular polymorphism of the *DAT1* gene, which encodes the dopamine transporter protein (Curatolo et al., 2009).

Pathophysiology

Neuroimaging studies suggest smaller brain volumes in children with ADHD, particularly at the right caudate nucleus, the frontal cortex, and the cerebellum (Valera et al., 2007). White matter tracts seem disrupted in the posterior corpus callosum (*splenium*). In adults, evidence for smaller volume seems restricted to the *dorsolateral prefrontal* and *anterior cingulate cortices* (Seidman et al., 2006). Functional neuroimaging revealed impairment of memory encoding of neutral pictures, which in healthy control subjects involves the *anterior cingulate cortex*, and did not show activation in this region in adolescent patients with ADHD (Krauel et al., 2007).

Steven Stahl (2008) has proposed a convincing model to explain the relationship between various symptoms of ADHD and different corresponding neural structures and circuits. According to Stahl, attention is regulated by a dorsal anterior cingulate cortex→striatum→thalamus loop, while emotional reinforcement for sustaining attention is regulated through a subgenual anterior cingulate cortex→nucleus accumbens→thalamus loop. Executive function is hypothesized by Stahl to be regulated by a dorsolateral prefrontal cortex→striatum→thalamus loop, while impulsivity and compulsivity are regulated by an orbital frontal cortex→striatum→thalamus loop.

Pharmacotherapy

Current treatments include psychostimulants such as amphetamine and methylphenidate, which promote the release of norepinephrine and dopamine and block their reuptake; the highly selective norepinephrine reuptake inhibitor atomoxetine; and (off-label) modafinil. Bupropion, which acts as a reuptake inhibitor for dopamine, is also indicated for the treatment of ADHD. All four of these types of medication seem to improve response inhibition (Chamberlain, Robbins, & Sabakian, 2007). Methylphenidate and amphetamine can increase the development of secondary reinforcers, presumably by enhancing the phasic release of dopamine (Hill, 1970; Robbins, 1978).

MOVEMENT DISORDERS

Movement disorders are neurologically based conditions that affect ease of movement, resulting in abnormal speed of movement (*dyskinesia*), excessive movement (*hyperkinesia*), or slowed voluntary movement (*hypokinesia*) (Deuschl , Bain, & Brin, 1998). *Dystonia* (prolonged muscle contractions), tics (involuntary muscle contractions), and *myoclonus* (brief irregular movements) are primarily caused, as are all movement disorders, by interruptions in circuitry within the basal ganglia. Other locomotion disorders, which are caused primarily by interruption of normal functioning in the cerebellum, motor cortex, inner ear, and spinal cord, are not generally classified as *movement disorders*. Table 4.3 lists conditions that fall under the rubric movement disorders. The list of pharmacological agents in the table represents only an indication of some of the approaches used to treat these disorders and is not meant to be exhaustive. It should be remembered that some movement disorders (such as *Tourette's syndrome*) are often best treated behaviorally, with or without adjunctive medication, whereas others (such as Parkinson's disease) may require physical and speech therapy along with medication; still other conditions (such as mild restless-legs syndrome) do not always justify the use of medication.

Huntington's Disease (Chorea)

Huntington's disease (HD) is transmitted in an *autosomal dominant* pattern and has *complete penetrance*. It is thought that increased glutamatergic transmission at NMDA receptors produces neurodegenerative changes through *excitotoxicity* (Rohkamm, 2004). HD typically appears between ages 35 and 45. In early-stage HD, akinesia and cognitive impairment are prominent, with depression, impulse dyscontrol, and poor frustration tolerance. In the intermediate stage, progressive

Table 4.3   Major Movement Disorders

Disorder	Description	Etiology	Pharmacotherapy
Huntington's disease	Involuntary *chorea* characterized by brief, abrupt, irregular, unpredictable, nonstereotyped movements	Dysregulation of the basal ganglia motor circuit; final thalamocortical output is increased, resulting in hyperkinesis	Symptomatic treatment of chorea includes the use of dopamine antagonist and benzodiazepines
Parkinson's disease	Resting tremor, rigidity, akinesia, and impairment of postural reflexes	Lesions in the basal ganglia, predominantly in the substantia nigra, where final thalamocortical output is decreased, resulting in hypokinesis	Levodopa, dopamine agonists, monoamine oxidase type B (MAO-B) inhibitors
Restless-legs syndrome (RLS)	Compelling urge to move the legs; worse during periods of rest or inactivity	Dopaminergic dysfunction; possible hypoactivity in basal ganglia dopaminergic neurons	Dopamine agonists and L-dopa; gabapentin, benzodiazepines. Agents that block the dopaminergic system aggravate RLS symptoms
Tourette's syndrome	Involuntary vocalization; usually brief, and stereotyped	Genetic predisposition; hypoactivity in striatal dopaminergic involvement	Dopamine-receptor blocking agents (haloperidol, pimozide, and fluphenazine)

dementia is apparent, as is the appearance of *choreiform* movements. In late-stage HD, chorea is displaced by akinesia and muscle atrophy associated with *cachectia*.

Parkinson's Disease

The etiology of *Parkinson's disease* (PD) is unknown. Its progression is associated with loss of neurons in the substantia nigra (pars compacta) and the formation of *Lewy bodies*. Loss of pigmentation in the substantia nigra is correlated with deficient dopamine projection to the striatum (putamen and caudate nucleus). The effect of deficient dopaminergic synapses in the striatum, where dopamine neurons serve an inhibitory function, is an increase in striatal activity, which in turn disinhibits the subthalamic nucleus via the *indirect pathway* (via the external *globus pallidus*). The subthalamic projection to the internal globus pallidus increases the inhibitory effect of the globus pallidus on the thalamus. A simultaneous decrease in striatal inhibition of the globus pallidus (internal segment) along the *direct pathway* enhances the inhibitory influence of the globus pallidus on the thalamus, which subsequently further reduces activity in the thalamocortical projection (Nolte & Angevine, 2000). The end result is reduced voluntary movement and a potentiation of involuntary movement, with the manifestation of the classic symptoms of PD: akinesia, rigidity, and postural instability. Although it would be impossible to depict all known pathways involved in the fine regulation of movement through basal ganglia involvement, Figure 4.2 depicts a simplified version of the various pathways involved in PD and contrasts them with normal neural activity in this area of motor regulation.

Restless-Legs Syndrome (RLS)

A single cause for *restless-legs syndrome* has not been isolated or adequately demonstrated to date. There would appear to be a dopamine-deficient aspect to its dynamics, but investigations have not been able to define one particular mechanism, although dopaminergic hypoactivity appears to have been demonstrated (Cervenka et al., 2004). RLS has been conceptualized by some as a mild form of Parkinson's disease, but voluntary movement is not compromised. Another theory suggests that the CNS iron deficiency found in RLS patients points to reduced functioning of dopaminergic neurons when iron-deprived (Hening, Buchfuhrer, & Lee, 2008).

Tourette's Syndrome

This syndrome has in common with other tics the intermittent, rapid involuntary behavior that interrupts normal volitional action but can be suppressed by voluntary effort, yet this behavior rebounds with greater intensity once the effort is relaxed. The tic involved in Tourette's syndrome is vocalization, and it frequently occurs along with OCD (Frankel et al., 1986) and ADHD (Denckla, 2006). A person with Tourette's syndrome has about a 50% chance of passing the gene to one of his or her children, yet Tourette's is a condition of variable expression and *incomplete penetrance* (van de Wetering & Heutink, 1993); not every genotype will become phenotypic. Albin (2006) has emphasized the importance of the ventral striatum in the formation of habits and its implication in Tourette's syndrome, mediated by dopaminergic hyperactivation in the basal ganglia.

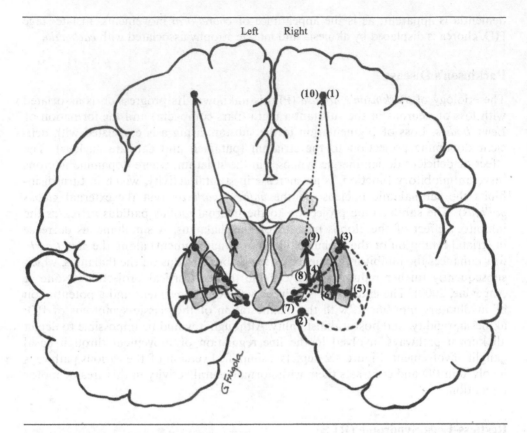

Figure 4.2   Neuropathways in Parkinson's Disease

The left hemisphere represents normal basal ganglia motor circuitry, while the right hemisphere represents weakened signals from the substantia nigra to the striatum, as seen in Parkinson's disease. Disruption of the excitatory/inhibitory modulating circuits in the basal ganglia ultimately reduces its moderating input on the motor cortex. The descending excitatory glutamatergic efferent from the motor cortex (1) converges in the striatum (3) with the dual-function (inhibition/excitation) dopaminergic projections from the substantia nigra (2). All these actions increase, with cholinergic complicity, inhibition of the cortical impact on the globus pallidus internus (4) while simultaneously potentiating GABAergic and enkephalin inhibitory projections to the globus pallidus externus (5). The inhibitory GABAergic projection (6) from the globus pallidus externus to the subthalamic nucleus (via the globus pallidus internus) is decreased (7), which increases the glutamatergic excitatory projections from the subthalamic nucleus to the globus pallidus internus (8). Coupled with the weakened GABAergic inhibitory projections from the globus pallidus internus to the striatum (4), the GABAergic tonic inhibition (9) of the thalamus is increased, which in turn decreases regulation of the cortex as a result of reduced neural input (10).

EXTRAPYRAMIDAL DYSFUNCTIONS

The *extrapyramidal* pathways play an important role in movement by regulating motor responses without directly innervating muscles. The extrapyramidal tracts are located in the reticular formation of the pons and medulla and connect downward to the spinal cord and upward toward the basal ganglia. The word *extrapyramidal* refers to pathways "other than" the tracts of the motor cortex that travel through the "pyramids" of the medulla. The extrapyramidal pathway is modulated by higher-order brain structures from the diencephalon and encephalon, including the *nigrostriatal pathway*, the basal ganglia, the cerebellum, the vestibular nuclei, and areas of the cerebral cortex. Yet, the extrapyramidal tract is more than a passive conduit; it is a structure with functions of its own.

The term *extrapyramidal dysfunctions* refers to a class of movement disorders that includes dystonia, dyskinesia/tardive dyskinesia, akinesia/hypokinesia, and *akathisia*. These disorders have their origins in the basal ganglia, but, unlike the movement disorders just discussed, they are largely induced side effects of medications. Factor analysis of the Extrapyramidal Rating Scale (Chouinard & Margolese, 2006) found six factors that constitute induced movement disorders of the basal ganglia/extrapyramidal tract: (1) hypokinesia, (2) orofacial dyskinesia, (3) trunk/limb dyskinesia, (4) akathisia, (5) tremor, and (6) tardive dystonia.

In Table 4.4, we have grouped the dyskinesias together, separating out tardive dyskinesia, and provide descriptions of three other major extrapyramidal dysfunctions: dystonia, hypokinesia/akinesia, and akathisia.

Table 4.4   Extrapyramidal Dysfunctions

Disorder	Description	Etiology	Pharmacotherapy
Dystonia	*Tonic* muscular contractions in eyes, mouth, throat, neck, and limbs	Nigrostriatal dopamine receptor D_2 blockade	Discontinue neuroleptic; start anticholinergic (e.g., diphenhydramine, benztropine, trihexyphenidyl; start benzodiazepine
Hypokinesia: (a) akinesia (b) bradykinesia (c) rigidity	Slow movements and reduced facial expression: (a) slow to initiate movement, (b) slowness in continued execution, (c) resistance to passive movement	Diminished dopaminergic-cell activity in the basal ganglia direct pathway	Change neuroleptic to one with less D_2 blockage (e.g., aripiprazole)
Dyskinesia/ tardive dyskinesia/ rabbit syndrome	Involuntary choreiform movements affecting the orofacial region and extremities	Extrapyramidal side effects from blockade of D_2 receptors in the striatum	Discontinue neuroleptic, switch to alternative MOA; administer cholinergic or anticholinergic agent according to type of dyskinesia.
Akathisia	Subjective feeling of unrest, difficulty remaining seated, agitation, restlessness	Extrapyramidal side effects associated with blockade of D_2 receptors and serotonin-reuptake inhibition	Symptoms may persist after agent is discontinued; may be treated with antiparkinsonian agents in addition to benzodiazepines

Dystonia

Focal dystonia, in which a specific part of the body exhibits twitching, is thought to be the result of malfunction in the sensorimotor cortex, whereas the spasticity in *cerebral palsy* is primarily associated with cerebellar pathology; a parallel basal ganglia involvement may contribute to *athetoid* or dyskinetic cerebral palsy, in which mixed muscle tone results in difficulty standing or sitting up straight. Nonetheless, dystonias generally associated with psychotropic medication are bilateral, affect a larger area, and originate from the basal ganglia. Extrapyramidal dystonic reactions are characterized by spasmodic, involuntary contractions of muscles in the face, neck, trunk, pelvis, and extremities (Fahn, 1984). Most drugs produce dystonic reactions by blocking nigrostriatal dopamine D_2 receptors, with a resulting excess of striatal cholinergic output. Corrective strategies attempt to reduce the impact of D_2 blockade by withdrawing the neuroleptic and switching to an agent with less affinity for this receptor or adding an agent that mitigates the concomitant increase in acetylcholine activity (Marsden & Jenner, 1980).

Hypokinesia

Hypokinesia is a slowing down of movement, resulting in gait or reaching movements that occur in slow motion, like movements in zero gravity. Diminished dopaminergic cell activity in the basal ganglia's direct pathway is believed to be the origin of the disorder (Nambu, 2004). *Akinesia* refers to slowness in initiating movements, *bradykinesia* refers to slowness in continuing a movement during execution, and rigidity refers to resistance to passive movement.

Dyskinesias

Dyskinesias ("abnormal movements" in Greek) refer to involuntary anomalies in performing voluntary movements, resulting in tic, chorea, spasm, or myoclonus. The term is generally used to refer to any dysfunctional movement, but it is more specifically used in psychopharmacology in relation to iatrogenic extrapyramidal disorders. More pertinent to our purposes is tardive dyskinesia, which makes a delayed appearance after neuroleptics are initiated and may include grimacing, jaw-swinging, repetitive chewing, tongue protrusion, lip-smacking, and rapid blinking. Tardive dyskinesia is believed to result from extrapyramidal side effects of D_2-receptor blockade in the striatum (Missale et al., 1998), although recent research suggests that, along with dopamine-receptor hypersensitivity, there may also be gamma-aminobutyric acid insufficiency as well as neuroleptic-induced neuronal toxicity through free radical and excitotoxic mechanisms (Sachdev, 2001). One convincing explanation for tardive dyskinesia's delayed onset is provided by Stephen Stahl (2010). According to Stahl, D_2 blockade progressively leads to an upregulation of the D_2 receptors, making these receptors in the nigrostriatal pathway more sensitive to diminished amounts of dopamine and eventually leading to decreased coordination of involuntary movement.

The *rabbit syndrome,* sometimes considered to be a distinct syndrome which incorporates components of tardive dyskinesia and parkinsonism (Villeneuve, 1972), is a rare extrapyramidal side effect of antipsychotic drugs in which tremors around the mouth produce involuntary, fine, rhythmic motions, without involvement of the tongue (Catena Dell'osso et al., 2007; Goswami, 1994).

The preferred approach to drug-induced dyskinesia is early detection, withdrawal of the offending drug, and switching to another drug known to have fewer extrapyramidal side effects, such as clozapine, or at least switching to a neuroleptic with a different mechanism of action profile (e.g., from a conventional antipsychotic to an atypical one). Adding an anticholinergic agent, such as benztropine or diphenhydramine, is recommended for rabbit syndrome, as well as for other extrapyramidal disorders (Hocaoglu, 2009), but not for tardive dyskinesia (Klawans & Rubovits, 1974) because preventative anticholinergic therapy to relieve extrapyramidal disorders has been shown to lower the threshold for tardive dyskinesia. In fact, cholinergic-enhancing agents such as donepezil prove useful in mitigating tardive dyskinesia, although this is a trade-off, because the stronger the cholinesterase inhibitor is, the greater the potential for inducing other *extrapyramidal symptoms* (Nasello, Gidalis, & Felicio, 2003).

Akathisia

Akathisia consists of a subjective experience of internal tension and the need to relieve the tension through movement. The outward manifestation of akathisia is pacing or other kinds of movement-oriented behaviors, such as fidgeting, or purposelessly alternating sitting and standing in rapid succession. Akathisia may not always be observable, as in the case of a mixed hypokinetic-akathetic state (Tuisku et al., 2000), or when the affected person makes an effort to suppress the outward signs of internal distress. *Tardive akathisia* is a form of persistent akathisia and may continue even after antipsychotic medication has been withdrawn (Dufresne & Wagner, 1988). Akathisia is associated with neuroleptic use, but it is also seen with SSRIs and SNRIs (Akagi, 2002).

NEUROLEPTIC MALIGNANCY SYNDROME

Neuroleptic malignancy syndrome (NMS) is not a movement disorder per se, but movement dysfunction is associated with it—mainly rigidity and bradykinesia. In fact, these movement components and their associated muscle correlates are what distinguish this syndrome from *serotonin syndrome*. Neuroleptic malignancy syndrome is unpredictable and can be caused by overdosing on neuroleptics as well as by individual sensitivity to D_2-receptor blockade; nearly all cases appear within the first 30 days of exposure to neuroleptics. NMS results in five central symptoms, often arranged in the mnemonic FEVER:

F = fever
E = encephalopathy
V = vital instability
E = elevated *creatine phosphokinase* (CPK)
R = rigidity

While the serotonin syndrome affects autonomic regulation, especially temperature, NMS involves severe muscle activity, leading to rhabdomyolysis and increased serum creatine kinase (Ladds et al., 2009). The treatment for NMS requires the immediate withdrawal of the perpetrating agent, as well as supportive care. Muscle relaxants such as benzodiazepine have also been used. NMS is a self-limiting, iatrogenic disorder that can be reversed upon withdrawal of the antipsychotic medication. Nonetheless, one problem with achieving rapid withdrawal from the offending antipsychotic is that the depot preparations of neuroleptics may linger for weeks. Hyperthermia is treated with topical cooling agents. Aggressive hydration is indicated to reduce the kidney-damaging effects of rhabdomyolysis (*myoglobinuric renal failure*), and benzodiazepine may reduce agitation and mitigate muscle rigidity. Dopamine agonists, such as amantadine, may reset D_2 receptors and reduce mortality by 50% (Sakkas et al., 1991). Although the majority of patients survive NMS, this syndrome earned the designation "malignancy" because it is associated with a mortality rate of about 10% (Strawn, Keck, & Caroff, 2007).

SLEEP DISORDERS

Behavioral sleep medicine is a prime example of the contribution of medical psychology—in this case health psychology—to the research, diagnosis, and treatment of biopsychosocial syndromes within a medical context (Stepanski & Perlis, 2003). With the advent of prescriptive authority for psychologists, pharmacotherapy has become an additional competency for the pharmacologically trained medical psychologist working in the area of sleep disorders (Morris, 2011).

Sleep disorders are diagnosed when the normal *sleep architecture* is interrupted, with resulting distress to the patient. Although sleep patterns vary considerably from person to person, the sleep-wakefulness template from which aberrations might be initially detected includes uninterrupted alertness during wakefulness, with relative ease of sleep onset when desired and ensuing continuous, uninterrupted sleep, characterized by cyclical alterations in the level of brain activity, good oxygenation, and minimum limb movement other than during repositioning.

For our purposes, sleep disorders may be divided into two broad categories: those which affect sleep onset and sleep continuance owing to inherent changes in sleep architecture, such as *insomnia* or *narcolepsy*, and those that interrupt sleep because of epiphenomena, which is the case with *parasomnias*.

Sleep Onset/Continuance Disorders

Insomnia

Delayed sleep onset and poor quality sleep caused by multiple awakenings are common clinical complaints, yet insomnia is uncommonly complex in its classification, categorization, and diagnosis, according to the nosological systems used (Lichstein & Riedel, 1994), with more than a dozen subcategories recognized. Insomnia might be profitably understood by separating, albeit arbitrarily, onset problems from continuance problems.

Onset of sleep is consensually understood to be governed neurochemically by the suppression of excitatory neurotransmitters and the potentiation of inhibiting transmitters within structures of the brain that are most involved in maintaining alertness or, conversely, promoting a resting, vegetative state. Although a "sleep center" as such has not yet been identified, some areas are more associated with vigilance and alertness, such as the raphe nucleus, the locus coeruleus, the perifornical lateral hypothalamus, and the tuberomammillary nucleus, whereas other structures appear to be involved in promoting slumber, such as the median preoptic nucleus, the ventrolateral preoptic nucleus, and the pineal gland (Brown, 2006). Nonetheless, since Michel Jouvet's groundbreaking work on the neurotransmitters involved in sleeping and dreaming (Jouvet, 1967), efforts to elucidate the specific action of these neurotransmitters and the implication of particular brain anatomy in sleep phenomena have led to mixed results. Jouvet originally introduced serotonin as the primary sleep hormone and implicated norepinephrine in dreaming, but he later denounced his serotonin hypothesis after decades of research had failed to isolate this hormone as responsible for sleep (Jouvet, 1999). More recently, the ventrolateral part of the preoptic area or, more generally, the basal forebrain with cholinergic projections and the GABAergic thalamic reticular nucleus have been postulated as sleep-onset pacemakers (Steriade & McCarley, 2005). Other transmitters, mainly melatonin and *hypocretin*, have been proposed as essential for the onset and maintenance of sleep,[9] yet no single structure or combination of structures or transmitters has been unequivocally shown to house the "sleep center."

Clinically, *insomnia* is divided into problems with the onset and maintenance of sleep, since patient complaints usually take one form or the other. Anecdotally, clinicians may make a distinction between the impact of anxiety and depression on insomnia, but research has shown that both onset and continuance are disturbed by either anxiety or depression. The severity of insomnia correlates with the intensity of anxiety and/or depression, yet there are few differences in the manifestations of insomnia for these two conditions. One exception appears to be the greater number of nocturnal awakenings for depressed patients when compared with anxious patients (Taylor et al., 2005).

Insomnia is treated effectively with cognitive behavioral approaches that emphasize reestablishing sleep hygiene by shaping sleep behavior to occur during the nocturnal hours (Morin, Batien, & Savard, 2003). When pharmacotherapy is indicated for insomnia, GABAergic agents that agonize $GABA_A$ receptors (benzodiazepines and non-benzodiazepine hypnotics) or agents with antihistaminergic actions (diphenhydramine) are prescribed. Different drugs affect the sleep architecture in different ways; the profile of sleep induced by an anticholinergic agent, for example, differents from that of sleep induced by an antihistaminergic or a GABAergic agent (Itil, 1968). These differences are not always appreciated or taken into consideration in clinical decision-making.

Narcolepsy

Narcolepsy is a chronic sleep disorder of unknown neurological origin that is characterized by excessive daytime sleepiness and intermittent *sleep attacks*. Other narcoleptic phenomena include features of dissociated REM, sleep such as *cataplexy*, *sleep paralysis*, and *hypnagogic hallucination* (American Academy of Sleep Medicine, 2005). Although the cause of narcolepsy has not yet been determined, much research points in the direction of hypocretins. The neurons that produce hypocretins are located largely in the hypothalamus. They are active during wakefulness and may keep the neuropathways needed for wakefulness from shutting down unexpectedly. The role of hypocretins in narcolepsy appears better established than the role of the

---

[9]*Orexins*, alternatively referred to as hypocretins, are highly excitatory neuropeptides synthesized in the lateral hypothalamus and appear to be suppressed for the onset and continuance of sleep (Hungs & Mignot, 2001). Levels of melatonin, the substance which appears to regulate the biological clock and hence to facilitate sleep onset, decline gradually as we age (Shafii, 1998).

hypocretin system in normal sleep regulation. It has been speculated, however, that hypocretin cells may drive cholinergic and monoaminergic activity across the sleep cycle. Input from the suprachiasmatic nucleus to hypocretin-containing neurons may explain the occurrence of clock-dependent alertness and may also be relevant to seasonal affective disorder (SAD) (Taheri, Zeitzer, & Mignot, 2002). (See also footnote 10 concerning SAD and melatonin.)

Narcolepsy has been treated for decades with *analeptics*, such as amphetamine, but in 1999 the FDA approved modafinil, a non-amphetamine–based stimulant, for the treatment of narcolepsy; tricyclic antidepressants have also been used to control cataplexy. In 2002, the FDA approved a drug with a very different mechanism of action to treat narcolepsy. *Sodium oxybate* (*gamma-hydroxybutyric acid*) is a naturally occurring substance in the mammalian brain that acts as an agonist to inhibitory $GABA_B$ receptors (Black et al., 2010) while also acting as an agonist at excitatory G-protein–coupled *GHB (gamma-hydroxybutyrate) receptors* (Snead, 2000).

Parasomnias

During the night, brain activity moves progressively in cycles of 90 to 110 minutes on average (Hobson, Lydic, & Baghdoyan, 1986; Swierzewsky, 2007) from light sleep, with comparatively greater neuronal firing, to deeper levels of sleep, with corresponding slowing of brain activity (slow-wave sleep or SWS). Essentially, five levels have been identified as composing normal sleep architecture: *non-REM* stages 1 through 4 and stage 1 *REM*. Excluding normal dreaming, which occurs during REM sleep, certain other behavioral correlates associated with the different levels of sleep may be problematic: *Nocturnal myoclonus* or periodic leg movement and hypnagogic hallucinations may appear during stage 1 non-REM; *night terrors* and sleep-walking appear mainly in stage 4; *enuresis* and sodium oxybate production are common to all stages. Figure 4.3 is an EEG tracing depicting the different levels of sleep.

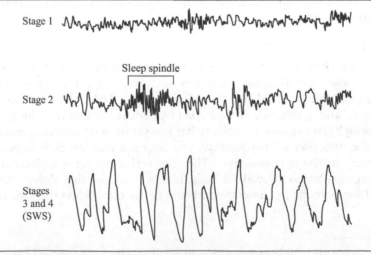

Figure 4.3   EEG Tracings Showing the Stages of Sleep
From Perlis, M., & Lichstein, K. (2003). *Treating sleep disorders: The principles and practice of behavioral sleep medicine* (p. 47). Philadelphia, PA: Wiley.

Nocturnal Myoclonus

The stereotypical, repetitive movements of the extremities in nocturnal myoclonus are reminiscent of those seen in the restless-legs syndrome, except that these periodic limb movements occur during sleep. It should be noted, nonetheless, that pharmacological agents that tend to improve restless-legs syndrome or akathisia tend to worsen nocturnal myoclonus (Cortese et al., 2005). Some researchers have implicated a subcortical contribution to this sleep disorder, although a precise circuit has not been identified; indeed, it may turn out that no specific CNS pathology exists; rather, the symptom may represent the unmasking of normal brain pacemaker activity that is typically suppressed in those with normal, undisturbed sleep function (Edinger, 2003). Comorbidity for periodic leg movements is found with ADHD and with various movement disorders; nocturnal myoclonus is also associated with the use of SSRIs and tricyclic antidepressants, as well as with alcohol consumption. Pharmacological treatment has emphasized dopamine agonists or dopamine precursors, such as *pergolide* and *carbidopa-levodopa* compounds, with the drawback of possibly exacerbating restless-legs syndrome (Montplaisir et al., 2000).

Enuresis

Antidiuretic hormone (ADH) secretion during sleep leads to urine concentration and decreased volume which, together with increased bladder capacity and acquired requisite motor control, allow children to remain dry at night by the age of 6. Failure to gain bladder control while asleep by age 6 is diagnosed as nocturnal enuresis. Nocturnal enuresis has an inherited component and is a developmental disorder that tends to resolve with time (Lawless, 2001); the prevalence of nocturnal enuresis is approximately 15% for boys and 10% for girls at 6 years of age but is only 1% by age 15. Abnormal ADH levels are not significantly associated with nocturnal enuresis in the majority of children (Riillig et al., 1989). Therefore, treatment does not generally warrant long-term use of hormonal therapy. Pharmacotherapy for nocturnal enuresis is only rarely recommended, with anticholinergic agents occasionally prescribed with the rationale that they block muscarinic receptors on the *detrusor muscle* and consequently decrease the bladder's ability to contract (Abrams & Andersson, 2007). Treatment of enuresis, as is true with most sleep-onset disorders or parasomnias, entails a psychobiosocial approach, with emphasis on the psychosocial reeducation of contributory problematic behavior.

Other Parasomnias

Obstructive sleep apnea, *somnambulism* (sleep-walking), night terrors, *sleep soliloquy* (sleep-talking), REM-sleep behavior disorder, and *circadian rhythm disorders* are other forms of parasomnias (Arlin, 1981). Sleep apnea, or short periods during which air flow to the lungs ceases during sleep, may occur at any of the different levels of sleep. The risk of obstructive sleep apnea increases with smoking, obesity, and age. Sleep-walking and night terrors tend to occur in non-REM sleep, usually in stages 3 and 4, and can be precipitated or exacerbated by sleep deprivation as well as by agents that induce deeper levels of sleep, such as alcohol, sedative-hypnotics, and neuroleptics (Bazil, 2004). Sleep soliloquy may occur in non-REM and REM sleep and is very common in children; speech content is random in sleep soliloquy. REM-sleep behavior disorder is the most common REM-sleep parasomnia and involves physically acting out dreams owing to the absence of normal REM-related muscle atonia. Circadian rhythm sleep disorders (Dagan, 2002) are characterized by malsynchronization between a person's biological clock and the standard 24-hour environmental schedule. They can be extrinsic disorders, as in jetlag, or intrinsic disorders, which may affect sleep onset or awakening rhythm.[10]

CHRONIC PAIN

There is no area of psychology where the interface with medicine has been better accomplished than in pain management. Health and rehabilitation psychologists have long played an integral role in the management of *chronic pain*, forming part of the *multidisciplinary* pain management team found in many hospitals and outpatient clinics (Muse et al., 1991). The involvement of the pharmacologically trained medical psychologist in such a context is especially pressing, since there is a mounting need to address psychopharmacological treatment of chronic pain more responsibly than has been done in the past. But what role could a medical psychologist possibly play in pain management when the nature of prescribing medical psychologists' prescriptive authority rules out the use of opioid-based *analgesics*?[11]

The answer to this question lies in differentiating between acute pain and chronic pain. Whereas *acute pain* is short-lived, eliciting apprehension and anxiety in the sufferer, chronic pain is persistent and prolonged and tends to cultivate a depressive reaction in those affected (Sternbach, 1980). Unlike acute pain, which corresponds in great part to a circumscribed lesion, *nonmalignant (benign) chronic pain* persists beyond the initial injury and might best be conceived of as a secondary correlate to the original injury; it becomes, in fact, a *functionally autonomous* condition that bears little or no relationship to the original injury.

Neuropathology of Chronic Pain

The neuropathology of chronic pain has been theorized to include at least three mechanisms: neuromuscular spasm, spinal cord nerve hyperconduction, and cerebral perseveration.

Neuromuscular Spasm

The peripheral site of the body implicated in maintaining chronic pain involves the muscles and their tendency to spasm when exposed to prolonged tension. This tension originates, in most cases, from the initial body flinch that occurs as a protective

---

[10]Parenthetically, one intriguing theory (which is far from proved but which has had some heuristic value) links circadian rhythm and depression to seasonal sleep patterns and proposes that seasonal affective disorder (SAD) may be related to melatonin superproduction during periods of relative darkness and the consequent depletion of melatonin's precursor, serotonin. According to this theory, photosensitive retinal ganglion cells (ipRGCs) mediate circadian *photoentrainment* (Fu et al., 2005). With the onset of the fall season, dim light and darkness stimulate the ipRGCs to project, via the retinohypothalamic tract and the suprachiasmatic nucleus, to the pineal gland, where melatonin (which is associated with induced sleep) is released. Melatonin is produced from the precursor serotonin. The theory suggests that the onset of SAD may be triggered by light-sensitive cells in the retina, which stimulate greater melatonin release in the pineal gland and, consequently, deplete serotonin.
[11]The prescribing of narcotics was never requested by pharmacologically trained psychologists and is specifically excluded from the prescribing medical psychologist licensing laws of Louisiana and New Mexico.

reflex after the original injury. If the tension persists for a sufficient period of time, prolonged by acute pain or by confounding psychological tension, persistent spasm contributes to further pain by generating a buildup of *lactic acid* around *nociceptors* in the muscle (Bear et al., 2007; Hill, 1970),[12] as well as by causing fatigue and *myofasciitis*. Paradoxically, Pedersen, Connors, & Paradiso (2002) have recently demonstrated that lactic acid may be an irritant, but it is also essential in preventing muscle fatigue.[13] *Myofacial pain* syndrome refers to pain and inflammation in a muscle group and usually involves *trigger points* where localized spasm within the muscle group creates tender spots. The increase in discomfort associated with myofacial pain syndrome includes collateral contributors such as stress and depression. In terms of clinical management of skeletal muscle pain, gradual exercise is recommended to relieve tension, release spasms, and promote greater elasticity and flexibility and less of the "defensive posturing" inherent in muscle spasm (Muse et al., 1984).

Spinal Cord Nerve Conduction

Ronald Melzack first proposed his *Gate Control Theory of Pain* in 1965 (Melzack & Wall, 1965). It postulates that a "gate" exists at the spinal cord level that regulates access from the periphery to the *dorsal horn* and its ascending spinal tracts, determining how much nociception will reach the brain. Small-diameter pain nerve fibers and large-diameter tactile fibers carry information from the site of injury to two different intermediary cells (inhibitors and facilitators) in the dorsal horn of the spinal cord. Signals from fibers of both diameters excite the facilitator transmission cells, and when the output of the transmission exceeds a critical level, pain begins. While the facilitator transmission cells are the gate for pain, inhibitory cells shut the gate. When pain and touch fibers are activated, they affect both the facilitator and inhibitory cells; the smaller-diameter pain fibers impede the inhibitory cells, while the large-diameter fibers excite the inhibitory cells and tend to close the gate. The greater the small-fiber activity relative to the large-fiber activity, the greater the pain. This theory has led to clinical recommendations for greater activity, which may reduce the perception of pain to the extent that larger fibers (involved in touch, pressure, and stretch) are activated and inhibit access to ascending spinal column transmission. It has also led to the use of transcutaneous electrical nerve stimulation (TENS).

Cerebral Perseveration

Just as there are facilitator and inhibitory neurons in the periphery, there are activating and inhibiting mechanisms and pathways in the brain that work together to keep the organism in equilibrium. When this equilibrium is upset, one part of the brain may perseverate. It has been hypothesized that the somatosensory cortex, located in the postcentral gyrus, continues to fire after the loss of its peripheral connections, as in the case of *phantom limb*, largely because of an imbalance between excitatory and

---

[12]The buildup of lactic acid leads to an excess of hydrogen protons in the interstitial space. The hydrogen ions activate H^+-gated ion channels on adjacent nociceptors.

[13]Potassium ions accumulate extracellularly, making it harder for sodium ions to propagate the action potential. Lactic acid counters this fatigue by interfering with the flow of chloride ions, effectively lowering the amount of sodium current necessary for muscle activation. This mechanism, presumably, reduces fatigue but potentiates spasm.

inhibitory neurons.[14] One clinical outcome of the recognition of cerebral perseveration has been, in the case of phantom limb, the cross-training of the deprived area of the sensory cortex to "connect" to the ipsilateral surviving organ. In the case of a severed right hand, for example, training is achieved through providing mirrored virtual feedback from the left hand to the left hemisphere, which promotes the perception of input from the right hand and, presumably, satisfies the left somatosensory cortex's need for stimulation. The subjective experience of such retraining has been relief from "phantom" sensations in patients exposed to this novel therapy (Ramachandran & Rogers-Ramachandran, 1996; Yang et al., 1994).

Although it is instructive to separate the different neuropathological explanations of pain, it is usually not the case that a single component can fully explain any given case of chronic pain. Quite the contrary. Chronic pain affects the entire organism, and any explanation of its mechanisms will necessarily be multifaceted. Recognizing this fact, Ronald Melzack (1999) incorporated parts of his original Gate Control Theory into a farther-reaching conceptualization of chronic pain. In his *Neuromatrix Theory of Pain*, Melzack proposes that the body activates perceptual, homeostatic, and behavioral programs after injury, disease, or chronic stress (Melzack, 2005). Pain is produced by the output of a widely distributed neural network in the brain rather than directly by sensory input evoked by injury, inflammation, or other pathological conditions. The neuromatrix, which is genetically determined and modified by sensory experience, is the primary mechanism that generates the neural pattern that produces pain. Its output pattern is determined by multiple influences, of which the somatic sensory input is only a part, that converge on the neuromatrix. The neuromatrix, in turn, comprises a widely distributed neural network that includes parallel somatosensory, limbic, and thalamocortical components that subserve the sensory discriminative, affective-motivational, and evaluative-cognitive dimensions of the pain experience.

Multidisciplinary Diagnosis and Treatment of Chronic Pain

Psychologists have been a recognized part of the multidisciplinary treatment team for patients with chronic pain since Wilbert Fordyce's monumental book *Behavioral Methods for Chronic Pain and Illness* (1976). The past 40 years have seen psychologists contribute to differential diagnosing and multimodal treatment of pain syndromes. Because chronic pain is complex, an interdisciplinary, collaborative effort between the psychologist and other health professionals is the usual course of action. This coordinated approach includes didactic information-sharing with patients in order to educate them about the nature of chronic pain; exercise programs to promote greater activity; medication schedules aimed at reducing reliance on powerful and inappropriate drugs; relaxation techniques and biofeedback to encourage skeletal-muscle relaxation; and individual and family counseling aimed at resolving

---

[14]One of the effects of reduced stimulation of the brain, as occurs with the loss of input from a severed limb or in sensory deprivation studies, is increased self-stimulation of that area of the brain deprived of environmental or organ stimulation (Schultz & Melzack, 1991); presumably, as proposed in the *auditory plasticity theory of tinnitus* (Snow, 2004), the increase in spontaneous neuronal firing occurs as a secondary result of the disinhibition of minor or parallel pathways, and their subsequent amplification, in the vacuum left by the diminished or absent organ, resulting in the phenomenological proprioception/introception of sense organs in the absence of peripheral stimulation, as in the case of tinnitus associated with hearing loss.

issues of overdependence, vocational/financial concerns, and the emotional consequences of chronic pain in depression. Hypnosis, dietary counseling, and procedures
such as *nerve blocks*, physical therapy, and TENS are less frequent interventions. An
emphasis on avoiding unnecessary surgery is also a top priority in coordinated pain
management.

Psychologists play a pivotal role in diagnosing the emotional components of
chronic pain (Bruns & Disorbio, 2005). Some pain conditions, such as tension
headache, have their basis in emotional upset and tension, while other emotional
responses such as adjustment reaction with depressed mood may be the result
of dealing with the various aspects of chronic pain; still other conditions, such as
migraine, have a biological basis that is stress-reactive and triggered by emotional
responses. There is generally interplay between the biological origin of pain and its
exacerbation from emotional responses, yet in the case of somatoform disorder, pain
is exclusively or predominantly caused by psychological factors. Concurrent conditions such as injury-acquired PTSD (Muse & Frigola, 1986) and pain-related substance dependency (Streltzer & Johansen, 2006) also require the attention of the
pain psychologist. Indeed, McWilliams, Cox, and Enns (2003) found that PTSD
occurs three times more often in pain patients than in the general population, while
other anxiety-based disorders occur several times more often for pain patients, and
mood disorders are approximately twice as prevalent in the chronic pain population.
Gender differences are of interest to the medical psychologist, with all major pain
syndromes being more prevalent in women (Von Korff & LeResche, 2005).

Clinical Psychopharmacology in Pain Management

There is little place for the use of narcotics in the management of chronic pain (Hendler,
1981), although advocates for such drugs exist (France et al., 1984; Portenoy & Foley,
1986) and narcotics continue to be used for this purpose (Ballantyne & Mao, 2003;
McQuay, 1999), albeit not without controversy.[15] For example, the Oregon Health and
Science University Web site, "Where healing, teaching and discovery come together"
states unequivocally that "*opioid analgesics* are accepted as part of a comprehensive
management plan for chronic non-malignant pain" and that "no scientific evidence suggests that providing opioid analgesia worsens addictive disease" (Oregon Health and
Science University, 2010). In fact, in 2003 the Oregon legislature made it easier to give
opioids to patients with chronic pain unrelated to cancer by eliminating the need for
a specialist to prescribe these powerful drugs and by paving the way for the extended
use of narcotics by primary care providers for the treatment of chronic, nonmalignant,
intractable pain.

The reason pharmacologically trained medical psychologists place opioid treatment for chronic pain at the *end* of their list of options is threefold: (1) There are

---

[15]According to the Substance Abuse and Mental Health Services Administration (SAMHSA), "Increases
in the percentage of admissions reporting prescription pain reliever abuse in the United States underscore
the public health importance of the misuse of pain relievers in several respects. First, the increases from
1998 to 2008 were widespread, cutting across admissions by age, gender, race/ethnicity, education, employment, and region. Therefore, successful efforts to prevent pain reliever misuse and to treat addiction to
pain relievers need to cover a wide range of populations and need to be tailored appropriately to these
different populations." Parenthetically: "Among admissions for which medication-assisted opioid therapy
was planned, reports of pain reliever abuse more than tripled, from 6.8% in 1998 to 26.5% in 2008"
(SAMHSA, 2010).

more effective treatments available that have fewer unwanted secondary effects;[16] (2) the behavioral contingencies under which these drugs are prescribed to patients with pain encourage addictive behavior;[17] and (3) their use is not supported by evidence-based decision-making but by professional consensus.

Juxtaposed to the use of opioids in the management of chronic pain is the judicious prescribing of antidepressant medication within a multimodal approach to pain management. An established research history has established the efficacy of antidepressant medication in the treatment of pain (Ashburn & Staats, 1999; Magni, 1991; Mico et al., 2006; Ward, Bloom, & Friedel, 1979). A summary of numerous studies would suggest that antidepressant drugs are considered first-line medications for chronic pain and are effective in relieving pain even when no comorbid depression is present. The tricyclic antidepressants appear to be superior to the SSRIs in treating chronic pain (Saarto & Wiffen, 2007), as effective as gabapentin for treating chronic *neuropathic pain* (Moulin, Clark, & Gilron, 2007), and no more effective than stress-management therapy for treating tension headache (Holroyd, O'Donnell, & Stensland, 2001). On the other hand, side effects are greater for gabapentin than for tricyclic antidepressants in the treatment of neuropathic pain (Field & Swarm, 2008).

The second argument used by pharmacologically trained medical psychologists against the use of opioids in the treatment of chronic pain syndromes is the risk that such a practice sets the stage for a conditioned response that increases the likelihood of addiction. Fordyce (1976) spelled out, within the operant conditioning paradigm, the connection between pain and the highly motivating negative reinforcement associated with avoiding it. Narcotics are inherently reinforcing for the pleasure that they provide; this is the basis for the alarming addiction to prescription narcotics such as *OxyContin* in the population at large (Goodnough, 2011). If the additional reinforcing quality of reducing pain is added to opioids' attractiveness, the goal-seeking behavior of narcotic consumption will be that much higher. Since narcotics do not cure chronic pain, it is the short-term relief that predisposes a patient to future addiction. Many suffering patients will ask for pain relief, but it is irresponsible, in our opinion, for the clinician to lead them down a blind alley when other approaches are available. Much of what is accomplished in pain management is based upon the attitude that some amount of pain must be tolerated to regain functional behavior in important areas of life, such as vocational and social interactions. To prescribe

---

[16]Witness the effect not only on the user but also the fetus and newborn, in the case of the pregnant user (Jones et al., 2010).

[17]"Today [4/19/2011], the White House unveiled a multi-agency plan aimed at reducing the 'epidemic' of prescription drug abuse in the U.S. In concert with the White House plan, the Food and Drug Administration (FDA) is announcing a new risk reduction program—called a Risk Evaluation and Mitigation Strategy—for all extended-release and long-acting opioid medications. FDA experts say extended-release and long-acting opioids—including OxyContin, Avinza, Dolophine, Duragesic, and eight other brand names—are extensively misprescribed, misused, and abused, leading to overdoses, addiction, and even deaths across the United States. The FDA says a 2007 survey revealed that more than half of opioid abusers got the drug from a friend or relative. Opioids—such as morphine and oxycodone—are used to treat moderate and severe pain. Over the past few decades, drug makers have developed extended-release opioid formulas to treat people in pain over a long period. The new REMS plan focuses primarily on educating doctors about proper pain management, patient selection, and other requirements and improving patient awareness about how to use these drugs safely. As part of the plan, the FDA wants companies to give patients educational materials, including a medication guide that uses consumer friendly language to explain safe use and disposal" (DDI, 2011).

the false hope of achieving this goal without the effort and discomfort required is disingenuous.

Finally, a host of studies have pointed out that there is little evidence that opioid use in the treatment of non-cancer–related chronic pain is effective and without significant side effects (Ballantyne & Mao, 2003; Olsen & Daumit, 2002). In fact, although research findings have been inadequate, opinions and consensus positions abound (Chou et al., 2009a). For these reasons, there is growing agreement among clinicians involved in pain management to exercise prudence and to moderate the use of opioids in treating chronic nonmalignant pain syndromes (Colameco, Coren, & Ciervo, 2009; Trescot et al., 2008); this option is best held in reserve until other approaches have failed and should then be used only for selected, behaviorally monitored patients (Chou et al., 2009b).

In summary, pharmacologically trained medical psychologists have a great deal to contribute to pain management. That prescribing psychologists do not currently have authorization with the Drug Enforcement Agency to prescribe Schedule 2 or 3 narcotics poses little disadvantage when working with chronic pain patients.

CHAPTER 4 KEY TERMS

Absence seizures: Sometimes referred to as petit-mal seizures, these are characterized by an interruption in consciousness. They may appear alone (mostly in childhood) or may be accompanied by myoclonic and tonic-clonic seizures (mainly in adulthood).

Activated microglia: These are microglia that reconfigure themselves for immune defense in response to stimuli such as proinflammatory cytokines or constituents of cells that have died and broken apart. They proliferate, secrete cytotoxic and inflammatory chemicals, take on an ameboid shape to engulf pathogens, and migrate to a site of injury or invasion.

Activation ratio: The degree to which one copy (vs. the other copy) in a pair of chromosomes is used to transcribe proteins.

Acute pain: Sudden, often intense onset of pain after damage to tissues from disease or trauma.

Akathisia: The Greek translation of akathisia is "unable to sit." The term refers to a movement disorder in which a subjective experience of distress, associated with inactivity, propels the person to move about in order to reduce the feeling. It is manifest by "fidgety" behavior, such as pacing.

Akinesia: Literally, "unable to move"; refers to difficulties in initiating or starting a voluntary movement.

Alcohol-related neurodevelopmental disorders: A term originally suggested by the Institute of Medicine to replace the term *fetal alcohol effect*.

Alpha-synuclein: A protein found in neurons that may play a role in vesicle trafficking and the control of energy production by mitochondria. Its overproduction and/ or misfolding leads it to aggregate into Lewy bodies within neurons; thought to play a role in Parkinson's disease and dementia with Lewy bodies.

Amyloid beta (Aβ): A peptide whose abnormal level of production and coalescence into extracellular plaques is thought to play a role in Alzheimer's disease.

Amyloid precursor protein (APP): A membrane protein found in multiple tissues but associated primarily with the synapses. Its function is speculated to contribute to synapse configuration and neural plasticity.

Amyotrophic lateral sclerosis: A disease of progressive muscle weakness and atrophy caused by the degeneration of motor neurons in the cortex, brainstem, and spinal cord.

Analeptics: Central nervous system stimulant medications.

Analgesics: Literally, "without pain"; refers to any pharmacological agent whose primary action is to relieve pain.

Aneurysm: An abnormal ballooning of a portion of an artery due to weakness in the wall of the vessel.

Angelman syndrome: A neurogenetic disorder manifest as developmental delay, lack of speech, seizures, and walking/balance disorders.

Anterior cerebral arteries: A pair of arteries on the brain that supply oxygen to most medial portions of frontal lobes and superior medial parietal lobes.

Anterior cingulate cortex: An inner lobe of cortex, near the inner surface of the frontal lobe, involved in the processing of pain, affective tone, motivation, and the detection and correction of errors in performance.

Antidiuretic hormone: ADH, also known as vasopressin, is synthesized as a neuropeptide in the hypothalamus and secreted through the pituitary in greater quantities during sleep.

Arteriovenous malformations: An abnormal connection between veins and arteries, usually congenital.

Athetoid: Literally, "out of place"; refers to purposeless writhing movements, typically of the hands and feet.

Atonic seizure: A sudden loss of muscle tone due to seizure.

ATPase: A class of enzymes using adenosine triphosphate (ATP), including those enzymes used to make lysosomes acidic.

Auditory plasticity theory of tinnitus: According to the auditory plasticity theory, damage to the cochlea enhances neural activity in the temporal lobe, auditory association cortex, and inferior colliculus. Tinnitus might be considered to be the auditory system analog to phantom limb sensations in amputees.

Aura: A perceptual change that is prodromal to the onset of seizure.

Autism spectrum disorder: Term in the new edition of the *DSM-5* chosen to replace pervasive developmental disorder, autism, Asperger's syndrome, and childhood disintegrative disorder.

Autosomal dominant: The gene in question is located on one of the non-sex chromosomes. In contrast to recessive genes, a single copy is sufficient to transmit its trait, as in the case of Huntington's chorea.

Basal ganglia: Nuclei found on both sides of the thalamus, below the cingulate gyrus and within the temporal lobes. It includes the caudate nucleus, putamen, globus pallidus, and subthalamic nucleus and has connections with the substantia nigra.

Basilar artery: One of two arteries (the vertebral artery being the second) that supply blood to the circle of Willis.

Behavioral sleep medicine: Refers to the branch of clinical sleep medicine and health psychology that identifies psychological factors that contribute to sleep disorders. It also develops and applies behavioral interventions in the treatment of sleep disorders.

Brachycephaly: A cephalic disorder that occurs when the coronal suture fuses prematurely, causing the skull to have a shortened front-to-back diameter.

Bradykinesia: Literally, slow movement"; refers to slowness in performing a movement or in carrying out a movement once its execution has begun.

Cachectia: Literally, "bad state"; refers to atrophy with loss of weight and muscle mass due to disease.

Carbidopa-levodopa: Levodopa is the precursor for dopamine; if not buffered, it is converted by the enzyme DOPA decarboxylase and is spent in the peripheral nervous system. Carbidopa is a DOPA decarboxylase inhibitor that guards the levodopa through the peripheral nervous system to deliver it to the central nervous system where it is anabolized to dopamine.

Cataplexy: Sudden, transient loss of muscle tone.

Caudate nucleus: Part of the basal ganglia, the caudate nucleus curves around the thalamus, and is thought to be involved in learning and memory.

Cerebellar hypoplasia: A developmental disorder characterized by the incomplete development or underdevelopment of the cerebellum.

Cerebral atherosclerosis: Narrowing of cerebral blood vessels due to the buildup of fatty plaques within the lumen.

Cerebral embolism: Sudden blocking downstream of an artery by an embolus.

Cerebral palsy: A generic term referring to various movement disorders (including spasticity, dyskinesia, hypotonia, and ataxia) stemming largely from cerebellar dysfunction. The disorders are manifest early after birth and may have their origin in hypoxia or oxygen deficiency during a critical developmental period.

Cerebral peduncles: White matter tracts connecting the cerebellum with the brainstem.

Cerebral thrombosis: Blocking of blood flow by a blood clot dislodged from the vessel wall.

Cerebral vasculitis: Inflammation of blood vessel walls within the central nervous system.

Cerebrovascular accident: Interruption of blood supply to any part of the body: Stroke.

Cholinesterase inhibitors: Chemicals that increase cholinergic signaling by blocking the enzyme cholinesterase, which is responsible for breaking down acetylcholine in the synapse.

Chorea: Roughly translated from the Greek, chorea means "dance"; refers to an irregular, rapid, uncontrolled, involuntary movement.

Choreiform: Adjective, referring to chorea-like movement.

Chronic pain: Pain lasting several months.

Circadian rhythm disorders: The term *circadian* (from the Latin, meaning "around the day") refers to the 24-hour biological clock that guides the metabolic processes in most plants and animals. Disorders in this clock result in disruption of the rhythm inherent in the 24-hour circadian schedule.

Circle of Willis: Intersection of several arteries at the base of the brain.

Clonic: Abnormal neuromuscular activity characterized by a rapid, involuntary contraction-relaxation pattern.

Complete penetrance: Penetrance refers to the extent that a genotype is revealed in a phenotypical trait. Complete penetrance translates to 100% manifestation of the underlying gene, as in the case of Huntington's disease.

Complex (partial) seizure: The loss of consciousness during seizure. (See *Simple partial seizure.*)

Concussion: Brain injury caused by a blow to the head; a mild form of traumatic brain injury.

Corpus callosotomy: Surgical severing of the corpus callosum.

Creatine phosphokinase (CPK): Also known as creatine kinase (CK), CPK is an enzyme that catalyzes the conversion of creatine by consuming adenosine triphosphate (ATP) to create phosphocreatine and adenosine diphosphate (ADP). The enzyme is largely retained within the tissue (in situ) where it is recycled. In the case of dysfunction, such as in rhabdomyolysis, CPK may leak into the bloodstream, where it can be assayed. Measurement of CPK is a standard lab test in aiding the diagnosis of neuroleptic malignancy syndrome.

Cytokines: A family of chemicals produced widely in the body that modulates the immune system—promoting or suppressing inflammation, triggering fever, and attracting white blood cells to a site of injury.

Detrusor muscle: Bladder muscle that, when contracted, expels urine from the bladder.

Direct pathway: A neuronal circuit within the basal ganglia that facilitates the initiation and execution of voluntary movement. Within the central nervous system, the motor cortex sends activating signals to the striatum. The caudate and putamen play an inhibitory role within the direct pathway; once they become activated, they project to the globus pallidus internus and substantia nigra pars reticulata, suppressing these structures' activation, respectively. The globus pallidus internus and the substantia nigra reticulata normally inhibit activity within the ventrolateral nucleus of the thalamus, which modulates and prevents over-activation of the motor cortices, especially during periods of rest. When the direct pathway is activated, the ventrolateral nucleus of the thalamus is allowed to send uninhibited, activating signals to the motor cortex, amplifying muscle contractions. If the direct pathway is interrupted, as in Parkinson's disease, activation of the thalamus is reduced, resulting in hypokinesia.

Dorsal horn: A part of the spinal cord that receives projections from the dorsal root and plays an important role in nociception and pain. Neurons in the dorsal horn receive input from peripheral sensory neurons and transmit the signals to the brain.

Dorsolateral prefrontal cortex: The lateral region of the frontal lobes, involved in working memory and executive functioning.

Down syndrome: A genetic condition involving an extra copy of all or part of chromosome 21 (trisomy 21), which is associated with decreased physical growth and life expectancy, specific facial features and usually (but not invariably) mild-to-moderate mental retardation.

Dysbindin: Part of a protein complex found in muscles and neurons that may play a role in schizophrenia. Inadequate production of dysbindin may impair glutamate release and the growth of dendritic spines.

Dyskinesia: Literally, "difficult movement"; referring to diminished voluntary control of movement and increased involuntary movement.

Dystonia: Diminished muscle tone.

Ectoderm: One of the three primary germ cell layers that make up the very early embryo.

Embolus: An errant mass within a blood vessel.

Encephalopathy: Disease of the brain.

Enuresis: From the Greek, "abundance of water"; refers to loss of bladder control. Nocturnal enuresis refers to bedwetting.

Epigenetic factors: Factors that govern which genes are transcribed at which times, as during development and differentiation. Once set in motion, epigenetic changes may endure for the lifetime of the organism.

Epilepsia partialis continua: A rare type of seizure that consists of recurrent focal motor involvement of the hands and feet. It may last seconds to minutes during a period of weeks or years.

Epilepsy: A neurological disorder provoking convulsions and loss of consciousness as a result of disordered discharge of cerebral neurons.

Epileptic focus: A circumscribed area of the brain where desynchronized neuronal firing begins, leading to a seizure.

Excitotoxicity: The damage or destruction of nerve cells caused when excessive excitatory stimulation, typically by glutamate, abnormally increases the intracellular calcium concentration, activating enzymes and/or triggering apoptosis (cellular self-destruction).

Executive functioning: The intentional cognitive processes of self-regulation, including planning and goal-setting, maintaining and switching between cognitive sets, and selecting stimuli and responses in light of goals.

Extrapyramidal: Neural pathway, located in the anterior horn, that indirectly coordinates movement by modulating neuronal activity outside the cerebral-pyramidal tract.

Extrapyramidal symptoms: Disruption of the extrapyramidal system can lead to such disturbances of motor control as tremor, muscle rigidity, dystonic spasms, involuntary movements, slowed movements (bradykinesia), and the inability to initiate movement (akinesia). Collectively, these are termed *extrapyramidal dysfunctions*.

Febrile seizures: Convulsions associated with an increase in body temperature in children 6 months to 6 years of age.

Fetal alcohol spectrum disorders: A continuum of permanent birth defects caused by maternal consumption of alcohol during pregnancy.

Fibril: A thin filament. In Alzheimer's disease, fibrils are the abnormal, threadlike structures of the amyloid beta peptide that aggregate, forming extracellular plaques.

Focal dystonia: Involuntary contraction of muscles in a particular part of the body.

Focal seizure: See *Partial seizure.*

Fragile X syndrome: A genetic condition, caused by silencing of a specific gene (the FMR1 gene), associated with social anxiety, physical features such as an elongated face and poor muscle tone and, primarily in males, intellectual disability involving executive functioning, verbal working memory, arithmetic, and visuospatial skills.

Frontotemporal lobular degeneration: A form of neurodegenerative disease characterized by marked changes in personality, social functioning, and language and motor skills, with marked brain atrophy, usually concentrated in the frontal and/or temporal lobes. Also termed *frontotemporal dementia.*

Functional autonomy: A term attributed to the psychologist Gordon Allport; refers to an acquired function that exists independent of its origin. For example, pain that originated from injury continues after the resolution of the original injury.

Functional MRI: A magnetic resonance imaging technique in which the magnetic properties of hemoglobin are used to measure local changes in blood flow in the brain and, indirectly, neural activity.

Fusiform gyrus: A part of the temporal lobe, also known as the *occipitotemporal gyrus.* Neurons in the fusiform gyrus are fewer and smaller in autism.

Gametes: Reproductive cells that unite to form a zygote.

Gate Control Theory of Pain: Proposed by Ronald Melzack and Patrick Wall, the theory refutes the Cartesian notion that the sensation of pain travels in a direct pathway from the injured area to the brain; rather, it postulates that the perception of pain is mediated by intermediate neurons modulating the signal.

Generalized seizures: Seizures that affect the brain bilaterally from the onset. Loss of consciousness is present and may be accompanied, depending on the type of general seizure, by tonic-clonic, myoclonic, absence, and atonic symptoms.

GHB (gamma-hydroxybutyrate) receptors: A recently identified G-protein–coupled receptor, distributed widely in the cerebral cortex and subcortical locations. It facilitates the release of glutamate but may also modulate other neurons, including monoamine neurons.

Glasgow Coma Scale: Neurological scale that aims to give a reliable, objective way of recording the conscious state of a person during initial, as well as subsequent, assessment.

Globus pallidus: Structure within the basal ganglia that relays information from the striatum to the thalamus.

Grand-mal seizures: See *Tonic-clonic seizures.*

Hamartomas: A benign tumor composed of local mature cells.

Heritability coefficient: The ratio of concordance for a trait in monozygotic versus dizygotic twins; an estimate of the importance of genes plus gene-environment interactions in determining a trait.

Huntington's disease: Neurodegenerative disorder affecting diverse areas of the brain and manifest as movement disorders, dementia, and cognitive decline. The striatum is especially affected, with involvement of the direct and indirect movement pathways. Hyperkinesia is the dominant symptom, but hypokinesia is also common in the later stages.

Hypermethylation: Methylation is the attachment of a methyl group to a region of DNA, suppressing its transcription. In hypermethylation, sites that are not usually methylated become so.

Hyperkinesia: Extreme movement of a pathological origin. (See also *Huntington's disease.*)

Hypnagogic hallucination: Episode of hearing or seeing nonexistent stimuli while falling asleep.

Hypocretin (orexin): Excitatory neuropeptide. Hypocretin-containing neurons have widespread projections throughout the central nervous system, with particularly dense excitatory projections to monoaminergic centers such as the noradrenergic locus coeruleus, histaminergic tuberomammillary nucleus, serotonergic raphe nucleus, and dopaminergic ventral tegmental area.

Hypokinesia: Abnormally diminished motor activity. (See also *Parkinson's disease.*)

Ictal orgasms: Rare orgasm experienced by both genders during the aura of partial seizures located in the temporal lobe.

Inclusion bodies: Aggregates within a cell that form when foreign particles (e.g., viral) or misfolded proteins precipitate and coalesce from the cytosol.

Incomplete penetrance: When a heritable trait is manifest less than 100% of the time by individuals carrying the principal gene.

Indirect pathway: The indirect movement pathway operates in conjunction with the direct pathway. The indirect pathway passes through the striatum and external globus pallidus before passing through the subthalamic nucleus and projecting to the substantia nigra. Parallel to the activating influence of the direct pathway, the indirect pathway sends inhibitory signals to the globus pallidus externus, reducing inhibitory projections that this structure usually extends to the subthalamic nucleus. Cells of the subthalamic nucleus are then permitted to send more activating signals to globus pallidus internus and substantia nigra pars reticulata, which in turn project inhibitory signals to the ventrolateral nucleus of the thalamus, reducing activation of the motor cerebral cortex.

Infarction: Formation of dead tissue due to lack of oxygen.

Inflammatory cascade: A complex biochemical sequence that orchestrates the vasodilation, swelling, activation, and migration of white blood cells to a site of injury or infection.

Intracerebral hemorrhage: Leakage of a cerebral blood vessel into the brain.

Ipsilesional gaze shift: A symptom of stroke in the middle cerebral artery; the pupils of the eye tend to move toward the side of the body where the lesion is located.

Insomnia: Difficulty in getting to sleep, staying asleep, or feeling rested upon awakening.

Interleukin-10: A cytokine, secreted by white blood cells, that is anti-inflammatory and that shifts the immune response from an emphasis on the cytotoxic actions of macrophages (Th1) to an emphasis on antibody production (Th2).

Ischemia: Restriction in blood supply.

Islet amyloid polypeptide (or amylin): A hormone, secreted by pancreatic beta cells, that induces satiation and slows digestion in response to eating. Amylin molecules can bind to each other, forming complexes that are toxic to the beta cells and are likely contributors to diabetes.

Lactic acid (hydroxy carboxylic acid): During normal metabolism and exercise, lactate is produced. It does not increase in concentration, however, until the rate of lactate production exceeds the rate of lactate removal.

Lacunar disease: Occlusion of one of the penetrating arteries that provides blood to the brain's deep structures.

Laminae II and III: Two of the six layers of cerebral cortex. Laminae II and III are rich in pyramidal cells and show similar voltage oscillations.

Lewy bodies: Pathological aggregates of protein within the nerve cell. Lewy bodies are found in several neurodegenerative disorders, including Parkinson's, Alzheimer's, Pick's, and dementia with Lewy bodies.

Long-term synaptic depression: A persistent decrease in the strength of a synapse, brought about when the presynaptic neuron is firing while the postsynaptic neuron is not.

Long-term potentiation: A persistent increase in the strength of a synapse, brought about when the presynaptic and postsynaptic neurons fire simultaneously.

Lymphocytes: A class of white blood cells made up of natural killer cells (which attack pathogens by releasing granules of destructive enzymes), B cells (which produce antibodies), and T cells (which help orchestrate the immune response and in some cases also release cytotoxic granules).

Lysosomes: Sacs within the cell that are filled with acid and digestive enzymes. Lysosomes fuse with vacuoles containing food particles, pathogens, discarded protein, or other debris and break down their contents.

Macrophages: Large, ameba-like white blood cells that scavenge cellular debris, engulf pathogens, and display components of the pathogen to spur the production of antibodies.

Meiotic machinery: The intracellular structures, most notably spindle filaments, that draw two copies of a chromosome away from each other, so that each daughter cell contains only one copy. This process is used to produce sperm and egg cells.

Melatonin: N-acetyl-5-methoxytryptamine is a hormone, produced by the pineal gland, which is involved in regulating the circadian rhythm.

Meningoencephalitis: An often dangerous inflammation of the brain and meninges, caused by mumps, other viruses, bacteria, or protozoal infection.

Metabolic syndrome: The combined presence of several conditions, including abdominal obesity, reduced high-density lipoprotein (HDL) ("good") cholesterol, and increased triglycerides, blood pressure, and fasting glucose. Metabolic syndrome raises the odds of developing cardiovascular disease and diabetes.

Methylprednisolone: A synthetic hormone related to cortisol that is used as an anti-inflammatory and immune-modulating drug in autoimmune disorders.

Microglia: Cells in the brain and spinal cord that, like macrophages elsewhere in the body, recognize, engulf, and destroy pathogens.

Microtubules: Self-organizing cylindrical filaments that form part of the internal skeleton of cells and facilitate the movement of vesicles within the cell.

Middle cerebral arteries: A pair of arteries that project to many parts of the lateral cerebral cortex and to the anterior temporal lobes and insular cortices.

Movement disorder: Pathological condition that affects the speed, fluency, ease, and quality of movement.

Multidisciplinary: Several disciplines working together without necessarily integrating. In pain management, an interdisciplinary team may include a psychologist, anesthesiologist, neurologist, exercise physiologist, physical therapist, biofeedback technician, and dietitian.

Myoclonic epilepsy: Seizures characterized by jerking movements caused by contraction and sudden muscle relaxation.

Myoclonus: Sudden, involuntary jerking of a muscle or group of muscles.

Myofacial pain: Chronic muscular pain affecting the fascia, or connecting tissue of the muscles.

Myofasciitis: Inflammation of muscle and its fascia.

Myoglobinuric renal failure: Kidney disease in which muscle damage (e.g., rhabdomyolysis) causes a large quantity of myoglobin protein to accumulate in the tubules, leading to obstruction and renal ischemia with nephrosis.

Narcolepsy: A neurologically based dyssomnia of unknown origin that causes transient moments of sleeplike phenomena (e.g., sleep attack, cataplexy, sleep paralysis, and hypnagogic hallucinations).

Nerve blocks: The injection of a local anesthetic near nerves, usually spinal nerve roots, for temporary control of pain. Permanent nerve block can be produced by the destruction of nerve tissue.

Nerve growth factors: Signaling molecules that support the growth, survival, and elaborate branching structure of neurons.

Neural tube: Embryonic precursor to the central nervous system.

Neuritic plaques: Extracellular deposits of amyloid peptide surrounded by neurons whose dendrites and axons have deteriorated.

Neurofibrillary tangles: Within neurons, filamentous aggregates of the protein tau, to which an excessive number of phosphate groups have been attached. Neurofibrillary tangles are found in Alzheimer's disease and in most frontotemporal dementias and are probably toxic to neurons.

Neurofibromatosis: A genetically inherited disorder in which the nerve tissue grows tumors.

Neurofilament: A class of filaments, comprising protein subunits, within the axons of nerve cells. Neurofilaments repel each other and thus determine the diameter of axons and, through this, their electrical conduction velocity.

Neuroleptic malignancy syndrome (NMS): Refers to a constellation of symptoms, including hyperthermia, muscle rigidity, and autonomic dysregulation, caused as side effects to neuroleptic medication.

Neuromatrix Theory of Pain: According to the neuromatrix theory, mediating influences are present in pain perception at the periphery and spinal cord and there is an extensive pain network involving the thalamus, cortex, and limbic system, all of which contribute to an individual's final perception of pain.

Neuropathic pain: Pain arising as a direct result of damage to the somatosensory system.

Night terrors: A parasomnia in which the sleeper experiences intense fear while in non-REM slow-wave sleep. Dream content is rarely associated with the fear.

Nigrostriatal pathway: Neuropathway that connects the substantia nigra with the striatum and operates principally via dopaminergic neurons.

Nociceptors: A sensory receptor that signals pain in response to potentially injurious stimuli.

Nocturnal myoclonus: Periodic limb movement in sleep.

Nonmalignant (benign) chronic pain: In the absence of an active lesion or malignant process, benign chronic pain is pain that lasts several months beyond the normal healing period for an injury or disease.

Non-REM: Sleep that does not result in rapid eye movement and occupies about 80% of human sleep. It spans the four levels of sleep (stages 1 to 4) and is devoid of dream content.

Notch receptor: A receptor present in nearly all multicellular organisms that allows the differentiation of cells to be regulated by surface proteins on neighboring cells.

Oligodendrocytes: A type of glial cell that provides the insulating myelin sheath around certain axons in the central nervous system. In the peripheral nervous system, the same function is performed by Schwann cells.

Oligomers: A substance consisting of identical, repeated units attached together. If there is a large number of units, the term would be *polymer* instead.

Opioid analgesics: Narcotic-based pain killers.

Orbitofrontal cortex: A region of the cerebral cortex located just above the eyes and thought to be involved in intuition, planning, and the regulation of emotions and cravings.

Organochlorine pesticides: Chlorine-based, organic pesticide (e.g., DDT).

Orexin: See *Hypocretin.*

OxyContin: An opiate (narcotic) analgesic.

Palpebral fissures: Anatomical name for the separation between the upper and lower eyelids.

PANDAS: The term *Pediatric Autoimmune Neuropsychiatric Disorders Associated with Streptococcal infections* is used to describe rapid-onset childhood obsessive-compulsive disorder (OCD) and/or tic disorders such as Tourette's syndrome (TS) that occur after infection with group A beta-hemolytic streptococcus (GABHS) (e.g., strep throat and scarlet fever).

Parasomnias: Sleep disorders that disrupt sleep different from sleep onset disorders such as insomnia or narcolepsy.

Parkinson's disease: A neurodegeneration of the substantia nigra that affects both the direct and indirect movement pathways, creating a state of hypokinesia. Loss of dopaminergic neurons in the substantia nigra pars compacta reduces this structure's projection to the striatum. Dopamine from the pars compacta excites the direct pathway and inhibits the indirect pathway. The reduction of dopamine in the initial segments of these pathways creates a paradoxical end result: The excitatory nature of the direct pathway is reduced while the inhibitory nature of the indirect pathway is increased; both effects lead to fewer thalamic projections to the motor cortex, which causes hypokinesis.

Partial seizures: Seizures that affect only one area of the brain; can be either simple or complex.

Penicillamine: A drug of the chelator class, which sequesters heavy metals in the body.

Pentylenetetrazole: A GABA-receptor antagonist that increases neural excitability; used at one time as a circulatory and respiratory stimulant.

Pergolide: Medicine associated with the treatment of parkinsonism. It is an ergot alkaloid and acts as a dopamine agonist.

Pervasive developmental disorders: A group of disorders characterized by delays in the development of socialization and communication skills.

Petit-mal seizures: See *Absence seizures.*

Phantom limb: The sensation that a missing organ is still attached to the body.

Phenylketonuria (PKU): PKU is a condition in which a newborn is unable to properly break down an amino acid called phenylalanine, which is involved in the production of melanin. The buildup of phenylalanine is toxic and results in delayed mental and social skills, microcephalia, hyperactivity, mental retardation, and seizures.

Philtrum: A medial cleft extending from the nose to the upper lip.

Phonatory activation: Utterance of sounds through the vocal cords.

Phospholipidases: Excess accumulation of intracellular phospholipids.

Photoentrainment: Alignment of an organism's circadian rhythm to that of an external rhythm in its environment.

Photopsias: Perceived flashes of light. Also called *phosphenes.*

Plaques: Patches; for example, the abnormal deposits of amyloid peptides in extracellular spaces.

Positron emission tomography (PET): A three-dimensional imaging technique which detects radiation emitted from a biological active substance injected in the body.

Postconcussive syndrome: A common sequela of traumatic brain injury that includes headache, dizziness, neuropsychiatric symptoms, and cognitive impairment.

Posterior cerebral arteries: A pair of arteries that supply oxygenated blood to the occipital lobes.

Postictal sleep: Sleep following a seizure, usually lasting 5 to 30 minutes.

Prader-Willi syndrome: A congenital disease that involves obesity, decreased muscle tone, decreased mental capacity, and sex glands that produce little or no hormones.

Primary brain injury: Injury to the brain that is complete at the time of the original insult.

Prion protein: A specific protein on the outer surface of nerve cell membranes that may help to transport copper ions into the cell or play a role in synapse formation. When the prion protein is misfolded, it becomes toxic to nerve cells and can induce other proteins to similarly misfold. The misfolded protein has a large beta sheet that makes it resistant to the cells' protein-degrading machinery.

Prolactin: A pituitary hormone subserving lactation that in high amounts may reduce libido. Prolactin also causes the proliferation of oligodendritic precursor cells and may be responsible for the remyelination of white matter plaques in multiple sclerosis during pregnancy.

Proteolytic enzymes: A group of enzymes that break the long molecule of protein into its constituent peptides and eventually into amino acids.

Putamen: Part of the basal ganglia. Located at the lower, inner forebrain, the putamen is thought to be involved in the learning and control of motor behavior and perhaps in category learning.

Pyramidal neurons: Large, triangular-shaped, pyramidal neurons are the main excitatory cells in prefrontal cortex and use glutamate as a neurotransmitter. Because of the extensive branching of their dendrites and axons, they are well suited to integrate information.

Rabbit syndrome (RS): Rabbit syndrome was described in 1972 as a perioral hyperkinetic disorder, with a frequency of 5.0 to 5.5 Hz, in association with long-term neuroleptic drug therapy. It was differentiated from tardive dyskinesia with the help of two important features: its persistence in stage 1 non-REM sleep and sparing of tongue involvement.

Rapamycin: An immunosuppressant drug whose primary use is to prevent rejection in organ transplantation.

Reality distortion syndrome: Hallucinations, delusions associated with psychosis.

Reinforcer: A stimulus—the provision of a desired outcome or the removal of an aversive outcome—that increases the future probability of the behavior that preceded it.

REM: "Rapid-eye movement" refers to a stage of sleep in which major saccades or quick eye movements are visible together with heightened brain activity, as evidenced by alpha waves (8 to 13 cycles/ second) on EEG tracings. REM sleep is associated with dreaming.

Restless-legs syndrome: Neurological syndrome that results in an irresistible urge to move one's legs to reduce uncomfortable lower-limb sensations.

Rivastigmine: A cholinesterase inhibitor used in the treatment of dementia.

Second impact syndrome: A condition in which the brain swells after a person suffers a second concussion before recovering from the first.

Secondary brain injury: Indirect damage to the brain after the original insult or trauma.

Secondary reinforcer: A stimulus that acquires its reinforcing qualities through conditioning or repeated pairing with a stimulus that is already reinforcing.

Secretase: An enzyme that cleaves protein, especially amyloid precursor protein.

Serotonin syndrome: Potentially life-threatening reaction to excessive serotonin at the synaptic cleft, resulting in multiple autonomic, metabolic, and muscular dysfunctions.

Shaken-baby syndrome: Severe form of child abuse caused by violently shaking an infant or child. Injuries are most likely to happen when the baby is shaken and hits its head on something. Symptoms include convulsions and loss of consciousness.

Simple partial seizure (SPS): A partial seizure in which consciousness is not lost or impaired. Muscular, sensory, and psychic (emotional/perceptual) functioning may be affected.

Sleep architecture: The pattern of progression through the various phases of sleep across time.

Sleep attack: Irresistible urge to sleep that comes on suddenly.

Sleep paralysis: Inability to voluntarily move while remaining conscious during the onset of sleep or upon awakening.

Sleep soliloquy: Sleep-talking; a parasomnia that occurs during REM or transitional non-REM, just short of wakening.

Sodium oxybate: Also called gamma-hydroxybutyrate (GHB), sodium oxybate is a central nervous system depressant prescribed to treat cataplexy.

Somnambulism: Sleep-walking; a parasomnia occurring in stages 3 and 4 of sleep.

Sonic hedgehog: A signaling molecule involved in embryonic development, in the proliferation and differentiation of adult stem cells, and in the initiation of cancer. In the brain, the sonic hedgehog promotes the growth and branching of axons.

Single-photon emission computed tomography (SPECT): An imaging technique. Depending on the specific tracer, SPECT scans can show regional cerebral blood flow, rate of metabolism, the rate of reuptake of a specific neurotransmitter, or the concentration of neurotransmitter receptors.

Splenium: The most posterior region of the corpus callosum, involved in the transfer of information from the temporal, parietal, and occipital lobes between the two hemispheres.

Status epilepticus: A life-threatening episode of prolonged, uninterrupted seizures.

Striatum: Part of the basal ganglia at the lower, inner forebrain consisting of the caudate, putamen, and tracts of white matter termed the internal capsule. The striatum receives extensive input from the cortex, sending output to the other components of the basal ganglia, and indirectly to the thalamus and cortex. It is thought to be involved in executive functioning, the planning and control of movement, and the response to novelty and reward.

Subarachnoid hemorrhage: Bleeding into the subarachnoid space between the arachnoid membrane and the pia mater.

Substantia nigra pars compacta: Located in the midbrain and comprising part of the basal ganglia, the substantia nigra pars compacta appears to be involved in fine motor control, learned behaviors, the sleep-wake cycle, and perhaps the ability to sense the passage of time. Loss of dopaminergic neurons in this nucleus is responsible for Parkinson's disease.

Superior cerebellar peduncle: A tract of white matter connecting the cerebellum with the pons and midbrain.

Supplementary motor area (SMA): A part of the sensorimotor cortex.

Synaptic plasticity: The ability of neurons to change in order to modify the synapse in response to use or disuse of the synaptic connection.

Syntax: The way words are formed into a phrase or sentence.

Tardive akathisia: Delayed onset of inner restlessness after taking neuroleptic drugs, manifest as an inability to remain still.

Tardive dyskinesia: A syndrome of repetitive, involuntary, purposeless movements, often involving the mouth, face, or limbs. It can be idiopathic but is most often caused by neuroleptic medications. Its name derives from its late (tardive) onset.

Tau protein: A protein that supports the structure of nerve cells by promoting the assembly and stabilization of microtubules.

Tegmentum: A region at the base of the midbrain involved in oculomotor control.

Telomeric exchange: Sister-chromatid exchange is a form of genetic recombination in which two copies of the same chromosome exchange DNA during the formation of sperm and egg cells. When the exchange occurs near the ends of the chromosomes (telomeres), the two copies are then less likely to separate properly during meiosis.

Teratogen exposure: Exposure to toxic chemicals in vitro, producing birth defects.

Todd paralysis: Focal weakness in a part of the body after a seizure.

Tonic: In muscles, it refers to tonus or contraction.

Tonic-clonic seizures: A type of generalized seizure affecting the entire brain, which causes a convulsion characterized by two muscle phases: first, muscle rigidity (tonic), then muscle jerks (clonic). Also called "grand-mal seizures."

Tourette's syndrome: Tic disorder, usually first manifest in childhood, that may involve a facial tic, involuntary vocalizations, and other tics (e.g., shoulder shrugging and eye blinking).

Transcutaneous electrical nerve stimulation (TENS): Use of a device to electrically stimulate surface nerve endings to generate tactile sensations that compete with the perception of pain.

Transentorhinal cortex: A region in the medial temporal lobe, near the hippocampus, that appears to be involved in the formation of autobiographical memories. It is one of the first brain regions to be affected by neurofibrillary tangles and cell loss in Alzheimer's disease.

Transient ischemic attacks (TIAs): A transient stroke that lasts only a few minutes. It occurs when the blood supply to part of the brain is briefly interrupted.

Transporter protein: A protein that spans the cell membrane of a neuron, allowing the transfer of a specific substance into the cell. A subclass of transporter proteins allows for the reuptake of neurotransmitters into the presynaptic cell.

Trigger points: Hypersensitive points on skeletal muscle where nodules may form.

Trisomy: A condition in which the cells of the body contain three copies, rather than two, of a chromosome. This occurs when the two copies do not properly separate during the formation of the egg or sperm. (See also *Telomeric exchange.*)

Tuberous sclerosis: A group of genetic disorders that affect the skin, brain/nervous system, kidneys, and heart and cause tumors to grow. Neurodevelopmental symptoms include mental retardation, developmental delays, and seizure.

Tumor necrosis factor-α: A cytokine that promotes inflammation and an acute-phase response that directly inhibits viral replication.

Vacuoles: Sacks, surrounded by a membrane, within cells that are formed by the merger of many small vesicles. Vacuoles have various purposes within cells, including the segregation and export of harmful substances.

Vagus nerve stimulation (VNS): An implant in the neck that delivers electrical simulation to the vagus nerve.

Verbal short-term memory: Language-based memory of short duration.

Virus coat protein: The protein constituting the outer layer of a virus, protecting the infectious RNA or DNA core.

Volumetric MRI: The use of structural magnetic resonance imaging data, that is appropriately transformed so that all images are in the same orientation, to measure the volume of structures such as specific brain regions.

Weber's syndrome: A form of stroke characterized by the presence of an oculomotor nerve palsy and contralateral hemiparesis or hemiplegia.

Williams' syndrome: A genetic condition caused by 25 missing genes. Neurodevelopmental symptoms include mild-to-moderate mental retardation, ADHD-like distractibility, and gregarious personality.

Chapter 4 Questions

1. Which test might best discern the difference between neuroleptic malignant syndrome and serotonin syndrome?
   a. Electroencephalogram (EEG)
   b. Electrolyte profile
   c. Lithium serum level
   d. Creatine phosphokinase level
2. In Parkinson's disease, direct pathway activity_____ while the indirect pathway activity_____ thalamic projections to the motor cortices.
   a. Increase, decreases
   b. Decreases, increases
   c. Decreases, decreases
   d. Increases, increases
3. Tardive dyskinesia may be treated with_____ drugs, while rabbit syndrome is best treated with_____ drugs.
   a. Anticholinergic, cholinergic
   b. Cholinergic, anticholinergic
   c. Acetylcholinesterase, cholinergic
   d. Anticholinergic, anticholinergic

4. Excessive muscle tension leads to a buildup of lactic acid and causes pain because
    a. Hydrogen ions build up outside the neuron.
    b. Potassium ions build up inside the neuron.
    c. Chloride ions build up inside the neuron.
    d. Sodium ions build up outside the neuron.

5. Developmental delay, resulting in enuresis, is more prevalent in
    a. Hispanics.
    b. Asians.
    c. Boys.
    d. Girls.

6. Amyloid beta (Aβ) is associated with
    a. Alzheimer's disease.
    b. Dementia with Lewy bodies.
    c. Frontotemporal dementias.
    d. All of the above

7. Trisomy 21 is associated with
    a. Fragile X syndrome.
    b. Down syndrome.
    c. Williams' syndrome.
    d. All of the above

8. Neurodevelopmental disorders may be
    a. Genetic/congenital.
    b. Endogenous/exogenous.
    c. Metabolic or chromosomal.
    d. All of the above

9. Which of the following is not subsumed under autism spectrum disorder in the *DSM-5*?
    a. Pervasive developmental disorder
    b. Asperger's syndrome
    c. Angelman syndrome
    d. Childhood disintegrative disorder

10. Abnormal growth of benign tumors that affect the nervous system occurs in
    a. Smith-Magenis syndrome.
    b. Neurofibromatosis.
    c. Tuberous scoliosis.
    d. Both b and c

11. Weakness in the contralateral lower limb and incontinence may indicate
    a. Anterior cerebral artery infarct.
    b. Posterior cerebral artery infarct.
    c. Middle cerebral artery infarct.
    d. None of the above

12. Demyelination, although associated with other neurodegenerative diseases, is the hallmark of
   a. Huntington's disease.
   b. Multiple sclerosis.
   c. Cerebral palsy.
   d. Parkinsonism.
13. Second impact syndrome
   a. Refers to re-experiencing traumatic events by persons with posttraumatic stress disorder (PTSD).
   b. Psychological exposure to the same trauma repeatedly.
   c. Reinjury of the brain shortly after an original traumatic brain injury (TBI).
   d. Indirect pathologic conditions subsequent to direct insult to the brain.
14. What percentage of Americans will experience a seizure in their lifetime?
   a. Less than 1%
   b. 1%
   c. 5%
   d. 10%
15. Psychomotor syndrome of schizophrenia refers to
   a. Positive symptoms.
   b. Negative symptoms.
   c. Psychosocial signs.
   d. Biological signs.
16. Insomnia
   a. Is effectively treated with behavioral approaches.
   b. Generally requires the use of benzodiazepines.
   c. Is pharmacologically best treated with antihistamines.
   d. Should always be directly treated.
17. The use of opioids in the treatment of chronic pain
   a. Has increased.
   b. Is controversial.
   c. Is linked to drug addiction.
   d. All of the above

   Answers: (1) d, (2) c, (3) b, (4) a, (5) c, (6) d, (7) b, (8) d, (9) c, (10) d, (11) a, (12) b, (13) c, (14) d, (15) b, (16) a, (17) d.

REFERENCES

Abel, E., & Sokol, R. (1987). Incidence of fetal alcohol syndrome and economic impact of FAS-related anomalies. *Drug and Alcohol Dependence, 19*, 51–70.

Abrams, P., & Andersson, K. E. (2007). Muscarinic receptor antagonists for overactive bladder. *British Journal of Urology International, 100*, 987.

Adams, R., Chimowitz, M., Alpert, J., Awad, I., Cerqueria, M., Fayad, P., & Taubert, K. (2003). Coronary risk evaluation in patients with transient ischemic attack and ischemic stroke: A scientific statement for healthcare professionals from the Stroke Council and the Council on Clinical Cardiology of the American Heart Association/American Stroke Association. *Circulation, 108,* 1278.

Ajmone-Marsan, C., & Goldhammer, L. (1973). Clinical patterns and electrographic data in cases of partial seizures of fronto-central-parietal origin. In M. Brazier (Ed.), *Epilepsy, its phenomenon in man.* San Diego, CA: Academic Press.

Akagi, H. (2002). Akathisia: Overlooked at a cost. *British Medical Journal, 324,* 1506–1507.

Ala, A., Walker, A., Ashkan, K., Dooley, J., & Schilsky, M. (2007). Wilson's disease. *Lancet, 369,* 397–408.

Albin, R. (2006). Neurobiology of basal ganglia and Tourette syndrome: Striatal and dopamine function. In J. T. Walkup, J. W. Mink, & P. J. Hollenbeck (Eds.), *Advances in neurology: Tourette syndrome.* Philadelphia, PA: Lippincott.

Allen, R. (2004). Dopamine and iron in the pathophysiology of restless legs syndrome (RLS). *Sleep Medicine, 5,* 385–391.

American Academy of Sleep Medicine (2005). *The international classification of sleep disorders: Diagnostic and coding manual.* Rochester, MN: Author.

American Congress of Rehabilitation Medicine. (1993). Mild Traumatic Brain Injury Committee of the Head Injury Interdisciplinary Special Interest Group. *Journal of Head Trauma and Rehabilitation, 8,* 86–87.

American Heart Association. (2010). Heart Stroke Update. *Journal of the American Heart Association, 121,* e46–e215.

American Psychiatric Association. (1994). *Diagnostic and statistical manual of mental disorders* (4th ed.) (*DSM-IV*). Washington, DC: American Psychiatric Press.

American Psychiatric Association. (2000). *Diagnostic and statistical manual of mental disorders* (4th ed., text revision) (*DSM-IV, TR*). Washington, DC: Author.

American Psychiatric Association. (2011). Autism spectrum disorder. *DSM-IV Work Group.* http://www.dsm5.org/ProposedRevisions/Pages/proposedrevision.aspx?rid=94

Amminger, G. P., Schafer, M. R., Papageorgiou, K., Klier, C. M., Cotton, S. M., Harrigan, S. M. (2010). Long-chain omega-3 fatty acids for indicated prevention of psychotic disorders. *Archives of General Psychiatry, 67,* 146–154.

Arlin, A. (1981). *Sleep talking: Psychology and psychophysiology.* Hillsdale, NJ: Erlbaum.

Arundine, M., Aarts, M., Lau, A., & Tymianski, M. (2004). Vulnerability of central neurons to secondary insults after in vitro mechanical stretch. *Journal of Euroscience, 23,* 8106–8123.

Ashburn, M., & Staats, P. (1999). Management of chronic pain. *Lancet, 353,* 1865–1869.

Ballantyne, J., & Mao, J. (2003). Opioid therapy for chronic pain. *New England Journal of Medicine, 349,* 1943–1953.

Bazil, C. (2004). Nocturnal seizures. *Seminars in Neurology, 24,* 293–300.

Bear, M., Connors, B., & Paradiso, M. (2007). *Neuroscience: Exploring the brain.* Baltimore, MD: Lippincott Williams & Wilkins.

Bellettato, C. M., & Scarpa, M. (2010). Pathophysiology of neuropathic lysosomal storage disorders. *Journal of Inherited Metabolic Disease, 33,* 347–362.

Bhasin, M., Rowan, E., Edwards, K., & McKeith, I. (2007). Cholinesterase inhibitors in dementia with Lewy bodies—A comparative analysis. *International Journal of Geriatric Psychiatry, 22,* 890–895.

Black, J., Pardi, D., Homfeldt, C., & Inhaber, N. (2010). The nightly use of sodium oxybate is associated with a reduction in nocturnal sleep disruption: A double-blind, placebo-controlled study in patients with narcolepsy. *Journal of Clinical Sleep Medicine, 6,* 596–602.

Block, M. L., & Hong, J. S. (2005). Microglia and inflammation-mediated neurodegeneration: Multiple triggers with a common mechanism. *Progress in Neurobiology, 76,* 77–98.

Block, M. L., Zecca, L., & Hong, J. S. (2007). Microglia-mediated neurotoxicity: Uncovering the molecular mechanisms. *Nature Reviews Neuroscience, 8*, 57–69.

Boake, C., McCauley, S., & Levin, H. (2004). Limited agreement between criteria-based diagnosis of post-concussional syndrome. *Journal of Neuropsychiatry and Clinical Neuroscience, 16*, 493–499.

Bowler, J. (2003). Acetylcholinesterase inhibitors for vascular dementia and Alzheimer's disease combined with cerebrovascular disease. *Stroke, 34*, 584–586.

Brodaty, H., McGilchrist, C., Harris, L., & Peters, K. (1993). Time until institutionalization and death in patients with dementia: Role of caregiver training and risk factors. *Archives of Neurology, 50*, 643–560.

Brodie, M., & Kwan, P. (2002). Staged approach to epilepsy management. *Neurology, 58*, S2–S8.

Brown, C. (2006). *The neural mechanism for sleep initiation in the mammalian brain*. Thesis: Stephen F. Austin State University.

Brown, T., & Holmes, G. (2008). *Handbook of epilepsy*. Philadelphia, PA: Lippincott Williams & Wilkins.

Bruns, D., & Disorbio, J. (2005, Nov/Dec). Chronic pain and biopsychosocial disorders: The BHI-2 approach to classification and assessment. *Practical Pain Management*, 2–9.

Butterfield, D. A., & Sultana, R. (2007). Proteomics analysis in Alzheimer's disease: New insights into mechanisms of neurodegeneration. In M. B. H. Youdim, P. Riederer, S. A. Mandel, & L. Battistin (Eds.), *Handbook of neurochemistry and molecular neurobiology: Degenerative diseases of the nervous system* (pp. 233–252). New York, NY: Springer.

Byne, W., Hazlett, E. A., Buchsbaum, M. S., & Kemether, E. (2009). The thalamus and schizophrenia: Current status of research. *Acta Neuropathologica, 117*, 347–368.

Calleja, J., Carpizo, R., Berciano, J. (1988). Orgasmic epilepsy. *Epilepsia, 29*, 635–639.

Cardoso, S. M., Pereira, C. F., Moreira, P. I., Arduino, D. M., Esteves, A. R., & Oliveira, C. R. (2010). Mitochondrial control of autophagic lysosomal pathway in Alzheimer's disease. *Experimental Neurology, 223*, 294–298.

Catena Dell'osso, M., Fagiolini, A., Ducci, F., Masalehdan, A., Ciapparelli, A., & Frank, E. (2007). Newer antipsychotics and the rabbit syndrome. *Clinical Practice and Epidemiology in Mental Health, 3*, 6.

CDC. (2009). Drinking while pregnant still a problem: Alcohol use during pregnancy can cause birth defects and developmental disabilities. Women who are pregnant or might get pregnant should abstain from using alcohol. *Morbidity and Mortality Weekly Report, 58*, 529–532.

Cervenka, S., Palhagen, S., Comley, R, Panagiotidis, G., Cselényi, Z., & Matthews, J. (2004). Support for dopaminergic hypoactivity in restless legs syndrome: A PET study on D_2-receptor binding. *Brain: A Journal of Neurology, 129*, 2017–2028.

Chamberlain, S. R., Robbins, T. W., & Sabakian, B. J. (2007). The neurobiology of attention-deficit/hyperactivity disorder. *Biological Psychiatry, 61*, 1317–1319.

Chen, C.-M., Lin, J.-K., Liu, S.-H., & Lin-Shiau, S.-Y. (2008). Novel regimen through combination of memantine and tea polyphenol for neuroprotection against brain excitotoxicity. *Journal of Neuroscience Research, 86*, 2696–2704.

Chou, R., Ballantyne, J., Fanciullo, G., Fine, P., & Miaskowski, C. (2009a). Research gaps on use of opioids for chronic noncancer pain: Findings from a review of the evidence for an American Pain Society and American Academy of Pain Medicine clinical practice guideline. *Journal of Pain, 10*, 147–159.

Chou, R., Fanciullo, G., Fine, P., et al. (2009b). Clinical guidelines for the use of chronic opioid therapy in chronic noncancer pain. *Journal of Pain, 10*, 113–130.

Chouinard, G., & Margolese, H. (2006). Manual for the Extrapyramidal Symptom Rating Scale (ESRS). *Schizophrenia Research, 85*, 305.

Chugani, D., Muzik, O., Behen, M., Rothermel, R., Janisse, J., Lee, J., & Chugani, H. (1999). Developmental changes in brain serotonin synthesis capacity in autistic and nonautistic children. *Annals of Neurology, 45*, 287–295.

Cohen, T., Leister, E., Ajo, D., Leuthardt, E., & Genin, G. (2005). Deformation of the human brain induced by mild acceleration. *Journal of Neurotrauma, 22*, 845–856.

Colameco, S., Coren, J., & Ciervo, C. (2009). Continuous opioid treatment for chronic non-cancerous pain: A time for moderation in prescribing. *Postgraduate Medicine, 121*, 61–66.

Comper, P., Bisschop, S., Carnide, N., & Tricco, A. (2005). A systematic review of treatments for mild traumatic brain injury. *Brain Injury, 19*, 863–880.

Correll, C. U., Leucht, S., & Kane, J. M. (2004). Lower risk for tardive dyskinesia associated with second-generation antipsychotics: A systematic review of 1-year studies. *American Journal of Psychiatry, 161*, 414–425.

Cortese, S., Konofal, E., Lecendreux, M., Arnulf, I., Mouren, M., Darra, F., & Dalla Bernardina, B. (2005). Restless legs syndrome and attention-deficit/hyperactivity disorder: A review of the literature. *Sleep: Journal of Sleep and Sleep Disorders Research, 28*, 1007–1013.

Crownshaw, T. (2004). The role of pharmacotherapy in the management of behaviour disorders in traumatic brain injury patients. *Brain Injury, 18*, 1–31.

Cuccaro, M. L., Wright, H. H., Abramson, R. K., Marstellar, F. A., & Valentine, J. (1993). Whole-blood serotonin and cognitive functioning in autistic individuals and their first-degree relatives. *Journal of Neuropsychiatry and Clinical Neurosciences, 5*, 94–101.

Curatolo, P., Paloscia, C., D'Agati, E., Moavero, R., & Pasini, A. (2009). The neurobiology of attention deficit/hyperactivity disorder. *European Journal of Paediatric Neurology, 13*, 299–304.

Dagan, Y. (2002). Circadian rhythm sleep disorders (CRSD). *Sleep Medicine Reviews, 6*, 45–54.

Das, S., & Ray, K. (2006). Wilson's disease: An update. *Nature Clinical Practice: Neurology, 2*, 482–493. 12doi:10.1038/ncpneuro0291

Daumit, G. L., Goff, D. C., Meyer, J. M., Davis, V. G., Nasrallah, H. A., & McEvoy, J. P. (2008). Antipsychotic effects on estimated 10-year coronary heart disease risk in the CATIE schizophrenia study. *Schizophrenia Research, 105*, 175–187.

Daviglus, M. L., Bell, C. C., Berrettini, W., Bowen, P. E., Connolly, E. S., Jr., Cox, N. J., & Dunbar-Jacob, J. (2010). National Institutes of Health State-of-the-Science Conference statement: Preventing Alzheimer disease and cognitive decline. *Annals of Internal Medicine, 153*, 176–181.

Denckla, M. (2006). Attention deficit hyperactivity disorder: the childhood co-morbidity that most influences the disability burden in Tourette syndrome. *Advances in Neurology, 99*, 17–21.

Deuschl, G., Bain, P., & Brin, M. (1998). Consensus Statement of the Movement Disorder Society on Tremor. *Movement Disorders, 13*, 2–23.

Dierssen, M., & Ramakers, G. J. A. (2006). Dendritic pathology in mental retardation: From molecular genetics to neurobiology. *Genes, Brain and Behavior, 5* (Suppl. 2), 48–60.

Duara, R., Barker, W., Loewenstein, D., & Bain, L. (2009). The basis for disease-modifying treatments for Alzheimer's disease: The Sixth Annual Mild Cognitive Impairment Symposium. *Alzheimer's and Dementia, 5*, 66–74.

Dufresne, R., & Wagner, R. L. (1988). Antipsychotic-withdrawal akathisia versus antipsychotic-induced akathisia: Further evidence for the existence of tardive akathisia. *Journal of Clinical Psychiatry, 49*, 435–438.

Easton, J., Saver, J., Albers, G., Alberts, M., Chaturvedi, S., Feldmann, E., . . . & Sacco, R. (2009). Definition and evaluation of transient ischemic attack: A scientific statement for healthcare professionals from the American Heart Association/American Stroke Association Stroke Council; Council on Cardiovascular Surgery and Anesthesia; Council on Cardiovascular Radiology and Intervention; Council on Cardiovascular Nursing; and the Interdisciplinary Council on Peripheral Vascular Disease. [The American Academy of Neurology affirms the value of this statement as an educational tool for neurologists.] *Stroke, 40,* 2276–2293.

Edinger, J. (2003). Periodic limb movement: Assessment and management techniques. In M. Perlis & K. Lichstein (Eds.), *Treating sleep disorders: Principles and practice of behavioral sleep medicine.* Hobokon, NJ: Wiley.

Emre, M., Aarsland, D., Albanese, A., Byrne, E. J., Deuschl, G., & De Deyn, P. (2004). Rivastigmine for dementia associated with Parkinson's disease. *New England Journal of Medicine, 351,* 2509–2518.

Engel, J., & Pedley, T. (Eds.). (1998). *Epilepsy: A comprehensive textbook.* Philadelphia, PA: Lippincott-Raven.

Epilepsy Foundation. (2011). http://www.epilepsyfoundation.org/about/statistics.cfm

Fahn, S. (1984). The varied clinical expressions of dystonia. *Neurologic Clinics, 2,* 541–554.

Fallahzadeh, M. K., Borhani Haghighi, A., & Namazi, M. R. (2010). Proton pump inhibitors: Predisposers to Alzheimer disease? *Journal of Clinical Pharmacy and Therapeutics, 35,* 125–126.

Farlow, M. R., Miller, M. L., & Pejovic, V. (2008). Treatment options in Alzheimer's disease: Maximizing benefit, managing expectations. *Dementia and Geriatric Cognitive Disorders, 25,* 108–122.

Fernandez, F., Morishita, W., Zuniga, E., Nguyen, J., Blank, M., Malenka, R. C., & Gardner, C. (2007). Pharmacotherapy for cognitive impairment in a mouse model of Down syndrome. *Nature Neuroscience, 10,* 411–413.

Field, B., & Swarm, R. (2008). *Chronic pain.* Cambridge, MA: Hogrefe.

Fordyce, W. E. (1976). *Behavioral methods for chronic pain and illness.* St Louis, MO: C.V. Mosby.

Foussias, G., & Remington, G. (2010). Antipsychotics and schizophrenia: From efficacy and effectiveness to clinical decision-making. *Canadian Journal of Psychiatry, 55,* 117–125.

Frank-Cannon, T. C., Alto, L. T., McAlpine, F. E., & Tansey, M. G. (2009). Does neuroinflammation fan the flame in neurodegenerative diseases? *Molecular Neurodegeneration, 4*(47). doi:10.1186/1750-1326-4-47

France, R., Urban, B., & Keefe, F. (1984). Long-term use of narcotic analgesics in chronic pain. *Social Science and Medicine, 19,* 1379–1382.

Frankel, M., Cummings, J., Robertson, M., Trimble, M., Hill, M., & Benson, F. (1986). Obsessions and compulsions in Gilles de la Tourette's syndrome. *Neurology, 36,* 378–382.

Fu, Y., Zhong, H., Wang, M., Luo, D., Liao, H., Maeda, . . . & Yau, K. (2005). Intrinsically photosensitive retinal ganglion cells detect light with a vitamin A–based photopigment, melanopsin. *Proceedings of the National Academy of Sciences, 102,* 10339–10344.

Gardiner, K., Herault, Y., Lott, I. T., Antonarakis, S. E., Reeves, R. H., & Dierssen, M. (2010). Down syndrome: From understanding the neurobiology to therapy. *Journal of Neuroscience, 30,* 14943–14945.

Garey, L. (2010). When cortical development goes wrong: Schizophrenia as a neurodevelopmental disease of microcircuits. *Journal of Anatomy, 217,* 324–333.

Gasperini, C., & Ruggieri, S. (2009). New oral drugs for multiple sclerosis. *Neurological Sciences, 30*(Suppl. 2), s179–s183.

Geschwind, D. (2009). Advances in autism. *Annual Review of Medicine, 60,* 367–380.

Ghanem, T., & Early, S. (2006). Vagal nerve stimulator implantation: An otolaryngologist's perspective. *Otolaryngology–Head and Neck Surgery, 135,* 46–51.

Goodnough, A. (2011, February 6). Pharmacies besieged by addicted thieves. *New York Times.*

Goswami, U,, Gangadhar, B., Chandra, P., Channavabasavanna, S., & Sundararajan, R. (1994). A prospective study of the rabbit syndrome. *Neuropsychopharmacology, 11*, 271.

Gothelf, D., Furfaro, J. A., Penniman, L. C., Glover, G. H., & Reiss, A. L. (2005). The contributions of novel brain imaging techniques to understanding the neurobiology of mental retardation and developmental disabilities. *Mental Retardation and Developmental Disabilities Research Reviews, 11*, 331–339.

Haass, C., & Selkoe, D. J. (2007). Soluble protein oligomers in neurodegeneration: Lessons from the Alzheimer's amyloid beta-peptide. *Nature Reviews Molecular Cell Biology, 8*, 101–112.

Hagerman, R. J. (2006). Lessons from fragile X regarding neurobiology, autism, and neurodegeneration. *Developmental and Behavioral Pediatrics, 27*, 63–74.

Hanson, E., Healy, K., Wolf, D., & Kohler, C. (2010). Assessment of pharmacotherapy for negative symptoms of schizophrenia. *Current Psychiatry Reports, 12*, 563–571.

Hanson, J. E., Blank, M., Valenzuela, R. A., Garner, C. C., & Madison, D. V. (2007). The functional nature of synaptic circuitry is altered in area CA3 of the hippocampus in a mouse model of Down's syndrome. *Journal of Physiology, 579*, 53–67.

Harrison, J., & Bolton, P. (1997). Annotation: Tuberous sclerosis. *Journal of Child Psychology and Psychiatry, 38*, 603–614.

Hendler, N. (1981). *Diagnosis and nonsurgical management of chronic pain*. New York, NY: Raven Press.

Hening, W., Buchfuhrer, M., & Lee, H. (2008). *Clinical management of restless leg syndrome*. New York, NY: Professional Communications.

Hill, R. (1970). Facilitation of conditioned reinforcement as a mechanism of psychomotor stimulation. In E. Costa & S. Garattini (Eds.), *International symposium on amphetamines and related compounds* (pp. 781–795). New York, NY: Raven Press.

Hobson, J., Lydic, R., & Baghdoyan, H. (1986). Evolving concepts of sleep cycle generation: From brain centers to neuronal populations. *Behavioral and Brain Sciences, 9*, 370–400.

Hocaoglu, C. (2009). Clozapine-induced rabbit syndrome: A case report. *Mental Health, 1*, 1–3.

Hock, C., Konietzko, U., Streffer, J. R., Tracy, J., Signorell, A., Muller-Tillmanns, B., . . . & Garcia, E., (2003). Antibodies against beta-amyloid slow cognitive decline in Alzheimer's disease. *Neuron, 38*, 547–554.

Hoge, C., McGurk, D., Thomas, J., Cox, A., Engel, C., & Castro, C. (2008). Mild traumatic brain injury in U.S. soldiers returning from Iraq. *New England Journal of Medicine, 358*, 453–463.

Holroyd, K., O'Donnell, F., & Stensland, M. (2001). Management of chronic tension-type headache with tricyclic antidepressant medication, stress management therapy, and their combination: A randomized controlled trial. *Journal of the American Medical Association*, 286, 1969–1970.

Honea, R. A., Meyer-Lindenberg, A., Hobbs, K. B., Pezawas, L., Mattay, V. S., Egan, M., . . . & Callicott, J. (2008). Is gray matter volume an intermediate phenotype for schizophrenia? A voxel-based morphometry study of patients with schizophrenia and their healthy siblings. *Biological Psychiatry, 63*, 465–474.

Hungs, M., & Mignot, E. (2001). Hypocretin/orexin: Sleep and narcolepsy. *BioEssays 23*, 397–408.

ILAE. Commission on Classification and Terminology of the International League Against Epilepsy (1981). Proposal for revised clinical and electroencephalographic classification of epileptic seizures. *Epilepsia, 22*, 489–501.

Itil, T. (1968). Anticholinergic drug-induced sleep-like EEG pattern in man. *Psychopharmacology, 14*, 383–398.

Iverson, G., Zasler, N., & Lange, R. (2006). Post-concussive disorder. In N. D. Zasler, D. I. Katz, & R. D. Zafonta (Eds.), *Brain injury medicine: Principles and practice*. New York, NY: Demos Medical Publishing.

Janszkyab, J., Ebnera, A., Szuperac, Z., Schulz, R., Hollo A., Szücs, A., & Clemens, B. (2004). Orgasmic aura—A report of seven cases. *Seizure, 13*, 441–444.

Jellinger, K. A. (2007). Lewy body disorders. In M. B. H. Youdim, P. Riederer, S. A. Mandel, & L. Battistin (Eds.), *Handbook of neurochemistry and molecular neurobiology: Degenerative diseases of the nervous system* (pp. 267–343). New York, NY: Springer.

Johnsen, E., & Jørgensen, H. A. (2008). Effectiveness of second generation antipsychotics: A systematic review of randomized trials. *BMC Psychiatry, 8*, 31.

Jones, H. E., Kaltenbach, K., Heil, S., Stine, S., Coyle, M., Arria, A., . . . & Fischer, G. (2010). Neonatal abstinence syndrome after methadone or buprenorphine exposure. *New England Journal of Medicine, 363*, 2320–2331.

Josephs, K. A. (2008). Frontotemporal dementia and related disorders: Deciphering the enigma. *Annals of Neurology, 64*, 4–14.

Jouvet, M. (1967). The states of sleep. *Scientific American, 216*, 62–68.

Jouvet, M. (1999). Sleep and serotonin: An unfinished story. *Neuropsychopharmacology, 21*, 245–275.

Kaada, B., & Jasper, H. (1949). Respiratory responses to stimulation of the temporal pole, insula and hippocampal and limbic gyri in man. *Journal of Neurophysiology, 12*, 385.

Kane, J. M., Woerner, M., Weinhold, P., Wegner, J., & Kinon, B. A. (1982). A prospective study of tardive dyskinesia development: Preliminary results. *Journal of Clinical Psychopharmacology, 2*, 345–349.

Keilson, M., Hauser, W., & Magrill, J. (1989). Electrocardiographic changes during electrographic seizures. *Archives of Neurology, 46*, 1169–1170.

Keshavan, M. S., Tandon, R., Boutros, N. N., & Nasrallah, H. A. (2008). Schizophrenia, "just the facts": What we know in 2008. Part 3: Neurobiology. *Schizophrenia Research, 106*, 89–107.

Klawans, H. L., & Rubovits, R. (1974). Effects of cholinergic and anticholinergic agents on tardive dyskinesia. *Journal of Neurology, Neurosurgery, and Psychiatry, 27*, 941–947.

Knopman, D., Rocca, W., & Cha, R. (2002). Incidence of vascular dementia in Rochester, Minn., 1985–1989. *Archives of Neurology, 59*, 1605–1610.

Koenigsknecht-Talboo, J., & Landreth, G. E. (2005). Microglial phagocytosis induced by fibrillar beta-amyloid and IgGs are differentially regulated by proinflammatory cytokines. *Journal of Neuroscience, 25*, 8240–8249.

Kotagal, P., & Lüders, H. (1998). Simple motor seizures. In J. Engel & T. A. Pedley (Eds.), *Epilepsy: A comprehensive textbook*. Philadelphia, PA: Lippincott-Raven.

Koutsilieri, E., Arendt, G., Neuen-Jacob, E., Scheller, C., Grünblatt, E., & Riederer, P. (2007). HIV dementia: A neurodegenerative disorder with viral etiology. In M. B. H. Youdim, P. Riederer, S. A. Mandel, & L. Battistin (Eds.), *Handbook of neurochemistry and molecular neurobiology: Degenerative diseases of the nervous system* (pp. 359–371). New York, NY: Springer.

Kövari, E., Horvath, J., & Bouras, C. (2009). Neuropathology of Lewy body disorders. *Brain Research Bulletin, 80*, 203–210.

Krauel, K., Duzel, E., Hinrichs, H., Santel, S., Rellum, T., & Baving, L. (2007). Impact of emotional salience on episodic memory in attention-deficit/hyperactivity disorder: A functional magnetic resonance imaging study. *Biological Psychiatry, 61*, 1370–1379.

Ladds, B., Thomas, P., Mejia, C., & Hauser, D. (2009). Extreme elevation of creatinine phosphokinase levels in neuroleptic malignant syndrome associated with atypical antipsychotics. *American Journal of Psychiatry, 166*, 114–115.

Lane, H.-Y., Lin, C.-H., Huang, Y.-J., Liao, C.-H., Chang, Y.-C., & Tsai, G. E. (2010). A randomized, double-blind, placebo-controlled comparison study of sarcosine (N-methylglycine) and D-serine add-on treatment for schizophrenia. *International Journal of Neuropsychopharmacology, 13*, 451–460.

Laruelle, M., Frankle, W. G., Narendran, R., Kegeles, L. S., & Abi-Dargham, A. (2005). Mechanism of action of antipsychotic drugs: From dopamine D2 receptor antagonism to glutamate NMDA facilitation. *Clinical Therapeutics, 27*(Suppl. A), s16–s24.

Lassmman, H., Niedobitek, G., Aloisi, F., & Middledorp, J. (2011). Epstein–Barr virus in the multiple sclerosis brain: A controversial issue. *Brain: A Journal of Neurology*, 1–15. Advance published online: doi:10.1093/brain/awr197

Lawless, R. (2001). Nocturnal enuresis: Current concepts. *Pediatrics in Review, 22*, 399–406.

Ledbetter, D., Riccardi, V., Airhart, S., et al. (1981). Deletions of chromosome 15 as a cause of the Prader-Willi syndrome. *New England Journal of Medicine, 304*, 325–329.

Leucht, S., Corves, C., Arbter, D., Engel, R. R., Li, C., & Davis, J. M. (2009a). Second-generation versus first-generation antipsychotic drugs for schizophrenia: A meta-analysis. *Lancet, 373*, 31–41.

Leucht, S., Komossa, K., Rummel-Kluge, C., Corves, C., Hunger, H., Schmid, F., . . . & Davis, J. (2009b). A meta-analysis of head-to-head comparisons of second-generation antipsychotics in the treatment of schizophrenia. *American Journal of Psychiatry, 166*, 152–163.

Levkovitz, Y., Mendlovich, S., Riwkes, S., Braw, Y., Levkovitch-Verbin, H., Gal, G., . . . & Kron S. (2010). A double-blind, randomized study of minocycline for the treatment of negative and cognitive symptoms in early-phase schizophrenia. *Journal of Clinical Psychiatry, 71*, 138–149.

Lichstein, K. L., & Riedel, B. W. (1994). Behavioral assessment and treatment of insomnia: A review with an emphasis on clinical application. *Behavioral Therapy, 25*, 659–688.

Liddle, P. (1987). The symptoms of chronic schizophrenia: A reexamination of the positive-negative dichotomy. *British Journal of Psychiatry, 151*, 145–151.

Lieberman, J. A., Stroup, T. S., McEvoy, J. P., Swartz, M. S., Rosenheck, R. A., Perkins, D. O., . . . & Hsiao, J. (2005). Effectiveness of antipsychotic drugs in patients with chronic schizophrenia. *New England Journal of Medicine, 353*, 1209–1223.

Lovel, M., & Fazio, V. (2008). Concussion management in the child and adolescent athlete. *Current Sports Medicine Report, 7*, 12–15.

Maezawa, I., Swanberg, S., Harvey, D., LaSalle, J., & Jin, L. (2009). Rett syndrome astrocytes are abnormal and spread MeCP2 deficiency through gap junctions. *Journal of Neuroscience, 29*, 5051–5056.

Magni, G. (1991). The use of antidepressants in the treatment of chronic pain. A review of the current evidence. *Drugs, 42*, 730–48.

Mangas, A., Coveñas, R., & Geffard, M. (2010). New drug therapies for multiple sclerosis. *Current Opinion in Neurology, 23*, 287–292.

Mangialasche, F., Solomon, A., Winblad, B., Mecocci, P., & Kivipelto, M. (2010). Alzheimer's disease: Clinical trials and drug development. *Lancet Neurology, 9*, 702–716.

Mapstone, T. (2008). Vagus nerve stimulation: Current concepts. *Neurosurgery Focus, 25*, E9.

Margolese, H. C., Chouinard, G., Kolivakis, T. T., Beauclair, L., & Miller, R. (2005). Tardive dyskinesia in the era of typical and atypical antipsychotics. Part 1: Pathophysiology and mechanisms of induction. *Canadian Journal of Psychiatry, 50*, 541–547.

Marsden, C., & Jenner, P. (1980). The pathophysiology of extrapyramidal side-effects of neuroleptic drugs. *Psychological Medicine, 10*, 55–72.

Martinelli Boneschi, F., Rovaris, M., & Johnson, K. (2003). Effect of glatiramer acetate on relapse rate and accumulated disability in multiple sclerosis: Meta-analysis of three double-blind, randomized, placebo-controlled clinical trials. *Multiple Sclerosis, 9*, 349–355.

Matsuoka, Y., Jouroukhin, Y., Gray, A. J., Ma, L., Hirata-Fukae, C., & Li, H. F. (2008). A neuronal microtubule-interacting agent, NAPVSIPQ, reduces tau pathology and enhances cognitive function in a mouse model of Alzheimer's disease. *Journal of Pharmacology and Experimental Therapeutics, 325*, 146–153.

Mayo Clinic. (2011). http://www.mayoclinic.com/health/epilepsy/DS00342

McCrea, M. (2008). *Mild traumatic brain injury and postconcussion syndrome: The new evidence base of diagnosis and treatment.* New York, NY: Oxford University Press.

McEvoy, J. P., Lieberman, J. A., Stroup, T. S., Davis, S. M., Meltzer, H. Y., & Rosenheck, R. A. (2006). Effectiveness of clozapine versus olanzapine, quetiapine, and risperidone in patients with chronic schizophrenia who did not respond to prior atypical antipsychotic treatment. *American Journal of Psychiatry, 163*, 600–610.

McKeith, I., Del-Ser, T., Spano, P. F., Emre, M., Wesnes, K., & Anand, R. (2000). Efficacy of rivastigmine in dementia with Lewy bodies: A randomised, double-blind, placebo-controlled international study. *Lancet, 356*, 2031–2036.

McKeith, I. G., Dickson, D. W., Lowe, J., Emre, M., O'Brien, J. T., & Feldman, H. (2005). Diagnosis and management of dementia with Lewy bodies. Third report of the DLB consortium. *Neurology, 65*, 1863–1872.

McKeith, I., Mintzer, J., Aarsland, D., Burn, D., Chiu, H., & Cohen-Mansfield, J. (2004). Dementia with Lewy bodies. *Lancet Neurology, 3*, 19–28.

McQuay, H. (1999). Opioids in pain management. *Lancet, 353*, 2229–2232.

McWilliams, L., Cox, B., & Enns, M. (2003). Mood and anxiety disorders associated with chronic pain: An examination of a nationally representative sample. *Pain, 106*, 127–133.

Medina, D. X., Caccamo, A., & Oddo, S. (2011). Methylene blue reduces Aβ levels and rescues early cognitive deficit by increasing proteasome activity. *Brain Pathology, 21*, 140–149.

Melzack, R. (1999). From the gate to the neuromatrix. *Pain Supplement, 6*, S121–S126.

Melzack, R. (2005). Evolution of the neuromatrix theory of pain. *Pain Practice, 5*, 85–94.

Melzack, R., & Wall, P. D. (1965). Pain mechanisms: A new theory. *Science, 150*, 971–979.

Mico, J., Ardid, D., Berrocoso, E., & Eschalier, A. (2006). Antidepressants and pain. *Trends in Psychopharmacological Sciences, 27*, 348–354.

Milligan, E. D., & Watkins, L. R. (2009). Pathological and protective roles of glia in chronic pain. *Nature Reviews Neuroscience, 10*, 23–36.

Milo, R., & Kahana, E. (2010). Multiple sclerosis: Geoepidemiology, genetics and the environment. *Autoimmunity Reviews, 9*, A387–A394.

Missale, C., Nash, R., Robinson, S., Jaber, M., & Caron, M. (1998). Dopamine receptors: From structure to function. *Physiological Reviews, 78*, 190–225.

Montplaisir, J. A., Nicolas, R., Godbout, R., & Walters, A. (2000). Restless legs syndrome and periodic limb movement disorder. In M. H. Kryger, T. Roth, & W. C. Dements (Eds.), *Principles and practice of sleep medicine.* Philadelphia, PA: Saunders.

Moreira, P. I., Cardoso, S. M., Santos, M. S., & Oliveira, C. R. (2006). The key role of mitochondria in Alzheimer's disease. *Journal of Alzheimer's Disease, 9*, 101–110.

Morin, C., Batien, C., & Savard, J. (2003). Current status of cognitive-behavior therapy for insomnia: Evidence for treatment effectiveness and feasibility. In M. Perils & K. Lichstein (Eds.), *Treating sleep disorders: Principles and practice of behavioral sleep medicine.* Hoboken, NJ: Wiley.

Morris, N. (2011). *Treating sleep disorders in primary care.* American Psychological Association 119th annual convention. Washington, DC.

Moulin, D., Clark, A., & Gilron, I. (2007). Pharmacological management of chronic neuropathic pain: Consensus statement and guideline from the Canadian Pain Society. *Pain Research Management, 12*, 13–21.

Muse, M., & Frigola, G. (1986). Development of a quick screening instrument for detecting posttraumatic stress in the chronic pain patient: Construction of the "Posttraumatic Chronic Pain Test" (PCPT). *Clinical Journal of Pain, 2*, 155.

Muse, M., Frigola, G., del Río, R., & Viñas, F. (1991). Algology: The integration of psychology and medicine. *Journal of Integrative and Eclectic Psychotherapy, 10*, 265–274.

Muse, M., LeFew, B., Shafiei, M., & Frigola, G. (1984). *Exercise for the chronic pain patient.* New York, NY: Mouvement Publications.

Myhr, K. (2008). Diagnosis and treatment of multiple sclerosis. *Acta Neurologica Scandinavica, 117*, 12–21.

Nambu, A. (2004). A new dynamic model of the cortico-basal ganglia loop. *Progress in Brain Research, 143*, 461–466.

Nasello, A. G., Gidali, D., & Felicio, L. F. (2003). A comparative study of the anticholinesterase activity of several antipsychotic agents. *Pharmacology Biochemistry and Behavior, 75*, 895–901.

Neugroschl, J., & Sano, M. (2010). Current treatment and recent clinical research in Alzheimer's disease. *Mount Sinai Journal of Medicine, 77*, 3–16.

Newschaffer, C., Croen, L., Daniels, J., Giarelli, E., Grether, J., Levy, S., & Mandell, D. (2007). The epidemiology of autism spectrum disorders. *Annual Review of Public Health, 28*, 235–258.

Nigg, J. T. (2005). Neuropsychologic theory and findings in attention-deficit/hyperactivity disorder: The state of the field and salient challenges for the coming decade. *Biological Psychiatry, 57*, 1424–1435.

Nolte, J., & Angevine, J. (2000). *The human brain in photographs and diagrams.* St. Louis, MO: C.V. Mosby.

Oblak, A., Gibbs, T., & Blatt, G. (2010). Decreased GABA(B) receptors in the cingulate cortex and fusiform gyrus in autism. *Journal of Neurochemistry, 12*, 1414–1423.

Oostra, B. A., & Chiurazzi, P. (2001). The fragile X gene and its function. *Clinical Genetics, 60*, 399–408.

Opar, A. (2008). Mixed results for disease-modification strategies for Alzheimer's disease. *Nature Reviews Drug Discovery, 7*, 717–718.

Oregon Health and Science University. (2010). *Opioids and chronic non-malignant pain: A clinician's handbook.* http://www.ohsu.edu/ahec/pain/painmanual.html?WT_rank=1

Orgogozo, J. M., Gilman, S., Dartigues, J. F., Laurent, B., Puel, M., Kirby, L. C., . . . & Hock, C. (2003). Subacute meningoencephalitis in a subset of patients with AD after Abeta42 immunization. *Neurology, 61*, 46–54.

Pedersen, T., Nielsen, O., Lamb, G., & Stephenson, D. (2002). Intracellular acidosis enhances the excitability of working muscle. *Science, 305*, 1144–1147.

Piguet, O., Hornberger, M., Mioshi, E., & Hodges, J. R. (2010). Behavioural-variant frontotemporal dementia: Diagnosis, clinical staging, and management. *Lancet Neurology, 10*, 162–172. doi:10.1016/S1474-4422(10)70299-4

Pimplikar, S. W., Nixon, R. A., Robakis, N. K., Shen, J., & Tsai, L.-H. (2010). Amyloid-independent mechanisms in Alzheimer's disease pathogenesis. *Journal of Neuroscience, 30*, 14946–14954.

Policies Committee and the Clinical Policies Subcommittee on Seizures. (2004). Clinical policy: Critical issues in the evaluation and management of adult patients presenting to the emergency department with seizures. *Annals of Emergency Medicine, 43*, 605–625.

Portenoy, R., & Foley, K. (1986). Chronic use of opioid analgesics in non-malignant pain: Report of 38 cases. *Pain, 25*, 171–186.

Potkin, S. G., Litman, R. E., Torres, R., & Wolfgang, C. D. (2008). Efficacy of iloperidone in the treatment of schizophrenia: Initial phase 3 studies. *Journal of Clinical Psychopharmacology, 28*, s4–s11.

Ramachandran, V. S., & Rogers-Ramachandran, D. C. (1996). Synaesthesia in phantom limbs induced with mirrors. *Proceedings of the Royal Society of London, 263*, 377–386.

Reeves, R. H., & Garner, C. C. (2007). A year of unprecedented progress in Down syndrome basic research. *Mental Retardation and Developmental Disabilities Research Reviews, 13*, 215–220.

Remington, G. (2007). Tardive dyskinesia: Eliminated, forgotten, or overshadowed? *Current Opinion in Psychiatry, 20*, 131–137.

Rezai-Zadeh, K., Ehrhart, J., Bai, Y., Sanberg, P. R., Bickford, P., Tan, J., & Shytle, R. D. (2008). Apignenin and luteolin modulate microglial activation via inhibition of STAT I-induced CD40 expression. *Journal of Neuroinflammation, 5*, 41. doi: 10.1186/1742-2094-5-41

Riillig, S., Knudsen, U., Norgaard, J., Pedersen, E., & Djurhuus, J. (1989). Abnormal diurnal rhythm of plasma vasopressin and urinary output in patients with enuresis. *American Journal of Physiology, 256*, 664–671.

Robbins, T. W. (1978). The acquisition of responding with conditioned reinforcement: Effects of pipradol, methylphenidate, d-amphetamine, and nomifensine. *Psychopharmacology, 58*, 79–87.

Roberson, E. D. (2006). Frontotemporal dementia. *Current Neurology and Neuroscience Reports, 6*, 481–489.

Roberson, E. D. (2011). Contemporary approaches to Alzheimer's disease and frontotemporal dementia. In E. D. Roberson (Ed.), *Alzheimer's disease and frontotemporal dementia: Methods and protocols* (pp. 1–9). New York, NY: Humana.

Rohkamm, R. (2004). *Color atlas of neurology.* New York, NY: Thieme.

Roper, R. J., Baxter, L. L., Saran, N. G., Klinedinst, D. K., Beachy, P. A., & Reeves, R. H. (2006). Defective cerebellar response to mitogenic Hedgehog signaling in Down syndrome mice. *Proceedings of the National Academy of Sciences (USA), 103*, 1452–1456.

Rummel-Kluge, C., Komossa, K., Schwarz, S., Hunger, H., Schmid, F., Asenjo Lobos, C., . . . & Leucht, S. (2010). Head-to-head comparisons of metabolic side effects of second generation antipsychotics in the treatment of schizophrenia: A systematic review and meta-analysis. *Schizophrenia Research, 123*, 225–233.

Rutherford, W., Merrett, J., & McDonald, J. (1979). Symptoms at one year following concussion from minor head injury. *Injuries, 10*, 225–230.

Saarto, T., & Wiffen, P. (2007). Antidepressants for neuropathic pain. *Cochrane Database System*, Published online November 10, 2010.

Sachdev, P. (2001). The current status of tardive dyskinesia. *Australian and New Zealand Journal of Psychiatry, 34*, 355–369.

Sakkas, P., Davis, J., Janicak, P., & Wang, Z. (1991). Drug treatment of the neuroleptic malignancy syndrome. *Psychopharmacology Bulletin, 27*, 381–384.

Salehi, A., Delcroix, J.-D., Belichenko, P. V., Zhan, K., Wu, C., & Valletta, J. S. (2006). Increased App expression in a mouse model of Down's syndrome disrupts NGF transport and causes cholinergic neuron degeneration. *Neuron, 51*, 29–42.

SAMHSA. (2010, July). Substance abuse treatment admissions involving abuse of pain relievers: 1998 and 2008. *The TEDS Report.*

Sampson, P., Streissguth, A., & Bookstein, F. (1997). Incidence of fetal alcohol syndrome and prevalence of alcohol-related neurodevelopmental disorder. *Teratology, 56*, 317–326.

Samson, K. (2007). CDC-backed study suggests possible link between autistic disorders and maternal pesticide exposure in California. *Neurology Today, 7*, 7.

Samuel, W., Caligiuri, M., Galasko, D., Lacro, J., Marini, M., McClure, F. S., & Jeste, W. (2000). Better cognitive and psychopathologic response to donepezil in patients prospectively diagnosed as dementia with Lewy bodies: A preliminary study. *International Journal of Geriatric Psychiatry, 15*, 794–802.

Schultz, G., & Melzack, R. (1991). The Charles Bonnet syndrome: Phantom visual images. *Perception, 20*, 809–825.

Seeman, P. (2002). Atypical antipsychotics: Mechanism of action. *Canadian Journal of Psychiatry, 47*, 27–38.

Seeman, P., & Lee, T. (1975). Antipsychotic drugs: Direct correlation between clinical potency and presynaptic action on dopamine neurons. *Science, 188*, 1217–1219.

Seidman, L. J., Valera, E. M., Makris, N., Monuteaux, M. C., Boriel, D. L., & Kelkar, K. (2006). Dorsolateral prefrontal and anterior cingulate cortex volumetric abnormalities in adults with attention-deficit/hyperactivity disorder identified by magnetic resonance imaging. *Biological Psychiatry, 60*, 1071–1080.

Selkoe, D. J. (2004). Alzheimer disease: Mechanistic understanding predicts novel therapies. *Annals of Internal Medicine, 140*, 627–638.

Sellenbjerg, F., Barnes, D., Filippini, G., Midgard, R., Montalban, X., Rieckmann, P. (2005). EFNS guideline on treatment of multiple sclerosis relapses: Report of an EFNS task force on treatment of multiple sclerosis relapses. *European Journal of Neurology, 12*, 939–946.

Sepehry, A. A., Potvin, S., Élie, R., & Stip, E. (2007). SSRI add-on therapy for the negative symptoms of schizophrenia: A meta-analysis. *Journal of Clinical Psychiatry, 68*, 604–610.

Shafii, M. (1998). *Melatonin in psychiatric and neoplastic disorders*. Washington, DC. American Psychiatric Press.

Sherman, S. L., Allen, E. G., Bean, L. H., & Freeman, S. B. (2007). Epidemiology of Down syndrome. *Mental Retardation and Developmental Disabilities Research Reviews, 13*, 221–227.

Shirzadi, A. A., & Ghaemi, S. N. (2006). Side effects of atypical antipsychotics: Extrapyramidal symptoms and the metabolic syndrome. *Harvard Review of Psychiatry, 14*, 152–164.

Sitzer, D. I., Twamley, E. W., & Jeste, D. V. (2006). Cognitive training in Alzheimer's disease: A meta-analysis of the literature. *Acta Psychiatrica Scandinavica, 114*, 75–90.

Smith, A., McGavran, L., Robinson, J., Waldstein, G., Macfarlane, J., Zonona, J., . . . & Lahr, M., (1986). Interstitial deletion of (17)(p11.2p11.2) in nine patients. *American Journal of Medical Genetics, 24*, 393–414.

Smith, D., & Meaney, D. (2000). Axonal damage in traumatic brain injury. *Neuroscientist, 6*, 483–495.

Snead, O. (2000). Evidence for a G protein-coupled gamma-hydroxybutyric acid receptor. *Journal of Neurochemistry, 75*, 1986–1996.

Snow, J. B. (2004). *Tinnitus: Theory and management*. Toronto, ON: B. C. Decker.

Song, H. R., Cheng, J. J., Miao, H., & Shang, Q. Z. (2009). Scutellaria flavonoid supplementation reverses aging-related cognitive impairment and neuronal changes in aged rats. *Brain Injury, 23*, 146–153

Spector, A., Orrell, M., Davies, S., & Woods, B. (2000). Reality orientation for dementia. *Cochrane Database of Systematic Reviews*: CD001119.

Spilman, P., Podlutskaya, N., Hart, M. J., Debnath, J., Gorostiza, O., & Bredesen, D. (2010). Inhibition of mTOR by rapamycin abolishes cognitive deficits and reduces amyloid-beta levels in a mouse model of Alzheimer's disease. *PLoS One, 5*:e9979.

Stahl, S. (2007). *Essential psychopharmacology: Neuroscientific basis and practical applications*. Boston, MA: Cambridge University Press.

Stahl, S. (2008). *Everything you wanted to know about ADHD*. Carlsbad, CA: NEI Press.

Stahl, S. (2009). *Stahl's illustrated antipsychotics*. New York, NY: Cambridge University Press.

Stahl, S. (2010). *Psychosis and schizophrenia: Thinking it through*. Carlsbad, CA: Neuroscience Education Institute.

Stepanski, E. J., & Perlis, M. L. (2003). A historical perspective and commentary on practice issues. In M. L. Perlis & K. Lichstein (Eds.), *Treating sleep disorders: Principles and practice of behavioral sleep medicine*. Hoboken, NJ: Wiley.

Steriade, M., & McCarley, R. (2005). *Brain control of wakefulness and sleep*. New York, NY: Kluwer Academic/Plenum.

Sternbach, R. (1980). *The psychology of pain*. New York, NY: Raven Press.

Stratton, K., Howe, C., & Battaglia, F. (1996). *Fetal alcohol syndrome: Diagnosis, epidemiology, prevention, and treatment*. Washington, DC: National Academy Press.

Strawn, J., Keck, P., Jr., & Caroff, S. (2007). Neuroleptic malignant syndrome. *American Journal of Psychiatry, 164*, 870–876.

Streissguth, A. P., Barr, H. M., Kogan, J., & Bookstein, F. L. (1996). *Understanding the occurrence of secondary disabilities in clients with fetal alcohol syndrome (FAS) and fetal alcohol effects (FAE): Final report to the Centers for Disease Control and Prevention*. Seattle, WA: University of Washington.

Streltzer, J., & Johansen, L. (2006). Prescription drug dependence and evolving beliefs about chronic pain management. *American Journal of Psychiatry, 163*, 594–598.

Swartz, B., Brown, C., Mandelkern, M., Khonsari, A., Patell, A., Thomas, K., . . . & Walsh, G. (2002). The use of 2-deoxy-2-[18F]fluoro-D-glucose positron emission tomography (FDG-PET) in the routine diagnosis of epilepsy. *Molecular Imaging and Biology, 4*, 245–252.

Swerdlow, R. H., & Khan, S. M. (2004). A "mitochondrial cascade hypothesis" for sporadic Alzheimer's disease. *Medical Hypotheses, 63*, 8–20.

Swierzewski, S. (2007). Sleep stages overview: Waking, non-REM, REM, sleep cycle, factors, age. *Sleep Channel*, Healthcommunities.com

Tachida, Y., Nakagawa, K., Saito, T., Saido, T. C., Honda, T., Saito, Y., . . . & Hashimoto, Y. (2008). Interleukin-1 beta up-regulates TACE to enhance alpha cleavage of APP in neurons: Resulting decrease in Abeta production. *Journal of Neurochemistry, 104*, 1387–1393.

Taheri, S., Zeitzer, J., & Mignot, E. (2002). The role of hypocretins in sleep regulation and narcolepsy. *Annual Review of Neuroscience, 25*, 283–313.

Tandon, R., Keshavan, M. S., & Nasrallah, H. A. (2008). Schizophrenia, "just the facts": What we know in 2008. 2. Epidemiology and etiology. *Schizophrenia Research, 102*, 1–18.

Tateno, M., Kobayashi, S., & Saito, T. (2009). Imaging improves diagnosis of dementia with Lewy bodies. *Psychiatry Investigation, 6*, 233–240.

Taylor, D., Lichstein, K., Durrence, H., Reidel, B., & Bush, A. (2005). Epidemiology of insomnia, depression and anxiety. *Sleep, 28*, 1457–1464.

Taylor-Flusberg, H. (1999) *Neurodevelopmental disorders*. Boston, MA: MIT Press.

Teasdale, G., & Jennett, B. (1974). Assessment of coma and impaired consciousness. A practical scale. *Lancet, 2*, 81–84.

Trescot, A., Helm, S., Hansen, H., Benyamin, R., Glasser, S., Adlaka, R., . . . & Manchikanti, L. (2008). Opioids in the management of chronic non-cancer pain: An update of American Society of the Interventional Pain Physicians' (ASIPP) Guidelines. *Pain Physician, 11*, S5–S62.

Tripp, G., & Wickens, J. R. (2009). Neurobiology of ADHD. *Neuropharmacology, 57*, 579–589.

Tuberous Sclerosis Alliance. (2009). *Current clinical trials*. http://www.tsalliance.org/pages.aspx?content=370

Tuisku, K., Lauerma, H., Holi, M., Honkonen, T., & Rimon, R. (2000). Akathisia masked by hypokinesia. *Pharmacopsychiatry, 33*, 147–1499.

Valera, E. M., Faraone, S. V., Murray, K. E., & Seidman, L. J. (2007). Meta-analysis of structural imaging findings in attention-deficit/hyperactivity disorder. *Biological Psychiatry, 61*, 1361–1369.

van de Wetering, B. J., & Heutink, P. (1993). The genetics of the Gilles de la Tourette syndrome: A review. *Journal of Laboratory and Clinical Medicine, 121*, 638–645.

Villeneuve, A. (1972). The rabbit syndrome: A peculiar extrapyramidal reaction. *Canadian Psychiatric Association Journal, 17(Suppl. 2)*, 69–72.

Von Korff, M., & LeResche, L. (2005). Epidemiology of pain. In H. Merskey & J. D. Loser (Eds.), *The paths of pain 1975–2005*. Seattle, WA: IASP Press.

Wakefield, A. J., Murch, S. H., Anthony, A., Linnell, J., Casson, D. M., Malik, M., . . . & Walker-Smith, J. A. (1998). Ileal-lymphoid-nodular hyperplasia, non-specific colitis, and pervasive developmental disorder in children. *Lancet, 351*, 637–641.

Wang, Y. J., Thomas, P., Zhong, J. H., Bi, F. F., Kosaraju, S., Pollard, A., . . . & Zhou, X. (2009). Consumption of grape seed extract prevents amyloid-beta deposition and attenuates inflammation in brain of an Alzheimer's disease mouse. *Neurotoxicity Research, 15*, 3–14.

Ward, N., Bloom, V., & Friedel, R. (1979). The effectiveness of tricyclic antidepressants in the treatment of coexisting pain and depression. *Pain, 7*, 331–341.

Weber, J., & McCormack, P. L. (2009). Asenapine. *CNS Drugs, 23*, 781–792.

Weinstein, A., & Swanson, R. (1998). Cerebrovascular disease. In P. J. Snyder & P. D. Nussbaum (Eds.), *Clinical neuropsychology: A pocket handbook for assessment*. Washington, DC: American Psychological Association.

WHO (World Health Organization). (2011). http://www.who.int/mediacentre/factsheets/fs999/en

Wiederholt, W. (2000). *Neurology for non-neurologists*. Philadelphia, PA: Saunders.

Willcutt, E. G., Doyle, A. E., Nigg, J. T., Faraone, S. V., & Pennington, B. F. (2005). Validity of the executive function theory of attention-deficit/hyperactivity disorder: A meta-analytic review. *Biological Psychiatry, 57*, 1336–1346.

Wirrell, E., Camfield, C., Camfield, P., & Dooley, J. (1996). Long-term prognosis of typical childhood absence epilepsy: Remission or progression to juvenile myoclonic epilepsy. *Neurology, 47*, 912–918.

Yang, T. T., Gallen, C. C., Ramachandran, V. S., & Cobb, S. (1994). Noninvasive detection of cerebral plasticity in adult human somatosensory cortex. *NeuroReport, 5*, 701–704.

Zhao, B. (2009). Natural antioxidants protect neurons in Alzheimer's disease and Parkinson's disease. *Neurochemistry Research, 34*, 630–638.

Chapter 5

PHYSIOLOGY AND PATHOPHYSIOLOGY

Lawrence R. Kotkin

This chapter provides a concise overview of physiology and pathophysiology. As lifespan development affects each of these, the most salient issues in pediatrics and gerontology are presented at the end of each system. Further, the structure of this chapter begins with features of cell biology (cytology), genetics, defense processes, and interactions. This is followed by an analysis of the human body, system by system, which is made clinically relevant by review of systems, physical examination, and laboratory information. While we review the major systems of the body in this chapter, an exception is made for the nervous system, which has been addressed in the previous chapters on neuroscience and neuropathology. To the extent that space permits, the chapter presents common pathologies and medical *iatrogenic* issues that may be encountered in clinical psychopharmacology.

PRELIMINARIES

Physiology and pathophysiology would not exist without their respective anatomical bases. In addition to an understanding of the anatomy involved in the body's different functional systems, it is wise to learn and differentiate certain technical terms. A sampling of some essential positional and directional terms is found in Table 5.1. These terms are used to locate organs and parts of organs throughout the body. They are especially useful in referring to otherwise difficult-to-define neurostructures in the brain.

THE CELL

Human cells are defined by deoxyribonucleic acid (DNA), the genetically transmitted template from which structure and function are created. Ribonucleic acid (RNA), the functional template, is created from DNA, and is the source from which all physiology emerges.

Structure

The *nucleus* is the structure in which most of the DNA resides, with binding proteins (*histones*) that fold into chromosomes; it is also the citadel from which RNA is sent forth to carry out DNA's design to ensure the survival of the organism. (See Figure 5.1.)

   Cytoplasmic organelles, comprised of *cytosol* or *cytoplasm*, carry out chemical processes directed by nucleic RNA, and are encased in proteinic membranes. They

Table 5.1   Terms Denoting the Location of Organs Relative to the Entire Body

Anterior	The front.
Anteroposterior	From front to back.
Caudal	Toward the feet or tail.
Cephalic or cranial	Toward the head, deep; away from the surface.
Coronal	A coronal plane is any vertical plane that divides the body into ventral and dorsal sections.
Distal	Away from the origin or center (used as compared to medial).
Dorsal	The back (may not correspond to posterior as, for example, with the head, which tilts forward thereby changing the orientation).
Inferior	Below, inferolateral—below and to one side.
Infra	Below (used as a prefix).
Ipsilateral	On the same side as
Lateral	Toward the left or right side and away from.
Medial	Toward the center line of the body.
Posterior	Toward the back.
Pronate	Rotating so that the palm or sole are moving toward the down position.
Prone	Lying, so the ventral surface faces down.
Proximal	Toward the origin.
Sagittal	A vertical plane from anterior to posterior when the body is standing (mid-sagittal divides the body into right and left halves).
Superficial	Toward the surface; superior; over or above.
Supinate	Rotating hand or foot so the palm or sole moves toward the upward position.
Supra	Over (used as a prefix).
Transverse horizontal	A plane through a standing person.
Ventral	The front of the body or abdomen.*
Vertical	Orthogonal to horizontal.

*Not to be confused with anterior and cephalic, as the head changes the orientation by tilting forward.

are chemical factories, storage facilities, with waste removal operations. The cell is held together with a network of fibers and membranes whose function determines the structure and operation of the space they either enclose or permeate.

Ribosomes (nucleoproteins) are synthesized by RNA-directed operations in the nucleus and are released into the cytoplasm. Most of their function is directed at protein synthesis.

Endoplasmic reticulum takes the products of the organelles and produces a network of protein and lipids to create membranes. Within the network are tubes (cisternae) that permeate the cytoplasm to the outer membrane. The membrane is variously rough (because of attached protein particles) or smooth (without attached

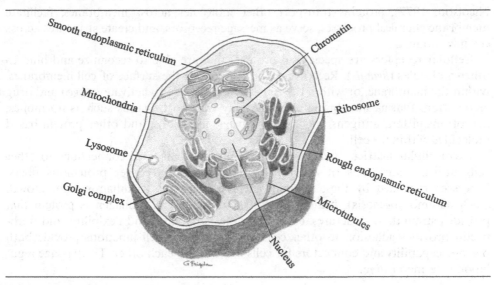

Figure 5.1   The Cell

ribosomes or riboneucleoproteins). The *Golgi complex* or Golgi apparatus is a network of proteins formed from the endoplasmic reticulum into small sacs (vesicles) that break off to deliver products to other structures or to the cell membrane for release outside of the cell.

Lysosomes are the sacs that contain digestive proteins that operate within the cell. They merge with vesicles to create digestive vacuoles. Among the digestive functions is the elimination of debris from cells that have completed their life cycles and died (via autophagosomes). This latter process is termed *autophagy*.

Similar to lysosomes are peroxisomes, which provide an enzyme (catalase) that then oxidizes hydrogen atoms to produce peroxides. These powerful chemicals provide oxygen for other chemical processes.

Mitochondria operate for cellular energy production via enzymes that produce much of the cell's ATP (*adenosine triphosphate*).

The membranes that compose organelles are composed of protein and lipid (fat) molecules, which establish membrane integrity and are themselves dependent on phospholipids, glycolipids, and cholesterol. The polarity of the lipid molecules (antipathy) determines which part is hydrophobic (prevents passage of ion-charged or water-soluble molecules, allowing only lipid-soluble molecules to pass through) or hydrophilic (allows ion-charged molecules through). The polarity further creates organization into a bilayer of molecules. This provides a variably permeable membrane, depending on the composition of the molecules attempting passage.[1]

Proteins, because of their ability to chemically combine with lipids, can attach to surfaces or cross membranes. Also, proteins can combine with carbohydrates and thereby allow the latter to be part of membrane composition. Their functions include recognition of cell markers on other cells. In the fluid mosaic model (Singer &

[1]See Figure 5.6.

Nicolson, 1972), proteins transport other molecules across membranes, facilitate membrane chemical processes, serve as message receptors, and create structures across cell membranes.

Cellular receptors are specialized proteins that are able to recognize and bind to other molecules (*ligands*). Receptors can be found on the surface of cell membranes, within the membrane, or within the cell. They may serve to activate *antigen* and drug recognition. Plasma membrane receptors may transport ligands such as hormones, neurotransmitters, antigens, metabolites, drugs, infections, and other protein-based molecules within the cell.

Extracellular matrices and basement membranes can form connections to other cells utilizing secretions of the cells with *collagen* and other proteinous fibers. Processes regulated by these proteins include responses to inflammation, growth (such as embryogenesis), healing, and structure creation. Collagen is protein that provides strength to structures, elastin provides stretching and flexibility, and fibronectin provides adhesion to other cells and structures. Cell junctions provide both passage capability and connectors for cells to join with each other. The passage regulation is termed *gating*.

Function

Eight possible functions exhaustively include all cellular operations: (a) movement (typically, muscles); (b) conductivity (neurons); (c) metabolic absorption (intake and use of nutrients and other substances from their environs); (d) secretion (production and release of substances used elsewhere); (e) excretion (ridding of wastes following other operations); (f) respiration (intake of oxygen used in producing energy and chemical transformation); (g) reproduction (growth and replication of cells); and (h) communication (many cells operate to communicate with others, such as nerve cells, endocrine cells, and muscle cells) (Albert et al., 2002).

Structure Meets Function

Communication among cells, necessary for homeostasis, is accomplished via hormones passing in the blood (endocrine), neural signaling, *paracrine* signaling, and *autocrine* signaling. Second messengers operate within cells after activation at the cell membrane (cyclic adenosine monophosphate [cAMP] and calcium ions). Most cell membrane protein activation occurs at ion-channel, G-protein, or enzyme-linked receptors. G-proteins serve as intermediaries in intracellular communication, oftentimes receiving information about cellular function and transmitting it to the nucleus, where gene transcription provides the cell with a response to developing conditions reported via G-proteins. Problematic communications in cells serve as the bases for many pathologies such as the cancers (neoplasms).

Cellular metabolism refers to the process whereby energy is either consumed (*anabolism*) or released (catabolism). Food is hydrolyzed to produce ATP via enzymes with affinities for specific substances, or *substrates*. Three stages occur during metabolism:

1. Food is broken down into smaller units (proteins into amino acids, *polysaccharides* into simple sugars such as glucose, and fats into fatty acids).
2. Small molecules are broken down within the cytoplasm for glycolysis via oxidation.

3. Degradation of acetyl CoA into CO_2 and H_2O occurs. In the latter, the *Krebs cycle* (citric acid cycle) occurs followed by *oxidative phosphorylation* (Wellen et al., 2009).

Membrane transport can take the form of passive transport when water and uncharged molecules pass through semipermeable membranes via osmosis, hydrostatic pressure, and *diffusion*. These are processes that don't require energy created by biological activity. On the other hand, *active transport* requires metabolic activity, as well as receptor involvement. While passive transport requires hydrostatic pressure for filtration of dissolved substance and relies a great deal on osmosis, or the process by which water flows from a low-solute concentration to a high-solute concentration, mediated transport occurs when proteins with receptors function to identify and move specific substances across membranes. These might be charged ions (e.g., Na^+ and K^+) transported by the action of ATPase[2] or organic molecules (e.g., glucose transported by insulin). Active transport relies on mediated transport to move against concentration gradients and therefore requires the expenditure of energy.

Reproduction occurs when cell division (mitosis) occurs followed by *cytokinesis*. Growth of the mass occurs during interphase (G_1, S, and G_2 phases), prior to cell division. The cell cycle includes a prophase (new chromosomes appear), metaphase (spindle fibers separate with newly created chromosomes), anaphase (separation of chromatids), and, last, telophase (new cell membrane formation). Regulation of cell growth and development is by cytokines (peptides) or growth factors. Cells then move via migration processes.

Tissues are formed during a second level of organization where cells recognize each other and subsequently form a unit through adhesion. Connective tissue comes in many forms, including loose, elastic, reticular, cartilage, bone, vascular, *adipose* (fat), tendons, and ligaments, as well as three type of muscle: smooth (gastrointestinal [GI] tract, heart, bladder, blood vessels); cardiac; and skeletal or striate.

Cellular and Tissue Dysfunction

Apoptosis is programmed self-destruction of cells resulting from normal as well as pathological processes. The resulting cell remnants are disposed of by phagocytosis or shedding. It is *not* the destruction of cells that occurs by action of outside agents.

Cell Changes in Morphology

The cell life cycle includes response to injury, aging, and eventual cell death. Part of the cycle includes adaptation, as well as maladaptation, and may change the shape of the cell's morphology, evolving into *atrophy*, hypertrophy, hyperplasia, dysplasia, or metaplasia.

Atrophy refers to a decrease in cell size. This may take the form of physiologic atrophy occurring during early stages of development, or pathological atrophy that occurs from disuse, poor nutrition, or aging. Hypertrophy refers to increased cell mass due to hormonal stimulation or adaptive demand, such as muscle enlargement from demand in striatal cells in the heart and skeletal muscles. Pathological hypertrophy may occur secondary to hypertension or valve problems. Hyperplasia is an

---

[2]Note that for every ATP molecule processed, three molecules of Na move out of the cell and two molecules of K move in.

increase in cell division. It may occur secondary to severe injury with cell death, causing overcompensation and regeneration. Hormonal hyperplasia is most often specific to estrogen-stimulated organs such as in the uterus and breast. Pathologic hyperplasia is a proliferation of cells that may be either hormonally induced or due to growth factors that may become malignant. Dysplasia is a transitory change in cell morphology and is graded as mild, moderate, or severe. Most often occurring in *epithelial cells*, dysplasia may reverse if the provoking stimuli are removed, but it may also be a harbinger and precursor for cancer. Metaplasia is a replacement process of a mature cell, likely to be less differentiated and often having less protective capacity.

Cellular injury is due to failure of resilience in accommodating injurious stimuli. Injurious agents may include chemical agents, *hypoxia*, *anoxia*, infections, free radicals, physical and mechanical stimuli, immunological reactions, genetics, and nutritional factors. Hypoxia (inadequate oxygen) or *ischemia* (obstruction of blood flow), damages, but might not kill, cells (autodigestion). Anoxia (an absence of oxygen) may be lethal to cells.

Mechanical, Chemical, and Bacterial Injury

Any microorganism such as bacteria, viruses, and funguses that are unsuccessfully fought can lead to cell death. Parasites may deplete defenses as well as directly attack organisms. Free radicals are the result of chemical reactions in which portions of compounds no longer attached to the other portion of the molecule, now with unpaired electrons, seek to combine with other portions of molecules and compete with the existing counterpart in a stable molecule. The result is a damaged (previously functional) molecule, which may be any protein, lipid, or carbohydrate; this may lead to dysfunction of the affected membrane or loss of phospholipids, structural damage, inflammation, and irreversible release of enzymes (CPK, LDH) and calcium ions, eventually resulting in cellular instability and subsequent cell death.

Physical and mechanical injuries may damage any cell portion and disrupt the structure of the cell; elicit inflammation, immunological reactions, and genetic errors; and impair nutritional functions. Note that reduced ATP production resulting from impaired mitochondrial oxygenation leads to a cascade of reversible processes, but may even lead to cell death once lysosomes have swollen from increased acidity. The body, it should be noted, creates free radicals through a variety of mechanisms, including absorption of energy (radiation, including ultraviolet [UV]); oxidative processes from digestion; and enzyme action on ingested chemicals or drugs. Peroxidation, fragmentation of proteins, and DNA breakage are part of the reactive chain.

Chemical injury results from biochemical interactions with a resulting increased cell membrane permeability. This may occur through a chemical directly combining with the membrane and damaging linkages, as well as through the promotion of lipid peroxidation. Reactive oxygen species (ROS) is a term referring to free radicals that are more likely to combine chemically with other organic compounds in a manner that damages cells. ROS may be the source that creates disease processes such as atherosclerosis, various brain disorders, cancer, and a variety of deteriorative processes. Antioxidants (e.g., vitamins E and C, cysteine) function to remove free radicals from the system by either inactivating or blocking synthesis, or by enzymes that modulate destruction of free radicals (Noguchi, Watanabe, & Shi, 2000).

While many chemically active substances can cause destruction of cells immediately if trace amounts are potent, cell death is more likely to occur following long-term exposure with larger volumes; of particular concern are those substances that create direct injury via chemical combination with cell structures, or through the propagation of reactive free radicals and lipid peroxidation (Parke & Sapota, 1996). Chemical agents that we consider poisons common in the environment include many hydrocarbons. Also of particular concern are street drugs (such as heroin), not just because of inherent toxicity but because of adulterants used to cut or dilute the drugs (Cole et al., 2011).

Injuries such as blunt force (contusion), abrasion (scrape), laceration (tears), and bone fractures may result in blood accumulation (hematoma) that cause damage by pressure on surrounding tissue. Intrusive injury may take the form of incision, stabbing, or chopping.

Asphyxia can take the form of suffocation as the result of smothering, strangulation, *aspiration*, or drowning. Other assaults on the body include infections, immune response with resulting inflammation, genetic factors, and nutritional problems. A common example of nutritional assault is unregulated glucose: hyperglycemia (high blood sugar or diabetes) or hypoglycemia (low blood sugar). Diabetes mellitus may be the most complex disease process known, as all body systems are adversely affected (see section on endocrine disorders). Secondary complications are the primary concern in hyperglycemia, whereas hypoglycemia is, itself, an acute complication. Both are sources of tissue damage. Diabetes is just one example of disorders of cell storage. Other such conditions include difficulty in storing and eliminating water, lipids, carbohydrates, glycogen, proteins, bilirubin, and calcium.

Inflammation is the cellular response to injury. The suffix -*itis* refers to a tissue inflammatory process. Each tissue may have a characteristic inflammatory response, and whole-body responses may be well systematized to respond in an orchestrated manner according to antibody identification.

The inflammatory process involves a sequence of programmed biological reactions to tissue damage (Castellheim, Brekke, Espevik, Harboe, & Mollnes, 2009). Once assault on the body's integrity is perceived, *mast cells* and platelets release a variety of mediators such as prostaglandin, histamine, *leukotrienes*, and serotonin (5HT).[3] Responses to inflammation include transient vasoconstriction, subsequent local vasodilation, and increased permeability (the latter constituting the vascular response to injury). Additionally, *leukocytes* are attracted (first neutrophils, then *monocytes* and macrophages) to eventually destroy and finally remove debris. Accumulated fluid and protein subsequently inhibit blood flow and induce damage to surrounding tissues. As part of the inflammatory response, a systemic effect might be fever (caused by release of *pyrogens* such as interleukin-1 from white cells and macrophages); increase in body temperature is achieved through metabolic increase. The time sequence for acute, reversible inflammation is usually complete in about 48 hours. Chronic inflammation may cause serious damage, such as seen in stomach ulcers, and may persist until the etiological agents are removed.

If the tissue damage persists and becomes breached, the possibility of infection increases. Both removal of the inflammatory agent (including infections) and resolution or suppression of the inflammation may be necessary. The latter may be accomplished by anti-inflammatory drugs such as aspirin or prednisone. At the end of the process, scar tissue resulting from accumulation of collagen may develop and remain. Healing may occur via resolution in which minimally damaged cells recover and initially regenerate, requiring eventual replacement via mitosis.

---

[3]Note that anti-inflammatory drugs antagonize these receptors to reduce their effects.

Electrolyte imbalances (e.g., Na^+, Ca^{2+}, H^+, OH^-, Cl^-, Mg^{2+}, K^+, HPO_4^-) may occur during illness. Aldosterone, a hormone secreted by the adrenal cortex, regulates concentrations of sodium (reabsorption) and potassium (secretion) by acting on the distal tubule of the kidneys.[4] Hypernatremia (excessive sodium) levels may result from dehydration, iatrogenic treatment of cardiac arrest via sodium bicarbonate, oversecretion of aldosterone, or *Cushing syndrome* (ACTH hypersecretion). Hyponatremia (low sodium) may result from *hyperhydration*, polydipsia, ACTH hyposecretion, *hypovolemia*, brain swelling (edema), and *nephrotic syndrome*. Hypochloremia (chloride loss) may be associated with hyponatremia or elevated bicarbonate as with alkalosis (high pH). Diseases associated with hypochloremia include cystic *fibrosis*.

Changes in pH (acidity vs. alkalinity) may affect K^+ and Mg^{2+} concentrations. For example, magnesium concentrations may complicate postcoma recovery from diabetic *ketoacidosis* (DKA). Insulin also affects potassium levels through stimulation of the Na^+, K^+, ATPase pump. Hypokalemia (low potassium) interacts with insulin by suppression of secretion, glycogen synthesis, and impaired renal function. A further problematic effect involves cardiac function via hyperpolarization. Diseases associated with hyperkalemia include renal failure, trauma, any insulin deficiencies, and *Addison disease*.

Calcium and phosphate (HPO_4^-) concentrations are related to levels of parathyroid (PTH) hormone, vitamin D, and calcitonin. These regulate absorption from the intestines, bone deposition, and renal absorption and excretion. Disease processes associated with *hypocalcemia* include vitamin D deficiency and may relate to fat malabsorption (vitamin D is fat soluble) or inadequate sunlight exposure and hypoalbuminemia (low bound calcium in plasma). Conversely, hypercalcemia may occur with hyperparathyroidism, bone metastases, sarcoidosis, and excessive vitamin D. Of note are behavioral manifestations as well as fatigue, weakness, lethargy, and anorexia. Electrocardiogram (ECG) changes may demonstrate heart block and bradycardia.

CO_2 levels reflect saturation of oxygen and are present in the bicarbonate (HCO_3^- radical). Hydrogen ion (H^+) values reflect pH (acidity vs. alkalinity) levels. It should be noted that changes in pH (reflected in hydrogen concentration) are associated with, among other contingencies, K^+ balance. Extremes of acid and base in the blood may be found as a result of loss of bicarbonate or presence of noncarbonic acids for acidosis (e.g., see DKA) or alkalosis (e.g., see hyperaldosteronism), and may reflect failure or loss of buffers (compounds that moderate acidity/alkalinity).

DNA and Genetic Disorders

Deoxyribonucleic acid (DNA) is the template from which RNA (ribonucleic acid), a second-level messenger, transmits structural changes within the organism. Errors (mutations) may occur in the replication process in the nucleus or in the cytoplasm.

DNA is arranged or folded into chromosomes. Humans have 23 pairs, 22 of which are called autosomes with the 23rd determining sex. There are an estimated 50,000 to 100,000 genes on the chromosomes. Errors on these chromosomes and their component genes may be classed as single-gene disorders (classed mostly as recessive, dominant, and X-linked recessive) such as the autosomal recessive cystic fibrosis, the autosomal dominant Huntington's disease, and the X-linked recessive fragile X syndrome. For the latter, interestingly, men cannot pass an X-linked gene to their sons, though they can do so to their daughters.

---

[4]See Figure 5.4.

Chromosomal disorders involve abnormalities in duplication or reassembly of chromosomes causing abnormal placement, structure, or number of chromosomes. Down syndrome is a trisomy on the 21st pair of chromosomes, resulting in an excess of chromosomes, while Turner's syndrome, where there is only one X present on what would ordinarily be a pair of chromosomes, results in an impoverished number of chromosomes.

As the basis for phenotype (gene expression in the living organism) is our DNA, it is not surprising that most congenital abnormalities stem from that structure. Exposure to toxins, ionizing radiation, and inherited errors create the inborn risk factors that lead to most disorders, as well as provide the resilience that resists them. Schizophrenia and the various forms of diabetes derive from a compilation of risk factors that, taken together, find expression when that combination is sufficient.

Two terms associated with genetic traits are penetrance and expressivity. *Penetrance* refers to the percentage of people with the genotype who show the phenotype. *Expressivity* refers to the variability in form of phenotype and may affect the degree of damage shown, even if the penetrance is complete. An entire science is devoted to tracking and analyzing the impact of the pedigrees of genetically linked disorders. Probably the most famous of these is the hemophilia-A trait that affected many of the royal families of Europe, historically associated with British, Russian, Spanish, and Prussian houses.

Multifactorial inheritance has found expression in many disease risk factors. Relative risk is shown by dividing the incidence of those exposed to a risk factor by the incidence of those not exposed. Many diseases with genetic bases are polygenic: The more genes accumulated for an individual, the greater the liability, until some threshold is reached. One example of such a disease is pyloric stenosis, found among young children and expressed as a narrowing of the pylorus (channel between the stomach and intestine).

SURVIVAL: THE BODY'S INTERPLAY WITH THE ENVIRONMENT

The incidence rate of a disease refers to the number of new cases in a particular time period, most commonly a year, divided by the total N in that population. The prevalence rate is the total number of cases existing in that population, again divided by the total N. While incident rates may best reflect acute increases in infectious disease, prevalence rates reflect more long-term lifestyle influences. In modern times, prevalence rates are significantly affected by health and hygiene practices as well as by advances in medicine.

Genetic Interactions With the Environment

Relative risk (incidence rate of those exposed to a risk divided by incidence rate of those not exposed) helps examine the impact of risk factors. Genetic risk factors assume a liability distribution in a population. Given a genetic loading for a disease, a threshold of liability must be reached before the disease is expressed. This may be expressed as concordance rate where there is a variable contribution of genetics and the environment. A disease process such as type 2 diabetes, where there is a 0.90 concordance for monozygotic twins, is heavily dependent on environmental factors such as food intake and body mass or fat percentage, physical activity, and emotional stress. A chicken-and-egg situation may arise where the very high incidence of depression among diabetics exacerbates both the incidence and the morbidity associated with its management, and vice versa.

Congenital diseases are present at birth, even though they may have multiple factors affecting their expression. Some may be purely genetic, such as Tay-Sachs disease, and some may have occasion to be iatrogenic, such as neural tube defects possibly caused by valproate sodium administered during pregnancy. The major multiple risk factor of *hypercholesteremia*, implicated in coronary artery disease, appears to also have multiple gene variants producing problematic lipoproteins. Relative risk load will likely determine the expression of any disease with a heritable component.

Inflammation and Immunity

The body has an automatic response to attacks and damage. This includes both physical, mechanical, and chemical barriers and the inflammatory response. The latter is activated when the former set of barriers is attacked and breached.

Once the body's initial defenses have been passed, the body responds with a characteristic inflammation. Inflammation is a nonspecific response to irritation, injury, or attack. When activated, there is a vascular response, including dilation, increased permeability and leaking of fluids, and white blood cells moving to the site and sticking to the walls. The response time for this process is seconds. After these events occur, inflammation self-limits the process via plasma proteins (proenzymes) that prevent spread, draw fluid to the area to prevent infection and damage, activate the adaptive immune system, and remove the products of inflammation to assist healing. In this process, the clotting cascade is activated (Hageman factor) and fibrin and fibrinogen form.

Multiple systems operate to elicit this inflammatory response. Phagocytes at inflammatory sites die and release enzymes, having gone through the process of adhering to, engulfing, and destroying the foreign body. Those enzymes digest connective tissue, which causes tissue destruction as part of the inflammatory process. Other cells noted in this process include neutrophils (the most frequent phagocyte in the early stages of inflammatory response), followed by macrophages and lymphocytes. Cytokines enhance the destructive effects of macrophages on bacteria. Eosinophils, though less phagocytic, defend against parasites and mediate mast cell inflammatory products. Natural killer (NK) cells recognize and eliminate cells infected by viruses and abnormal cells such as neoplasms (cancer). Platelets are cell fragments that circulate freely until an injury occurs, when they migrate to the location, adhere, and aggregate. The result is coagulation and *degranulation*.

Immune Deficiency

Primary immunodeficiency (inborn or congenital) is a genetic defect as opposed to secondary immunodeficiency, which is acquired. Such acquisition may be iatrogenic, the result of treating such disorders as lupus erythematosus or other lupoid diseases with immunosuppressants (prednisone, azathioprene, etc.), or may be due to infections such as human immunodeficiency virus (HIV).

Primary immunodeficiencies originating from lymphoid stem cells may be B-lymphocyte (defense cells developing in the bone marrow) defects, or may involve T-lymphocytes (from the thymus). Of the latter, helper T-lymphocytes are often essential to development of B-lymphocyte immune responses. The reverse, where B-cells might be deficient, is unlikely to affect T-cells. A deficiency of B-cells is termed hypo- or agammaglobulinemia. A variety of genetic causes, some auto-somal, such as hyperIgM syndrome, affect the B-cells. The combination T- and B-lymphocyte deficiencies can be the most severe, and like other deficiencies are multitudinous.

Other deficiencies fall in the complement (protection) and the phagocytic and bacteria killing (in combination with IgG or C3b) classes. They initiate cascades of operation with a variety of causal factors generally characterized by operational anomalies (such as C3 deficiency) or inadequate cell production, such as when myeloid cells don't mature. The latter results in recurrent, milder neutropenias that adversely affect recovery from infections. Other manifestations of inadequate cell presence may be more severe, such as chronic granulomatous disease. As noted, these tend to be congenital.

Secondary deficiencies run the gamut of causes, including normal transient physiologic processes and events (e.g., pregnancy, infancy, aging); emotional and physical stresses; poor diet and/or metabolic inadequacies; infections; malignan-cies; physical and physiological traumas; and iatrogenic interventions (psychotro-pic, antibiotic, surgery with anesthesia, corticosteroid, or other immunosuppressive medications).

Finally, HIV (a form of retrovirus that carries RNA instead of DNA) provokes a secondary immunodeficiency syndrome that depletes Th cells and otherwise targets dendritic cells, macrophages, CD8-positive Tc cells, natural killer cells, and certain neural cells. It is, however, depletion of CD-4+ cells that has a large effect on the immune system.

Stress

Chronic stress reduces the body's defenses. Physiological vulnerability due to disease process can be exacerbated and coping capacity reduced by both physical and psy-chological stressors. The General Adaptation Syndrome (Selye, 1936), defined by the sequence of alarm, resistance, and exhaustion, mobilizes the sympathetic branch of the autonomic nervous system along the hypothalamus-pituitary-adrenal axis. Physiologic stress, enmeshed with psychological factors, comprises aspects of psy-choneuroimmunology (see also discussion of endocrine system) and homeostasis. A significant hormone, released along with the neurotransmitters epinephrine and norepinephrine, is corticotropin-releasing hormone (including endorphins, ACTH, prolactin, and growth hormone, among others), affecting release of cortisol. The result of endocrine activation under stress results in blood pressure increase, arteriole smooth muscle contraction, lipolysis with release of free fatty acids, and the complex effect of gluconeogenesis plus glycogenolysis. Other effects include reduced inflam-matory response and immunosuppression, and fluid retention via release of vaso-pressin and antidiuretic hormone (ADH).

Psychopharmacology Considerations

Cells in general, and the human organism as a whole, are vulnerable during the first nine months of life, particularly so during the first trimester of pregnancy. Certain psychotropic medications are known to be teratogenic, whereas others are known to be relatively safe, but the majority have unknown effects on fetal development: Temazepam and flurazepam are known to cause birth defects, while some tricyclics, paroxetine, lithium, valproate, and carbamazepine, as well as benzodiazepines are

Table 5.2   Teratogenic Classification of Psychotropics

FDA Pregnancy Rating*	Psychotropic
Category X	Benzodiazepines/benzodiazepine derivatives: estazolam, temazepam, flurazepam, triazolam, quazepam.
Category D	SSRI: paroxetine. Mood stabilizers: lithium, valproic acid, carbamazepine, topiramate. Benzodiazepines: alprazolam, lorazepam, diazepam, clonazepam, oxazepam, chlordiazepoxide.
Category C	SSRIs: fluoxetine, sertraline, citalopram, escitalopram, fluvoxamine. SNRIs: duloxetine, venlafaxine. MAOIs: phenelzine, isocarboxazid, tranylcypromine, selegiline. Tricyclics**: amitriptyline, amoxapine, clomipramine. Conventional and atypical antipsychotics: chlorpromazine, fluphenazine, haloperidol; olanzapine, quetiapine, resperidone, ziprasidone, aripiprazole. Mood stabilizer: lamotrigine. Sleep aid: zaleplon, zolpidem. Stimulants: methylphenidate, amphetamine, atomoxetine.
Category B**	Antidepressant: maprotiline. Antipsychotic: clozapine. Anxiolytic: buspirone. Sleep aid: diphenhydramine. ADHD: guanfacine.

*X = Contraindicated in pregnancy; D = Positive evidence of risk; C = Risk not ruled out; B = No evidence of risk to humans.
**Note: With the exception of mood stabilizers, there is one pregnancy-safe medication for each class.
Source: Muse (2010).

suspected of causing birth defects; other medications have insufficient studies done to conclude their relative teratogenicity, such as clonazepam, selective serotonin reuptake inhibitors (SSRI), monoamine oxidase inhibitors (MAOI), most conventional and atypical antipsychotics, methylphenidate, and amphetamine. Still, a few medications have been shown to be relatively safe for use during pregnancy, such as clozapine, buspirone, zolpidem, and guanfacine (Shepard & Lamire, 2004). (See Table 5.2.)

FUNCTIONAL SYSTEMS OF THE BODY

This section reviews the major systems of the body, including (a) the endocrine system, (b) the hematological systems, (c) the cardiovascular and lymphatic systems, (d) the pulmonary system, (e) the kidneys and urological system, (f) the digestive system, (g) the musculoskeletal system, and (h) the integument system. We also take a brief look at multiple system pathologies. We defer the nervous system, however, to special emphasis in previous sections of this book, and refer the reader to Chapters 3 and 4.

The Endocrine System: Hormones

The endocrine system, comprised of glands spread throughout the body, creates regulatory chemicals called hormones. Their functions involve (a) preparing the body for creation and maintenance of new life, (b) differentiation of the developing fetus's nervous and reproductive system, (c) controlling development during childhood and adolescence, (d) maintaining optimal homeostasis, and (e) responding to emergencies with corrective and/or adaptive changes. These actions involve communication among the cells in three manners: (1) autocrine (intracellular), (2) paracrine (between adjacent cells), and (3) endocrine (among unconnected cells).

The endocrine system operates by releasing hormones into the circulatory system, which, in turn, effect systemic changes downstream. This is achieved through mechanisms peculiar to the endocrine system, which include timed rhythms, feedback systems, systems for targeting distant cells and organs with specific receptors, and inactivation methods whereby the liver metabolizes hormones and the kidneys excrete them. As with neural cells, receptors may up or down regulate.[5]

The Pituitary

The pituitary is also called the "master gland" because it influences the secretions of other glands. It is functionally and anatomically divided into an anterior section and a posterior section. The anterior portion secretes somatotropin or growth hormone (GH), follicle-stimulating hormone (FSH), luteinizing hormone (LH), adrenocorticotropic hormone (ACTH), thyroid-stimulating hormone (TSH), alpha-melanocyte-stimulating hormone (MSH), and prolactin.[6]

Thyrotropin-releasing hormone (TRH) stimulates thyroid stimulating hormone (TSH), while stomatostatin inhibits TSH. GH stimulates and controls growth during development and metabolism. The effects are complex and include stimulation of insulin-like growth factor. Other effects include anabolism of protein, fat utilization by breakdown of triglycerides and adipocyte oxidation, and metabolism of carbohydrates. The latter is a complex process, sometimes likened to opposition of insulin effects, and includes suppressing insulin-instigated uptake of glucose, and the stimulation of gluconeogenesis in the liver. Insulin does not suppress GH production. LH (gonadotropins) and FSH regulate activity in the testes for males and ovaries for females, respectively. ACTH is released every few hours, but is increased under stress by the presence of cortisol in a negative feedback loop (high cortisol suppresses ACTH, high ACTH causes cortisol release, low cortisol levels lead to ACTH production). TSH stimulates T_3 (triiodothyronine) and T_4 (thyroxine), and is suppressed by somatotropin. MSH stimulates production of melanin in the skin and hair follicles. Prolactin secretion, which may be stimulated by TRH and suppressed by estrogens and dopamine, prepares pregnant women's breasts for milk production by stimulating milk synthesis.

Autoimmune processes against TSH receptors may result in binding that causes increased T_4 production or hyperthyroidism (Graves' disease). Decreased TSH, conversely, may result in hypothyroidism by inadequate production of T_4 or poor conversion of T_4 into T_3. Hypothyroidism may also be the end result of

---

[5]To avoid redundancy, plasma membrane receptors and first/second messengers are examined in the chapters on neurological communication.

[6]*FLAGTOP mnemonic:* *F*ollicle-stimulating hormone (FSH), *L*uteinizing hormone (LH), *A*drenocorticotropin hormone (ACTH), *G*rowth hormone (GH), *T*hyroid-stimulating hormone (TSH), *O*xytocin, *P*rolactin.

hyperthyroidism, once the thyroids have been damaged during autoimmune attack and no longer produce T_4 and T_3, as in Hashimoto's thyroiditis.

GH secretion abnormalities have their greatest effect during childhood: Hyposecretion of GH may result in a well-proportioned and physiologically normal, but very small, person termed a midget. Inability to respond to GH can also occur at the receptor sites, with resulting growth retardation. Hypersecretion of GH may result in gigantism. In adults, it may lead to acromegaly. It should also be noted that most forms of dwarfism are not caused by lack of GH, but instead have a variety of causes, most with a genetic basis.[7]

The posterior pituitary stimulates vasopressin or antidiuretic hormone (ADH), which regulates fluid retention. Deficient ADH, or problems at the receptor level, lead to excessive urine loss (diabetes insipidus).

Water-soluble hormones are most often first messengers (the glycoproteins, amines, small peptides) and find their receptors on plasma membranes. The lipid-soluble hormones such as the steroids may have receptors on plasma membranes or have nuclear receptors, and thyroid hormones may be nuclear or *cytosolic*. Second-messenger molecules such as cyclic adenosine monophosphate (cAMP), calcium ions (Ca^{2+}), and cyclic guanosine monophosphate (cGMP) provide the link to cytoplasmic functions for hormones.[8]

As much of the signaling for the endocrine system stems from the hypothalamus, located superior to the pituitary, the basic structural nuclei of the hypothalamus provide a guide to function. Blood pathways connect it to the anterior pituitary while nerve ducts connect the hypothalamus to the posterior pituitary. The portal hypophyseal connections to the pituitary provide both stimulating and inhibiting hormones such as corticotropin-releasing hormone (CRH), thyrotropin-releasing hormone (TRH), gonadotropins-releasing hormone (GnRH), and growth-hormone-releasing hormone (GHRH).

The Thyroid and Parathyroid Glands

Products from the follicles of the thyroid gland include calcitonin (lowers calcium levels in the blood) and somatostatin. The major product, however, is thyroid hormone. TRH acts to release thyroid hormone stores and increase iodide uptake for T_3 (triiodothyronine) and, subsequently, T_4 (tetraiodothyronine) synthesis. Transport of these is accomplished via binding to one of three proteins (thyroxine-binding globulin, thyroxine-binding albumen, and albumin). Thyroid hormone affects metabolism and growth of tissues throughout the body with a variety of effects, including cell metabolism of proteins, fats, and glucose, and influences body heat and oxygen usage. A secondary effect, resulting from glucose metabolism alteration, is increased insulin demand.

Parathyroid hormone (PTH) regulates serum calcium in a feedback loop.

The Endocrine Functions of the Pancreas

The pancreas acts as both an endocrine gland, producing hormones, and an exocrine gland, producing a variety of digestive enzymes. These enzymes will receive further treatment in the digestive system, to follow.

---

[7]Many genetic-driven hormone deficiencies are now treatable with replacement by hormones of recombinant DNA origin.

[8]Receptor regulation (up and down), and first (water-soluble) and second (lipid-soluble) messengers are reviewed in Chapter 3, Neuroscience.

It should be noted that the pancreas's production of insulin, if it fails, results in one of the most complex systemic disorders: diabetes mellitus. Insulin is synthesized by the beta cells of the pancreas by breakdown of a precursor made of A, B, and C peptide chains. The A and B chains remain together to become insulin, while the C peptide is removed. The level of serum C-peptide is differentially diagnostic for type 1 (absolute insulin deficiency with beta-cell destruction) versus type 2 (classified as predominantly insulin resistance with relative insulin deficiency to predominantly an insulin secretory defect with insulin resistance). Type 2 diabetes may be temporary, as a result of drug treatment (such as with prednisone) or other acute causes that are reversible. (Notkins, 2002; American Diabetes Association, 2011).

Insulin facilitates transport and uptake across certain cell membranes for metabolism. While insulin is produced in the pancreas, it is metabolized by the liver and kidneys. Its effects include suppression of gluconeogenesis in the liver and the storage of glucose as glycogen, primarily in the liver and muscle tissues. As muscle tissue is dependent on insulin for glucose transport, and receptors become more sensitive to insulin with increased muscle activity, serum glucose levels can drop dramatically with exercise, causing hypoglycemia (low blood glucose). Conversely, a lack of exercise may increase insulin resistance; increased adipose tissue can also contribute to insulin resistance. Cells dependent on insulin for glucose transport include muscle, the liver, and adipose tissues. Cells that do not require insulin for glucose transport include the blood, nerve cells, the eyes, kidneys, and skin. Hyperglycemia in these latter structures becomes problematic as insulin does not reduce glucose that finds its way into those tissues. As a result, damage from excessive glucose accumulates with reduced efficiency of blood cells, nerve cells, eyes, and kidneys. These processes are very complex and may take decades to appear.

Iatrogenic diabetes may result from a variety of drugs, including prednisone, ACTH therapy, and certain psychotropics (Beduin & de Haan, 2010; Marquina, Pena, Fernandez, & Baptista, in press). The risk of complications varies among the atypical antipsychotics including clozapine, olanzapine, risperidone, quetiapine, and to a lesser degree with aripiprazole and ziprasidone. The source of atypical antipsychotics' side effect relates to increased impaired glucose tolerance, and, rarely among type 2 diabetics, development of diabetic ketoacidosis (DKA). The incidence of neuroleptic-related tardive dyskinesia increases among diabetics.

Thyroid hormone replacement and other drugs may increase insulin requirements, while others may decrease it (e.g., ethanol suppresses gluconeogenesis in the liver at the same time it masks hypoglycemic symptoms, complicating management.). Hypoglycemia normally elicits counterregulatory hormones (cortisol, epinephrine) to raise serum glucose. Insulin also acts to reduce proteolysis in muscles and to increase lipid storage while synthesizing fatty acids and promoting *esterification*.

Alpha cells in the pancreas and GI tract secrete glucagon, which stimulates gluconeogenesis and glycolysis. Glucagon is antagonistic to insulin. It also stimulates lipolysis, which produces free fatty acids and ketones. There is evidence that destruction of alpha cells with diabetes may contribute to poor glucose regulation. Pancreatic somatostatin, produced by delta cells, assists with digestive homeostasis, but the pancreatic origin is not well understood. It may have a role in inhibiting both insulin and glucagon secretion.

Assessment of diabetes mellitus is usually accomplished with self-monitoring of blood glucose (SMBG); urinalysis for glucose should be zero. Many physicians also monitor insulin production by measuring C-peptide (product of insulin created from proinsulin), circulating insulin levels, and the percentage of glucose present in the blood insulin carrier hemoglobin A1c.

Adrenal Glands

The adrenal cortex, stimulated by ACTH, produces the *glucocorticoids* responsible for carbohydrate metabolism, increased appetite, anti-inflammatory actions, growth hormone suppression, and alertness/sleep. Cortisol is produced in the adrenal cortex, stimulated by CRH. Of the mineral corticoids, aldosterone is the most potent and, via regulation by *renin* and angiotensin, acts to maintain sodium levels by increasing sodium reabsorption in the *nephron ducts*. People with Cushing disease who comorbidly develop high aldosterone run the risk of hypertension, low potassium levels, parasthesias, muscle spasms, and periods of muscle paralysis. Hypoactive adrenals with low aldosterone (often autoimmune or due to infection) result in Addison's disease with weakness, postural hypotension, and feeling tired due to excessive sodium excretion, retention of potassium, and hypovolemia. Low cortisol levels may lead to hypoglycemia.

The adrenal medulla's *chromaffin cells* (pheochromocytes) produce epinephrine and norepinephrine. In this case they act as hormones, not neurotransmitters. They are the major source of the "fight or flight" response.

Aging Effects on the Endocrine System

Pathological changes in hormonal regulation may result in either increased or decreased hormonal production. There is often a complex positive and/or negative feedback mechanism that is disrupted.

Some age-related changes include:

Thyroid—may experience cumulative autoimmune damage.

Parathyroid—PTH may be decreased with age with lower calcium intake and resulting *osteopenia*/osteoporosis.

Adrenals—decreased metabolic clearance of cortisol results in lower secretion.

Posterior pituitary—the hyponatremia seen in elders does not appear related to changes in the posterior pituitary, as ADH secretion is supported by other mechanisms.

Anterior pituitary—fibrosis, necrosis, excess iron, microadenomas, and atrophy. GH secretion decreases, resulting in increased visceral fat deposits, decreased muscle, and decreased bone density.

Endocrine Pathologies

Various pathologies associated with the endocrine system are outlined below, according to the structures involved:

Thyroid Dysfunction

- *Hyperthyroidism.* The term reserved for increased levels of thyroid hormone in the blood is thyrotoxicosis or hyperthyroidism. Symptoms are typically metabolic and, morphologically, are often manifested as goiter. The most common cause is Graves' disease, an autoimmune disorder characterized by hyperthyroidism, goiter (enlarged thyroid), ophthalmopathy, and dermopathy.

- *Hypothyroidism.* A deficiency of thyroid function may be primary, with causes such as circulating autoimmune antibodies, iodine deficiency, thyroiditis, antithyroid drugs, and loss of thyroid tissue following treatment of hyperthyroidism. One such cause is Hashimoto's disease, which produces antibodies to thyroid gland tissue. Secondary causes of hypothyroidism include hypothalamus or pituitary dysfunction (Mayo Clinic Associates, 2010).

Parathyroid Dysfunction

- *Hyperparathyroidism.* Problems may be seen in hypercalcemia, *hyperphosphaturia*, bone *resorption*, metabolic acidosis, and renal disease. Also, gout may be present, resulting in renal failure. Symptoms may include renal colic, recurrent urinary tract infections (UTIs), renal failure, abdominal pain and peptic ulcers, pancreatitis, osteoporosis and other bone diseases, muscle weakness and pain, delirium, constipation, anorexia with nausea and vomiting, and inflammation and pain in joints as seen with gout.

- *Hypoparathyroidism.* Hypoparathyroidism usually occurs secondary to thyroid surgery. Most symptoms are related to hypocalcemia. The condition may also be caused from alcoholism, malnutrition, malabsorption, or increased renal clearance causing low magnesium levels. On an acute basis, diabetic ketoacidosis (DKA) may lower magnesium levels enough to, secondarily, cause hypoparathyroidism until levels are corrected.

Pancreas Dysfunction

- *Hyperglycemia.* (American Diabetes Association, 2011). Type 1 diabetes[9] is an autoimmune disorder in which beta cells are destroyed following onset of the disease subsequent to exposure to stressors such as emotional events, injury, and viruses.[10] While the autoimmune process may take 5 to 10 years for relatively complete destruction of beta cells, onset of symptoms is usually rapid with weight loss, *polyphagia*, polydipsia, increased urination, ketone production (with characteristic sweet, fruity breath similar to nail polish solvent), fatigue, blurred vision, itchy and dry skin, diarrhea or constipation, weakness, nausea, and vomiting.

  The primary defect in type 1 diabetes is an absence of insulin production as, eventually, all or most beta cells are destroyed. As some 75% affected are under the age of 30, the term *childhood onset diabetes* is also used to refer to type 1. If the pancreas is unable to produce insulin, other sources of energy than glucose must be provided; lipolysis forms ketones, which can substitute for glucose in the short term. The blood, however, becomes acidic (ketoacidosis) with excessive lipolysis, and progresses to coma and death if insulin and replacement metabolites are not provided.

  The increased blood glucose causes osmotic flow to build, with increased elimination via the kidneys. Typically, serum glucose levels will exceed the renal threshold at 180 mg/dL to show spilling of glucose into the urine. Because of this elimination vector, blood glucose would not usually extend to very high levels for healthy kidneys. High glucose levels (above 250 mg/dL) may prevent physical activity, as counterregulatory hormones (see hypoglycemia) are secreted when

---

[9]Type 2 diabetes is similar to type 1 but for the relative lack of insulin production by beta cells. The characteristic defect in this form is insulin resistance.

[10]Type 1A diabetes is associated with genetic risk factor and autoimmune dysfunction, while there is a rare, fulminating form of type 1 termed idiopathic (type 1B) diabetes. This nonimmune form (approximately 15% of type 1s) is secondary to other disease processes such as pancreatitis.

ordinary processes would suppress them. Cognitive impairment and depression are common effects in the short term, while long-term effects include peripheral neuropathy, characterized by parasthesias, pain, and ultimately absence of sensation.

- *Hypoglycemia.* Hypoglycemia is an acute emergency for those treated with *exogenous* insulin wherein blood glucose drops below 70 mg/dL. It requires immediate treatment by administration of carbohydrates to bring the blood glucose back to normal ranges (70 to 110 mg/dL). Ordinarily, low blood glucose will elicit counterregulatory hormones: cortisol and epinephrine, which stimulate release of glucagon and further stimulate the conversion of glycogen to glucose and the onset of gluconeogenesis. Administration of exogenous glucagon via intramuscular injection will temporarily do the same thing, but replacement carbohydrates must be provided, as glycogen stored in muscles and the liver is depleted. Untreated hypoglycemia, especially in young males, may lead to seizures, coma, and death. Symptoms vary with individuals but may include, for mild cases (approximately 60 to 70 mg/dL), nervousness, tingling, diaphoresis, fatigue, dizziness, poor coordination, headache, and anxiety. As blood glucose drops, all symptoms may increase with surges of anger, combativeness, and oppositionality, making treatment difficult; double vision, confusion, delayed response time for cognition and speech, slurred speech, mood swings, ataxia, muscle rigidity and spasms, seizures, and coma are symptoms of moderate to severe hypoglycemia.

Adrenal Pathologies

- *Hypoadrenal output.* Adrenal medulla disorders do not usually include low output. The exception to this is the impact of an adrenalectomy, which results in decrease catecholamines, although norepinephrine excretion remains normal.
- *Hyperadrenal output.* Hyperexcretion may occur with *pheochromocytomas*, a tumor with a low malignancy rate, and increased release of catecholamines (epinephrine and norepinephrine) may ensue, with resulting hypertension and persistently high feelings of anxiety.

Psychopharmacology Considerations

Acute signs of anxiety may be related to hyperthyroidism or, in rare cases, to pheochromocytomas. There is often a collateral rise in hypertension in the case of pheochromocytoma. While routine thyroid testing is indicated for anxiety disorders, testing for a pheochromocytoma is done only when adrenal implication is suspected. For bipolar patients, thyroid testing is done to establish a baseline before starting lithium treatment; testing is continued periodically throughout the period that lithium is taken, which may be years.

Hematological Systems

Approximately 60% of blood volume consists of plasma, while the rest of the blood is formed of components like red cells and white cells. Ninety percent is water and much of the solute is protein. Within the plasma are water; various electrolytes (e.g., Na^+, Ca^{2+}, H^+, OH^-, Cl^-, Mg^{2+}, K^+, HPO_4^-); proteins (albumin, globulins, fibrinogen, *transferrin*, and ferritin); gases (carbonate, O_2, and N_2); nutrients; and waste products (including urea, creatinine, uric acid, and bilirubin), as well as transported hormones. Cells present in the blood include erythrocytes (red blood cells), leukocytes (white blood cells),[11] and platelets (which are not cells but, rather, fragments). Present also are mast cells, which function to make blood vessels permeable and are intimately involved in initiating inflammation.

Blood cells begin with *hematopoiesis* in the bone marrow. The process involves mitosis and differentiation (maturation). Stem cells are the originating undifferentiated cells leading to bone marrow (B-cell) and thymus (T-cell) lymphocytes or to other blood components, including natural killer (NK) cells. Red cells, stimulated by erythropoietin, develop into mature erythrocytes. Erythrocytes contain hemoglobin, which carries oxygen attached to a single iron ion, which is in turn attached to a polypeptide chain. The attachment and release mechanisms for oxygen are affected by the charge of the Fe ion.

Erythropoiesis requires protein plus a number of vitamins, including B_{12}, folate, B_6, riboflavin, *pantothenic acid*, niacin, ascorbic acid, and vitamin E. Deficiencies in any of these components result in various anemias and failure in cell production.

Older erythrocytes have enzymes to facilitate glycolysis and adenosine triphosphate (ATP) synthesis. This ATP keeps the cell alive but gradually fails as the erythrocyte ages, resulting in deformities and membrane damage as it passes through the small openings in the capillaries. Geriatric populations are prone to a variety of deficiencies that affect blood cell production; many of these deficiencies have their origins in impaired ability of elders to digest nutrients, stemming in part from aging epithelium and mucous membranes in the digestive tract.

Platelets (thrombocytes) develop from *megakaryocytes* via *endomitosis*; platelets form when the karyocyte divides initially (mitosis) but fails to separate into cells with complete DNA, but evolves, instead, into fragments. Platelets are involved in the inflammatory response and coagulation. This is achieved by the presence of clotting factor. After creation, a clot is removed at the final stage of hemostasis by first sealing the wound, retracting fibrous tissue, and then *lysis*.

Dysfunctions in Red Cells

Red blood cell pathologies take the form of anemia—defined as decreased number of erythrocytes and/or decreased volume or quality of hemoglobin. The many anemias can be caused by decreased or defective production or increased destruction. Subcategories of anemia include (a) blood loss due to trauma or hemorrhage; (b) nutritional deficiencies leading to such conditions as pernicious anemia due to inadequate B_{12} as a result of atrophic gastritis with a lack of intrinsic factor (IF), and anemia due to folate deficiency or iron deficiency; (c) sideroblastic anemia caused by defective mitochondrial metabolism; (d) aplastic anemia, resulting in reduced or absent blood of all types as bone marrow fails to produce blood cells: and (e) hemolytic anemia, with early destruction of erythrocytes by immune process.

Apart from anemia, red blood cell *pathology* also includes polycythemia—a disorder in which red blood cell production is increased. Causes may include abnormality of bone marrow stem cells, increased erythropoietin due to secreting tumors, and environmental stimuli such as high-altitude living, smoking, and chronic obstructive pulmonary disease (COPD).

---

[11]White blood cells are further divided into (a) agranulocytes (lymphocytes, monocytes, and macrophages) and (b) granulocytes (eosinophils, neutrophils, and basophils).

Dysfunctions in White Blood Cells

Leukocyte alterations include increased production (leukocytosis) or decreased production (leukopenia). Causes of leukocytosis and leucopenia are varied: Neutropenia is a loss of normal neutrophils. If neutrophils are not produced, *granulopenia* or *agranulocytosis* occurs, and may be life threatening. Causes may be drugs, irradiation, infections, genetic disorders, or immune processes. Eosinophilia (high levels of eosinophils) may be due to allergies, dermatologic disorders, or parasitic invasion. Eosiopenia (low levels) may be due to migration to inflamed areas. Basophilia (high basophils) may be due to inflammatory responses or hypersensitivity reactions. Basopenia (low) may be due to hyperthyroidism, acute infection, or steroid therapies. Basopenia is also noted during ovulation and in pregnancy. Monocytosis (increased monocytes) is transient and goes along with neutropenic response to infections. Monocytopenia (decreased monocytes) may occur with leukemia and prednisone treatment.

Conditions associated with white blood cell abnormalities include (a) lymphocytosis, stimulated by antigens (viruses), but rarely from bacteria; (b) lymphocytopenia, most often attributed to low production associated with neoplasias, but also associated with heart failure and other diseases due to elevated cortisol, especially AIDS; (c) infectious mononucleosis; (d) leukemias; and (e) myeloma.

Psychopharmacology Considerations

A host of conditions may present with symptoms that mimic depression.[12] Infection, anemia, and electrolyte imbalance are just a few. Standard laboratory tests for screening out such conditions include a complete blood count (CBC) (which includes red blood cells for testing anemia and white blood cells for screening infection) and an electrolyte panel (which is usually included in a comprehensive metabolic panel). Of particular concern in prescribing psychotropics is the possible side effect of clozapine and carbamazepine in inducing iatrogenic agranulocytosis. Lab testing for agranulocytosis (also called neutropenia) forms part of the complete blood count, specifically the neutrophil count.

Cardiovascular and Lymphatic Systems

The circulatory system consists of the heart; its activating nervous system and hormones; peripheral vasculature (arteries, veins, capillaries, and intermediary vessels); and lymphatic system.

Coronary Function

The heart, sitting at an angle in the mediatinum, is a muscular pump consisting of four chambers: the right atrium, right ventricle, left atrium, and left ventricle. The ventricles have thicker walls than the atria as they do most of the pumping (right ventricle to the lungs and left ventricle to the rest of the body), while the atria receive blood from the body (right atrium) and the lungs (left atrium). (See Figure 5.2.) The heart wall consists of the pericardium (outside protective and interactive layer), myocardium (cardiac muscle attached to cardiac skeleton), and endocardium (layer with blood vessels supplying the heart and which forms the chamber walls). The skeleton to which these walls are attached consists of connective tissue at the center.

---

[12]See Chapter 6 for a further discussion of assessment and monitoring procedures.

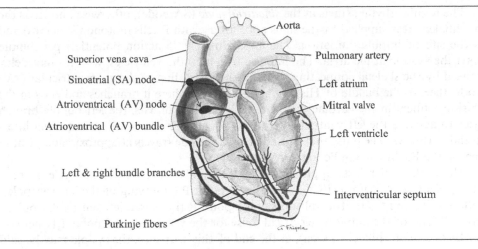

Figure 5.2   The Heart

As the heart is a pump, there is also a set of valves so that blood flows in only one direction. In between ventricular pulses, two atrioventricular (AV) valves separate the atria and ventricles. This allows the ventricles to fill while the atria are relaxed. The right atrioventricular valve is tricuspid, and the left (also called the mitral valve) is bicuspid. Semiluminar valves open to permit both pulmonary (from the right ventricle) and systemic (from the left ventricle) blood flow, then closing to prevent backflow. All valves and tissues function as a unit, so damage to any part affects the whole.

Blood returns to the heart via the superior and inferior venae cavae into the right atrium. After emptying into the right ventricle, contraction of the ventricle pushes blood through the pulmonary artery, where it bifurcates to deliver blood to both lungs. Pulmonary veins, after exchanges of gases in the lungs, bring the blood back to the left atrium, where it then fills the left ventricle for a higher pressure pulse to the rest of the circulatory system via the aorta.[13] The next step, when the ventricles contract, corresponds to the systolic pressure. Four phases constitute ventricular contraction: (a) a slight rise in pressure closes the atrioventricular valves, (b) the aortic valve opens with a lowering of pressure in the ventricles, (c) the aortic valve closes, and (d) the mitral valve opens and the ventricle refills from the atrium.

Cardiac function is supported by arteries and veins that supply blood, nutrients, and electrolytes to the heart and without which the heart dies. Branching of the right and left coronary arteries is complex and varies. Collateral arteries (*anastomoses*) connect the branches and function to protect the heart from occlusions (myocardial infarction), while the coronary capillary network is vast.

In spite of the apparent simplicity of the heart, regulation of function is complex. The heart has its own neural conduction system with nodes self-initiating and maintaining the cycle in the absence of stimulation from the autonomic nervous system. Nonetheless, the sympathetic and parasympathetic systems regulate the rhythm of the cycle (heart rate), and the heart is also affected by endocrine releases to the circulatory system.

---

[13]Note that there is a resting phase during which the baseline pressure in the blood vessels corresponds to the diastolic period when the ventricles are filled.

The regular rhythm starts at the *sinoatrial node* (SA node), otherwise known as the pacemaker. It is supplied by the sinus node artery with P cells (autonomic nerves) and is the site of impulse initiation. The approximately 75 action potentials per minute start the systole at the atria. The impulse travels to the ventricles, with a slight delay caused by the skeletal connecting tissue of the heart, first to the atrioventricular (AV) node, then to the bundle of His (common bundle), where it branches and ends in the Purkinje fibers in the cardiac wall. From the bundle of His, the left bundle branch rises to activate the left ventricular wall. Various other nodes are activated via internodal pathways. The pulse that started at the SA node travels at approximately 1 mm/sec via the Bachman bundle to the AV node.

The cycle, which lasts approximately 0.8 seconds for a ventricular cycle, as seen on an electrocardiogram (ECG), consists of point P (emptying of the left ventricle), followed by point Q (mitral valve opening), point R (increased left ventricular pulse), point S (end of the initiating electrical pulse for the ventricle), and point T (where on an ECG a slight hillock is seen); at the end of this sequence, the systole may be said to end and the aortic valve closes with an increase in left atrial pressure followed by the mitral valve opening and a resting phase of decreasing aortic pressure, followed by a repeat of another SA pulse at point P. (See Figure 5.3.)

It should be noted that the heart is perfused only during rest so that when a ventricular contraction occurs, the heart is not getting blood. A rapid heartbeat may, therefore, prevent cardiac perfusion, as that part of the cycle shortens and ventricular contractions constrict coronary arteries. A normal ECG follows a predictable set of patterns: P (atrial depolarization), the PR interval (time from SA stimulus to ventricular stimulus), QRS complex (the sum of ventricular muscle depolarizations), the ST interval (approximately 0.10 seconds), and the QT interval (approximately 0.4 seconds), electrical systole of the ventricles.

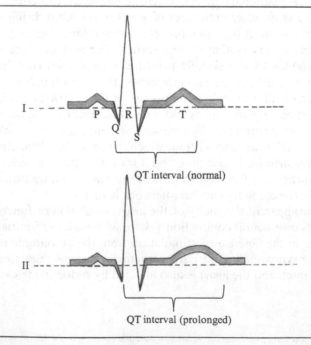

Figure 5.3   QT Interval

Regulation by the sympathetic and parasympathetic systems moderates coronary function, with sympathetic innervations associated with acceleration and parasympathetic fibers involved with slowing the heart pace. The sympathetic fibers innervate the entire coronary atria and ventricles, and increase performance via beta-adrenergic receptors stimulated by norepinephrine and an increase in Ca^{2+} ions. Conversely, stimulation by parasympathetic fibers (vagus nerve) decreases heart rate by releasing acetylcholine.

Adrenergic receptors respond to sympathetic stimuli, and their action depends on the relative presence of alpha and beta receptors in the heart and whether the neurotransmitter is epinephrine or norepinephrine. Note that both will stimulate the heart ($beta_1$) and constrict some vessels ($alpha_1$), but epinephrine differentially dilates specific vessels ($beta_2$). $Alpha_2$, when stimulated by norepinephrine, autoinhibits norepinephrine, promoting vasodilation.

Myocardial cells are similar to skeletal muscle, but differ in that cardiac muscle consists of branching networks (versus parallel organization), have only one nucleus, can transmit impulses from cell to cell, maintain energy synthesis, and have access to more ions. Cardiac muscle, unlike skeletal muscle, must work continually while mitochondria supply ATP. Last, cardiac muscles contain more T tubules, allowing transport of Na^+ and K^+ across their walls. Metabolism is, therefore, a constant demand with less than 30% available in reserve, requiring increased circulation during exercise. Following contraction, like skeletal muscle, relaxation ensues with calcium removed from the cells.[14]

Control of cardiac activity occurs in the medulla, but also in the hypothalamus, cerebral cortex, thalamus, and interneuron networks. The medulla adjusts heart rate and blood pressure through the autonomic nerves with reciprocal inhibition of sympathetic system (suppression of the SA node) and parasympathetic system (stimulating the SA node). The hypothalamus responds to temperature, and the cerebral cortex adjusts cardiac rate though the endocrine system in accordance with emotions. Further, the baroreceptor (mechanical muscle reflex) responds to blood pressure changes (increasing/decreasing heart rate if blood pressure drops/rises and adjusting vasodilation/constriction). Atrial receptors adjust blood pressure via a peptide (atrial natriuretic peptide) that increases or decreases diuretic influences. Likewise, hormones can influence the vasculature as well as cardiac contractility.

Vascular System

The peripheral vasculature consists of arteries, veins, arterioles, venules, and capillaries. Each blood vessel's structure varies according to its respective function. Arteries are comparatively thick-walled as opposed to veins, while veins have a system of valves that prevent backup of blood. Blood vessel lining consists of endothelial cells that adjust to local conditions via growth, contraction/relaxation/movement, repair, prevention of clots, and breakdown of fibrous tissue. Blood flow is determined by blood pressure and peripheral resistance. Dilated arteries reduce blood pressure whereas constricted arteries increase blood pressure, affecting blood flow through

---

[14]Cardiac performance is affected by the preload (pressure following diastole), contractility, heart rate, and afterload (resistance against the systole). Two laws to remember: Frank-Starling law shows a relationship between volume of blood in the heart at the preload to ventricular pressure, and Laplace's law relates muscle wall tension to intraventricular pressure and internal radius, but inversely with wall thickness.

peripheral resistance. Viscosity also affects blood flow, and may be regulated via diuretic and antidiuretic systems.

Arterial *chemoreceptors* in areas of the medulla and in the major arteries (carotid and aorta) respond to oxygen saturation, carbon dioxide, and pH via control of respiration and blood pressure. Arterial pressure, whose purpose is to perfuse the tissues of the body via capillaries, is expressed as mean arterial pressure (MAP): MAP = systolic + ½(systolic − diastolic).

The effects of aging on the heart are unclear because confounding disease processes accelerate with age. However, arterial stiffening and blood pressure increase while perfusion declines. Afterload increases as well as contraction. Heart rate decreases with age, and women sometimes experience a decrease in cardiac output.

Major cardiac disorders include arteriosclerosis (thickened and hardened walls), atherosclerosis (accumulation of lipid plaque), hypertension (sustained increase in baseline arterial pressure—primary or essential and secondary with malignant hypertension—diastolic over 140 mmHg). Causes of secondary hypertension include renal disorders, endocrine disorders, arteriosclerosis, coarctation of the aorta (low distal perfusion elicits high peripheral resistance), pregnancy, intracranial pressure and other neurologic disorders, and drugs such as MAOIs and stimulants. The effect of high blood pressure includes direct damage to the kidneys, brain, retina, heart, and distal arteries.

Coronary artery disease is a leading source of mortality in the United States, usually caused by atherosclerosis. The disease ranges from ischemia (temporary loss of perfusion) to coronary infarction with death of cardiac tissue. Risk factors include dyslipidemia (elevated lipoproteins such as cholesterol), hypertension, nicotine, diabetes mellitus, obesity, sedentary lifestyle, various inflammatory processes, lack of *homocysteine*-degrading enzyme, and infections. Myocardial ischemia may be seen as angina pectoris, transient ischemia of the myocardium, silent ischemia, and mental stress. Unstable angina (a reversible myocardial ischemia) may occur as a presage of heart attack. Myocardial infarction results in necrotic heart tissue.

Heart disease may result in congestive heart failure (left heart failure) with systolic heart failure causing inadequate distribution into the systemic arteries. Diastolic heart failure can occur with systolic heart failure or independently, and is defined as pulmonary congestion with normal stroke volume and output.

Lymphatic System

The lymphatic system collects tissue fluid for return to the bloodstream. Lymphatic fluid is mostly water, but solids are primarily albumen. The lymphatic system drains through the thoracic duct into the subclavian veins. Like veins, lymph vessels are thin-walled and contain valves allowing flow in only one direction. The lymphatic system circulates lymphatic fluid along a route, to some extent paralleling the venous system. Its two primary mobile organs are the thymus (T-cells) and bone marrow (B-cells), while stationary structure is provided by the spleen, lymph nodes, tonsils, and *Peyer patches* of the small intestine. The lymphatic system joins the arteriovenous system with the immune system. The lymphoid organs include:

- The spleen, which is responsible for filtering and cleaning the blood of microorganisms, and as a site of blood storage and creation. Destruction of the spleen may increase circulating lymphocytes, decrease iron, and impair the immune system.

- The lymph nodes, which form part of the lymphatic system cluster and connect with lymphatic veins. These vessels are too fragile to tolerate arterial pressure, and return blood to the heart via the same route as veins.
- The mononuclear phagocyte system, which begins in the bone marrow and promotes cell migration of macrophages throughout the body to destroy and digest waste material, debris, and foreign matter, including microorganisms.

While the spleen is the largest organ of the lymphatic system, splenic functions are complex and not well understood. However, in spite of involvement in blood regulation and infection controls, a person can live without one. An enlarged spleen (splenomegaly) may be palpated just below the ribs on the left side. Splenomegaly may precipitate anemia, leukopenia, thrombocytopenia, or combinations. The enlarged spleen can be fragile and prone to hemorrhage if injured. The congestive form of splenomegaly is associated with neoplasias, hepatic cirrhosis, hemolytic anemia, and *myeloproliferations*. The infiltrative form occurs when macrophages become clogged with material they can't digest. People of geriatric age do not appear prone to any special category of splenic dysfunction.

Psychopharmacology Considerations

Some cardiovascular drugs, such as beta blockers, are used for their psychotropic secondary effects. It is always prudent to clear up any doubt of cardiovascular contraindications for patients before prescribing such medication for the relief of emotional symptoms. Here, a phone consultation with the primary care physician (PCP) or cardiologist is indicated. As mentioned before, beta blockers are also a concern for the asthmatic patient. Among psychotropics, tricyclic antidepressant medication and neuroleptic antipsychotics carry one of the greatest cardiovascular risks due to the potential for iatrogenic *prolonged QT interval* (Pellinen, Färkkilä, & Heikkilä, 1987; Julien, 2005). *Torsades de pointes*, a particularly lethal form of prolonged QT interval, has been associated with lithium, phenothiazines, and tricyclic antidepressants. While the exact mechanism of action is not completely understood, the phenothiazines' and tricyclics' action has been called "quinidine-like" inasmuch as they tend to slow the induction of sodium in the myocardium while retaining potassium, which results in a delay in repolarization after an action potential.[15]

The Pulmonary System

The pulmonary system consists of the lungs (upper and lower), the chest cavity, and pulmonary circulation. Its purposes are ventilation, diffusion of gases between the lungs and the blood, and perfusion of blood between the capillaries of the lungs and the body's tissues. There is a space (*mediastinum*) between the lungs where the heart, great blood vessels, and esophagus reside. The lungs, being fragile, are protected from contaminants by the upper respiratory mucosa, nasal hairs, cilia, alveolar macrophages, and irritant receptors in the nostrils and trachea, which trigger cough.

---

[15]Quinidine is a stereoisomer of quinine. As an antiarrhythmic agent, quinidine primarily works by blocking the fast inward sodium current as well as the outward current of potassium. The effect of blocking these currents during the rapid depolarization phase is a prolongation of the action potential and a delay in the subsequent repolarization. The resulting effect of quinidine on the ion channels prolongs the QT interval (Camm, Malik, & Yap, 2004).

Gas-exchange airways include the bronchioles, alveolar ducts, and alveoli. Pulmonary and bronchial circulation supports gas exchange via blood-filled vessels that are part of systemic circulation, sensitive to systemic blood pressure. The chest wall both protects the lungs and, when expanded via the diaphragm and intercostal muscles, expands the lungs. The *pleura*, a sac encasing the lungs, is also attached to the chest wall and allows the wall to pull on the lungs directly.

Ventilation, the mechanical movement of air and gases between the lungs and the environment, permits the exchange of O_2 and CO_2. The rate of ventilation is controlled by a variety of homeostatic mechanisms centered in the brain stem, affecting respiratory muscles. Peripheral chemoreceptors in the brain stem receive information on gaseous levels from receptors in the aorta and carotid arteries. Innervation of the lungs is an autonomic function, but may be modified by cortical controls. Chemoreceptors monitor arterial blood gases via pH in cerebrospinal fluid (CSF). They control the major muscles (diaphragm and intercostal) and the sternocleidomastoid and scalene muscles. Other factors in the mechanical process of respiration and ventilation include airway resistance and muscular effort involved in breathing. Gas pressure affects absorption and transfer of oxygen and carbon dioxide. Ambient temperature and barometric air pressure also affect this transfer. The sequence follows the lung ventilation, diffusion of oxygen into capillaries, perfusion of oxygen into systemic capillaries, and then diffusion of that oxygen into cells. The elimination of carbon dioxide follows a reverse process of diffusion of CO_2 into capillaries, perfusion by venous blood, diffusion of CO_2 into the lung alveoli, and ventilation of CO_2 out of the lungs. Oxygen attaches to, and dissociates from, hemoglobin (Hb) with a direct associate for arterial pressure (PaO_2)

As people age, several normal alterations adversely affect the pulmonary system: loss of elastic recoil, chest wall stiffening, changes in gas exchange, and increased flow resistance. Pathology in pulmonary function is most often shown by coughing and dyspnea (shortness of breath), but also chest pain, changes in sputum, hemoptysis (coughing up blood), changes in breathing, cyanosis, and hypoventilation.

Pleural problems may include pneumothorax (air in the pleural sac, which can lead to collapse of the lungs as the pressure that adheres the lungs to the walls decreases) or pleural effusion (fluid in the pleural sac, which may be exudates: pleurisy, blood, pus, or lymphatic fluid called chyle). Abscesses may form and cause obstructions. Pulmonary fibrosis refers to an excess of connective tissue in the lung. Furthermore, when the chest wall is burdened by fat, is immobilized, or has malformation, breathing becomes labored.

Specific pulmonary syndromes include acute respiratory distress (lung inflammation and capillary injury to the *alveoli*), postoperative respiratory failure (a potential complication for all major surgery), and obstructive pulmonary disease (airway blockage that presents as worse on exhaling, with wheezing sounds). Common causes of obstructive pulmonary disease are asthma, chronic bronchitis, and emphysema, with the latter two highly comorbid and sharing the term chronic obstructive pulmonary disease (COPD). Asthma attacks tend to be of short duration but with chronically inflamed airways and involvement of the bronchia. Emphysema involves enlarged gas-exchange airways with destruction of alveolar walls but without fibrosis. Respiratory infections include pneumonia (lower respiratory tract—fungal, viral, or bacterial) and tuberculosis (caused by mycobacterium).

Pulmonary embolism is due to a thrombus, fat particle, air bubble, or pieces of tissue causing blockage of the pulmonary circulatory bed, with the most frequent source being blood clots from veins in the thighs (deep vein thrombosis). Risk factors include immobilization with stagnant venous flow, hypercoagulation, and injured vessel walls.

In children, congestion and other obstructions are considered emergencies due to the small size of their airways and limited tolerance. Basal rates are higher than in adults with concomitant demands, immunological response may be lower, and physiological controls of respiration may be less stable. In adults, sleep apnea can be caused by multiple factors but is most associated with a collapsed soft palate as a result of obesity. Elders are more prone to chronic pulmonary disorders that may culminate in pneumonia for which they may have little defense (Hart & Millard, 2010).

Of particular concern for prescribing medical psychologists is the effect that various psychotropics may have on pulmonary function. Beta blockers, for example, prescribed for the control of performance anxiety may be contraindicated in the patient with asthma or COPD because blocking beta receptors in the bronchi tends to constrict them and may complicate preexisting breathing problems. Likewise, benzodiazepines may not be a good sleep aid for someone with obstructive sleep apnea because they tend to promote deeper levels of sleep and may reduce the awakening reflex that prevents severe oxygen deprivation during sleep.

Psychopharmacologic Considerations

Anxiety and panic are associated with shortness of breath (SOB), and may indicate an underlying asthma or COPD condition (Livermore, Sharpe, & McKenzie, 2010). Here, the medical psychologist is at an advantage for being able to screen for physiological causes of anxiety before making a differential diagnosis. Also of concern for pharmacotherapy for anxiety-related insomnia is the presence of obstructive sleep apnea, which is generally a contraindication for the use of hypnotics as sleep aids. While benzodiazepine-based tranquilizers like alprazolam and lorazepam are usually avoided as sleeping aids for patients with sleep apnea, zolpidem has been shown not to impede the efficacy of the *continuous positive airway pressure (CPAP)* machine for nocturnal treatment of obstructive sleep apnea (Berry & Patel, 2006).

The Kidneys and Urological System

The kidneys maintain homeostasis via control of solute and water transport or retention, metabolic excretion, disposal of many wastes, conservation of many nutrients, and regulation of pH. Kidneys include the renal capsule within which are the renal cortex and renal medulla. The cortex houses the tubules and *glomeruli*, and the medulla holds the distal and proximal tubules plus the collecting ducts. The basic unit of the kidney is the nephron, a tubular structure that includes the renal corpuscle, proximal convoluted tubule, *loop of Henle*, distal convoluted tubule, and the collecting duct. (See Figure 5.4.)

The distal tubule, made of straight and convoluted segments, with a collecting duct made of principal cells that reabsorb sodium and water and secrete potassium, and intercalated cells that secrete hydrogen or bicarbonate and secrete potassium, is highly vascularized with arterial flow from the abdominal aorta. It empties reabsorbed solutes into the renal vein, which then transports to the *vena cava*. Liquid that is not reabsorbed—that is, urine—is transported to the ureters from the distal tubules and deposited into the bladder. As it fills, the bladder's detrusor muscle is distended and parasympathetic innervations subsequently stimulate a spinal reflex to begin *micturition*.

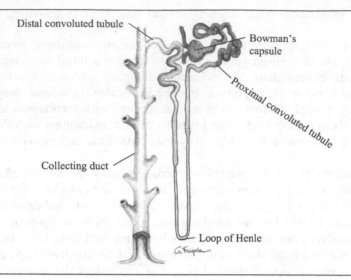

Figure 5.4 Nephron

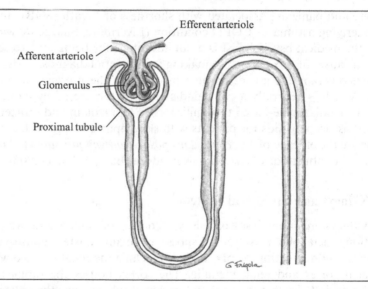

Figure 5.5 Glomerular Filter

Nephrons function as filters with the fluid being protein free, but containing sodium, chloride, and potassium ions as well as creatinine, urea, and glucose. *Glomerular filtration rate (GFR)* excretes 1 to 2 liters per day with the rest reabsorbed by active transport. (See Figure 5.5.) Obstructions may increase pressure at the Bowman's capsule, decreasing GFR. Glucose, normally not transported into urine, may cross the barrier when the concentration exceeds 180 mg/dL.

The proximal tubule operates to reabsorb sodium (generating osmotic pressure) along with proteins, water, electrolytes, and organic materials. The absorbed water increases concentration of urea in the tubular lumen. Sodium (Na^+) ions are reabsorbed along with chloride (Cl^-) ions, but with a lag as the tubule is less permeable to chloride. Hydrogen (H^+) ions replace the Na^+ by combining with HCO_3, to subsequently reconfigure as CO_2 and H_2O, which are able to diffuse.

The pass through the loop of Henle follows the proximal tubule in the fluid flow and accounts for much of any changes in concentration or dilution of urine, a function of the length of the loops and how far they insert in the medulla. The loop of Henle's main function is to create *hyperosmolar* pressure in the medulla, which it does by reabsorbing more solute than water. ADH controls the reabsorption of water in the distal tubule with sodium. Potassium is secreted, with control by aldosterone. Hydrogen compound elimination is achieved via the distal tubule, which in turn regulates pH balance by reducing acid balance. Overall, the kidneys do not normally reabsorb or excrete excessive volumes of water and sodium, and the tubules adjust their function to reflect changes in GFR (sodium/water reabsorption in the proximal tubule and excretion in the distal tubule).

Urine is concentrated and diluted via countercurrents in parallel tubes. The loop of Henle magnifies this effect. The ascending part of this loop differentially transports sodium and chloride out, leaving water behind. The gradient reverses in the downward loop. Catecholamines cause sodium and water to reabsorb in the proximal tubule. ADH controls the final output by increasing water permeability in the distal tubule so that water reabsorption increases. This secretion can cause oliguria or lowered excretion of urine. Without ADH, urine would dilute from water excretion.

Diuretics may block sodium reabsorption and act on different structures: Osmotic diuretics and *carbonic anhydrase inhibitors* act on the proximal tubule. Sodium/chloride reabsorption inhibitors act either on the end of the ascending loop or on the ascending limb of the loop of Henle, or by cortical vasodilation to increase urine formation. Potassium-sparing diuretics act on the distal tubule.

Measures of kidney function include plasma creatinine, *cystatin C* concentration, and blood urea nitrogen (BUN). Urinalysis also yields color, pH, and specific gravity. Compromised kidney function might reveal sediments in the urine such as red blood cells, casts, crystals, and white blood cells or other substances such as glucose, bilirubin, *urobilinogen*, leukocyte esterase and nitrates, ketones, protein, hemoglobin, and *myoglobin* (Johnson et al., 2004).

With age, kidneys may respond to the efforts at regulation and filtration with hypertrophy, decreasing size, and decreased blood flow, all of which may reduce kidney function and have implications for pharmacokinetics (Baer, 2008). In the elderly, tubules normally maintain their function, but adaptation decreases and reabsorption of electrolytes, glucose, and bicarbonate decreases. Adjustment of pH changes may be delayed with potential for hypovolemia or hypervolemia. Also, bladder functions deteriorate with increased frequency of urination, urgency, and *nocturia*. Nocturia has been associated with a variety of conditions, including multiple sclerosis and increased mortality (PR Newswire, 2010). Leakage may occur as muscles lose their tonicity and resilience. Other problems include benign prostatic hypertrophy (BPH), and the retention of drugs ordinarily excreted at a higher rate with attendant potential for overdose.

Psychopharmacologic Considerations

Pharmacokinetics can be significantly affected with compromised kidney function (Lee, Lee, & Oh, 2006). Kidney disease, aging, or dehydration can lead to increased serum drug levels as drugs and metabolites are not excreted at an expected rate or the proportion of drug to other solutes increases as the result of dehydration. Lithium can precipitate dehydration by displacing sodium, thereby raising the levels of serum lithium to toxic levels, which can lead, in turn, to kidney damage. It is a good idea to run periodic kidney function tests such as GRF, BUN, and creatinine when prescribing any medication.

The Digestive System

The purpose of the digestive system is to mechanically and chemically break down ingested materials into molecules that can be processed for extraction of fluids, nutrients, vitamins, and minerals, and for production of energy.

Gastrointestinal Tract

The gastrointestinal (GI) tract includes the mouth, esophagus, stomach, small intestine, large intestine, rectum, and anus. Functions include (a) food ingestion and preparation (mechanical); (b) peristaltic movement through the tract; (c) secretion of enzymes, water, and mucus; (d) enzyme digestion; (e) absorption of processed food; and (f) elimination of wastes by defecation. The layers of the system include the mucosa, submucosa, muscularis, and adventitia from the center of the canal toward the outside. Functions of the mouth include salivation (mostly water, but also mucus, sodium, bicarbonate, chloride, potassium, and ptyalin, the enzyme responsible for carbohydrate breakdown in the mouth). The esophagus transports food from the mouth to the stomach via peristalsis, autonomically controlled rhythmic, coordinated muscular movement. Food passes from the esophagus into the fundus, the body of the stomach, through the *antrum* and the pylorus into the duodenum. In the stomach, digestive juices combine with food and water to make *chyme*, which is then pushed into the duodenum, where acid is neutralized by alkaline secretions of the pancreas. The stomach mucosa permits very little absorption into the bloodstream, although aspirin and alcohol will pass through the walls. A number of hormones are secreted in response to gastric stimuli in the stomach (gastrin, histamine, somatostatin, acetylcholine, and gastrin-releasing peptide) and intestine (motilin, secretin, cholecystokinin, enteroglucagon, gastric inhibitory peptide, peptide YY, pancreatic polypeptide, and vasoactive intestinal peptide). Hydrochloric acid stimulates release of pepsin, acts to kill bacteria, and breaks down proteins in the stomach. Pepsin breaks down proteins into peptides. Bile from the liver, accumulated and stored in the gallbladder, is delivered to the duodenum to break down fats.

The majority of absorption occurs in the digestive lumen of the intestines, where the inner lining is composed of a lipid bilayer, which preferentially selects certain molecules from the chyme that are permitted passage to the circulatory system. A lipid bilayer is a lining of phospholipids two molecules thick, laid out in such a manner that the hydrophilic phosphate heads point out on either side of the bilayer and the hydrophobic fatty acid tails point in to the core of the bilayer. (See Figure 5.6.) Lipid bilayers are impermeable to most water-soluble (hydrophilic) molecules and are particularly impermeable to ions; this allows cells to regulate salt concentrations and pH by pumping ions across their membranes using proteins called ion pumps.

The small intestine, beginning with the duodenum, progresses to the jejunum, and then to the ileum before emptying into the large intestine at the *ileocecal valve*, which prevents reflux. Segmentation (contractions of larger smooth muscle) and peristalsis (contraction of small segments) comprise the operation of motility in the small intestine.

The large intestine is composed of four different segments: the ascending colon, transverse colon, descending colon, and sigmoid colon. The colon terminates at the

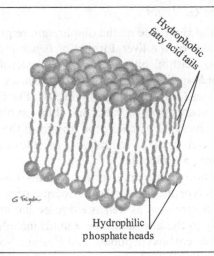

Hydrophobic fatty acid tails

Hydrophilic phosphate heads

Figure 5.6   Phospholipid Bilayer

juncture of the sigmoid colon and the rectum. The large intestine, beginning with the *cecum* with its vermiform appendix, receives chyme and transports it through the ascending, transverse, and descending colon into the sigmoid colon, where feces volume and weight stimulate the rectal reflex (rectum) for defecation via the anus. Intestinal bacteria in the colon[16] become colonized later in life (*E. coli,* clostridium, and streptococcus), and metabolize bile salts for reabsorption and detoxification, as well as conversion of hormones, lipids, and carbohydrates for absorption.

The entire abdominal and pelvic organs are separated from the rest of the body by a sac called the peritoneum, which has two layers separated by a fluid-filled cavity. *Villi,* covering the folds of the intestine, permit absorption. Cell membranes of epithelial tissue are hydrophobic, and do not allow absorption of water and electrolytes directly across cell membranes, but rather through intercellular spaces.

Nutrients are variably absorbed in the stomach (water and alcohol); duodenum (iron, fats, water, proteins, vitamins, calcium, *monosaccharides,* magnesium, and sodium); jejunum (sugars and proteins); ileum (bile salts, vitamin B_{12}, and chloride); and colon (water and electrolytes).

Carbohydrate metabolism first involves hydrolyzing complex carbohydrates using pancreatic and salivary amylases, and subsequently requires breaking saccharides down into galactose, glucose, and fructose. While fructose is absorbed passively (slowly), galactose and glucose use the sodium active transport. Both sugars and proteins are mostly absorbed in the proximal area of the small intestine.

Protein unfolding and hydrolysis to peptides occur in the small intestine and utilize brush-border enzymes (aminopeptidases found in microvilli) to hydrolyze proteins into small peptides that can cross cell membranes.

Fats are digested and absorbed via emulsification and lipolysis, leading to micelle formation into fat molecules and the absorption of these fat molecules before their final catabolism into triglycerides and phospholipids.

---

[16]Bacteria are specific to the large intestine, as acid kills bacteria in the stomach, as do enzymes and bile acids in the small intestine.

Peripheral Organs of the GI Tract

The liver, located under the right side of the diaphragm, requires an extensive blood supply. The multiple lobules of the liver, formed of *hepatocytes,* can regenerate and secrete electrolytes, lipids, lecithin, bile acids, and cholesterol. They also synthesize plasma protein, store lipids in lipocytes, and possess sinuses with highly permeable endothelium and phagocytes (Kupfer cells and pit cells). The liver secretes bile, which emulsifies and assists in absorption of fats. Bilirubin, coming from destroyed red blood cells in the spleen, gives bile its color; the iron from the dead red blood cells is recovered and stored for re-creation of red blood cells. Bile collects in the gallbladder for storage with cholesterol and bile salts.

The pancreas, in addition to its endocrine functions (insulin, glucagon, soma-tostatin, and pancreatic polypeptides), acts as a exocrine organ by supplying alkaline fluids containing various electrolytes, as well as enzymes that metabolize fats, proteins, and carbohydrates directly to the bile duct. These fluids include *trypsin* and its inhibi-tor, *chymotrypsin,* as well as carboxypeptidase and elastase (secreted in inactive form to protect the pancreas and activated by *enterokinase* in the duodenal mucosa). The pancreas also produces and supplies alpha-amylase and lipases, both activated by hor-mones and vagus innervations.

Dysfunctions of the Digestive System

Dysfunctions of the digestive system symptomatically may include anorexia (loss of desire to eat), vomiting, constipation, diarrhea, abdominal pain, and GI bleeding. Motility disorders include dysphagia (problems swallowing), gastroesophageal reflux disease (GERD), *hiatal hernia* (diaphragmatic hernia), pyloric obstruction (blocked opening from stomach to duodenum), intestinal obstruction and *ileus* (may be due to obstructive object or motility failure), gastritis (inflamed gastric or stomach mucosa), and peptic ulcer disease (ulceration of lower esophagus, stomach, and/or duode-num). Stress ulcers are usually acute and due to illness, trauma, or nerve injuries. Ulcerative colitis is a chronic inflammation of the colon, extending from the rectum into the colon. Diverticula are sacs that collect and form pouches in the colon. When inflamed, the condition is termed *diverticulitis.* Appendicitis is an inflammation of the vermiform appendix, which, in spite of there being little or no function of the organ, may present as an emergency.

Nutritional disorders include obesity, anorexia, bulimia nervosa, and starvation, as well as deficiencies in many substances required to promote or sustain life.

Ancillary organ dysfunction and disease include liver portal hypertension, hepatic encephalopathy, and multiple forms of hepatitis. Cirrhosis of the liver is due to an inflammation resulting in fibrosis and nodular regeneration, which disorganize liver tissue. Alcoholic liver disease, a prelude to cirrhosis, presents with inflammation, degeneration, and necrosis. *Biliary cirrhosis* results from inflammation starting in the *canaliculi* and bile ducts, rather than the liver. Gallbladder disorders result from obstruction (gallstones) and inflammation. When a stone lodges in a duct, it becomes *cholecystitis.*

The pancreas can present with pancreatitis, ranging from mild to severe inflam-mation. Chronic pancreatitis, most often caused by alcohol abuse, presents with pain from increased pressure, ischemia, neuritis, and further injury to tissues.

Cancers may occur in the esophagus (carcinoma), the stomach, the colon, and the rectum (the latter two are the second most common causes of cancer death in the United States) (American Cancer Society, 2005). The liver may present with cancer, usually from metastases. Gallbladder carcinoma has obesity as a primary risk factor. Pancreatic cancer carries a high mortality rate and is of unknown etiology.

Psychopharmacologic Considerations

The liver is the primary organ responsible for metabolizing medication; therefore, any compromised liver function is important to take into account when prescribing. If liver disease is confirmed, alternative medications that do not use the cytochrome P450 (CYP 450) enzyme system for metabolism may be indicated, or the dose may be adjusted downward if the liver's ability to break down active ingredients is reduced. Liver function laboratory test should be available for review by the prescribing psychologist or, if not, should be ordered. A standard liver panel includes albumin (Alb), alanine transaminase (ALT), aspartate transaminase (AST), alkaline phosphatase (ALP), and total bilirubin (TBIL).

The Musculoskeletal System

Bone is made of connective tissue with cells, *ground substance*, fibers, and minerals that provide rigidity (mostly calcium). Bone cells grow and self-repair, change morphology, and reabsorb old damaged bone tissue. Bone is made of osteoblasts, osteocytes, osteoclasts, and with a structure (matrix) consisting of *collagen*, proteoglycans, morphogenic proteins, glycoproteins, and minerals. A variety of cytokines stimulate either formation or resorption of bone. Two types of bone tissue exist: osseous compact and spongy tissue. Compact bone has a central canal, layers called lamellae, spaces between the layers, bone cells, and channels (canaliculi). All bone is covered with a double layer of connective tissue (periosteum), which contains blood vessels and nerves, and the inner layer, which attaches to the bone, tendons, and ligaments. There are 206 bones in the human body.

Skeletal (striate) muscles, by either relaxing or contracting, move the body's bones. Most muscles are paired in opposition and come in two forms: fusiform (elongated) and pennate (flat). Muscles are encased in a framework called fascia that protects the muscle, attaches to *prominences* on bones, and provides framework for nerves and blood/lymphatic circulation. These muscle fibers are organized into *sarcomeres*. The anterior horns of the spinal cord provide innervation to muscle fibers, forming the motor unit. This unit contracts as a whole. Within the muscle are stretch sensors called spindles. Cells have a muscle membrane, myofibrils, sarcotubular system, sarcoplasm, and mitochondria. Muscle contraction begins at the sarcomere, a part of the myofibril that is the contracting unit. Muscle contraction involves activation, coupling (depolarization of transverse tubules), contraction, and relaxation (calcium removal to the sarcoplasmic reticulum). The neurotransmitter responsible for activation is acetylcholine.

Muscle Function

To operate, muscles utilize ATP and phosphocreatine to provide energy for contraction, transport, and combining actin and myosin. The stored glycogen is converted to glucose to provide brief anaerobic energy. Sustained activity requires aerobic glycolysis. All muscle contraction is all-or-none with maximal effort; sustained activity involves adding motor units via repetitive discharge. Two forms are sustained (isometric) and moving (isotonic). At maximum effort, the muscle is fully contracted (tetanus).

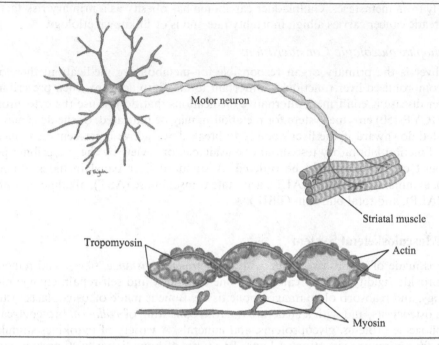

Figure 5.7   Motor Neuron and Myosin Cross Bridge

Actin and myosin are ATP-based motor proteins that work in unison to achieve activation and cessation of muscle fiber motility, leading to skeletal movement. Muscle fiber generates contraction through the action of actin and myosin cross-bridge cycling. (See Figure 5.7.) Upon nerve stimulation at the muscle plate, myosin binds to actin, releasing adenosine diphosphate (ADP). Motility occurs when the myosin head returns to its low-energy conformation, generating force that pulls the thin filament toward the center of the sarcomere. Binding of another ATP molecule causes dissociation of myosin from actin, and the cycle repeats itself.

Musculoskeletal Disorders

Disorders of bone include trauma with fractures, which may be complete or incomplete and open or closed. Dislocation (displacement of bone from a joint) and subluxation (partial displacement) may occur with fractures. Sprains and strains may occur with tendons and ligaments. The tendon attaches muscle to bone, whereas a ligament connects bones at joints. A tendon tear is called a strain, whereas ligament tears are termed sprains. If the tear is complete and separated, it is termed an avulsion. Inflammation from trauma and repeated stresses can result in joint deterioration (tendenosis) or inflammation of the bursal sac (bursitis). Muscle strains, usually from sports or trauma, refer to muscle damage. *Rhabdomyolysis*, a potentially fatal complication, may occur with severe muscle trauma, especially as crush syndrome, but may also occur with prolonged immobilization.

Bone diseases include bone loss or osteoporosis with cortical bone becoming porous and thin. If decreased, it may be termed osteopenia. Causes may be menopause, iatrogenic (e.g., chronic treatment with cortisone), or regional (localized loss with known etiology such as immobilization). Age-related loss begins around age 40.

Kyphosis or spinal curvature may progress with chronic degeneration. Osteomalacia refers to inadequate mineralization in mature bone where replaced bone is spongy. Paget disease occurs with an escalation in the rate of bone remodeling, which softens and enlarges bones. Osteomyelitis occurs with infection of bone, most often bacterial, with both endogenous (infections from other parts of the body, e.g., sinusitis) and exogenous sources. Bone tumors may have bone cells, cartilage, fibrous tissue, marrow, or vascular tissue as origins. Malignant tumors show increases in nuclear/cytoplasmic ratio, irregular nuclear border, excess *chromatin*, prominent nucleolus, and increased cells showing mitosis.

Children show low rates of bone tumors, with incidence in adults gradually increasing with age. Forms of tumors include osteosarcoma, chondrosarcoma, fibrosarcoma (collagenic), and myelogenic tumor. Giant cell tumors tend to be benign and affect mostly adults in the 20- to 40-year age range.

Joints may experience osteoarthritis (degenerative with inflammation), which increases with age and is characterized by loss of *articular* cartilage. Classic arthritis involves destruction of *synovial* membranes or articular cartilage with systemic inflammation. It may have infectious or noninfectious causes. Rheumatoid arthritis (RA) is an autoimmune disorder creating inflammation with swelling and joint destruction, nodules, and subluxation of joints. Infections associated with it include Lyme disease, tuberculosis, *suppurative* (various infections), and viral arthritis. *Ankylosing spondylitis*, an inflammatory disease, results in stiffness and fusion of the joint in the spine and sacroiliac junctures. Gout inflammation results from excessive uric acid production in the blood, subsequently inflaming the synovial tissues.

Muscle disorders, especially those involving lipids (Liang & Nishina, 2010; Xue, 2011), are characterized by weakness and fatigue. Myopathies may be caused by congenital defect, infection, trauma, malnutrition, and a multitude of diseases. Pathologic contractures may have adequate ATP but, due to a disease process such as muscular dystrophy, show progressive muscle degeneration and atrophy. Movement disorders such as Parkinsonism, tardive dyskinesia, and Huntington's chorea represent neural signaling problems rather than *myopathy* per se.

Psychopharmacologic Considerations

Rhabdomyolysis may be precipitated by several recreational drugs, including amphetamine, phencyclidine (PCP), alcohol, cocaine, ecstasy, heroin, and narcotics (Vanholder, Sever, Erek, & Lameire, 2000). The breakdown of muscle tissue leads to an accumulation of protein by-products in the blood, which blocks the glomerular filter and eventually leads to kidney failure. Laboratory tests that assay serum protein (serum creatine phosphokinase, serum myoglobulin, and urinary myoglobulin levels) should be ordered when rhabdomyolysis is suspected.

The Integument (Skin, Hair, and Nails)

Skin, the major protection against microorganisms for the body, has three layers: epidermis, dermis, and subcutaneous layer. The epidermis grows, shedding the upper layer with its *keratinocytes* and *melanocytes*. The dermis consists of collagen, elastin, and reticulin, and the gel-like ground substance. These flexible, mobile cells include hair follicles, sebaceous glands, sweat glands, blood vessels, lymphatic vessels, and nerves. Also present are fibroblasts, mast cells, and macrophages, as well as papillary projections into the epidermis. The subcutaneous layer contains fat and *adiocytes* with fibrous walls of collagen and large blood vessels.

Attached to the skin are nails, hair, sebaceous glands, *eccrine glands*, and apocrine sweat glands. Nails consist of keratin plates on fingers and toes with a proximal nail fold, matrix that grows the nail, nail bed, and nail plate. Fingernails and toenails grow approximately 1 mm per day.

Hair follicles and sebaceous glands work together as a unit, supplying color, density, grain, and distribution pattern to hair-covered skin. Sebaceous glands open to the skin surface via a canal secreting a lipid called sebum. Eccrine sweat glands secrete fluids that help regulate body temperature through evaporation. Apocrine sweat glands, less generalized in distribution, have limited functions. Papillary capillaries supply blood to the dermal layer of the skin.

Skin lesion forms may present as macules (freckles, petechae, measles); papules (warts, moles); patches (vitiligo, port wine stains); plaques (psoriasis, seborrheic and actinic keratoses); wheals (urticaria); nodules (lipomas); tumors (neoplasms); vesicles (chicken pox); bullae (blisters); pustules (acne); cysts (cystic acne); telangiectasia (rosacea); scale (flaking of the skin as with scarlet fever); lichenification (chronic dermatitis); keloid (keloid scarring after surgery); scars (healed wounds or incisions); excoriation (abrasions and scratches); fissures (cracks at the corners of the mouth); erosions (varicella); ulcers (decubiti); and atrophy (striae and aged skin) (Thomson & Wilson, 2002).

With aging, skin becomes thinner, drier, and wrinkled with changes in pigmentation. Decrease in vasculature and lymphatic drainage causes loss of the protective barriers and the atrophy of glands that moisturize the skin. Wrinkling occurs with loss of elastin. Wound healing decreases with loss of blood supply, cell multiplication, and immune response.

Skin dysfunctions include lesions from pressure ulcers, most common among immobilized people, especially elders who are bedridden.

Psychopharmacological Considerations

Of particular relevance and concern for prescribing medical psychologists is Stevens-Johnson syndrome, a severe allergic rash that may be provoked by certain psychotropics. (See Figure 5.8.) Stevens-Johnson syndrome is due to a drug reaction with generalized epidermal apoptosis and detachment. It is associated with many classes of medications, including antibiotics, but it is linked in particular to psychotropic medications belonging to the mood stabilizer class. Lamotrigine, oxcarbazepine, and carbamazepine are well-known risks for developing Stevens-Johnson syndrome. The syndrome usually begins with fever, sore throat, and fatigue, which is often misdiagnosed and usually treated with antibiotics. Ulcers and other lesions begin to appear in the mucous membranes, almost always in the mouth and lips but also in the genital and anal regions. A rash of round lesions about an inch across arises on the face, trunk, arms, legs, and soles of the feet (Tigchelaar, Kannikeswaran, & Kamat, 2008). Stevens-Johnson syndrome, with less than 10% of body surface area involved, has a mortality rate of around 5%. Other outcomes include organ damage and failure, cornea scratching, and blindness.

Multiple System Dysfunctions

Shock is classified by cause: *cardiogenic, neurogenic, vasogenic, anaphylactic, septic*, or hypovolemic. Traumatic shock combines hypovolemic and septic shock, in which case cells do not receive, or are unable to utilize, adequate oxygen, causing a shift to anaerobic metabolism. Water and sodium enter the cells. Glucose may not be delivered or

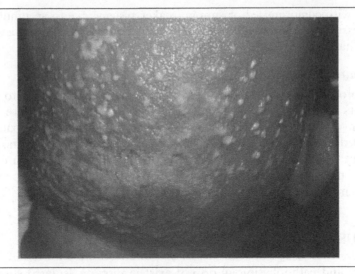

Figure 5.8   Stevens-Johnson Syndrome (Back of Scalp)
From Kandil, Dvorak, Mignano, Wu, & Zhu (2010). Reproduced with permission from BioMed Central.

may not be able to enter cells due to hormonal actions (growth hormone, cortisol, catecholamines, etc.). Muscle wasting may ensue as protein is broken down for energy, and breathing is impaired. Blood pressure may drop precipitously, and metabolic end products build up while tissue perfusion degrades.

Multiple organ dysfunction syndromes (MODS) involve two or more systems due to an uncontrolled inflammatory response to injury or illness. MODS may progress to organ failure and death. Etiology is severe sepsis.

Severe burns affect multiple organ systems. In third-degree burns, skin integrity (all layers) and sensation are absent, and severely damaged tissue will not heal but will require skin graft. Extracellular fluid causes hypovolemia, and other alterations cause generalized dysfunctions. Caution is exercised with fluid replacement, as recovery may result in intravenous fluids returning to areas previously depleted, causing edemas, including pulmonary edema. Damaged skin may exacerbate fluid loss via evaporation.

Differential effects of shock, burns, and MODS with children may manifest differently (Tantallein, Leon, Santos, & Sanchez, 2003). Shock most often is due to hemorrhage, dehydration, heart failure, or sepsis. Shock can complicate treatment of other problems. MODS may lead to organ failure. Sepsis occurs when cytokines and proteins cause vasodilation, increased capillary permeability, cardiovascular dysfunction, and poor distribution of blood perfusion. Vital signs vary for children, and blood pressure may need to be estimated. Burns in children differ because of thinner skin, likelihood of longer exposure as children fail to remove the source, and susceptibility to abuse. Children also may be exposed to corrosive agents. Again, the depth of the burn is often a determinant of effect with higher risk for shock and MODS. Cardiovascular functioning is affected by the lower fluid volume, effects of peripheral resistance, effect on the renal and GI systems due to blood flow impairment, metabolism, and immune suppression. Scars are likely to affect developmental adjustment. Susceptibility to infection and hypovolemia is greater.

Elders, with compromised or simply weaker systems due to accumulation of disease processes, represent a high risk for mortality in the event of multisystem pathology (Pandharipande, Jackson, & Ely, 2005).

Psychopharmacological Considerations

The compromise of entire organ systems is of particular concern to psychopharmacologists (Trzepacz, Levenson, & Tringali, 1991). As every effective psychotropic medication can have adverse effects, the medically compromised patient presents an increased mortality risk. It is likely that such events will occur almost exclusively in inpatient settings; nonetheless, being alert for the advent of such crises is vital. Awareness, prevention, and planning, together with close collaboration with medical specialists, may be the best defense against such catastrophes.

CONCLUSION

Physiology and pathophysiology do not exist in discrete, isolated static states. All systems interface. Good clinical practice takes the entire person into account when diagnosing and treating dysfunction. It is important that the prescribing medical psychologist continues to review his or her knowledge of the entire body's functioning, respecting the mutual impact of the various systems. While the emphasis is rightfully on the nervous system and the psychosocial environment in which mental health patients interact, it behooves the medical psychologist to be alert to signs and symptoms of distress in other systems, and to refer to specialists when appropriate.

CHAPTER 5 KEY TERMS

Active transport: A process by which material is moved against a gradient requiring expenditure of energy, usually ATP.

Addison disease: Adrenal insufficiency of steroid hormone production, resulting in hypocortisolism.

Adenosine triphosphate (ATP): A nucleotide that serves as an energy source for the body as well as a building block of RNA.

Adiocytes: Cells that comprise and store fat tissue.

Adipose: Pertaining to fat.

Agranulocytosis: Refers to the bone marrow being unable to produce white cells. Associated symptoms include a high fever, mucous membrane and skin lesions, a swollen neck, and chills.

Alveolus: An anatomical structure with a hollow cavity, such as found in the lungs.

Anabolism: The process of biosynthesis or creation of complex molecules from simpler ones.

Anaphylactic: Refers to a serious, often life-threatening, allergic reaction to a foreign protein.

Anastomosis: Network that connects two hollow tubes such as arteries, veins, ducts, or intestinal tracts.

Ankylosing spondylitis: A form of autoimmune arthritis of the spine in which the cartilage between vertebrae is attacked and may result in vertebrae fusing together.

Anoxia: An absence of oxygenation of tissues.

Antigen: Any substance that can elicit an immune response and combine with the product of that response, typically an antibody and/or sensitized T-lymphocytes.

Antrum: A cavity or chamber. With respect to the digestive system, it is near the pyloric end of the stomach and closed off during digestion.

Apoptosis: A programmed self-destruction of cells into fragments. The resulting cell remnants are disposed of by phagocytosis or shedding.

Articular: Refers to any joint.

Asphyxia: A severe decrease in oxygen concentration in the body with increased CO_2, and a loss of consciousness that may be fatal. Causes can include smothering, drowning, electric shock, choking, injury to air passages, or inhaling toxins.

Aspiration: Entry of foreign particles or liquids into air passages. May also refer to removal of fluid or air using suction.

Atrophy: Refers to a decrease in cell size. This may take the form of physiologic atrophy occurring during early stages of development or pathological atrophy that occurs from disuse, poor nutrition, or aging.

Autocrine: Secretion that acts on the cell that produced it.

Biliary cirrhosis: Swelling and irritation of the liver bile ducts with resultant scarring.

Canaliculi: Small ducts.

Carbonic anhydrase inhibitors: Drugs that make fluids more alkaline. They may be used to treat glaucoma and to change the pH of urine.

Cardiogenic: Originating with the heart, and with normal or abnormal functioning.

Cecum: A pouch that marks the beginning of the large intestine.

Chemoreceptors: Any sensory receptor sensitive to chemical stimuli.

Cholecystitis: Inflammation of the gallbladder.

Chromaffin cells (pheochromocytes): Special cells that compose the paraganglia and are connected to the ganglia of the celiac, renal, suprarenal, aortic, and hypogastric plexuses. The chromaffin cells of the adrenal medulla secrete two catecholamines, epinephrine and norepinephrine, which affect smooth muscle, cardiac muscle, and glands in the same way as sympathetic stimulation by increasing and prolonging sympathetic effects.

Chromatin: The genetic material from which chromosomes are made. They get their name from their ability to stain during cell division.

Chyme: A mass of partially digested food that passes from the stomach to the duodenum.

Chymotrypsin: A pancreatic extract that catalyzes the hydrolysis of certain peptide bonds such as tyrosine, tryptophan, and phenylalanine.

Collagen: Fibrous protein that supports other tissue in the body.

Continuous positive airway pressure (CPAP) machine: A treatment for sleep apnea in which a continuous positive air pressure is provided to maintain open airways.

Cushing syndrome: A disorder caused by high levels of cortisol in the blood.

Cystatin C: A low-molecular-weight protein found in serum and produced by all nucleated cells. Because it passes freely through glomeruli, it is a good measure of renal clearance and correlates well with GFR.

Cytokinesis: The cell, after forming two nuclei, begins to divide, after puckering and forming a furrow, followed by forming a cell wall and then completion of mitosis.

Cytoplasm: All of the material inside a cell with the exception of the nucleus.

Cytoplasmic organelles: Structures in the cytoplasm (e.g., mitochondria) that perform functions.

Cytosol: The liquid part of the cytoplasm.

Cytosolic: Refers to the liquid part of the cytoplasm, excluding organelles and particulates that don't dissolve.

Degranulation: The process of losing granules as cells dispose of their contents.

Diffusion: A process of mingling of molecules by random motion. Affected by local conditions such as temperature (e.g., higher temperatures increase the rate of diffusion).

Eccrine glands: Glands that secrete outwardly to the skin, mainly for temperature regulation.

Endomitosis: A form of mitosis in which the nucleus and cell do not divide but result in identical chromosomal copies within one nucleus.

Endoplasmic reticulum: An organelle with tubules and sacs existing as a network or web in the cytoplasm with connections to the membrane of the nucleus.

Enterokinase: In the upper small intestine, the mucus membrane secretes enterokinase to convert trypsinogen to trypsin.

Epithelial cells: Cells that line the interior surfaces within the body and its exterior surfaces.

Erythropoiesis: The process by which red blood cells (erythrocytes) are created in bone marrow.

Esterification: A process by which an acid is converted to an alkyl or aryl compound. It may be done via enzyme action, or when an acid reacts with an alcohol in the presence of minerals that can be catalytic.

Exogenous: Anything entering the local environment from an exterior source (e.g., insulin injection is exogenous in origin rather than created by the pancreatic cells).

Fibrosis: Scarring.

FLAGTOP mnemonic: Follicle-stimulating hormone (FSH), Luteinizing hormone (LH), Adrenocorticotropin hormone (ACTH), Growth hormone (GH), Thyroid-stimulating hormone (TSH), Oxytocin, Prolactin.

Glomerular filtration rate (GFR): The rate at which blood passes through the glomeruli each minute. In the lab, it is estimated from the creatinine level in the blood. The formula includes predictors such as age, gender, height, weight, and racial identification.

Glomeruli: Tufts of capillaries in the kidneys that provide for filtration of blood.

Glucocorticoids: A class of hormones secreted mostly by the adrenal cortex and primarily affecting metabolism. The best known is cortisol or hydrocortisone, which is synthesized from cholesterol.

Golgi complex or apparatus: A network of proteins formed from the endoplasmic reticulum into small sacs (vesicles), which break off to deliver products to other structures or to the cell membrane for release outside the cell. The complex also builds lysosomes, which digest cells.

Granulopenia: A severe lowering of white blood cell production (see *Agranulocytosis*).

Ground substance: A material in the body within which fibers and connective tissues are embedded.

Hematopoiesis: Formation and development of blood cells.

Hepatocytes: Liver cells.

Hiatal hernia: A breach in the diaphragm allowing visceral organs such as the stomach to protrude into the chest cavity.

Histones: Proteins associated with DNA, found in the chromatin of eukaryotes.

Homocysteine: A sulfur-containing amino acid found in the blood.

Hypercholesteremia: A syndrome of excessive levels of serum cholesterol.

Hyperhydration: Excess water content in the body.

Hyperosmolar: An increase beyond normal osmolarity expressed as number of osmoles of solute per liter of solution.

Hyperphosphaturia: An excessive secretion of phosphates into the urine.

Hypocalcemia: Low serum calcium level.

Hypovolemia: Low blood volume (also, hypovolemic).

Hypoxia: Reduced or inadequate oxygenation of tissues.

Iatrogenic: Caused by treatment.

Ileocecal valve: A sphincter muscle located at the juncture of the small and large intestines to prevent the backflow of fecal matter into the small intestine from the large intestine. This prevents feces from entering the blood.

Ileus: A bowel obstruction, often defined as a lack of motility in the intestines.

Ischemia: Any decrease in blood supply to tissues.

Keratinocytes: The most common epidermal cells. They are part of the living tissue but differentiate into dead cells and form a protective layer. They are replenished by cells underneath them.

Ketoacidosis: A life-threatening change in blood acid levels. Seen among some alcoholics with poor diets, but more often presents as diabetic ketoacidosis. The latter occurs from inadequate insulin supplies, seen most often among type 1 diabetics (and sick type 2s), as a result of low or absent insulin coverage, excess carbohydrate intake, and/or physical illness. It can lead to coma and carries a high mortality rate.

Krebs cycle: A two-stage process in which glucose enters the cell and through glycolysis is broken down into two pyruvate molecules from which acetyl-CoA is created.

Leukocytes: White blood cells whose function is to kill microorganisms.

Leukotrienes: Chemicals produced in response to allergen exposure that elicits an inflammatory response.

Ligand: Any ion (element or combination of elements with a positive or negative charge), molecule (a combination of elements, which may be the same element, such as oxygen, which results in a neutral charge), or group of molecules that can bind to another chemical to make an even larger structure.

Loop of Henle: The nephron loop. A blood vessel that goes into the renal medulla where it is variously permeable to interstitial fluid. The filtrate is hypotonic (lower concentration of solute) to the interstitial fluid.

Lysis: Cell breakdown.

Mast cells: Large cells found in connective tissue that contain (and release in response to inflammation) heparin and histamine.

Mediastinum: The middle part of the chest cavity.

Megakaryocyte: A bone marrow cell that produces platelets.

Melanocytes: Cells of the gingival tissue that produce melanin (pigmentation) in all people. Race does not affect this production.

Micturition: Urination.

Monocytes: White blood cells with a single nucleus that act as phagocytes. They may later become differentiated into more targeted macrophages.

Monosaccharides: Simple sugars such as glucose, fructose, and galactose. Two bonded together, such as sucrose or table sugar, are termed disaccharides.

Myeloproliferations: A chronic excessive creation of blood cells in the bone marrow.

Myoglobin: Contents of muscle fibers.

Myopathy: Disease of muscle tissue not of innervation or neuromuscular origin.

Nephron ducts: The collecting ducts of the kidneys from the various tubules.

Nephrotic syndrome: A group of symptoms characterized by protein in the urine greater than 3.5 g/day, low serum protein, high serum cholesterol and triglycerides, and edema of periphery, face, and abdomen.

Neurogenic: Originating with the nervous system or from a lesion or dysfunction within it.

Nocturia: A condition defined as more than two urinary voids per night.

Nucleus: The part of the cell within which are held operating instructions (DNA and RNA) that control replication of DNA.

Osteopenia: Lower than normal bone mineral density, but not low enough to warrant a classification of osteoporosis.

Oxidative phosphorylation: The creation of energy-holding chemicals (ATP production) through oxidizing (as if burning) fuel sources, such as glucose.

Pantothenic acid: Vitamin B5, a water-soluble vitamin essential for synthesis of enzyme CoA, as well as many carbohydrates, fats, and proteins.

Paracrine: Secretions that act on nearby cells without needing to enter the bloodstream.

Pathology: Study of disease.

Peroxidation: A chemical reaction in which toxic or infectious damage creates peroxides.

Peyer patches: Organized lymphoid nodules found in the small intestine.

Pheochromocytoma: A benign tumor found among chromaffin cells in the adrenal gland.

Pleura: Blood-perfused membrane enclosing the lungs and thoracic cavity with two sections separated by fluid.

Polyphagia: Uncontrolled eating, also known as hyperphagia.

Polysaccharides: Complex carbohydrates such as glycogen formed from monosaccharides and disaccharides.

Prolonged QT interval: An ECG marker for ventricular tachyarrhythmias like torsades de pointes; a risk factor for sudden death.

Prominence: A raised area on a bone created by deposits of minerals.

Pyrogens: Chemicals that increase the local or systemic temperature.

Renin: Part of the renin-angiotensin-aldosterone system that regulates fluid balance. Renin, an enzyme, is produced by the kidneys and acts to produce angiotensin, which then acts on the adrenal cortex to release aldosterone. The sequence raises blood pressure by retaining fluid.

Resorption: Lysis and reuptake leading to loss of substance in the body, such as minerals in bone.

Rhabdomyolysis: A breakdown of muscle fibers, which then releases myoglobin. This product may produce kidney damage.

Ribosomes: Nucleoproteins synthesized by RNA-directed operations in the nucleus and then released into the cytoplasm. Most of their function is directed at protein synthesis.

Sarcomeres: Basic units of muscle tissue that act in unison.

Septic (shock): An infection that has overwhelmed the system with a severe inflammatory response causing a drop in blood pressure.

Sinoatrial node: A bundle of nerves located in the upper part of the right atrium of the heart that initiates the automatic impulse rhythm.

Spondylitis: Inflammation of vertebrae.

Substrates: Any material or substance acted on by an enzyme.

Suppurative: Refers to any infection that forms pus.

Synovial: Refers to tissue secreting the lubricating fluid in a joint.

Torsades de pointes: A potentially fatal condition in which the QT interval is markedly increased and a ventricular tachycardia occurs in which the QRS complex varies from beat to beat.

Transferrin: A transport glycoprotein that carries iron from food to the liver and spleen.

Trypsin: A pancreatic enzyme that digests proteins. It has a role in cystic fibrosis and chronic pancreatitis.

Urobilinogen: A colorless compound formed in the intestines by reduction of bilirubin. Determination of the amount of urobilinogen excreted in a given period makes it possible to evaluate certain types of hemolytic anemia and also is of help in diagnosing liver dysfunction such as hepatocellular damage.

Vasogenic: Originating with the circulatory system or from a vascular lesion or dysfunction.

Venae cavae: The major veins that return blood from the system (excluding the lungs) to the right atrium of the heart. There are two venae cavae, superior and inferior. The former collects blood from the head and arms and enters at the top of the atrium.

Villi: Tiny hairlike projections that cover the wall of the small intestine. Their purpose is to slow down the progress of digested food to facilitate absorption of nutrients.

Chapter 5 Questions

1. A persistently high blood glucose (above 180 mg/dL) will most affect the immediate measurement of
   a. Liver enzymes.
   b. Serum pH.
   c. Specific gravity of urine.
   d. ATP production.

2. Lipophobic substances are best absorbed in
   a. The mouth.
   b. The esophagus.
   c. The stomach.
   d. The duodenum.

3. Viruses require _____ in order to reproduce in an organism.
   a. Host cells
   b. DNA strands
   c. Chromosomes
   d. Adenosine triphosphate

4. The major characteristics of cancers that distinguish them from normal tissue are
   a. Size, color, rate of metabolism, and tendency toward metastasis.
   b. Structure, rate of growth, invasive growth, and tendency toward metastasis.
   c. Structure, density, rate of metabolism, and tendency toward metastasis.
   d. Size, structure, color, and tendency toward metastasis.

5. The Golgi complex or apparatus refers to the
   a. Interconnections between cells to form stable matrices.
   b. Renal tubule loops that regulate fluid content of the blood.
   c. System by which proteins form vesicles in the endoplasmic reticulum.
   d. System for production of control hormones in the pituitary.

6. Cellular receptors operate by
   a. Opening and closing gates to ions floating in interstitial fluids.
   b. Matching ions on the cell membranes to ions present in released vesicles.
   c. Binding proteins to chemicals (ligands).
   d. Accepting proteins into cells for attachment to vesicles in the cytoplasm.

7. Atrophy of tissue is characterized by
   a. Apoptosis.
   b. Toxins from the environment.
   c. Changes in morphology of cells.
   d. Decrease in cell size.

8. The acute inflammatory process involves a sequence of reactions to tissue damage with
   a. Changes in blood flow and vascular permeability, release of chemical mediators controlling local and systemic responses, and attempts to return to homeostasis.
   b. Phagocytosis, catabolism, systemic increase in basal temperature, and apoptosis.
   c. A sequence of reactions to tissue damage and release of systemic pyrogens followed by mitosis of damaged tissue.
   d. A sequence of reactions to tissue damage and increases in local temperature, decrease in blood flow to the damaged tissue, release of antihistamines, and development of scar tissue.

9. An autosomal recessive trait error is one that appears
   a. Less often than a dominant trait.
   b. Alone among other recessive traits.
   c. On non-sex-transmitting chromosomes and requires contributions from both parents.
   d. Only on self-generating chromosomes and stays hidden.

10. An excess of thyroid-stimulating hormone (TSH) signals
    a. An overdose of exogenous thyroxine.
    b. Iodine toxicity.
    c. Inadequate output of TRH.
    d. Excessive output of T3 and T4.

11. Autoimmune disorders attack
    a. The immune system.
    b. A specific organ.
    c. Any healthy tissue misidentified by the body as antigenic.
    d. Any self-regulating body system.

12. T and B lymphocytes mature in the _____ and _____.
    a. Thyroid gland, bone end plates
    b. Thymus gland, bone marrow
    c. Thyroid gland, basilar membranes
    d. Thymus gland, basilar membranes

13. Peripheral vascular disease may contribute to
  a. Hypoglycemia, essential hypertension, leg pain, and stroke.
  b. Stenosis of leg arteries, intermittent claudication, and gangrene.
  c. Loss of arterial plaque, thinning of arterial basal membranes, and mitral valve prolapse.
  d. Hyperglycemia, essential claudication, and analgesias.
14. Protein in urine is consistent with
  a. A diet too high in amino acids.
  b. Renal disease.
  c. Vitamin K deficiency.
  d. Excessive erythropoietin production.
15. Drug-induced prolongation of the QT interval may cause
  a. Atrial bradycardia resulting in torsades de pointes.
  b. Ventricular tachycardia resulting in torsades de pointes.
  c. Atrial tachycardia resulting in CHF.
  d. Atrial bradycardia resulting in pulmonary edema.

Answers: (1) c, (2) d, (3) a, (4) b, (5) c, (6) c, (7) d, (8) a, (9) c, (10) c, (11) c, (12) b, (13) b, (14) b, and (15) c.

REFERENCES

Albert, B., Johnson, A., Lewis, J., Raff, M., Roberts, K., & Walter, P. (2002). *Molecular biology of the cell* (4th ed.). New York, NY: Garland.

American Cancer Society. (2005). *Cancer facts and figures—2005*. Atlanta, GA: Author.

American Diabetes Association. (2011). Diagnosis and classification of diabetes mellitus. *Diabetes Care, Supplement 1, Vol. 34*, 562–569.

Baer, Daniel M. (2008, November 1). UA and culture do not agree. *The free library*. Retrieved February 22, 2011 from http://www.thefreelibrary.com

Beduin, S., & de Haan, L. (2010). Off-label second generation antipsychotics for impulse regulation disorders: A review. *Psychopharmacology Bulletin, 43*(3), 45–81.

Berry, R. B., & Patel, P. B. (2006). Effect of zolpidem on the efficacy of continuous positive airway pressure as treatment for obstructive sleep apnea. *Sleep, 29*, 1052–1056.

Brubaker, L. (2000). Abnormalities of pelvic support. In L. J. Copeland & J. F. Farrell (Eds.), *Textbook of gynecology* (2nd ed.). Philadelphia, PA: Saunders.

Camm, J., Malik, M., & Yap, Y. (2004). *Acquired long QT syndrome*. Oxford, UK: Blackwell Publishing.

Castellheim, A., Brekke, O., Espevik, T., Harboe, M., & Mollnes, T. (2009). Innate immune responses to danger signals in systemic inflammatory response syndrome and sepsis. *Scandinavian Journal of Immunology, 69*, 479–491.

Cole, C., Jones, L., McVeigh, J., Kicman, A., Syed, Q., & Bellis, M. (2011). Adulterants in illicit drugs: Review of empirical evidence. *Drug Testing and Analysis, 3*, 89–96.

Hart, M., & Millard, M. (2010). Approaches to chronic disease management for asthma and chronic obstructive pulmonary disease: Strategies through the continuum of care. *Proceedings of the Baylor University Medical Center, 23*, 223–229.

Johnson, C., Levey, A., Coresh, J., Levin, A., Lau, J., & Eknoyan, G. (2004). Clinical practice guidelines for chronic kidney disease in adults: Part II. Glomerular filtration rate, proteinuria, and other markers. *American Family Physician, 70,* 1091–1097.

Julien, R. (2005). *A primer of drug action.* New York, NY: Worth Publishers.

Kandil, A.O, Dvorak, T., Mignano, Wu, J. K., & Zhu, J-J. (2010). Multifocal Stevens-Johnson syndrome after concurrent phenytoin and cranial and thoracic radiation treatment: A case study. *Radiation Oncology, 5,* 49–54.

Lee, M., Lee, J., & Oh, J. (2006). Pharmacokinetic changes of drugs in rat model of acute renal failure induced by uranyl nitrate: Correlation between drug metabolism and hepatic microsomal cytochrome P450 isozymes. *Current Clinical Pharmacology, 1,* 193–205.

Liang, W., & Nishina, I. (2010). State of the art in muscle lipid diseases. *Acta Myologica, 29,* 351–356.

Livermore, N., Sharpe, L., & McKenzie, D. (2010). Panic attacks and panic disorder in chronic obstructive pulmonary disease: A cognitive behavioral perspective. *Respiratory Medicine, 104,* 371–385.

Marquina, D., Pena, R., Fernandez, E., & Baptista, T. (in press). Abnormal correlation between serum leptin levels and body mass index may predict metabolic dysfunction irrespective of the psychopharmacological treatment. *International Clinical Psychopharmacology.*

Mayo Clinic Associates. (2010). *Hypothyroidism (signs and symptoms).* Mayo Foundation for Medical Education and Research (MFER).

Muse, M. (2010). *Clinical psychopharmacology for non-mental health prescribers.* Rockville, MD: Mensana Publications.

Noguchi, N., Watanabe, A., & Shi, H. (2000). Diverse functions of antioxidants. *Free Radical Research, 33*(6), 809–817.

Notkins, A. L. (2002). Immunologic and genetic factors in type 1 diabetes. *Journal of Biological Chemistry, 277,* 43545–43548.

Pandharipande, P., Jackson, J., & Ely, E. W. (2005). Delirium: Acute cognitive dysfunction in the critically ill. *Current Opinion in Critical Care, 11,* 360–368.

Parke, D., & Sapota, A. (1996). Chemical toxicity and reactive oxygen species. *International Journal of Occupational Medicine and Environmental Health, 9,* 331–340.

Pellinen, T., Färkkilä, M., Heikkilä, J., & Luomanmäki, K. (1987). Electrocardiographic and clinical features of tricyclic antidepressant intoxication: A survey of 88 cases and outlines of therapy. *Annals of Clinical Research, 19,* 12–17.

PR Newswire. (2010). Studies report nocturia was associated with risk of death and represented a significant economic burden to U.S. society. *The Free Library.*

Selye, H. (1936). A syndrome produced by diverse nocuous agents. *Nature, 138,* 32. Reproduced in 1998 in *Journal of Neuropsychiatry and Clinical Neurosciences, 10,* 230–231.

Shepard, T., & Lamire, R. (2004). *Catalog of teratogenic agents.* Baltimore, MD: Johns Hopkins University Press.

Singer, S., & Nicolson, J. (1972). The fluid mosaic model of the structure of cell membranes. *Science, 175,* 720–731.

Tantallein, J., Leon, R., Santos, A., & Sanchez, E. (2003). Multiple organ dysfunction syndrome in children. *Pediatric Critical Care Medicine, 4,* 263–264.

Thomson, J. M., & Wilson, S. F. (2002). *Health assessment for nursing practice.* St. Louis, MO: Mosby.

Tigchelaar, H., Kannikeswaran, N., & Kamat, D. (2008). Stevens-Johnson syndrome: An intriguing diagnosis. *Consultant for Pediatricians.* http://www.consultantlive.com/consultant-for-pediatricians/article/1145470/1403936

Trzepacz, P., Levenson, J., & Tringali, R. (1991). Psychopharmacology and neuropsychiatric syndromes in organ transplantation. *General Hospital Psychiatry, 13*, 233–245.

Vanholder, R., Sever, M., Erek, E., & Lameire, N. (2000). Rhabdomyolysis. *Journal of the American Society of Nephrology, 11*, 1553–1561.

Wellen, K., Hatzivassiliou, G., Sachdeva, U., Bui, T., Cross, J., & Thompson, C. B. (2009). ATP-citrate lyase links cellular metabolism to histone acetylation. *Science, 22*, 1076–1080.

Xue, Q. L. (2011). The frailty syndrome: Definition and natural history. *Clinical Geriatric Medicine, 27*, 1–15.

Chapter 6

BIOPSYCHOSOCIAL AND PHARMACOLOGICAL ASSESSMENT AND MONITORING

Robert D. Younger

A central component of prescribing medical psychology is the safe and effective use of medications. Assessing the need for medication and monitoring the evolution of pharmacotherapy comprise an essential tenet of clinical psychopharmacology. Apart from the ability of the medical psychologist (MP) to diagnose accurately through clinical interviewing and the use of psychometrics, to safely and effectively prescribe medications the pharmacologically trained medical psychologist must know how to assess the biomedical status of patients, including ongoing assessment of iatrogenic affects of medications in general. This chapter outlines common psychological and medical procedures employed to assess and monitor patients, including *physical examination* and *neurological examination*, as well as laboratory and other technologies, with emphasis on the biomedical aspects of practice.

GOAL OF ASSESSING THE WHOLE PERSON

Medical psychologists are uniquely qualified to assess the "whole person"; that is, they are able to assay the range of psychological, social and biological/medical aspects that make up the person, and to integrate these aspects into an appreciation for the unique individual. As first proposed by George Engle (1977), *biopsychosocial assessment* was intended for medical practice, but medical psychologists have expanded this concept and have successfully integrated the "bio" within the psychosocial. Moreover, the practicing prescribing medical psychologist integrates psychosocial knowledge and practice with biomedical assessment and pharmacological assessment and monitoring.

SCOPE OF PRACTICE AND LEVEL OF KNOWLEDGE AND EXPERTISE

The executive board of the American Psychological Association (APA)'s Division 55, the American Society for the Advancement of Pharmacotherapy, defines prescriptive authority relative to medical psychology: "Medical psychology is that branch of psychology that integrates somatic and psychotherapeutic modalities into the management of mental illness and emotional, cognitive, behavioral and substance use disorders. Medical psychologists may, where legally authorized, prescribe, order or consult regarding prescriptions of somatic treatment modalities, and monitor medications and/or other somatic treatment interventions, as well as order and interpret laboratory studies or other medical diagnostic studies such as might be consistent with enabling statutes" (Quillin, 2007). One could argue that the definition seems rather broad in that the medical psychologist with prescriptive authority could, theoretically, order varying types of "somatic treatment modalities," perhaps including *electrocardiogram* (*ECG*), *magnetic resonance imaging* (*MRI*), *functional magnetic resonance imaging* (*fMRI*), and *computerized tomography* (*CT*) scans. However, at least three caveats limit extensive use of these procedures beyond unusual cases: (a) just as physicians are theoretically prepared to perform everything from surgery to delivery of babies, most do not do so because of specialization in specific, limited competency areas, the recognition of other colleagues better prepared in adjacent specialty areas, and liability issues;[1] (b) it would be clinically unwise or imprudent, if not arguably unethical, for a medical psychologist to order testing or therapeutics for which a better option exists (e.g., why perform a physical examination when primary care medical providers are available?); and (c) liability issues as well as licensing board oversight would restrain prescribing medical psychologists from working beyond their scope of their expertise. Perhaps these three reasons, of which prescribing medical psychologists are cognizant, offer the rationale for the lack of malpractice suits despite years of practice and many thousands of prescriptions written and tests performed by prescribing medical psychologists.

The current two prescribing states, Louisiana and New Mexico, offer *scope of practice* in accordance with the preceding. Similarly, the U.S. Department of Defense military medical departments grant military and civilian psychologists prescriptive authority under these three caveats, and the Public Health Service and Indian Health Service currently recognize the competencies of prescribing medical psychologists with similar understandings. All jurisdictions and entities that grant prescriptive authority to medical psychologists (MPs) provide for essentially the same scope of practice and grant the same privileges and limitations.

And finally, although the American Psychological Association does not currently endorse *clinical treatment guidelines*, an interdivisional task force developed *practice guidelines* for psychologists involved in psychopharmacological issues (American Psychological Association, 2009). These guidelines offer the parameters of practice for pharmacologically trained MPs, including specified knowledge base for medical and pharmacological monitoring and management.[2]

HISTORY TAKING PROCEDURES

In medicine, an initial interview or assessment is still sometimes euphemistically termed "taking a history." This critical skill in both the practice of medicine and the practice of medical psychology serves as the bedrock of good care because it establishes the clinical baseline with which to compare the patient to others, as well as to monitor changes within the same individual across time. Both comparisons apply to other forms of assessment, such as laboratory studies and imaging,

[1]With reference to the practice of medical psychology, just because a prescribing medical psychologist could theoretically order medical tests such as an MRI or EKG does not mean the medical psychologist would do so.
[2]See Chapter 1 for a full discussion of the APA practice guidelines regarding psychologists' involvement in pharmacological issues.

as well as more esoteric assessment such as *pharmacogenetics*. This section focuses on information gathering relevant to medical psychology through general psychological assessment and *history taking*, while later sections speak to differential diagnosis.

Extending Psychological Assessment to the Practice of Medical Psychology

Clinical psychology traditionally gathers data directly from the patient via a questionnaire and then a clinical interview, with psychological testing or other studies to follow. This section focuses on psychological assessment and history taking for medical psychologists; medical psychology differs from traditional clinical psychology in its relative emphasis on the biomedical aspects of the complaints. Practicing psychology has been recently criticized for moving away from the traditional strength in the mental health field of assessment, with some graduate programs eliminating the study of projective techniques and placing a corresponding greater emphasis on psychotherapy. Similarly, and perhaps more dramatically, some observers have noted that medicine has moved away from direct physical examination and history gained from the patient to a more objective assessment such as laboratory studies and radiological and other assessment techniques, including the recent advent of complex genetic evaluation. Lamenting such moves, Chahl (2005) cited a 2002 survey of 78 psychiatric inpatients, which found that 17 percent received incomplete physical examinations while 35 percent were not examined at all. Although it is difficult to contemplate a psychiatric evaluation without a clinical interview—which includes the history—the lack of a complete physical examination in more than half of patients under psychiatric inpatient treatment points to the dangers of an inadequate knowledge base, as the "bio" aspect of diagnosis and treatment is compromised to the extent that all physical systems and organs are not properly assessed. Besides the risk of questionable outcomes due to inadequate initial assessment, the prescribing mental health professional, be that person a physician, nurse, or psychologist, who does not ensure that adequate psychological and medical assessments have been performed opens himself or herself up to risk of unanticipated medication events and potential malpractice. This section addresses the need to meaningfully conduct a psychological evaluation in conjunction with a medical evaluation.

Importance of a Standardized Assessment

The *Institute of Medicine* (*IOM*) and other public policy bodies increasingly point to standardized practices as lessening the possibility of poor medical outcomes, including medical errors. Standardized assessments contribute to a unified database to make probability statements as to causality as well as to measure change (Gawande, 2009).

Medical psychology has not seen a specific standardized assessment developed, but some adaptation of the traditional medical examination as well as the usual psychological evaluation has occurred within the field. As discussed earlier, the advantage of medical psychology over other disciplines is the assessment of the complete person by incorporating the biomedical aspects without neglecting psychological and social aspects.

Components of a Standardized Medical Psychology Assessment

Although medical psychology has existed in one form or another for more than half a century, referring to itself by many rubrics that include health psychology and rehabilitation psychology as well as medical psychology per se, prescribing medical psychology, the specialty that incorporates clinical psychopharmacology within the biopsychosocial paradigm of general medical psychology, is a relatively new specialty. It therefore does not have a rote series of questions to ask patients, although the components of a good psychology assessment remain unchanged. These include assessing the *presenting complaint* and taking a history of presenting symptoms. Beginning the assessment by focusing on the presenting complaint reinforces the patient's perception of what brought the patient to the consultation and what he or she seeks from the provider. Usually, the documentation of the presenting complaint quotes the patient, although some evaluators paraphrase. The history of the complaint includes the circumstances of its origins, such as when and where it began (particularly important for children), including the circumstances from which it sprang. A primary *review of systems* (*ROS*) includes initially attending to the organ system (usually in this case the central nervous system [CNS]) where problems seem to focus; a later, more global ROS will be done to cover all the organ systems.

Physical examination texts (e.g., Bickley, 2008) and medical history taking instructions (University of Florida, 2010a) suggest the importance of stating the presenting complaint in the patient's own words, without judgment; such texts also elaborate on model history taking of the complaint (e.g., who, what, when, where questions; presumably leading, in time, to how and why). One beginning medical text suggests that both physician and patient may have different agendas in focus (biomedical versus symptom), and intermediate outcome (gathering pertinent data versus telling one's story). Experienced clinicians can direct patients into gathering necessary information without alienating patients to allow the examination to proceed to consideration of a differential diagnosis. Medical psychologists often veer from the strict medical model (Engel, 1977) by encouraging their patients to tell their stories; this is done not only to gain symptom data, but also to promote insight into the patient by eliciting his or her phenomenological understanding of why the person has the symptom and, presumably, what would be the solution. Allowing the patient to talk unimpeded is, as clinical psychologists know, a fine way of building rapport and establishing a collaborative, therapeutic relationship with the patient.

Other Sources of Psychological and Medical History Taking

Gaining additional information from sources other than the patient, often essential in the case of children and adolescents but also the elderly and those unable or unwilling to give a good history, broadens the information available from which to make a decision. Such sources may be other persons familiar with the patient or they may be other avenues, such as laboratory testing, imaging procedures, psychometrics, or past clinical notes from previous providers.

Information derived from the initial interview with the patient as well as from supplementary sources would include:

- *Important medical systems.* The initial verbal history for the medical psychologist focuses on CNS, endocrine, renal, heart, and respiratory disease (those systems that can prove lethal or that more directly impact psychopharmacology). Other medical information is derived from documents related to history of accidents, illness, and surgeries.
- *Genetic history.* Family history particularly focuses on those psychiatric disorders with the highest genetic loading—depression, anxiety, schizophrenia, and

arguably bipolar disorder. Heritability of some forms of mental illness will be closer to the origins of the patient, so concentration is on first-order relatives.

- *Alcohol/drug history.* Medical psychologists assess use of alcohol and drugs, but it becomes even more incumbent upon the prescribing medical psychologist, and at times is critical due to effects of these chemicals on the body and the interactions of the chemicals on prescribed medications and other agents.[3]

- *Activities of daily living (ADLs).* Although this section is sometimes included in the family history or personal history section, as a medical psychologist you will want to ask the patient to describe the usual daily activities, from getting up in the morning to going to sleep. ADLs include what is usually done during the day, such as work or school, going from place to place, driving, and dietary habits. It may be helpful to ask about a day of work or school contrasted to a nonworkday. Social history can be gained at this time.

- *Illegal substances.* Similar to the information on common legal substances (see alcohol/drug history, above), the pharmacologically trained medical psychologist should take a detailed and careful history of the use of Drug Enforcement Administration (DEA)–controlled substances such as steroids and recreational drugs, over-the-counter preparations, as well as illegally obtained prescription medications. The prescribing medical psychologist is well advised to investigate drug–drug interactions through a variety of computer databases such as *Epocrates*, *Medline*, and *Rxlist*, just to name a few.[4] Ignoring or discounting drug–drug interactions not only leads to poor practice but dramatically increases liability risk. It is also essential to assess allergies and drug reactions when inquiring into the use of illegal substances.

- *Neurocognitive and mental status examinations.* The *neurocognitive assessment* is generally more in-depth for the medical psychologist than for other psychologists. For example, symptoms and signs of dysfunction of the 12 cranial nerves could be gained here as well as the physical examination and neurological examinations, to be discussed in the next section. The value of checklists, as Gawande (2009) advocates, comes more into play. Although clinical psychologists routinely

---

[3]For example, before prescribing a benzodiazepine, the medical psychologist would fully assess what other respiratory suppression substances might be onboard, as well as the likelihood of illegal psychostimulants. Legal and common substances include nicotine and caffeine, which speed metabolism and therefore affect the plasma levels of medications. Smoking can cut the effectiveness of conventional antipsychotic medication as well as the atypicals clozapine and olanzapine by half, while drinking two cups of coffee can reduce serum lithium levels by 50% (Sandson, 2011). The approximately 400 chemicals found in cigarette smoke produce uncertain effects; and more recently the prevalence of marijuana use, including prescription medical marijuana, adds a layer of complexity. Persons with schizophrenia and bipolar disorder often use both tobacco and marijuana, and therefore affect the metabolism of prescribed medications and their subsequent blood levels. Alcohol, of course, has a long and rich history in mental health assessment and since it is one of the most widely used psychoactive substances, and one of the most preventable causes of death and disability, it merits the medical psychologist's special attention. More specifically, the amount and timing of alcohol use impacts several classes of medications, including benzodiazepines. Alcohol use can decrease the seizure threshold and, with inherent compromising cognitive effects, lead to overdose and other untoward effects.

Most recently, states have begun to restrict newer, so-called *designer drugs* such as "spice." We can only anticipate that continued efforts to synthesize psychoactive substances and avoid governmental or regulatory restriction will lead to an increase in unanticipated chemical effects upon prescribed substances.

[4]Some of these drug lookup services are offered at a discount through professional organizations such as APA's Division 55, and some offer a free, but restricted, version that is useful for RxP students.

perform mental status examinations, the assessment of cranial nerve function and differentiation of central versus peripheral issues (e.g., shaking or vertigo) require knowledge of anatomy, physiology, and clinical medicine that is more inherent to the medical psychologist's training. Any symptom that goes unexplained can be referred to a neurologist or deferred for a subsequent follow-up assessment.

In summary, the prescribing MP combines the traditional psychological assessment, including a mental status examination, with a more focused medical history taken in preparation for subsequent physical and neurological examinations. Of course, some of this information could be taken by the MP while performing the physical and neurological exams, but such exams are likely to follow later in the assessment, after therapeutic rapport is established in the initial interview.

Review of Systems (ROS)

After completing the psychobiosocial interview in which specific complaints and symptoms are reviewed and background information is obtained, each biological system of the body is reviewed with the patient verbally in preparation for the physical examination. Although the review of systems can be done before the physical examination or during it, the ROS provides for patient verbal reporting of symptoms across all major organ systems. It includes asking basic questions of any current symptoms in these organ systems and any history of problems with them. Table 6.1 presents the systems reviewed in the ROS.

Table 6.1   Review of Systems (ROS)

As Reported by Patient

1. *General/Constitutional:* Fevers, sweats, weight change.
2. *Skin/Breast:* Rashes, pruritus, changing moles, lumps, lesions.
3. *Eyes/Ears/Nose/Mouth/Throat:* Headache, glasses, tinnitus, vertigo, sinusitis, dentures, mouth sores, sore throat.
4. *Cardiovascular:* Chest pain, angina, dyspnea on exertion, peripheral edema, history of murmur, palpitations, claudication, leg cramping.
5. *Respiratory:* Dyspnea, pleuritic pain, cough, sputum, wheezing, asthma.
6. *Gastrointestinal:* Dysphagia, heartburn, nausea, constipation, change in bowel habits or color of stool.
7. *Genitourinary:* Dysuria, nocturia, hematuria, urgency, urinary incontinence, urethral discharge, sores, dyspareunia, testicular pain, swelling.
8. *Musculoskeletal:* Joint or back pain, swelling, stiffness, deformity, muscle aches, locking of joint.
9. *Neurologic/Psychiatric:* Dizziness, involuntary movements, syncope, loss of coordination, motor weakness or paralysis, memory changes, speech difficulties, seizures, parasthesias, depression, sleep disturbance, crying spells, anorexia or hyperphagia, anhedonia, suicidal/homicidal ideation, loss of libido, anxiety, hallucinations, delusions, behavioral changes, substance abuse.
10. *Allergic/Immunologic/Lymphatic/Endocrine:* Reactions to drugs, food, insects, anemia, bleeding tendency, local or general lymph node enlargement or tenderness, polydipsia, asthenia, hormone therapy, secondary sexual development, intolerance to heat or cold, hot or cold flashes.

PHYSICAL AND NEUROLOGICAL EXAMINATIONS

Knowledge and ability to perform basic physical and neurological examinations are considered essential skills to safely and effectively prescribe. Most psychologists—indeed, most nonprescribing medical psychologists—are not trained or experienced in conducting these examinations and therefore such competency assumes having successfully completed an established curriculum with emphasis on clinical psychopharmacology.

Knowledge of Basic Physical and Neurological Examination Procedures

It is important here to make a distinction between knowledge of and performance of physical and neurological exams. While the pharmacologically trained medical psychologist is exposed to these procedures and, indeed, performs them under supervision during practicum, it will not become standard practice to perform them in the course of daily prescribing activity. Such examinations are, in most cases, better left to the primary care physician and neurologist to perform. Familiarity with these procedures, however, is essential for the prescribing medical psychologist to be able to read and interpret the importance of these examinations when performed by medical colleagues. It also sensitizes the prescribing psychologist to the need to refer for such exams if they are missing in the patient's medical history.

The *Psychopharmacology Examination for Psychologists* (*PEP*) requires the knowledge of "basic physical and neurological examination procedures" (American Psychological Association, 2010), but not necessarily the competence to perform them. Conducting physical examinations or presumably certifying them as accurate and sufficient, and certainly evaluating them, would be contingent upon the state or federal law or regulation authorizing them. The ability to conduct the examination does not require the medical psychologist to do so. The author, who is a prescribing medical psychologist, does not perform physical examinations himself but typically uses primary care providers to conduct them. Similarly, neurological examinations, which in large measure involve examination of the central nervous system and are more closely aligned to traditional clinical neuropsychology, probably would be delegated to other providers as well—mainly, neurologists. That being said, it would be difficult to develop sufficient knowledge in interpreting the results of these examinations without at some point conducting them, and it behooves the prescribing medical psychologist to conduct sufficient physical and neurological exams in training to arrive at a knowledge-based competency that allows confidence in incorporating the results of the exams into one's clinical decision making.

Developing Expertise in Physical and Neurological Examinations: How Much Is Enough?

Developing basic knowledge in these examinations requires knowledge of anatomy, physiology, and disease states (i.e., *clinical medicine*). In working with various medical professionals over many years, it seems reasonable to this author to gauge the level of required knowledge and skill that a prescribing medical psychologist might be expected to acquire to that of a psychiatrist and/or psychiatric nurse practitioner. Although some may argue that these are in fact two different standards, studies comparing the efficacy of nurse practitioners to physicians in those domains assessed have found them to be comparable. Just as with his or her psychiatric counterparts, the prescribing medical psychologist probably will not possess the knowledge and skill to become a consulting medical diagnostician, but that should not be the standard. In a note concerning managing risk, as of late 2010, no medical psychologist has been sued or otherwise disciplined for malpractice of clinical psychopharmacology. Similarly, it has not been alleged in the published media that there is evidence of unsafe practice by prescribing medical psychologists who routinely evaluate medical evidence and order medical tests.

While the prescribing medical psychologist will have had hands-on training in physical and neurological exams as part of the classroom curriculum, extending this training during the practicum and maintaining the skills once in the field are aided by further didactic material. Bates (Bickley, 2008) and Mosby (Seidel, Ball, Dains, & Benedict, 2010) offer texts, while CDs with detailed information on the physical exam as well as the classic neurology examination are also available (Kaufman, 2006). Video demonstration of these techniques can be invaluable because they can serve as a reference when one's knowledge begins to degrade through time. References should combine anatomy, physiology, and disease states (i.e., clinical medicine). *Emedicine* from WebMD is an example of the online programs to provide current examples and information across a range of medical issues (Emedicine, 2011). It is incumbent upon the prescribing medical psychologist to include periodic refresher courses on medical diagnostics, including physical and neurological examinations, as part of the continuing education requirements associated with specialization in clinical psychopharmacology.

PHYSICAL EXAMINATIONS

The following section assumes that the history taking portion of the examination, including the clinical interview and ROS, has already been done, with the physical examination and biomedical or laboratory studies to follow. The physical examination begins with general observation of the patient (Bickley, 2008). Without becoming too simplistic, observing the patient's general posture, speech, gait, and so on provides a wealth of information. Psychologists are well-versed in how to observe and describe one's mental state, verbal behaviors, and social relating, yet the medical psychologist takes the evaluation further to assess biomedical elements such as grip strength (as in shaking hands), body posture, gait, and discolorations in the skin. Much of this information can be gained without having the patient disrobe.

Medical psychologists have typically worked in hospitals or such medical settings and are familiar with standard precautions, which basically limit risk of exposure to pathogens or unsafe and unsanitary conditions for both the patient and the practitioner. Limiting exposure can be done by imposing barriers and following standard precautions and procedures. For example, wearing proper gloves, whether latex or other material, protects the hands from blood, body fluids, and so on, just as washing after gloves are removed and between patient contacts does. Presumably, medical psychologists will rarely need to wear a mask, face shield, or eye protection, but working with infectious diseases could require them. Besides shielding the patient and the practitioner from harmful substances, standard precautions also reduce risk of accident or injury. These include environmental controls such as cleaning and disinfection of the health care environment (equipment, beds, chairs, even restrooms), and attempts to prevent injuries ("sharps" disposal or necessary protections for confused or uncooperative patients). More broadly, reducing risk could include procedures such as keeping a patient in a private room and away from other patients.

Medical Equipment

The medical equipment required for conducting physical examinations depends upon the organ systems being examined. Again, most psychiatrists and psychiatric nurse practitioners do not conduct their own physical examinations, but rely on the examinations of specialists. The medical psychologist is likely to follow suit and only rarely conducts full or partial physical and/or neurological exams. The list of equipment used in physical examinations found in Table 6.2 is not meant to be an exhaustive list or even a required list of equipment, as that depends upon the examination's purpose.

Conducting the Examination

Prescribing medical psychologists observe physical and neurological exams performed by medical colleagues during their course work toward the postdoctoral master of science in clinical psychopharmacology. They will have also performed several exams on fellow students during the same course of studies before they begin their postdegree internship, at which time experience in conducting the physical and neurological exams is extended in the clinical setting, where the RxP psychologist-in-training typically rotates through medical departments and clinics as well as working directly within mental health settings.

Physical Examination

The following is not meant to be an exemplary procedure for conducting a physical examination but, rather, provides a general description and indicates routine guidelines. Most examiners proceed systematically by organ system using the method they learned during their educational and professional training. Vital signs and quick screening interview techniques that incorporate elements of the *Folstein Mini Mental Status Examination* may precede the physical exam.

Table 6.2   Equipment Used in Physical Exams

Instrument	Purpose
Platform scale	Measures height and weight but may be superseded by electronic versions.
Stethoscopes	Three types are available: magnetic, acoustic, and electronic. Acoustic is the most commonly used.
Ophthalmoscope	Looks into the eye for assessing pathology. Several apertures are available, depending upon type of examination.
Snellen Visual Acuity Chart	Standard "eye chart."
Near vision chart	Can use common reading materials.
Tympanometer	To introduce sound and air pressure tone to the middle ear.
Nasal speculum	To examine nose or other openings.
Tuning fork	Produces tone to assess hearing.
Hammer	Neurological and percussion (reflex).
Monofilament	Test skin sensitivity as in diabetic foot ulcers.

Organ systems include:

- *Musculoskeletal system:* Conducted head to toe testing for strength based on normative values (somewhat hard to find but can be done, especially tests like hand *dynamometer*). Besides weakness, one looks for effects of spinal lesions, inconsistence of effort, and other indications, including significantly unequal strengths across sides.
- *Cardiovascular system:* Heart sounds and rhythms using stethoscope. ECG data may be gained prior to or posterior to the physical exam. This is a critical area due to the primary life-sustaining nature of the system.
- *Chest examination:* Breathing, *auscultation*, and *percussion*, bilaterality.
- *Head, ear, eye, nose, and throat (HEENT) exam:* Hearing is tested for normal human voice, while the eyes may be tested for pupillary reflects as well as for acuity of vision. Much of the head, including smell, hearing, and eye function, is explored in the neurological exam to the extent that these sensory organs involve cranial nerve function.
- *Abdomen:* Explores all *quadrants*; listens for bowel sounds.
- *Skin:* Checks for skin pathology as well as signs of underlying pathology.[5]
- *Neurological:* Described in more detail later in this section.

An example of a completed physical examination is presented in Figure 6.1.

Neurological Examination

Due to a specialty emphasis on brain disorders and neuropathology, medical psychologists are generally more concerned with the neurological examination than the overall physical examination. Evaluation of the 12 cranial nerves should be a primary focus, but also differentiation of central versus peripheral neurological problems will help to differentiate symptoms that might be medication-related. The University of Florida's (2010b) teaching website displays excellent demonstrations of the neurological examination. Emphases of the primary neurological examination include (a) cranial nerves, (b) motor function, (c) coordination and gait, (d) reflex function, and (e) sensory examination. Of course, any abnormal findings need to be further evaluated through extensive neurological diagnostics, which might range from *nerve conduction studies* to *electroencephalogram* studies and various *imaging studies*.

The cranial nerves are tested individually, as indicated in Table 6.3.

LABORATORY TESTS

In order to meaningfully outline the use of normal laboratory values, it is useful to reinforce four terms used to measure the utility of laboratory tests: precision, *accuracy, sensitivity*, and *specificity* (American Association for Clinical Chemistry, 2010b). Precision roughly translates into repeatability, which most psychologists refer to as reliability. That is, does repeated measurement of the same sample yield the same results? In contrast, accuracy roughly translates for psychologists as validity. In this

---

[5]Note that the examination of skin or the integumentary system can be one of the most useful, partly because it's so visible and so accessible. Signs include yellow skin, possibly indicative of hepatic conditions, and bluish skin, indicating bruising or blood problems.

Physical Exam

Age: 17; Gender: Male

Vitals:

BP 119/62 /Pulse 53/ Temp 98.2 F (36.8 C) Ht 5' 10'' (1.784 m)/ weight 164 lbs (74.39 kg).

General: No acute distress, normal development, affect appropriate.

Skin: Normal color, no lesions. No rashes appreciated. No suspect moles.

Head: Normal appearance. Normal scalp and hair.

Eyes: Normal eyes, normal lids, and no strabismus or nystagmus. Visual acuity 20/20 bilaterally with Snellen card. Pupils 5mm, reactive equally to light and accommodation. Funduscopic exam shows no papilledema.

Ears: Normal shape and location. TMs and canals without erythema or exudates. Hearing intact to whisper test.

Nose: Mucosa moist with no erythema. No septal deviation/perforation. No polyps appreciated. No audible congestion, and no discharge.

Mouth, Throat, Neck: Lips, tongue, and buccal mucosa unremarkable. Normal hard/soft palate. Mucous membranes moist. Normal tonsils. Neck normal, supple with full range of motion and no thyroid enlargement.

Chest: Inspection normal, no chest wall deformity. Breasts normal for male, no discharge or tenderness.

Respiratory: Normal air exchange, no rales, no rhonchi, no wheeze. Respiration effort normal with no retractions.

Cardiac: Regular rate and rhythm, no murmurs.

Gastrointestinal: Nondistended abdomen. Normal active bowel sounds without renal or aortic bruits. Liver span 12 cm in midclavicular line. Spleen nonpalpable and does not extend beyond ribs to percussion in right lateral decubitus position. Bladder is not percussable. On palpation, no tenderness, masses, guarding, rebound, ascites.

Musculoskeletal: No scoliosis. Full ROM of extremities. No joint swelling.

Neurological:

MMSE: 30/30

Cranial nerves I–XII intact

Gross motor exam normal. Gait normal. Reflexes: Biceps 2+, triceps 1+, knee 2+, Achilles 2+ equal and symmetrical. No Babinski present. Rhomberg normal, gait normal (heel/toe tandem), able to walk on toes and heels.

Genitalia: Normal male, testes descended bilaterally, no hernia/varicocele, no mass.

Figure 6.1   Sample Physical Examination

case, accuracy means that a sample compares to a gold standard or comparison sample, or, in other words, the test measures what it is supposed to measure. Sensitivity and specificity work together in that sensitivity is the test's ability to correctly identify individuals with a particular condition (i.e., true positives) while specificity correctly excludes individuals without a condition (i.e., true negatives). Errors in sensitivity and specificity, analogous to Type I and Type II error in psychometrics, are understood to occur within a certain probability. Errors in sensitivity include persons falsely identified as having a condition (i.e., false positives) while an error in specificity incorrectly identifies an individual as not having a condition when, in fact, the person has it (i.e., false negatives). It may not be immediately obvious, but specificity is more important in some diseases, such as HIV, when the consequences of not identifying the condition can be more important than falsely excluding it.

The medical psychologist is cognizant of the need for multiple sources of information in arriving at a working diagnosis. In addition to the clinical interview and physical/neurological examinations (whether performed or reviewed), laboratory tests provide invaluable data. Laboratory studies produce values in the normal range for most patients. When this is not the case, however, abnormal lab values could be

Table 6.3   Sample Cranial Nerves Exam

Cranial Nerve	Testing Procedures
I—Olfactory	Have patients close both eyes and plug one nostril. Hold an orange under the open nostril and ask him or her to identify it. Test the other nostril with a lemon.
II—Optic	Ask the patient to cover one eye. The patient is asked to read progressively smaller lines on the near card or Snellen chart. Peripheral vision is tested as you sit 2 feet in front of your patients. Your eyes should be at the same level as theirs. Ask the patient to cover his or her right eye. You should cover your left eye as well, allowing you to reproduce a visual field similar to your patient's. Extend your right arm to the side, raise your forefinger, and position it about the same distance from your face and your patient's head. Your patient should let you know when he or she sees your finger.
III—Oculomotor IV—Trochlear VI—Abducens	To check for extraocular muscle movement, hold your forefinger about 18 inches away from your patient's eyes. Ask your patient to follow your finger with his or her eyes as you draw the letter H. Your partner's eyes should move together as they follow your finger with their eyes. His or her head should not move. Next, shine a penlight into your patient's eye from approximately 8 inches away. Pupil should constrict immediately. Repeat with other eye.
V—Trigeminal	To evaluate the strength and symmetry of the temporal muscles, put your fingertips on your patient's temples and ask him or her to clench the jaw. To assess the masseter muscles, place your fingertips on the patient's jaw and ask the patient to clench the jaw. The muscles should feel strong and even on both sides of the head and face. To test for the sensory function (ophthalmic, maxillary, and mandibular sensations): Have your patient close both eyes. Lightly touch his or her forehead, cheek, and jaw, on both sides of the face, using a cotton ball. Have the patient tell you when he or she feels the cotton touching them.
VII—Facial	Sensory: Assess the taste buds by touching a cotton applicator dipped in a sugar solution on to the tongue of your patient. Have them tell you where on the tongue they taste the sugar. Motor function: Have your patient raise the eyebrows, frown, smile and puff out the cheeks. Also, have your patient tightly close the eyes and resist your attempts to (gently) open them.
VIII—Vestibulocochlear	To test for hearing, stand 2 feet behind your patient's right side. Whisper several numbers and see if they can repeat them. Repeat the test on the left side. To test the balance portion of this nerve, have the person spin around 10 times. Watch the response of their eyes. A normal response to the spinning movement is vertigo. (A sense that the subject is dizzy or that the room is moving.) Do NOT allow your patient to fall or permit him or her to walk until the dizziness is completely gone!
IX—Glossopharyngeal X—Vagus	Sensory function: Place a piece of bitter-tasting chocolate on the tip, sides, and back of your patient's tongue. Have him or her let you know when they taste it. Motor function: Place your hand on your patient's throat and ask him or her to swallow. Check the gag reflex by gently touching the back of their throat with a cotton swab.

Cranial Nerve	Testing Procedures
XI—Accessory	Test the strength of the sternocleidomastoid muscle by placing your hand against your patient's cheek and having them turn their head as you apply resistance. Note the force they are able to apply against your hand. To assess the strength of the trapezius muscle, place your hands on your patient's shoulders and have him or her shrug the shoulders as you apply resistance.
XII—Hypoglossal	Have your patient stick out the tongue. Note any deviations from the midline. Ask your patient to move the tongue from side to side while you use the tongue depressor to prevent the movement. Note any lack of strength.

Sources: Jarvis (2004); Texas Health Science, University of North Texas.

due to a variety of factors, including actual pathology or disease, abnormal but incidental findings, *tail-end distributions* or results outside normative values but clinically insignificant (normative variants), indications of possible illness that are actually *subsyndromal,* and technique or timing error (Janicak, Davis, Preskorn, & Ayd, 2001).

Normal Results and Laboratory Panels

To ease the ordering of laboratory tests, and perhaps at least initially save resources by bundling tests into commonly used groups, hospitals and other users of laboratory services have developed shortcuts. These include *testing panels*, or a series of tests that would address common clinical scenarios. The *basic metabolic panel* shown in Table 6.4 illustrates common laboratory values, usually shown by a patient's result followed by the reference range for that individual's gender and age. Oftentimes automated or computerized reports do not take into account conditions such as pregnancy or disease states such as hepatic or heart disease. Therefore, the clinician will need to factor outside influences, such as alcohol ingestion or nicotine, into the reported results.[6]

Common Considerations in Ordering and Using Laboratory Tests

Beyond the considerations of gender and age, many other factors need to be weighed in interpreting laboratory test results. Race, body mass, disease, and a host of other factors can influence the reading of the results.

Sample Timing and Developing a Steady State

When ordering some tests, such as will be discussed later in therapeutic drug monitoring, drawing the sample too early or perhaps too late in the drug's assimilation

---

[6]Usually recognizing and understanding normal laboratory values is fairly straightforward, especially when an automated measurement system is used. Nonetheless, just because a patient has normal values doesn't mean that he or she is not sick: This would be arguing from the negative (i.e., your values are in the normal range so there's nothing wrong with you) and ignores, to some extent, individual differences as well as subsyndromal conditions or occult problems. Psychologists know, from their extensive background in research, that failing to reject the null hypothesis does not prove the nonexistence of a phenomenon; rather, it simply shows that the measurement used did not confirm the existence of the phenomenon.

Table 6.4   Normal Basic Metabolic Panel Results

Test	Normal Value Range
BUN	7 to 20 mg/dL
CO_2	20 to 29 mmol/L
Creatinine	0.8 to 1.4 mg/dL
Glucose	64 to 128 mg/dL
Serum chloride	101 to 111 mmol/L
Serum potassium	3.7 to 5.2 mEq/L
Serum sodium	136 to 144 mEq/L

Source: MedlinePlus (2010b).

produces several potential errors (Janicak et al., 2001). For example, if the drug level has not reached a *steady state*, usually after four to five *half-lives* of the drug, then the sample will not accurately reflect the amount of drug available to the tissue in question (usually the CNS, for mental health). If the sample is drawn too soon—before a steady state has been achieved—then the clinician may judge that the dose is ineffective and prematurely increase the dose. Conversely, when ordering a valproic acid blood sample, drawing the blood too late in the half-life cycle would yield a misleadingly small value and might erroneously lead to the conclusion that the prescribed dose is insufficient (Reed & Dutta, 2006). Knowledge of the half-life of various medications is essential.

Effects of Body Size and Adipose Tissue

Chapter 8 discusses pharmacokinetics in detail, but for our purposes suffice it to say that the goal of clinical pharmacokinetics is to deliver the medication to the appropriate target, whether individual cell or organ system (Howland, Mycek, Harvey, & Champe, 2005). Increasing body size increases the volume of blood and therefore can decrease the amount of drug delivered to the targeted organ system by increasing the amount of blood proteins, such as serum albumin, that bind to the drug molecule, and consequently reduce the freely circulating drug, which would otherwise be available to bind to target receptors. It also increases, in the case of lipophilic drug compounds, the rate of distribution from blood into adipose tissue. Adipose tissue, when abundant, can serve as a repository of the drug and, after the drug has been discontinued, the drug may continue to achieve an effect while it leaches from the adipose tissue back into the blood.

Drug–Drug Interactions

Enzyme inducers reduce plasma levels of the drug, and therefore its effects, by influencing the cytochrome P450 (CYP450) system to induce or accelerate the metabolism of the drug in question (Fann, 2004). This important system theoretically helps to protect the organism by speeding the departure of unneeded or unwanted chemicals, through oxidative metabolism and conjugation, to which the organism is exposed. From this viewpoint, the CYP450 system would serve an evolutionary function by protecting the organism from accidental poisonings. Understanding the CYP450 system and which drugs serve to induce or inhibit other enzymatic reactions allows the prescriber to anticipate drug–drug interactions. (See Table 6.5.)

Table 6.5 CYP450 Drug Interactions for Commonly Prescribed Medications

CYP450	Inducers	Inhibitors	"Victim Drugs" (Substrates)	Symptoms When Inhibited	Symptoms When Induced
1A2	Carbamazepine	Fluvoxamine	Asenapine	Insomnia/EPS[1]	Psychosis
	Cigarette smoke	Ciprofloxacin	Caffeine	Jitteriness	Withdrawal headaches
		Norfloxacin	Clomipramine	Seizures/arrhythmia/anticholinergic effects	Depression
		Ketoconazole	Clozapine	Seizures/sedation/anticholinergic effects	Psychosis
			Duloxetine	Increased blood pressure	Depression
			Mirtazapine	Somnolence	Depression
2C9/19	Ginkgo biloba	Fluoxetine	Diazepam	Intoxication	Anxiety/seizures
		Fluvoxamine	Tricyclics	Seizures/arrhythmia/anticholinergic	Depression
		Carbamazepine	Oral hypoglycemics	Hypoglycemia	Diabetes complications
		Modafinil	Warfarin	Hemorrhage	Pulmonary embolism/MI/stroke
		Oxcarbazepine			
		Valproate			
		Fluconazole			
2D6	None	Bupropion	Aripiprazole	EPS/akathisia/dystonia	Psychosis
		Fluoxetine	Duloxetine	Increased blood pressure	Depression
		Fluvoxamine	Mirtazapine	Somnolence	Depression/insomnia
		Paroxetine	Iloperidone	Tachycardia/hypotension/stiffness	Psychosis
		Quinidine	Tricyclics	Seizures/arrhythmia/anticholinergic	Depression
			Venlafaxine	Increased blood pressure	Depression
			Beta blockers	Hypotension	Hypertension
			Codeine/tramadol/hydrocodone	Less/no analgesia	Somnolence
3A4	Phenytoin	Nefazodone	Alprazolam	Sedation/intoxication	Panic/anxiety
	Carbamazepine	Grapefruit juice	Aripiprazole	EPS/akathisia/dystonia	Psychosis
	Oxcarbazepine	Protease inhibitors	Buspirone	Nausea/vomiting/dizziness/sedation	Anxiety
	Phenobarbital	Ketoconazole	Carbamazepine	Sedation/arrhythmia	Seizures
	Ginkgo biloba	Clarithromycin	Diazepam	Sedation/intoxication	Anxiety
	St. John's wort		Quetiapine	Sedation	Psychosis
			Methadone	Sedation	Opiate withdrawal
			Oral contraceptives	GI upset	Pregnancy
			Calcium channel blockers	Hypotension	Hypertension
			Statins (not pravastatin)	Rhabdomyolysis	Hyperlipidemia

Source: Sandson (2011).
1. EPS = Extrapyramidal symptoms.

The knowledgeable and diligent prescriber can also avoid drug–food interactions and genetic differences in response to drug administration.

Although an extensive discussion of drug–drug interactions is outside the scope of this chapter, the prescribing medical psychologist must be acutely aware of which chemicals can induce *cytochrome P450 enzymes* and which can inhibit or decrease them. For example, nicotine, alcohol, and most anticonvulsants induce several CYP enzymes (Janicak et al., 2001), whereas fluoxetine, bupropion, nefazodone, paroxetine, quinidine, and some antipsychotics can inhibit CYP enzymes (Janicak et al., 2001). A patient who is a heavy smoker, therefore, may require more frequent laboratory testing to determine the actual serum levels of, for example, an antipsychotic. The same patient on an increased dose of, say, clozapine who stops smoking may experience toxic levels of the drug as it accumulates over time because the CYP450 enzymes (in this case CYP1A2) are no longer induced by nicotine and cannot metabolize at the previously higher rate (DeLeon, 2004). In this case, therapeutic drug monitoring (see Table 6.9 later in this chapter) for clozapine could pick up the increase in serum concentrations, as compared to baselines taken while the patient was smoking, and avert a medical crisis.

Implications of Disease States

Hepatic or renal compromised patients can be identified and the progression of their disorder monitored by lab tests.[7] Renal disease can produce many pharmacological changes in blood levels, often through reduced urinary elimination. Renal disease affects clearance of drugs from the body and therefore is highly relevant to the safe practice of psychopharmacology. Two of the most pertinent renal laboratory tests are (a) *creatinine clearance*, which is a combination measurement of creatinine in the blood and urine, and (b) *glomerular filtration rate (GFR)*. Both measures indicate how well waste substances can be removed from the body. Creatinine clearance compares the level of creatinine in the urine with residual creatinine in the blood. With impaired renal function, the levels of creatinine in the blood build up relative to the amount that is eliminated by the kidneys and subsequently found in urine.

Renal disease leads to increased blood levels of drugs, and can therefore promote drug overdose. In addition, some diseases directly affect hepatic integrity, including viral infections, cirrhosis, and collagen vascular disease, and can affect the blood levels of medications that are metabolized in the liver. Other diseases, such as cardiac disease with right ventricular failure, can reduce the *first pass* effect and therefore delay biotransformation. While it is outside the scope of the chapter to detail all of the potential diseases that could affect laboratory values, endocrine disease merits mention because of its widespread effects, especially those that mimic psychiatric disorders. Also, autoimmune diseases such as systemic lupus erythematosus can produce psychiatric-like symptoms such as chronic fatigue and anhedonia and delusions. Also of considerable importance is the fact that autoimmune disorders, including those that affect the endocrine system such as Hashimoto's thyroiditis, can be precipitated by psychotropics, and may be picked up early by the astute clinician.

---

[7]One of the greatest contributions of medical psychologists to the field of clinical medicine, in the author's opinion, is their continual discovery of abnormal medical findings in the course of their examinations, and the subsequent referral of the affected person for further evaluation by medical specialists.

Laboratory Testing

The prescribing MP selects laboratory tests based partly on the patient characteristics such as age, sex, first exposure to a given treatment, and, for females, reproductive capacity. In addition, the prescribing clinician also selects tests based on the presumed disorder being evaluated, because the diagnosis—whether by diagnostic system (*Diagnostic and Statistical Manual of Mental Disorders, 4th edition [DSM-IV]* or *International Classification of Diseases, 10th Revsion [ICD 10]*) or by target symptoms—determines which medication to consider. Different medications place different demands on various organ systems; likewise, diseases or weaknesses of some organ systems could preclude using certain medications. Therefore, to adequately assess most patients, the provider would conduct, or have conducted, a physical examination as well as a history and then select laboratory tests depending on patient characteristics and the presenting problem.

Common Laboratory Test Panels

To ease the ordering of laboratory tests and initially save resources by bundling tests into commonly used groups, hospitals and other users of laboratory services have developed shortcuts for the ordering of such tests; as mentioned previously, these include testing panels, or a series of tests that would address common clinical scenarios.

Concept of Panels   It is standard practice in clinical or counseling psychology to employ psychometrics to answer specific questions, such as assessing for anxiety or depression, or perhaps detecting a psychotic process. Such tests augment the clinical interview, aid in ruling out initial impressions, and help the psychologist arrive at a working differential diagnosis, which will guide subsequent treatment. Differential diagnosing often requires administering more than one type of test, such as differentiating depression from dementia. Similarly, in medicine some laboratory tests yield information more applicable to prescribing psychotropic medications. Such tests include measures of metabolism (basic metabolic panel), liver function, kidney function, and thyroid function. For healthy young patients, the history (which contains the physical exam) and mental status examination may provide the vast majority of the information needed to consider pharmacotherapy. However, best practices dictate that providers order laboratory tests to assure that the patient is "medically cleared" (an archaic term to indicate that there is no overt medical pathology such as renal, metabolic/endocrine, respiratory, or heart disease) and to rule out an incipient, covert, or occult process. Such disease might be subclinical, but nevertheless needs to be taken into account.

Most patients will receive laboratory testing for complete blood count (CBC); *electrolytes, hematocrit,* and *hemoglobin*; renal, liver, and thyroid function; and lipids/ *blood sugar*. For the healthy patient, these standard tests will be all that are ordered, whereas a mental health patient with comorbid physical ailments might require far more extensive laboratory work.

Basic Metabolic Panel   The basic metabolic panel (BMP) includes measures related to kidney function (*blood urea nitrogen* [BUN] and creatinine); blood sugar (glucose to measure for hyperglycemia, hypoglycemia, diabetes, and prediabetes); metabolic disturbance with carbon dioxide (CO_2) or carbonate; and electrolytes (serum chloride, serum potassium, serum sodium) (American Association for Clinical Chemistry, 2010a).

One metabolic measure is the acidity or alkalinity of the blood, the acid–base balance. The acid–base state or equilibrium buffers the blood to maintain pH of approximately 7.35 to 7.45 under normal conditions in arterial blood (MedlinePlus, 2010b). Most pharmacological agents are designed to interact with a standard blood pH, and change in the acid–base equilibrium may theoretically affect pharmacokinetics, although the effect is likely to be nominal since actual changes in blood pH, although clinically significant, tend to be less than 0.5. Of more importance may be the effect that shifts in pH could have on permeability on psychotropic drug penetration at the blood–brain barrier (Oldendorf, 1974; Nagy, Szabo, & Huttner, 1985).[8] Nonetheless, while pH is important to catch if it becomes abnormal, there are few clinical guidelines for converting such variations into pharmacokinetic recommendations concerning drug indication/contraindication or dosing. The fact that the clinician is aware of the abnormality, however, sensitizes him or her to be on the lookout for any unusual clinical manifestations.

Reduced alkaline in the blood and tissues or metabolic acidosis produces sweet sickly breath, headache, and nausea, while excessive alkaline in the blood and tissues produces alkalosis. Respiratory acidosis (e.g., "blowing off too much CO_2" due to respiratory disease) and metabolic acidosis are not only important clinically but directly relate to treating underlying medical disease and therefore to prescribing psychiatric medications. Uncontrolled diabetes is of particular concern. Its presentation may be insidious and thus undetected by the patient, yet the medical psychologist must be on the lookout for it because of its growing incidence in the population and because it can be exacerbated through metabolic disturbances inherent to some antipsychotic medications. Therefore, screening for diabetes and metabolic disturbance forms a part of the basic laboratory examination.

Comprehensive Metabolic Panel   The *comprehensive metabolic panel* (*CMP*) adds more information to the BMP, for a total of between 12 and 20 specific tests, including acid–base balance as well as electrolytes, blood proteins (*albumin* and total protein), enzymes related to metabolic function, and substrates associated with elimination. Among electrolytes, concentrations of sodium and potassium are highly regulated in the body, and disturbances could present critical problems. The CMP also includes renal tests as well as liver tests such as *alkaline phosphatase* (*ALP*), *alanine amino transferase* (*ALT*), *aspartate amino transferase* (*AST*), and *bilirubin*.

The components of the CMP, without reference to age or gender, are listed in Table 6.6.[9]

---

[8]Status epilepticus creates metabolic acidosis due to a host of factors, including increased catecholamines and increased glycolysis; pH drops are greater in the brain than in the general circulatory system (Engel & Pedley, 2008). Perhaps more of heuristic value than for clinical application (Broglin, 2003), it is interesting to note that some forms of epilepsy may make the blood–brain barrier more permeable to substances such as barbiturates, at least in animal models (Nagy et al., 1985).

[9]Note that the basic readings of the CMP can be expanded by subsequently ordering specialty panels when a problem is suspected. For example, an electrolyte panel can be ordered to expand measures of acidosis by adding the anion gap reading to the standard CO_2 and electrolyte reading found in the standard CMP.

Table 6.6   Comprehensive Metabolic Panel (CMP)

Test	Reference Value
Albumin	3.9 to 5.0 g/dL
Alkaline phosphatase	44 to 147 IU/L
ALT (alanine transaminase)	8 to 37 IU/L
AST (aspartate aminotransferase)	10 to 34 IU/L
BUN (blood urea nitrogen)	7 to 20 mg/dL
Calcium—serum	8.5 to 10.9 mg/dL
Serum chloride	96 to 106 mmol/L
CO_2	20 to 29 mmol/L
Creatinine	0.8 to 1.4 mg/dL
Direct bilirubin	0.0 to 0.3 mg/dL
Gamma—GT (gamma-glutamyl transpeptidase)	0 to 51 IU/L
Glucose test	100 mg/dL
LDH (lactate dehydrogenase)	105 to 333 IU/L
Phosphorus—serum	2.4 to 4.1 mg/dL
Potassium test	3.7 to 5.2 mEq/L
Serum sodium	136 to 144 mEq/
Total bilirubin	0.2 to 1.9 mg/dL
Total cholesterol	100 to 240 mg/dL
Total protein	6.3 to 7.9 g/dL
Uric acid	4.1 to 8.8 mg/dL

Source: MedlinePlus (2010a).

Thyroid Tests

Thyroid tests merit particular attention due to the thyroid gland's function in the metabolism of drugs,[10] its vulnerability to injury by certain psychotropics, and its ability to present symptoms reminiscent of psychiatric manifestations due to thyroid dysfunction. Thyroid diseases masquerading as psychiatric diseases include (a) Graves' disease (too much thyroid), with excess energy and acceleration, giving the impression of hypomania or anxiety, and (b) Hashimoto's thyroiditis (thyroid enlarged but ineffective), with lethargy and fatigue that can give the misimpression of vegetative depression. Of particular concern for the prescribing medical psychologist treating bipolar disorder is the tendency for the first-line pharmacological agent for this condition, lithium, to induce autoimmune changes in the thyroid that may eventually lead to hypothyroidism if the changes are not detected and treatment stopped.

Low levels of circulating *triiodothyronine* (*T3*) and *thyroxine* (*T4*) stimulate the hypothalamus to secrete thyroid-releasing hormone, which, in turn, stimulates

---

[10]While the thyroid does not directly metabolize drugs (this is largely the function of the liver), it can affect the half-life of drugs in some cases by its influence on metabolism rate in general and its indirect influence on kidney excretion (Eichelbaum. 1976).

Table 6.7   Length of Time After Ingestion That Drug Can Be Detected in Urine

Drug	Detection (After Introduction)
Alcohol	7–12 hours
Amphetamine	48–72 hours
Barbiturate	24 hours for short-acting, 3 weeks for long-acting
Benzodiazepine	3 days
Cocaine	6–8 hours, metabolites 2–4 days
Codeine	48 hours
Heroin	36–72 hours
Marijuana	2–4 days, longer for habitual user
Methadone	3 days
Morphine	48–72 hours

Sources: Council on Scientific Affairs (1987); Moeller, Lee, & Kissack (2008).

the pituitary to release *thyroid-stimulating hormone* (*TSH*). Thus, patients with underlying hypothyroidism (high TSH) can have low levels of T3 and T4 following surgical radiological ablation of the thyroid, thyroiditis, idiopathic hypothyroidism, or iatrogenic results of medication. T4 and TSH levels are often used to differentiate pituitary from thyroid dysfunction, and TSH is used to monitor the effects of exogenous thyroid replacement.

Common thyroid tests include thyroid-stimulating hormone, with a reference range of 2 to 10 μU/mL (Pagana & Pagana, 2010), as well as triiodothyronine and thyroxine, and several other minor tests. It is standard procedure in clinical psychopharmacology to establish a baseline TSH to rule out thyroid implications in mental health symptoms as well as to refer back to the baseline, if lithium is prescribed, to identify major shifts or progressive trends toward iatrogenic hypothyroidism.

Other Common Tests

Besides laboratory tests for general medical illnesses, the medical psychologist will sometimes need to assess for drugs of abuse. The latency between use and possible laboratory detection of different drugs of abuse ranges from a few hours in the case of alcohol to several days or even up to weeks in the case of barbiturates. Marijuana can be detected up to several days for the occasional user, but the latency period can be much longer for the habitual user.[11] Table 6.7 presents detection times for discerning drugs of abuse in the blood.

In addition to the BMP, CMP, and tests for substances of abuse, various other chemicals may be assessed. These include environmental toxins like aluminum, arsenic, manganese, mercury, and lead, which can be detected in urine or blood, while organic compounds have no specific laboratory testing (Sadock, Sadock, & Ruiz, 2009). Over-the-counter medications that merit assessment, especially in the case

---

[11]Marijuana can be detected for several months in urine analysis of habitual users. Note that urine tests do not detect the psychoactive component in marijuana, THC (delta-9-tetrahydrocannabinol); they detect the nonpsychoactive marijuana metabolite THC-COOH, which can linger in the body for days and weeks.

Table 6.8   Critical Drug Values in Overdose

Critical Drug Levels	
Test Name	Greater Than
Acetaminophen	40 mcg/mL
Amitriptyline/Nortriptyline Fractionation	500 ng/mL
Carbamazepine	12 mcg/mL
Chlorpromazine	500 ng/mL for adults 200 ng/mL for pediatrics
Clomipramine (Anafranil)	900 ng/mL
Clonazepam	100 ng/mL
Cyanide—potentially toxic	50 mcg/dL
Cyclobenzaprine (Flexeril)	100 ng/mL
Diazepam (Valium)	2.5 mcg/mL
Doxepin and Metabolite	400 ng/mL
Ethanol	300 mg/dL
Imipramine/Desipramine Fractionation	500 ng/mL
Lithium	1.4 mEq/L
Lorazepam	300 ng/mL
Phenobarbital	60 ug/mL
Phenytoin	40 mcg/mL
Salicylate	40 mg/dL
Trazodone (Desyrel)	3.2 mcg/mL
Valproic acid	150 mcg/mL

Source: University of Iowa (2010).

of suspected overdose, include acetaminophen, which can cause liver toxicity, as well as salicylate (i.e., aspirin). See Table 6.8 for critical values associated with drug overdose.

Considerations for Specific Populations

Some populations, such as women, young males, the elderly, and patients newly introduced to psychotropics, may require differential testing or further deliberation. Janicak et al. (2001) and Jensvold, Halbreich, and Hamilton (1996), for example, outline differences in pharmacokinetics in females due to (a) absorption bioavailability, with increasing absorption of some weak bases (e.g., tricyclic antidepressants [TCAs]) since exogenous estrogen increases absorption, and slower transit time in the small intestine; (b) smaller volume of distribution and greater drug effect in females due to size and lower protein binding; (c) estadiol and progesterone in oral contraceptives, which reduce some specific CYP enzyme activity; and (d) various effects of pregnancy.

Greater muscle mass in young males may present more of a risk for neuroleptic malignant syndrome than those with less muscle mass. Neuroleptic malignancy syndrome develops 1.8 times as often in men as in women, probably due to the insulating effect of muscle and resultant potentiation of hyperthermia. Males with greater muscle mass may be further disposed to suffer from associated rhabdomyolysis (Curley & Irwin, 2008). Therefore, a general focus on medically relevant history, consideration of body composition, and possibly smaller doses with some antipsychotic medications may be in order.

Patients newly placed on antipsychotics, whether first- or second-generation antipsychotic medication, merit close examination for metabolic syndrome potential. In addition to the BMP and possibly CMP mentioned earlier, the usual physical examination, vital signs, and recording of weight, as well as laboratory studies that include glucose and lipid panels should be done serially to detect developing metabolic disease and other complications. Furthermore, some research suggests that schizophrenic patients tend to gain weight regardless of receiving antipsychotics. Patients with risk factors such as obesity, family history of metabolic disorder, or existing metabolic disease such as diabetes face increased risk of developing metabolic syndrome when placed on antipsychotic medications. The tendency for these medications to promote weight gain may lead to noncompliance in the form of prematurely discontinuing the medication, especially for women and young persons.

Specific Tests for Selected Medications

In addition to standard laboratory studies to establish the existence of preexisting conditions before prescribing psychotropics, some medications warrant specific testing shortly after the medication has been prescribed. Clozapine has been associated with agranulocytosis and therefore requires periodic complete blood counts. Lithium is associated with thyroid disease and requires periodic TSH testing. Some anticonvulsants are associated with kidney and liver disease and require periodic testing of renal and hepatic functions.

THERAPEUTIC DRUG MONITORING

The prescribing medical psychologist will soon recognize that all patients do not respond the same way to the same dose of the same drug. Because of the differences among patients, drugs can accumulate in the body or, conversely, metabolize quicker and produce less effect because there is less drug available at the site of action. To understand how drugs affect the body and how in turn the body influences how a medication is used, pharmacologists have developed methods, including *therapeutic drug monitoring (TDM)*, to measure these differences.

TDM uses both *pharmacodynamics*, defined as the "drug's affinity for its sites of action" (Janicak et al., 2001, p. 51) and pharmacokinetics, "the quantitative, time-dependent changes of both the plasma drug concentration and the total amount of drug in the body, following the drug's administration by various routes" (Howland et al., 2005), to measure drug effects in the body.[12]

Another way to differentiate pharmacodynamics from pharmacokinetics is to consider that pharmacodynamics measures the effect of the drug on the organism whereas pharmacokinetics measures the body's effect on the drug. Hiemke (2008) succinctly described the usefulness of TDM for understanding the pharmacokinetics

---

[12]Pharmacokinetics of the drug can be further divided into the following primary phases: absorption, distribution, metabolism, and elimination (see Chapter 8).

and pharmacodynamics of a drug in a given individual. TDM, although still in its infancy, promises to provide explanations of individual genetic responses to medications, leading to the possibility of tailoring medications to one's genetic background as well as one's individual responses to the drug.

Guidelines for TDM

The American Psychiatric Association (2000), as well as Europe's interdisciplinary therapeutic drug monitoring group of the Arbeitsgemeinschaft für Neuropsychopharmakologie und Pharmakopsychiatrie TDM-AGNP (Baumann et al., 2006) recommend specific measures for inclusion in standard TDM. Recommendations included baseline measurement and regular monitoring of body mass index, blood glucose, lipid profiles, signs of prolactin elevation or sexual dysfunction, and movement disorders. Europe emphasizes TDM more than the United States does (e.g., Hiemke, 2008).

Janicak et al. (2001) point out that some medications can be monitored in the body whereas others may not be amenable, due either to technical factors such as the first and second pass effects or to only slight usefulness. The following list shows the common classes of medications and indicates the relative usefulness of TDM.

- *Benzodiazepines.* Except for underlying disease, such as reduced clearance due to kidney disease, which may be monitored by GFR, TDM with benzodiazepines offers little benefit.

- *Antidepressants.* According to Janicak et al. (2001), TDM is not useful for many antidepressants, such as selective serotonin reuptake inhibitors (SSRIs), but tricyclic antidepressants (TCAs) deserve special mention due to accumulation leading to toxicity and death. The difference between effective dose and lethal dose can be narrow, leading to overdose. With TCAs, patients fall into three groups: the majority are normal metabolizers, while a smaller group, 5 to 10 percent, are poor metabolizers, and the smallest group of 0.5% are ultrarapid metabolizers. The linear relationship between dose and plasma drug levels in ultrarapid and normal metabolizers can predict dose needed for a specific plasma level. In poor metabolizers, TCAs will build up due to relative lack of CYP 2D6 metabolism (Janicak et al., 2001). TCAs studies showing a relationship between concentration and antidepressant response include nortriptyline, desipramine, amitriptyline, and imipramine (Janicak et al., 2001).[13]

    With monoamine oxidase inhibitors (MAOIs), TDM is employed "simply to determine how individual variability in pharmacokinetics could account for inter-individual variability in drug response" (Janicak et al., 2001, p. 268). This use is of greater utility when studying variability within a group and has less application in the clinical setting where the practitioner is more concerned with variability in a given individual, with a group of patients as reference. Platelet MAO inhibition might be used, but it is not readily available commercially, so TDM with MAOIs is infrequently used.

- *Antipsychotics.* Antipsychotics have received extensive coverage in TDM. Compared to the new antipsychotic medications, the first-generation antipsychotics receded in

---

[13]Procedurally, to use TDM with TCAs, initially prescribe a standard dose and after a week sample blood 10 to 12 hours after the last dose to assure absorption and distribution.

popularity due to greater side effects, especially attributable to D_2 blockade; still, the usefulness of TDM with the older, conventional antipsychotics is well established. TDM with second-generation antipsychotics is less well known. Within the first-generation antipsychotics, haloperidol, chlorpromazine, fluphenazine, trifluoperazine, and thiotixene all received TDM attention, with chlorpromazine having accumulated the greatest data (Janicak et al., 2001).

As mentioned, the more recent second-generation antipsychotics originally were thought to have far fewer side effects and to present less need for therapeutic monitoring. Notwithstanding this arguable difference with conventional antipsychotics, second-generation antipsychotics merit TDM due to metabolic syndrome (Janicak et al., 2001),[14] and prescribers may initially screen with CBC, glucose, prolactin level, and physical examination, while monitoring patients for weight gain and prolactin levels as opposed to monitoring actual therapeutic blood samples. Atypical and second-generation antipsychotics include risperidone and olanzapine, which are particularly associated with weight gain (Kantrowitz & Citrome, 2008). In addition, among the second-generation antipsychotics, olanzapine was found in one study (Chue & Singer, 2003) to be attributable to 29 deaths due to overdose; a potential for toxicity with plasma concentrations of as low as 100 ng/mL was found, with steady-state plasma concentrations rarely over 150 ng/mL.

Although categorized as an antipsychotic, but not a second-generation antipsychotic due to its unusual mechanism of action, Clozaril is useful for refractory schizophrenia (Kane & Correll, 2010). Clozapine, however, is an atypical antipsychotic that deserves special drug monitoring due to blood cell count changes and the possibility of agranulocytosis; for these reasons, clozapine requires periodic complete blood counts. Weekly *white blood cell count* (*WBC*) for the first six months is recommended and then every other week thereafter. If there is no abnormality after one year, a blood test can be done monthly. If a significant reduction occurs in neutrophil count (neutropenia) without agranulocytosis, the patient can be rechallenged once WBC and neutrophil counts recover.

Lithium has a long and well-researched history of use in affective disorder and particularly with mania. Lithium requires an initial renal function assessment, including creatinine and creatinine clearance.[15] Underdosing is ineffective, whereas overdosing leads to sweating and tremors, and can potentially be fatal. Jefferson (2010) offers practical prescribing advice on assessing usefulness of lithium, and the prescriber should be aware of lithium neuropathies (Raedler & Wiedemann, 2007).

---

[14]Metabolic monitoring of second-generation antipsychotics, however, is poorly followed by prescribers (Cassels, 2010).

[15]**Children's lab tests for lithium:** (a) Lithium monitoring: Every week until stable for 1 month, then every month for 3 months, then every 3 months thereafter. Blood drawn 12 hours after last dose. (b) Thyroid: Baseline, then 2 weeks after, then every month for 3 months, then every 3 months thereafter. TSH never to exceed 10 mU/L. (c) Renal: Baseline for creatinine and BUN, then 2 weeks after, then every month for 3 months, then every 3 months thereafter. (d) Cardiac: Baseline EKG, repeat in 2 months, then every year thereafter (Geller & DelBello, 2008).

Adult lab monitoring for lithium: Blood drawn to monitor lithium serum level every 3 to 6 months, thyroid function every 6 to 12 months, and renal function every 6 to 12 months for patients on maintenance regimens of lithium (Marcus, Olfson, Pincus, Zarin, & Kupfer, 1999).

Anticonvulsants usually carry a recommendation for periodic therapeutic drug monitoring, but the use of TDM for valproic acid has been categorized as controversial in at least one recent study (Haymond & Ensom, 2010). Still, valproic acid level checks may improve overall clinical care. Carbamazepine is more problematic for TDM due to the curvilinear relationship of dosage with drug effect. In general, older medications, including the older anticonvulsants, provide a rich history of accumulated data and clinical experience on which to base TDM.

Table 6.9 presents therapeutic monitoring indexes for various psychotropic drugs.

Special Population Considerations for TDM

TDM could be used with children and adolescents, but very few studies exist, with relatively more research on the psychokinetics of the psychostimulants. Compared with adults, lithium in children could have a shorter half-life and more rapid renal clearance (Janicak et al., 2001).

TDM may be more important with the elderly due to possible increased complications with lithium, especially due to compromised endocrine, CNS, or related systems. And dehydration must always be averted, especially in the elderly. For these reasons, valproate has been used with the elderly as a substitute for lithium.

Continuing Problem of the Missing TDM

While there is a dearth of data on which to base TDM for many drugs, and an even greater scarcity of recommendations for certain age groups, an arguably larger problem is the lack of TDM being performed when it is indicated, available, and recommended. For example, Kilbourne et al. (2007) found that less than 40% of 435 patients received a serum drug level for mood stabilizers and 38.8% received a thyroid function test for lithium, while slightly over 70% received complete blood counts and hepatic function tests for valproate or carbamazepine. About half of the patients prescribed atypical antipsychotics received cholesterol counts, and slightly less than 70% received serum glucose levels. Is there any reason, one might ask, why thyroid testing is not done on every patient receiving lithium, complete blood counts not ordered for every patient on clozapine, and metabolic panels, including glucose level, not monitored for all patients on olanzapine?

Adverse Drug Reactions

Differences Between Unwanted Side Effects and Adverse Events

Clarifying terms such as *adverse drug event* versus *adverse drug reaction* helps the prescribing medical psychologist anticipate bad outcomes and prepare a course of action to eliminate or ameliorate them. An adverse drug reaction or unwanted drug side effect can be defined as any unintended, undesired effect of a drug after its administration. With unwanted drug effects, the doctor might reduce the dosage, stop the drug, or switch to another drug.

Adverse drug events, in contrast, occur when injury has been caused by drugs; such events are usually serious reactions to a drug, outside the expected range of side effects. The following section focuses on signs of adverse events or reactions.

Assessing Types of Adverse Drug Reactions

Adverse drug reactions may affect anything from cardiac, hepatic, renal, and metabolic function to ophthalmic, gastrointestinal, and neurological function. Most assessment

Table 6.9   Therapeutic Drug Monitoring: Blood Monitoring Level for Selected Psychotropics

Drug	Optimal Range	Comment
Mood Stabilizers	Well-established serum levels which specify therapeutic window.	Need for continuous TDM throughout treatment.
Lithium	0.6–1.2 mEq/L.	Side effects: Induced hypothyroidism, cognitive blunting, fine tremors, bradycardia, malformations in first trimester of pregnancy: FDA Pregnancy Risk Rating: "D." Some risk of *torsades de pointes* and/or *prolonged QT interval.*
Valproic acid	50–125 mcg/mL.	Side effects: FDA Pregnancy Risk Rating: "D." Neural tube defects of up to 1.5% when valproate used in first semester of pregnancy.
Carbamazepine	4–12 mg/L.	Side effects: Agranulocytosis. Pregnancy Category: "D."
Antipsychotics	Little has been established concerning therapeutic and toxic blood levels of antipsychotic medication.	TDM is achieved by taking baseline and periodic readings. Significant intrapatient variations may have clinical significance. New FDA warning (2011) of movement disorders in newborn of mother treated during pregnancy.
Clozaril	Reference 200–400 ng/mL.	Routine serum testing not standard practice. Wide variation in therapeutic serum level and in toxicity level. Side effect: agranulocytosis/neutropenia; WBC required periodically. Low pregnancy rating of "B" for birth defects. Some risk of torsades de pointes.
Haloperidol	Reference: 4–25 ng/ml.	FDA Pregnancy rating "C" for birth defects. Risk of torsades de pointes.
Antidepressants	Little reference for SSRIs. TCA serum levels are better established.	TDM is underutilized in antidepressants, although studies show that dose is adjusted in >50% of cases when serum levels are obtained. As much as 20% of serum levels are found to be outside the therapeutic window (Kootstran-Ros, 2006).
Nortriptyline	50–150 or 170 ng/mL.	Some risk of prolonged QT interval.
Desipramine	110–160 nm/mL.	Some risk of prolonged QT interval.
Amitriptyline	80–160 ng/mL.	Some risk of prolonged QT interval.
Imipramine	For adults, min 265 ng/mL. For adolescents children much lower dose.	Some risk of prolonged QT interval. Effective dose close to cardiac and CNS complications.

Sources: Janicak et al. (2001); Preston (2010); Food and Drug Administration (2011); Centers for Education and Research on Therapeutics (2011).

techniques of drug side effects rely on the physical examination,[16] as well as laboratory results and imaging procedures. Behavior rating scales have been slow in developing to date, but a few exceptions include rating scales for movement disorders and sexual dysfunction. Although no single movement and behavior scale such as Apgar score (Apgar, 1953) for newborns or the Glasgow Coma Scale (Teasdale & Jennett, 1974) for head injury exists for movement disorders, the Abnormal Involuntary Movement Scale (AIMS) (Guy, 1976) has been extensively used for assessing anticholinergic and other reactions, primarily stemming from antipsychotic medication adverse side effects. The 12-item AIMS is easy to use and not as intrusive as some other measures. While less well known, the 10-item Rating Scale for Extrapyramidal Side Effects, also known as the Simpson-Angus Extrapyramidal Symptom Rating Scale (Psychiatry Online, 2011), has been used for research.

Sexual dysfunction is one of the more common side effects of antidepressant medication. Patients may prematurely stop taking the medications due to this pernicious side effect, and may subsequently relapse. McGahuey and associates developed and validated the five-item Arizona Sexual Experience Scale (McGahuey et al. 2000) to assess sexual satisfaction. A baseline reading on this scale before prescribing antidepressant medication allows the prescribing psychologist to periodically administer the quick scale during treatment to avert unwanted interruption in treatment.

BEHAVIORAL ASSESSMENT METHODS AND ASSESSING THE WHOLE PERSON

Combining all of the available information—biomedical and psychological—into a workable conceptualization that translates to a clinical formulation that guides the treatment of the individual patient should be one of the central strengths of the prescribing medical psychologist. Methods employed by the MP include direct observation of behaviors, rating scales, self-reports, and other psychometrics. This section concerns the use of behavioral assessment methods in baseline and ongoing monitoring of therapeutic effectiveness and quality of life, while a later section deals specifically with assessing the adverse effects of psychopharmacological agents.

In one of the more famous quotations in medicine, Sir William Osler proposed in 1904 that "It is much more important to know what sort of patient has a disease than what sort of disease a patient has" (Scherge, 2001). MPs can use the traditional strengths of psychological assessment to augment traditional medicine's focus on the more purely disease or biomedical model of mental illness and mental health.

Due to the domination of clinical psychopharmacology by psychiatry, not much has been written on using behavioral assessment methods, although behavioral assessment should be directly applicable to the assessment and monitoring of drug effects. The absence of data specific to the application of psychological measurements within the field of pharmacotherapy calls for professional humility among prescribing medical psychologists and for the determination to improve on the current state of affairs. Of particular concern is the lack of effectiveness data for demonstrating what, clinically, many psychologists see as overprescribing to children.

---

[16]Taking the patient's vitals, a part of the physical exam, can be extremely important in identifying cardiac and metabolic dysfunction.

Current controversy about the molding and, some would argue, pure invention of disease (Greenberg, 2011) through pharmaceutical companies' influence in *DSM-5* development points out the dangers of bias in diagnosing and recommending certain treatments and, ultimately, in monitoring treatment effectiveness when such evaluations are based merely on clinical impressions. All of these factors cry for external measures, often behavioral, of drug effectiveness.

Behavioral Assessment Methods

Direct Observation

Perhaps the most time-honored way to assess medication therapeutic effects is direct observation. At times it is difficult to separate direct observation from self-report. The tradition of psychology calls upon one to be skeptical of self-report at times, as direct observation theoretically yields more reliable data. All too often the patient's report differs from what is observed (van Noorden et al., 2010). Direct observation is obtained by frequent contact with the patient and familiarity with the patient's symptoms as they develop, or improve, across time. Direct observation argues for repeated and, oftentimes, frequent visits, which is far more the modus operandi of clinical psychology than it is of modern-day psychiatry.

Patient Self-Report

Self-report or patient estimate of drug effect vies with direct observation as favorite methods. The most common method for patient estimate is to simply ask how the patient is doing with the particular target symptom, comparing today's state with an earlier reference point in time. A somewhat more sophisticated and quasi-standardized form of self-report is found in self-report rating scales. For example, the patient rates current depression on a 1 to 10 scale, which is compared to the patient's rating on the same scale when therapy began. This introduces the familiar *global rating bias* (Piotrowski, Barnes-Farrell, & Srig, 1989), which is partly addressed by using self-rating scales that measure only one dimension of emotional status, such as the Beck Depression Inventory II or the Beck Anxiety Inventory. The advantage of using such inventories is to compare specific items, as in suicidality, across time.

Clinician Instruments

To address the inadequacies of patient self-report, clinicians often rate their patients on symptom scales such as the Brief Psychiatric Rating Scale for Schizophrenia (Psychiatric Times, 2011), Positive and Negative Affect Scale (Crawford & Henry, 2004), Hamilton Depression Rating Scale (Hamilton, 1960, 1997),[17] Clinical Global Impression (Guy, 1976), and several others. Many of these scales, nonetheless, are only slightly less subjective than the more transparent self-rating scales. Psychologists, in contrast, tend to develop and use tests in clinical practice that provide more objective psychometric measures of change, including vigilance testing for attention deficit disorder such as the Continuous Performance Test (CPT), across time.

---

[17]This is the scale that is used in the vast majority of pharmaceutical industry research on antidepressants. It has been criticized as psychometrically weak (Bagby, Ryder, Schuller, & Marshall, 2004), but it has a long history and is invariably used to compare new research data with findings in previous research using the Hamilton scale.

With controversy regarding possible overprescribing to children (Mathews, 2010), valid objective measures for diagnosing conditions such as Attention Deficit–Hyperactivity Disorder (ADHD) and for subsequently testing drug effects on the condition are more than warranted. However, with the exception of CPT testing for attention-deficit diagnosing and subsequent retesting for the efficacy of analeptics such as amphetamine and methylphenidate, relatively few objective measures of drug effect have been proposed. Depression measures focused on motor behavior would seem to provide a direction worth pursuing, especially since motor behavior is often assessed in animals to develop these drugs.

Measures of Function

Though the measurement of change occupies a long and occasionally troubled history in applied psychology, many practitioners see the goal of treatment as the improvement of life functions or in activities of daily living. While much maligned for multiple reasons, the *Diagnostic and Statistical Manual of Mental Disorders IV—Text Revision* (*DSM-IV-TR*) (American Psychiatric Association, 2000) provides ratings for an estimate of global functioning on Axis V, both for the patient's present functioning as well as for the same patient's highest level of functioning in the past year. Physical therapists and occupational therapists have long used measures of function to assess change; perhaps changes in daily functions such as ADLs could be adopted and standardized by medical psychologists to better measure the effects of pharmacotherapy and/or psychotherapy over the course of treatment.

Psychometrics at the Service of the Prescribing Medical Psychologist

In addition to biomedical testing and overall psychological assessment of patients, the medical psychologist can use specific psychometric measures, such as intellectual and neuropsychological tests, to aid in diagnosis and to direct overall treatment goals, including pharmacotherapy as well as psychosocial treatment modalities. These same measures can be used as indications for medication regimens, and finally to assist data on therapeutic effectiveness.

A historic strength, diagnostic prowess is a hallmark of clinical psychology. Building on this tradition, the medical psychologist appropriately assesses the full range of the patient's cognitive, behavioral, and affective functioning. MPs use standard psychological tests of psychopathology (e.g., Minnesota Multiphasic Personality Inventory [MMPI], Millon) as well as cognitive measures (e.g., Wechsler, Stanford-Binet), while those with training in neuropsychology also employ full neuropsychological batteries to differentiate conditions associated with organic factors (e.g., dementia, traumatic brain injury). Diagnosis is imperative to differential treatment, and it is here that the medical psychologist contributes a unique skill to the array of professionals currently prescribing for the mental health population. The strongest case for prescribing psychotropic medications is found when (a) a condition can be clearly differentiated, and (b) the condition has a known efficacious pharmacological treatment.

One of the most helpful uses of psychological assessment with respect to diagnosis and psychopharmacology is the ability to differentiate affective conditions from more specific brain disorders. Differentiation of the demented patient from the patient with major depression leads to very different treatment recommendations. Although both patients may be depressed, ignoring the relative contribution of each condition could lead to inadequate or wrong treatment. Similarly, differential diagnosis of attention deficit disorder from conduct disorder, oppositional defiant disorder, or learning disorder with comorbidities can lead to the underlying condition being adequately understood and, consequently, appropriately treated.

Psychological Assessment and Medication Monitoring

In addition to aiding diagnosis and providing for a more discriminating selection among psychobiosocial treatments, affective, personality, cognitive, and neuropsychological psychometric measures, when used serially, can assess continuous change and thereby monitor the effectiveness of therapy, including pharmacological treatment. As mentioned previously, since psychostimulant use is indicated with Attention Deficit–Hyperactivity Disorder (ADHD), it is important to serially measure its effect with the CPT and ADHD scales (DuPaul, Power, Anastopoulos, & Reed, 1998). Similarly, *acetylcholinesterase inhibitors*, such as donepezil and rivastigmine, prescribed for dementia, are another opportunity to measure medication effects on cognition and behavior across time on neuropsychological instruments. From that perspective, even the Folstein Mini Mental Status Examination offers a gross measure of cognitive function that can be administered periodically as treatment progresses.

Empirical Prescribing

Known in philosophy as circular logic, the idea that a drug that improves a condition also diagnoses the condition has been accepted by clinicians unknowledgeable in scientific deduction. To some, this was a form of empirical prescribing: I diagnosed you with ADHD and you improved with Ritalin; therefore, my diagnosis is empirically correct. The approach holds some intuitive appeal (i.e., it works), but it is conceptually erroneous, not only because it is based on a logical fallacy but because many psychotropics are broad-spectrum drugs (Stahl, 2008) and affect a variety of conditions.[18] Empirical prescribing, for the medical psychologist, means that treatment recommendations based on solid science are assigned to a given patient after a differential diagnosis indicates that the treatment is appropriate. Factors such as the patient's age, gender, race, and sociocultural beliefs are also taken into consideration to the extent that evidence-based guidelines provide for the relevance of such subject variables. If, indeed, pharmacotherapy is considered the first-line approach for the individual patient's needs, then careful note is made of the effectiveness of the medication, as well as its side effects, over time. Adjustments are made as the prescribing psychologist continues to collect feedback data.

Differential Diagnosis and Referral to Other Health Care Providers

To know when to seek assistance with differential diagnosis and subsequent referral to other health care providers necessitates that one knows what to look for (i.e., signs and symptoms of clinical medicine) and when those signs and symptoms necessitate a referral for subsequent evaluation. This implies that the condition is outside the

---

[18]Certain drugs are FDA approved for several conditions. For example, the selective serotonin reuptake inhibitor sertraline holds FDA approval for major depressive disorder, obsessive-compulsive disorder, panic disorder, posttraumatic stress disorder (PTSD), premenstrual dysphonic disorder (PMDD), and social anxiety disorder (Rxlist, 2010b). Similarly, the benzodiazepine diazepam may be used as an anxiolytic agent, but is it also used for management of acute alcohol withdrawal, for relief of skeletal muscle spasms, and as an adjunct in convulsive disorders (Rxlist, 2010a).

clinician's capacity to treat the symptom or disorder. Referral therefore stems from an accurate and timely diagnosis, based on training and scope of practice and combined with the knowledge of one's strengths and limitations as a clinician.

Techniques for Differential Diagnosis and Referral

The prescribing medical psychologist has not abrogated or given up traditional psychological assessment, although that assessment may be performed by others. In deciding to refer to other biomedical providers, the MP pursues the same goals and often uses the same tools for differential assessment as other psychologists. That is, after the initial evaluation has been performed by the medical psychologist, he or she must determine whether the clinical impression derived from the evaluation argues for the need for further assessment based on psychological as well as biomedical information available. If the physical examination and laboratory studies merited a referral to a physician or another health care provider before one gained psychopharmacological training, then they would continue to warrant that same referral after gaining prescriptive authority. Although the prescribing medical psychologist might competently take vital signs and order laboratory tests, if the results are abnormal the patient would be referred to the appropriate specialist.

While differential diagnosing within the specialty of prescribing medical psychology usually requires a detailed history, laboratory studies, and psychological assessment, the medical psychologist does not engage in the practice of medicine outside of his or her specialty; we would not anticipate that the MP would order genetic studies or engage in other medical "challenge" procedures due to the scope of practice of the specialty.

When to Refer

If a patient appears to have a specific disorder that can be treated better by a different specialty within or outside of psychology or mental health, then that patient would be referred to the indicated colleague. In this sense, most prescribing medical psychologists engaged in general practice will refer to specialty clinics for pain management, complex neuropsychological disorders (including traumatic brain injury), and special populations such as geriatrics, children, and adolescents.

What is more, some biomedical findings indicate immediate referral to specific health care specialists. Often, medical psychologists refer for further medical workup for unexplained physical findings (e.g., pain, weakness, gait disturbances, vision or hearing difficulties) or for obvious medical symptoms. Similarly, the prescribing medical psychologist often refers persons for further evaluation with abnormal basic and comprehensive metabolic panels. Not only does this ensure good treatment planning, but also the patient becomes aware of the MP's integrative role in comprehensive treatment. This provider also expeditiously refers any patients with respiratory, cardiac, or head injury issues due to the possibility of morbidity and mortality. And finally, any unexplained drug questions or drug–drug interactions can be referred to a clinical pharmacist or diagnostician, to explain the clinical circumstances and make suggestions. In this respect, it is advisable for the psychologist to make the effort to meet colleagues from various specialties and develop collegial relationships that facilitate telephone consultations when a question arises. These relationships quickly become reciprocal, as the prescribing psychologist often receives queries from his or her medical colleagues regarding clinical psychopharmacology.

Primary Care Psychology and the Prescribing Medical Psychologist

The primary care model of medical treatment and primary care psychology can be used to coax the treatment providers to work as a team. No one provider owns the patient; and physicians and others often greatly value the psychologist's expertise, especially if it involves prescribing or managing psychotropic medications. This kind of collaborative relationship is often seen between pediatricians and prescribing child psychologists (Muse, Brown, & Cothran-Ross, 2011).

ABILITY TO PROVIDE INFORMED CONSENT

For the prescribing medical psychologist, competency on the part of the patient is not a forensic question, but an operational one in which the psychologist determines whether the patient understands what medications are proposed, consents to their use, and is capable of understanding the consequences of that decision. This is undoubtedly an ethical question,[19] but it is also a clinical one: To what extent will compliance be compromised by a patient who is not fully capable of providing informed consent? A literature search of informed consent and medications most often finds the issue addressed through informed consent of subjects in a research protocol for medications. Prescribing medical psychologists will most certainly become more involved with research and the production of new medications, but our focus here is on the clinically active MP who is concerned with gaining informed consent from patients.

Although most adults presumably possess the ability to make an informed consent to take medications—especially adults and adolescents above the age to consent to medical treatment on their own—some groups either by law or by presumed limitation (e.g., age, intellectual limitation, disease process) require a more thorough investigation. The consent to take or decline medications might also require another responsible person such as a guardian or person tasked with consenting to medical care.

Children and adolescents, the elderly with diminished cognitive function, the mentally retarded, and the seriously mentally ill are subpopulations that require special consideration when attempting to form a therapeutic alliance and to enlist compliance through informed consent. Dell, Vaughan, & Kratochvil (2008) reviewed the many ethical and legal issues related to prescribing to children, and the prescribing medical psychologist who works with children and families would be well advised to consider such issues. While the information concerning the nature of the medication prescribed given to a young child need not be in technical detail, any effort to answer the child's concerns is certainly advisable in creating a collaborative relationship with the child and creating greater probability of compliance.

Mental retardation comes in many degrees, and the extent of the patient's understanding and ability to give consent, albeit partial, depends a great deal on the type of mental retardation in question. Recall that the diagnosis of mental retardation requires formal testing and an adaptive measure. One of the few studies in this area compared 50 mild mentally retarded persons with 50 moderately retarded and 50 controls (Fisher, Cea, Davidson, & Fried, 2006). About half of the mildly

---

[19]See Chapter 10 for a full discussion of the ethics of informed consent.

mentally retarded could comprehend concepts of human rights inherent in consent. The greater the mental retardation, the less the subjects were able to comprehend the concept of consent. In such cases, the perceptive psychologist not only works to gain the trust of the patient by therapeutic rapport, but also enlists the collaboration of the patient's caregiver by spending the time to answer all questions related to informed consent. The therapeutic alliance, in such circumstances, is a dual one in which the goal is to facilitate compliance on the part of the patient and the caregiver.

Most of the research in decisional capacity of the seriously mentally ill who take medication concerns schizophrenia (Paul & Oyebode, 1999), but other serious mental illnesses such as bipolar disorder or dementia have been investigated as well. In general, inpatient psychiatric patients demonstrate less consistency in their decision making than normal subjects do, and decision making among the hospitalized is further compromised by chronicity and degree of psychopathology (Rosenfeld & Turkheimer, 1995). Apart from the legal and ethical questions inherent in medicating the seriously mentally ill without their full consent, it is our argument that every attempt should be made to facilitate the patient's understanding of the recommendations being made and to enlist the greatest degree of cooperation and collaboration possible. It is a reasonable assumption that medication works in great part through the therapeutic alliance that ideally accompanies a collaborative relationship between patient and doctor.

CHAPTER 6 KEY TERMS

Accuracy: How a sample or test result compares to a gold standard or comparison sample or whether the test measures what it is supposed to measure.

Acetylcholinesterase inhibitors: Medications that inhibit the anabolism of the enzyme acetylcholinesterase, often used with dementing disorders to increase acetylcholine.

Activities of daily living (ADLs): Activities that one does to maintain a functional life, such as personal hygiene, housekeeping, and work.

Adverse drug event: An actual injury from a drug; any noxious, unintended, and undesired effect of a drug after its administration for prophylaxis or diagnosis.

Adverse drug reaction: Unwanted drug side effect, such as an allergy or immune response or a hypersensitivity reaction, which cannot be predicted from the known pharmacological properties of the drug.

Albumin: The main protein in human blood, responsible for maintaining osmotic pressure.

ALP (alkaline phosphatase): Blood test for detecting the presence of the liver enzyme alkaline phosphate in the blood, thereby detecting liver damage.

ALT (alanine amino transferase): Blood test for detecting the presence of the liver and heart enzyme alanine amino transferase, thereby detecting liver or heart damage.

AST (aspartate amino transferase): Blood test for detecting the presence of the liver and heart enzyme aspartate amino transferase, thereby detecting liver or heart damage.

Auscultation: From the Latin, to listen; auscultation is the technique of listening for body sounds, usually with a stethoscope.

Basic metabolic panel (BMP): Includes measures related to kidney function (blood urea nitrogen and creatinine); blood sugar (measure for hyperglycemia, hypoglycemia, diabetes, and prediabetes); metabolic disturbance with carbon dioxide or carbonate (CO_2); and electrolytes (serum chloride, serum potassium, serum sodium).

Bilirubin: Normal by-product of heme catabolism. Excessive amounts result in jaundice, and may indicate impaired liver function.

Biopsychosocial assessment: Based on psychiatrist George Engel's call for a "new medical model," the biopsychosocial approach includes a detailed assessment of the differential weight that biological, psychological, and social factors have on a given person's health and illness.

Blood sugar: The amount of blood glucose, a measure used to assess metabolic homeostasis.

Blood urea nitrogen (BUN): Lab test that measures the amount of nitrogen in the blood as an index of kidney function. Nitrogen is a by-product of protein breakdown in the liver and the production of urea. The kidneys' ability to rid the blood of BUN is an indication of their efficiency.

Clinical medicine: The study of disease by direct examination of the living patient.

Clinical treatment guidelines: Recommendations and protocols developed by a specialty to deal with aspects of the clinical management of the conditions treated within the specialty. Guidelines can be based on professional opinion (consensus) or can be evidence-based.

Comprehensive metabolic panel (CMP): In addition to the laboratory testing contained in the basic metabolic panel, the CMP adds albumin, alkaline phosphatase, ALT (alanine transaminase), AST (aspartate aminotransferase), calcium, direct bilirubin, gamma-GT (gamma-glutamyl transpeptidase), and LDH (lactate dehydrogenase). See also basic metabolic panel (BMP).

Computerized tomography (CT): Series of X-rays taken from different angles to produce cross-sectional images of soft tissues and bone; CT is an older imagery test, now often eclipsed by magnetic resonance imaging (MRI).

Creatinine clearance: Lab test that compares the amount of creatinine in the urine with creatinine levels in the blood. Creatinine is a by-product of normal creatine breakdown in the muscle, and its rate of clearance is an indicator of renal function.

Cytochrome P450 enzymes: Metabolic enzymes found in the liver that are responsible for catabolism of many drugs.

Designer drugs: Drugs that are produced to circumvent current drug laws pertaining to controlled substances.

Dynamometer: A handheld device for measuring force, strength, or power.

Electrocardiogram (ECG, EKG): Records cardiac activity such as heartbeat and electrical conduction through structure of the heart; provides information on heart attacks, arrhythmias, and heart failure.

Electroencephalogram: A recording of brain activity obtained by placing sensors on the scalp that read neural activity within the cranium.

Electrolytes: Substances that become ions in a solution and potentiate conductivity. Blood tests of electrolytes measure sodium, potassium, and chloride. CO_2 is also part of the electrolyte panel as an overall measure of pH in the blood resulting from the anion-cation balance of electrolytes. The anion gap (total sodium concentrates minus total chloride and CO_2 concentrates) is another index of electrolyte balance or, in the case of metabolic acidosis, imbalance.

Emedicine: Online clinical reference site for professionals: http://emedicine.medscape .com/

Epocrates: Online drug reference site for prescribing professionals: http://www .epocrates.com/

First pass: First pass effect or first pass metabolism refers to a process whereby a substantial part of a drug is metabolized by the liver, due to preferential shunting via the hepatic portal system, before the drug enters into the systemic circulatory system.

Folstein Mini Mental Status Examination: Brief 30-point questionnaire used for cognitive impairment screening.

Functional magnetic resonance imaging (fMRI): Functional MRI combines the information from the MRI with use of oxygen in the brain to indicate which regions are active and which are not; information is often shown in graphical, colored format, sometimes in real time. See also magnetic resonance imaging (MRI).

Global rating bias: The hypothesis that rater bias is a function of the rating instrument, and that multidimensional instruments run a greater risk of spillover bias from one dimension to another on the same instrument.

Glomerular filtration rate (GFR): A lab test to measure kidney function. The GFR is the volume of fluid filtered from the renal glomerular capillaries into the Bowman's capsule per unit time. The GFR can be determined by injecting inulin into the plasma. Since inulin is neither reabsorbed nor secreted by the kidney after glomerular filtration, its rate of excretion is directly proportional to the rate of filtration of water and solutes across the glomerular filter.

Half-lives: The elimination half-life is the time it takes for a drug to lose half of its pharmacological activity.

Hematocrit: A lab test that measures the percentage of blood volume that is made up of red blood cells. It is part of the complete blood count.

Hemoglobin: A red blood cell containing an iron ion, which transports oxygen.

History taking: As practiced by the medical psychologist, questioning the patient or significant other concerning the patient's psychobiosocial functioning, and documenting answers obtained.

Imaging studies: Tests performed with a variety of instruments for obtaining pictures of the inside of the patient's body.

Institute of Medicine (IOM): The Institute of Medicine, of the National Academy of Sciences, is an independent, nonprofit organization that works outside of government to provide unbiased and authoritative advice to decision makers and the public. http://resources.iom.edu/widgets/timeline/index.html

Magnetic resonance imaging (MRI): Uses a magnetic tube, which contains the patient, to create a magnetic field and produce detailed 3-D images of the organs and tissues; often used to image the brain and spinal cord as well as heart, MRI has superseded the older CT scan for much of medicine.

Medline: The National Library of Medicine's premier bibliographic database covering the fields of medicine, nursing, dentistry, veterinary medicine, the health care system, and the preclinical sciences. Online access at: http://www.nlm.nih.gov/databases/databases_medline.html

Mental status examination: An assessment of a patient's level of cognitive (knowledge-related) ability, behavior, emotional mood, and speech and thought patterns at the time of evaluation.

Nerve conduction studies: An electrophysiological test that evaluates the conduction of electrical impulses down peripheral nerves.

Neurocognitive assessment: A specialized evaluation that is primarily concerned with learning and behavior in relation to brain function.

Neurological examination: The assessment of sensory neuron and motor responses, especially reflexes, to determine whether the nervous system is impaired. In addition to peripheral nerves, it specifically tests the 12 pairs of cranial nerves that emanate from the nervous tissue of the brain.

Percussion: The examiner places one hand on the patient and then taps that hand with the index finger of the other hand. The examiner uses this technique to determine whether various organs are enlarged.

Pharmacodynamics: The study of the biochemical and physiological effects of drugs and the mechanisms of their actions.

Pharmacogenetics: The study of how genes influence an individual's response to drugs.

Pharmacokinetics: The movement of a drug through the body, involving four phases: absorption, distribution, metabolism, and excretion.

Physical examination: The process by which a doctor (health care professional) personally inspects the body of a patient for signs of disease.

Practice guidelines: Systematically developed statements to assist practitioners and patients in making decisions about appropriate health care. While some may pretend that such guidelines are evidence-based, this is more of a goal than a fact in medicine in general and clinical psychopharmacology in particular.

Presenting complaint: The reason the patient consults a health care professional, expressed in the patient's own words; for example, "I can't get out of bed in the morning because I feel hopeless and depressed."

Prolonged QT interval: An ECG marker for ventricular tachyarrhythmias like torsades de pointes; a risk factor for sudden death.

Psychopharmacology Examination for Psychologists (PEP): A 150-question, multiple-choice exam developed by the College of Professional Psychology of the American Psychological Association. The test has been adopted by different licensing jurisdictions as one of the many requisites for demonstrating that a medical psychologist is adequately trained to prescribe.

Quadrants: The four sections into which the x-y plane is divided by the x-axis and y-axis. For example, the abdomen is divided into upper left quadrant, upper right quadrant, lower left quadrant, and lower right quadrant.

Review of systems (ROS): A list of questions, arranged by organ system, designed to uncover dysfunction and disease.

Rxlist: An Internet drug index of prescription medications. Access at http://www.rxlist.com

Scope of practice: The activities that an individual health care provider performs in the delivery of patient care.

Sensitivity: A test's ability to correctly identify individuals with a particular condition (i.e., true positives).

Specificity: A test's ability to correctly exclude individuals without a condition (i.e., true negatives).

Steady state: Condition in which the introduction of substances keeps pace with their destruction or removal so that all volumes, concentrations, and pressures remain constant.

Subsyndromal: Presentation characterized by symptoms that are not severe enough for diagnosis as a clinically recognized syndrome.

Tail-end distribution: Sometimes referred to as long tail distribution; refers to a skewed distribution in which few cases are found at any one data point because there is no grouping of frequencies; thus low frequency does not necessarily indicate a data point outside of the norm.

Testing panels: A set of lab tests, standardized to investigate common function or disease, such as a liver panel to establish liver compromise or a white blood count to establish infection.

Therapeutic drug monitoring (TDM): The measurement of specific drugs at timed intervals in order to maintain a relatively constant concentration of the medication in the bloodstream.

Thyroid-stimulating hormone (TSH): A peptide hormone synthesized and secreted by thyrotrope cells in the anterior pituitary gland, which regulates the endocrine function of the thyroid gland.

Thyroxine (T4): Hormone made by the thyroid gland that has four iodine molecules attached to its molecular structure. T4 and other thyroid hormones help regulate growth and control the rate of chemical reactions (metabolism) in the body.

Torsades de pointes: A potentially fatal condition in which the QT interval is markedly increased and a ventricular tachycardia occurs in which the QRS complex varies from beat to beat.

Triiodothyronine (T3): A hormone made by the thyroid gland. It has three iodine molecules attached to its molecular structure. It is the most powerful thyroid hormone, and affects many metabolic processes in the body, including body temperature, growth, and heart rate.

White blood cell count (WBC): Measures the number of white blood cells: basophils, eosinophils, lymphocytes (T cells and B cells), monocytes, and neutrophils.

Chapter 6 Questions

1. Which of the following offers the most potential for therapeutic blood monitoring?
   a. Thiorizadine
   b. Olanzapine
   c. Lithium carbonate
   d. Fluoxetine

2. Which drug effect measure, theoretically, has the most potential in children?
   a. Positive and negative affect scale
   b. Teacher rating
   c. Direct observation of motoric behavior
   d. Verbal report by child

3. Which of the following findings is most consistent with uncontrolled diabetes?
   a. Elevated serum cholesterol
   b. Pain and sensitivity on soles of feet
   c. Elevated serum calcium
   d. Sweet, sickly breath

4. Which is *not* part of a WBC?
   a. Neutrophils
   b. Eosinophils
   c. Hemophils
   d. Basophils

5. The comprehensive metabolic panel includes all of the following except
   a. Electrolytes.
   b. Complete blood count.
   c. ANA.
   d. Glucose.

6. _____ and _____ hold the most promise in assessing changes due to administration of psychiatric medications.
   a. Teacher ratings, self-description
   b. Direct observation, neurocognitive evaluation
   c. Vigilance testing, affective measures
   d. Self-report, teacher report

7. Which patient potentially presents the greatest difficulty in gaining informed consent for taking psychiatric medications?
   a. Child with guardian
   b. Elderly patient with lupus
   c. Psychiatric patient recently involuntarily admitted to infectious disease ward
   d. Mildly mentally retarded patient

8. Which of the following is *not* a part of a renal panel?
   a. ALT
   b. BUN
   c. GFR
   d. Creatinine clearance

9. Which of the following is *not* in a standard electrolyte panel?
   a. Sodium
   b. Potassium
   c. Iron
   d. Chloride

10. Excessive bilirubin in the urine probably indicates
    a. Hepatic dysfunction.
    b. Renal dysfunction.
    c. Heart attack.
    d. Illicit drugs.
11. Review of systems (ROS)
    a. Refers to the physical exam.
    b. Is performed before the physical exam.
    c. Refers to the neurological exam.
    d. Is not required for children.
12. Basic metabolic panel tests for
    a. Kidney function.
    b. Liver function.
    c. Blood pH.
    d. All of the above.

    Answers: (1) c, (2) c, (3) d, (4) c, (5) c, (6) b, (7) c, (8) a, (9) c, (10) a,
    (11) b, and (12) d.

REFERENCES

American Association for Clinical Chemistry. (2010a, December 26). *Basic metabolic panel*. Retrieved from http://www.labtestsonline.org/understanding/analytes/bmp/glance.html

American Association for Clinical Chemistry. (2010b, December 26). *Laboratory tests online*. Retrieved from http://www.labtestsonline.org/understanding/features/reliability-2 .html

American Psychiatric Association. (2000). *Diagnostic and statistical manual of mental disorders* (4th ed., text rev.). Washington, DC: Author.

American Psychological Association. (2009). *Practice guidelines regarding psychologists' involvement in pharmacological issues*. Washington, DC: Author.

American Psychological Association. (2010, December 25). *Psychopharmacology Examination for Psychologists candidate application guide*. Retrieved from http://www.apapracticecentral .org/ce/courses/pep-application.pdf

Apgar, V. (1953). A proposal for a new method of evaluation of the newborn infant. *Current Research in Anesthesiology and Analgesia, 32*, 260–267.

Bagby, R., Ryder, A., Schuller, D., & Marshall, M. (2004). The Hamilton Depression Rating Scale: Has the gold standard become a lead weight? *American Journal of Psychiatry, 161*, 2163–2177.

Baumann, P., Hiemke, C., Ulrich, S., Eckermann, G., Kuss, H., Laux, G., Müller-Oerlingenhausen, B., Rao, M., Riederer, P., & Zernig, G. (2006). Arbeitsgemeinschaft fur Neuropsychopharmakologie und Pharmakopsychiatrie (AGNP)—Therapeutic Drug Monitoring (TDM). [Therapeutic drug monitoring (TDM) of psychotropic drugs: A consensus guideline of the AGNP-TDM group] [Article in French, abstract in English]. *Revue Medicale de la Suisse Romande, 24*, 1413–1418, 1420–1422, 1424–1426. PMID: 16786958 [PubMed—indexed for Medline]

Bickley, L. S. (2008) *Bates' guide to physical examination and history taking* (10th ed.). Philadelphia, PA: Lippincott.

Broglin, D. (2003). Status epilepticus: Pharmacokinetic basis of anticonvulsant treatment in adults. *Annales Françaises d'Anesthésie et de Réanimation, 20*, 159–170.

Cassels, C. (2010). Metabolic monitoring in patients taking second generation antipsychotics remains poor. *Medscape Today*, January 7, 2010.

Centers for Education and Research on Therapeutics. (2011). http://www.qtdrugs.org/

Chahl, P. (2005). A physical lesson for the clinicians? *Advances in Psychiatric Treatment, 11*, 31.

Chue, P., & Singer. P. (2003). A review of olanzapine-associated toxicity and fatality in overdose. *Journal of Psychiatry and Neuroscience, 28*, 253–261.

Council on Scientific Affairs. (1987). Scientific issues in drug testing. *Journal of the American Medical Association, 257*, 3110–3114.

Crawford, J. R., & Henry, J. D. (2004). The Positive and Negative Affect Schedule (PANAS): Construct validity, measurement properties and normative data in a large non-clinical sample. *British Journal of Clinical Psychology, 43*, 245–265.

Curley, F., & Irwin, R. (2008). Disorders of temperature control II: Hyperthermia. In R. S. Irwin & J. M. Ripp (Eds.), *Intensive care medicine*. Philadelphia, PA: Lippincott, Williams & Wilkins.

DeLeon, J. (2004). Psychopharmacology: Atypical antipsychotic doing: The effect of smoking and caffeine. *Psychiatric Service, 55*, 491–493.

Dell, M. L., Vaughan, B. S., & Kratochvil, C. J. (2008). Ethics and the prescription pad. *Child and Adolescent Psychiatric Clinics of North America, 17*(1), 93–111.

DuPaul, G., Power, T., Anastopoulos, A., & Reed, R. (1998). *ADHD Rating Scale—IV*. New York: Guilford.

Eichelbaum, M. (1976). Drug metabolism in thyroid disease. *Clinical Pharmacokinetics, 1*, 339–350.

Emedicine. (2011). Accessed from http://emedicine.medscape.com

Engel, G. (1977). The need for a new medical model: A challenge for biomedicine. *Science, 196*, 129–136.

Engel, J., & Pedley, T. (2008). *Epilepsy: A comprehensive textbook, Vol. 1*. Philadelphia, PA: Lippincott, Williams & Wilkins.

Fann, W. E. (2004). Drug interactions casebook: The cytochrome P450 system and beyond. *American Journal of Psychiatry, 161*, 2145–2146.

Fisher, C. B., Cea, C., Davidson, P. W., & Fried, A. L. (2006). Capacity of persons with mental retardation to consent to participate in randomized clinical trials. *American Journal of Psychiatry, 163*, 1813–1820.

Food and Drug Administration. (2011). *Antipsychotic drugs: Class labeling change—Treatment during pregnancy and potential risk to newborns*. Washington, DC: Author.

Gawande, A. (2009). *The checklist manifesto: How to get things right*. New York, NY: Picador.

Geller, B., & DelBello, M. (2008). *Treatment of bipolar disorder in children and adolescents*. New York, NY: Guilford.

Greenberg, G. (2010, December). Inside the battle to define mental health. *Wired*.

Guy, W. (1976). *ECDEU assessment manual for psychopharmacology*. Rockville, MD: Department of Health, Education, and Welfare.

Hamilton, M. (1960). A rating scale for depression. *Journal of Neurology, Neurosurgery and Psychiatry, 23*, 56–62.

Hamilton, M. (1997). *The Hamilton rating scale for depression*. Reproduced by GlaxoWellcome, Inc.

Haymond, J., & Ensom, M. H. H. (2010). Does valproic acid warrant therapeutic drug monitoring in bipolar affective disorder? *Therapeutic Drug Monitoring, 32*, 19–29.

Hiemke, C. (2008). Clinical utility of drug measurement and pharmacokinetics: Therapeutic drug monitoring in psychiatry. *European Journal of Clinical Pharmacology 64*, 159–166.

Howland, R. D., Mycek, M. J., Harvey, R. A., & Champe, P. C. (2005). *Lippincott's illustrated reviews: Pharmacology* (3rd ed.). Philadelphia, PA: Lippincott-Raven Publishers.

Janicak, P. G., Davis, J. M., Preskorn, S. H., & Ayd, F. J. (2001). *Principles and practice of psychopharmacotherapy* (3rd ed.). Philadelphia, PA: Lippincott, Williams & Wilkins.

Jarvis, C. (2004). *Physical examination & health assessment.* St. Louis, MO: Saunders.

Jefferson, J. (2010). A clinician's guide to monitoring kidney function in lithium-treated patients. *Journal of Clinical Psychiatry, 71*, 1153–1157.

Jensvold, M., Halbreich, U., & Hamilton, J. (1996). *Psychopharmacology and women: Sex, gender, and hormones.* Washington, DC: American Psychiatric Press.

Kane, J. M., & Correll, C. U. (2010). Past and present progress in the pharmacologic treatment of schizophrenia. *Journal of Clinical Psychiatry, 71*, 1115–1124.

Kantrowitz, J. T., & Citrome, L. (2008). Olanzapine: Review of safety 2008. *Expert Opinion Drug Safety, 7*, 761–769.

Kaufman, D. M. (2006). *Clinical neurology for psychiatrists* (4th ed.). Philadelphia, PA: Saunders.

Kilbourne, A. M., Post, E. P., Bauer, M. S., Zeber J. E., Copeland, L. A., Good, C. B., & Pincus, H. A. (2007). Therapeutic drug and cardiovascular disease risk monitoring in patients with bipolar disorder. *Journal of Affective Disorders, 102*, 145–151.

Marcus, S., Olfson, M., Pincus, H., Zarin, D., & Kupfer, D. (1999). Therapeutic drug monitoring of mood stabilizers in Medicaid patients with bipolar disorder. *American Journal of Psychiatry, 156*, 1014–1018.

Mathews, A. W. (2010). So young and so many pills. *Wall Street Journal.* Retrieved December 31, 2010.

McGahuey, C. A., Gelenberg, A. J., Laukes, C. A., Moreno, F. A., Delgado, P. L., McKnight, K. M., & Manber, R. (2000). Arizona Sexual Experience Scale. *Journal of Sex and Marital Therapy, 26*, 25–40.

MedlinePlus (2010a, November 30). Comprehensive metabolic panel. Retrieved from http://www.nlm.nih.gov/medlineplus/ency/article/003468.htm

MedlinePlus. (2010b, November 30). Creatine clearance. Retrieved from http://www.nlm.nih.gov/medlineplus/ency/article/003611.htm

Moeller, K., Lee, K., & Kissack, J. (2008). Urine drug screening: Practical guide for clinicians. *Mayo Clinic Proceedings, 83*, 66–76.

Muse, M., Brown, S., & Cothran-Ross, T. (2011). Psychology, psychopharmacology and pediatrics: When to treat and when to refer. In G. Kapalka (Ed.), *Pediatricians and pharmacologically trained psychologists: Practitioner's guide to collaborative treatment.* New York, NY: Springer.

Nagy, Z., Szabo, M., & Huttner, I. (1985). Blood-brain barrier impairment by low pH buffer perfusion via the internal carotid artery in rat. *Acta Neuropathologica, 68*, 160–163.

Pagana, K. D., & Pagana, T. J. (2010). *Mosby's diagnostic and laboratory test reference* (10th ed.). St. Louis, MO: Mosby.

Oldendorf, W. (1974). Blood-brain permeability to drugs. *Annual Review of Pharmacology, 14*, 239–248.

Paul, M., & Oyebode, F. (1999). Competence of voluntary psychiatric patients to give valid consent to neuroleptic medication. *Psychiatric Bulletin, 23*, 463–466.

Piotrowski, M., Barnes-Farrell, J., & Srig, F. (1989). Behavioral anchored bias: A replication and extension of Murphy and Constans. *Journal of Applied Psychology, 74*, 823–826.

Preston, J. (2010). *Handbook of clinical psychopharmacology for therapists.* Oakland, CA: New Harbinger.

Psychiatric Times. (2011, January 2). *Clinically useful scales: Brief psychiatric rating scale.* http://www.psychiatrictimes.com/clinical-scales/schizophrenia/

Psychiatry Online. (2011). *Examples of psychiatric rating scales.* Retrieved from http://www.psychiatryonline.com/popup.aspx?aID=137733

Quillin, J. (2007). Medical psychology defined. *ASAP Tablet, 5.*

Raedler, T., & Wiedemann, K. (2007). Lithium-induced nephropathies. *Psychopharmacology Bulletin, 40*, 134–149.

Reed, R., & Dutta, S. (2006). Does it really matter when a blood sample for valproic acid concentration is taken following once-daily administration of divalproex-ER? *Therapeutic Drug Monitoring, 28*, 413-418.

Rosenfeld, B. D., & Turkheimer, E. N. (1995). Modeling psychiatric patients' treatment decision making. *Law and Human Behavior, 19*, 389–405.

Rxlist. (2010a, December 9). *Diazepam.* Retrieved from http://www.rxlist.com/diazepam-drug.htm

Rxlist. (2010b, December 9). *Zoloft.* Retrieved from http://www.rxlist.com/zoloft-drug.htm

Sadock, B. J., Sadock, V. A., & Ruiz, P. (2009). *Kaplan & Sadock's comprehensive textbook of psychiatry* (9th ed.). Philadelphia, PA: Lippincott, Williams & Wilkins.

Sandson, N. (2011). Drug–drug interactions. *Carlat Psychiatric Report, 9*(2), 4–5.

Scherge, J. E. (2001). Commentary. *American Journal of Family Practice, 50.* Retrieved December 29, 2010, from citing Osler, W. (1904). *Aequanimitas.* Philadelphia, PA: Blakiston.

Seidel, H. M., Ball, J. M., Dains, J. E., & Benedict, G. W. (2010). *Mosby's guide to physical examination* (7th ed.). Philadelphia, PA: Mosby.

Stahl, S. M. (2008). *Stahl's essential psychopharmacology: Neuroscientific basis and practical applications* (3rd ed.). New York, NY: Cambridge Press.

Teasdale, G., & Jennett, B. (1974). Assessment of coma and impaired consciousness: A practical scale. *Lancet 2*, 81–84.

University of Florida. (2010a). *Medical history taking study guide.* Retrieved from http://medinfo.ufl.edu/year1/bcs/clist/history.html

University of Florida. (2010b). *Online physical exam teaching assistant.* Retrieved from http://opeta.medinfo.ufl.edu/neuro/NE_main.html

University of Iowa. (2010). *Laboratory services handbook.* Iowa City: Author.

van Noorden, M. S., Giltay, E. J., den Hollander-Gijsman, M. E., van der Wee, N. J., van Veen, T., & Zitman, F. G. (2010). Gender differences in clinical characteristics in a naturalistic sample of depressive outpatients: The Leiden Routine Outcome Monitoring Study. *Journal of Affective Disorders, 125*, 116–123.

Chapter 7

DIFFERENTIAL DIAGNOSIS IN MEDICAL PSYCHOLOGY

Kevin M. McGuinness
Michael R. Tilus
Erin M. McGuinness
Mary Y. Sa[1]

The importance of making an accurate differential diagnosis in medical psychology is undeniable when one considers that virtually all *DSM* symptoms can be caused by medical disorders (Madhusoodanan, Danan, & Moise 2007). It is as crucial and potentially life saving for psychologists to be skilled in the identification of patients with organic disorders, as it is essential that psychologists be informed on procedures for referring such patients for more definitive care.[2]

It is of particular importance for medical psychologists, especially prescribing medical psychologists, to be acutely aware of the differential diagnostic process when considering the broad array of health concerns that may be reported by their patients. Just as the family physician should ideally be able to sift through the psychological symptoms presented by patients who seek medical care, medical psychologists must be prepared to sort through the many physical symptoms that may be presented by patients seeking mental health care. Psychotropic medications, whether prescribed by physician or psychologist, can exacerbate or mask underlying physical health problems, causing profound and potentially dangerous consequences for patients.[3] It is incumbent on all practitioners who prescribe for the mental-health population to receive training on how to distinguish between physical and psychological sources of symptom complexes and to be familiar with the deleterious effects that medication can sometimes cause this population. Psychologists are specifically trained in the biopsychosocial model (Muse & McGrath, 2010) to be able to achieve such integration in diagnosis and treatment.

---

[1]Contributors to this chapter include Amandah-beth C. Tilus and Pamelah D. Tilus.

[2]Dr. Younger points out in the previous chapter that medical psychologists contribute to the early diagnosis of physical disease by noting suspect symptoms and referring to medical colleagues.

[3]Witness two recent cases of chemically induced dementia, as related by Dr. Robert Julien (2011), in which an institutionalized elderly patient's cognitive confusion and compromised memory cleared up when an offending tricyclic antidepressant, with anticholinergic actions, was discontinued; and a second patient in her late 80s was able to return to independent living after her clouded sensorium and amnesia were resolved once the offending benzodiazepine was discontinued.

MEDICAL DISORDERS THAT PRESENT AS PSYCHOLOGICAL DISORDERS

Fortunately, the process of proper evaluation and differential diagnosing need not be a guessing game. Table 7.1 lists presenting features that may initially alert the medical psychologist to potential underlying medical causes for psychological symptoms.

In consideration of the many possible presenting features outlined in Table 7.1, it is extremely important for the medical psychologist to initiate and maintain effective and timely communication with a patient's primary care practitioner. Such communication can provide the psychologist with invaluable information regarding a patient's medical history and may fill the information gaps common to the intake process. Ideally, new patients will have had a recent physical examination. Whenever possible, however, it is recommended that each patient's vital signs be recorded and reviewed as a standard part of the medical psychology visit.

Although the medical psychologist does not generally diagnose or treat organic medical conditions, familiarity with medical disorders that commonly present with psychological symptoms is indispensible. Table 7.2 presents a limited list of medical conditions that may masquerade as mental illness.

Although this list is not exhaustive, it provides a sampling of common medical conditions with correlative psychological and neuropsychological consequences. Medical psychologists should be familiar with such medical conditions and with their associated psychological corollaries.

In addition to presenting features that suggest a medical origin to psychological symptoms, there are cognitive, emotional, and behavioral symptoms that are associated with neurological disorders in particular. For example, *reduplicative paramnesia* (a rare condition in which patients believe they are in two locations at once), *denial of blindness*, and *denial of hemiparesis* are all potential psychological symptoms that may stem from neurological origin. Similarly, persecutory delusions and visual hallucinations frequently belie an organic condition. With respect to visual hallucinations,[4] an organic origin is more likely the case when such hallucinations occur in the absence of psychological symptoms. Perceptual distortions that are likely of organic origin include tinnitus, as well as gustatory and olfactory hallucinations. Parenthetically, mania is associated much less commonly with neurological disorders than with depression (Madhusudanan et al., 2007). Other neurological conditions, such as *PKU*[5] can be mistaken for ADHD or autism, and *Graves disease* may present as anxiety. When PKU is suspected, a quick review of the medical chart

---

[4]*Dementia with Lewy bodies* is associated with visual hallucinations in up to 75% of patients while reduplicative paramnesia, also associated with Lewy bodies, is far rarer. Lhermitte's hallucinosis, a mild form of dementia characterized by vivid visual hallucinations originating from lesions affecting the mid-brain and pons (Leo & Ahrens, 1998), is also rare.

[5]*Phenylketonuria (PKU)* is an autosomal recessive metabolic disorder that can mimic autism and ADHD inasmuch as the symptoms that accompany PKU are mental retardation, developmental delay, and hyperactivity. The enzyme phenylalanine hydroxylase, which is the rate-limiting enzyme for catecholamine anabolism, normally converts the amino acid phenylalanine into the amino acid tyrosine. If this reaction does not take place, phenylalanine accumulates and tyrosine is deficient. As phenylalanine builds, it competes for transport across the blood-brain barrier via amino acid transporters, eventually saturating the transporters and limiting access of other essential amino acid to the developing brain, resulting in brain damage and the symptoms associated with PKU.

Table 7.1   Critical Presenting Features Accompanying Psychological Symptoms That May Indicate Physical Etiology

- Late onset of initial presentation
- Known underlying medical conditions
- Atypical presentation of specific psychological disorders
- Absence of family history of mental illness
- Medication use
- Illicit drug use
- Treatment resistance or unusual response to treatment
- Sudden onset of psychological symptoms
- Abnormal vital signs
- Waxing and waning of mental status

Source: Chuang, 2009.

Table 7.2   Medical Conditions That May Present With Mental Health Symptoms

- Progressive neurological diseases such as Parkinson's disease, Huntington's disease, Alzheimer's disease, Picks disease, multiple sclerosis
- Central nervous system infections including neurosyphillis, HIV encephalopathy, encephalitis
- Brain lesions, including brain tumors, infarcts, calcification secondary to blunt force trauma
- Metabolic disorders such as electrolyte imbalances, cirrhosis, kidney disease, Wilson's disease, systemic lupus erythematosus
- Endocrine disorders such as parathyroid disorders, thyroid disease, adrenal disorders, pancreatic disorders
- Seizure disorders, including partial seizures and generalized seizures
- Deficiency states including vitamin deficiencies, electrolyte deficiencies, hormonal deficiencies
- Exogenous toxins
- Many others

may reveal previous diagnostic workups to rule the condition in or rule it out. PKU screening is standard procedure on newborns in the United States. However, there is a growing number of children in this country who are adopted from foreign countries, and one cannot assume that such testing was done. Although the prescribing medical psychologist might order lab tests to screen for PKU, this is a good example of a situation in which the psychologist would most properly collaborate with the patient's primary-care physician; it would more appropriately be the primary-care provider who orders screening since he or she is in a position to counsel the patient on dietary management of PKU, if confirmed.

The case of Graves hyperthyroidism versus anxiety, when working toward a differential diagnosis of psychomotor agitation, racing thoughts, and feelings of panic, demonstrates how conditions with a psychological etiology are difficult to differentiate from those with physical etiology based on presenting symptoms alone.

Table 7.3   Presumptive Clues of Physical Involvement

- Head injury
- Change in headache pattern
- Visual disturbances
- Sudden speech deficits
- Abnormal body movements*
- Abnormal vital signs
- Changes in consciousness

*Unrelated to neuroleptic use

Once again, a physical exam and laboratory work up are essential in this type of determination.

Some clues for identifying underlying medical causes for panic symptoms stemming from cerebral involvement from trauma, infection, or vascular accident include atypical features such as ataxia, alterations in consciousness or bladder control, or precipitous onset of a panic disorder in the elderly. Additionally, apathy is reportedly one of the most frequent personality alterations seen in cerebral disorders (Bózzola, Gorelick, & Freels 1992; Van Reekum, Stuss, & Ostrander, 2005).

According to Madhusoodanan et al. (2007), brain tumors can cause any and all psychiatric symptoms, but may not have accompanying localized signs, which can make the mental status exam less effective in identifying neurological disorders. Therefore, abnormalities of presentation and other inconsistencies in the evaluation process must be closely evaluated by the medical psychologist; when in doubt, it is recommended that the psychologist refer the patient for further medical assessment.

Although a patient may present with abnormal features that can alert the medical psychologist to an underlying medical condition (Chuang, 2009), there are also what Taylor (2007) calls *presumptive clues,* which can lead the psychologist to suspect an underlying medical disorder and prompt a referral for further medical assessment. Table 7.3 presents such clues.

In addition to a thorough patient examination upon intake, an exhaustive history of significant family health issues (complete with collateral input, when possible) is essential. A comprehensive family history can be vital in distinguishing between hereditary patterns of medical illness that tend to present with psychological symptoms and those symptom complexes that are separate from family genetic makeup, but are, instead, unique to the individual patient. Nonetheless, careful family history taking can reveal multigenerational patterns of family-specific symptomatology.

Although laboratory results may be available from previous providers, the prescribing medical psychologist often directly orders lab testing as standard procedure. The safe practice of prescribing often requires preliminary laboratory testing of urine and blood to establish baselines against which to monitor the patient's responses to medications. Such laboratory testing may be especially important in the more vulnerable populations such as children, older adults, patients with known comorbid physical illnesses, patients with some of the presenting features listed in Tables 7.1 to 7.3, or when prescribing medication with side-effect profiles, such as neuroleptics or mood stabilizers, which might upset blood chemistry. With regard to tricyclic amines (TCAs), a *baseline* electrocardiogram (*EKG*) is the standard recommendation, especially for children (Green-Hernandez, Singleton, and Aronzon, 2001), because of potential cardiac side effects. When administering neuroleptics, especially to children, Native Americans, obese adults, elders, or patients with diabetes, it is important to order a *comprehensive metabolic panel* (CMP) and EKG because of these medications' implications in metabolic syndrome. Also, when treating females of child-bearing years who may become pregnant, a pregnancy test is warranted, as many psychotropics carry a *teratogenic risk*. When considering administration of lithium, it is important to assess kidney and thyroid function, and to administer an EKG and metabolic panel. Although this list is not exhaustive, it addresses the more commonly prescribed psychotropic medications and the required baseline labs or tests.[6] When such a protocol is followed, it is more likely that an underlying medical disorder or an iatrogenic result will be properly identified.

In addition to gathering comprehensive family and medical histories and administering baseline tests and ordering lab work, it is also essential for the medical psychologist to include a complete *mental status examination* with acute attention paid to abnormalities in speech, gait, memory, motor skills, comprehension, or sensory perception. A thorough review of the patient's medical record is, of course, crucial, as is notifying the patient's primary health care practitioner of the addition of any psychotropic medications prescribed.

An accurate and comprehensive differential diagnosis by the prescribing medical psychologist is absolutely critical to safe and effective patient care. Overlooking a potential medical origin of a mental illness cannot only lead to poor treatment response but to serious exacerbation of an underlying medical disorder. The process of differential diagnosis is the cornerstone of proper treatment and appropriate referral. Table 7.4 presents a combination of possible physical and psychological bases for some of the symptoms most seen and treated by medical psychologists. Iatrogenic and *substance abuse* conditions, which can mimic psychological symptoms, are presented in Table 7.5.

PSYCHOLOGICAL DISORDERS THAT PRESENT AS MEDICAL DISORDERS

Just as medical disorders often present as mental illness, mental illness quite frequently masquerades in the form of physical symptoms. The differential diagnosis of psychological disorders that present as medical disease has a rich clinical history in *psychosomatic medicine* and *consultation-liaison (C-L) psychiatry* (Levenson, 2005).

Although the process of the psychosomatic consultation is rarely simple, following the process through a systematic procedural framework can be informative and may contribute incrementally to the validity of the eventual differential diagnosis. This chapter's second author often uses Levenson's (2005) outline as follows:

- Speak directly with the referring clinician.
- Review the current records and pertinent past records.
- Review the patient's medications.
- Gather collateral data.
- Interview and examine the patient.

---

[6]See Chapter 6 for a full discussion of laboratory testing and monitoring.

Table 7.4 Differential Diagnosis and Biopsychosocial Etiologies of Mental-Health Symptoms

Presented Symptoms	Associated Conditions	Differentiators	Discriminative Test
Hyperactivity/ motor agitation	1. ADHD 2. PKU 3. Mania 4. Hyperthyroidism	1. & 2. ADHD & Phenylketonuria (PKU) are developmental. 3. Mania has acute onset. 4. Hyperthyroidism = generalized increased energy, while maintaining goal directedness.	1. ADHD = CPT, normed psychometrics. 2. PKU = lab test (Phenylalanine hydroxylase). 3. History taking. 4. Lab test (TSH, T3, T4).
Mental retardation	1. Down syndrome 2. Williams syndrome 3. Fragile X syndrome 4. PKU	1. Distinctive facial physiognomy. 2. Gregariousness, attention deficit. 3. Social anxiety, perseveration. 4. Microcephalia, hyperactivity.	1. Genetic test (trisomy 21 = extra chromosome 21). 2. Genetic test (gene deletions of chromosome 7). 3. Genetic test (expansion of X chromosome). 4. HPLC: High-performance liquid chromatography.
Atypicality	1. Schizophrenia 2. Lewy body dementia 3. Amphetamine abuse 4. Korsakoff	1. Positive and negative symptoms. 2. Visual hallucination, parkinsonism. 3. Paranoia, formication. 4. Confabulation, retrograde and anteriograde amnesia.	1. Clinical interview, psychometrics (MMPI). 2. MR imaging and SPECT of neocortex. 3. Improvement with abstinence. 4. Clinical interview; MRI with contrast of atrophied mamillary bodies.
Anxiety	1. Psychosocial stressors 2. Endocrine disorders 3. Traumatic brain injury (TBI)	1. Significant life events: Immigration, loss of employment, loss of significant other. 2. (a) Hyperthyroidism, (b) hypoglycemia, (c) pheochromocytoma, (d) hyperadrencorticism (Cushings). 3. PTSD associated with injury vs. anxiety over residual effects of TBI.	1. Clinical interview, psychometrics. 2. Labs: (a) TSH, (b) blood glucose, (c) serum metanephrine, (d) dexamethasone suppression test. 3. Clinical interview to establish onset of anxiety.
Depression	1. Type of depression 2. Physical sequelae	1. Major depression vs. dysthymia vs. double depression vs. bipolar vs. adjustment disorder. 2. (a) Postpartum vs. (b) hypoglycemia vs. (c) hypothyroidism vs. (d) infection	1. Clinical interview, psychometrics. 2. (a) History taking, (b) blood glucose, (c) TSH, (d) CBC.
Suicidality	1. Depression 2. Physical malady 3. Alcohol abuse 4. Panic/PTSD	1. Approximately 60% of completed suicides. 2. Approximately 46% of completed suicides. 3. Approximately 43% of completed suicides. 4. Prevalent although stats not as refined.	Risk is higher in a person who reports suicide ideation and suffers from any of the listed co-occurring syndromes. Also, suicide risk significantly increases with the number of comorbid conditions.

- Formulate diagnostic and therapeutic strategies.
- Document with a clinical note.
- Speak directly with the referring clinician, again.
- Provide periodic follow-up.

Medical psychologists, whether working in the area of health, rehabilitation, pain management, or primary care are often called on to make differential diagnosis in the area of psychosomatic disorders. Such psychologists also have at their disposal psychological tests, screenings, and neuropsychological test batteries that often provide additional vital data. This topic will be discussed later in the chapter.

As explained in Chapter 6, a thorough mental status examination and *review of systems* (ROS) provides discrete, detailed and invaluable information about a patient's current condition. Those working in the field of psychosomatic medicine are cautioned against overlooking bona fide physical conditions when working with patients who present stress-related or somatoform symptoms. Just because a patient has a history of *somatization* does not mean that the same patient is not capable of developing a new, physically based, symptom that might be overlooked or minimized if every new condition is not considered on its own merit. James Morrison (1997) suggests clues that, in a psychosomatic presentation, may demand heightened clinical attention:

- New symptoms: These are often ignored, especially if they are relatively mild.
- More symptoms: These may include complaints of dysphoria combined with weight loss, difficulty thinking, sleep disturbance, and suicidal rumination.
- Symptom worsening: Symptom description may change from an occasional twinge of anxiety to outright panic attack; from mild heartburn to crushing substernal chest pain.
- Symptoms that persist: This is not the intermittent "blah" feeling of a bad day, but the persistent, intractable, day-after-day darkness that clouds someone's living.
- Alarming symptoms: Some physical or psychological symptoms automatically speak of serious disease such as a skin discoloration that could be melanoma or suicidal ideas within a depressed state.
- Symptom patterns: Symptoms that occur together tend to suggest a disorder with a common cause or for which a particular treatment may be effective.

In contrast to physically based somatic complaints, patients with psychosomatic illness often present with symptoms and symptom patterns that are often unusual or seemingly illogical. Such patients may mystify, frustrate, and sometimes irritate referring clinicians.

Somatization represents largely unsolved psychological conflict manifest in physical complaints (Lipowski, 1988). These are the patients who "frequently" complain of physical symptoms that either lack demonstrable organic bases or are judged to be grossly in excess of what one would expect on the grounds of objective medical findings. Such patients are ubiquitous in health-care settings worldwide and often present difficult diagnostic and management problems. They may or may not suffer from other mental-health disorders and tend to be high users of medical services, thus contributing to the growing costs of health care (Lipowski, 1988).

Catalina, Macias, and de Cos (2008) found that the prevalence of *factitious disorders* for hospitalized patients was 8%, with individuals most often female and at an average age of approximately 35 years. In the same study, Catalina et al. found that the most frequent symptoms were (a) nonconsistent response to treatment, (b) worsening of the symptoms when faced with the prospect of a discharge plan, (c) disappearance of the symptoms just after being admitted, and (d) intense relationships with other patients or staff during the hospitalization. These researchers noted that, of the patients suspected of factitious disorder, 25% were observed to report spurious physical and psychological symptoms. The challenge of working with factitious disorders is further complicated by high comorbidity rates with other psychological disorders (Catalina, Ugarte, & Moreno, 2009).

Van Dijke et al. (2010), looking for diagnostic determinants that may assist in understanding the symptomatology of somatization disordered patients, found an inverse correlation with *somatoform disorder (SoD)* and borderline personality disorder (BPD) along a continuum of affect dysregulation. After using clinical interviews to confirm or rule out the presence of BPD or SoD in 472 psychiatric inpatients, three qualitatively different forms of affect dysregulation were identified: (1) underregulation; (2) overregulation; and (3) combined under- and overregulation. BPD was associated with greater underregulation of affect, and SoD was associated with greater overregulation of affect. The comorbid BPD and SoD group reported more frequently both over- and underregulation than patients diagnosed with BPD or SoD alone or those with other psychiatric disorders.

In short, medical psychologists must utilize all their skills and abilities to effectively conceptualize the differential diagnosis of patients with medically unexplained symptoms. One of the challenges for the psychologist working in the medical setting is to protect high-utilizing patients from unnecessarily exposing themselves to medical and surgical procedures. Such patients may be at high risk for iatrogenic disease or secondary injury due to unnecessary diagnostic investigations, massive *polypharmacy*, and polysurgery. Further, such patients appear to be more likely to develop abuse and dependence on multiple classes of drugs prescribed for symptom control.

SUBSTANCES OF ABUSE

The ability to recognize and accurately diagnosis *substance use disorders (SUD)* is considered a core competency in psychosomatic and *addiction medicine,* with specialized proficiencies recognized in psychiatry, medicine, and psychology. The prescribing medical psychologist should take this to heart because there is probably no other diagnostic category in *DSM-IV-TR* (American Psychiatric Association, 2000) that depends as much on the psychologist's knowledge of pathophysiology, disease processes, pharmacology, and toxicology. When addressing SUDs, such knowledge must be interwoven with a comprehensive understanding of *substance-induced disorders* and their predictable sequelae of impaired mood, cognition, and behavior. For prescribing medical psychologists working in inpatient or outpatient addiction settings, specialization and subsequent certification in substance abuse by the American Psychological Association's *College of Professional Psychology* (Clay, 2000) is highly recommended. Such specialization, in addition to qualifications as a prescribing medical psychologist, includes competencies in accurate SUD diagnoses and SUD treatment-plan development, as well as collaborative consultation with attending physicians and treatment teams.

With the advent of *DSM-IV* (American Psychological Association, 1994), the category of Organic Mental Disorders was eliminated because the authors concluded that the application of the term *organic* to a select set of mental disorders might have implied that other psychiatric symptoms known as functional symptoms were somehow unrelated to biological factors. The psychiatric debate over structural versus functional notwithstanding, medical psychology, by its biopsychosocial orientation, strives for integration of the artificial dichotomy of mind-body, and maintains that one cannot reasonably pretend that psychological disorders exist disembodied from the physical domain. The balance between biological and genetic vulnerabilities on one hand and environmental/psychosocial stressors on the other hand is a convenient way to categorize etiologies within a *nosology*, but does not do justice to the interplay of the nature-nurture spectrum.

No place is this seen more clearly than in the area of drug-induced mental disorders. In the lead writer's clinical experience, different individuals react differently to the same drug. For example, this writer has seen people experience elation and increased energy under the influence of cocaine, and others develop paranoid delusions and hallucinations. The difference in their idiosyncratic responses is probably due to differences in biological vulnerabilities, genetic factors, and individual neurochemistry as well as personality traits, premorbid (latent or manifest) psychological conditions such as anxiety, depression, and psychosis, and situational factors such as the time, place, and company in which the drug was ingested. In the same way, some individuals with biological vulnerability toward mood disorders or psychosis generally remain stable under their normal life conditions, but, when exposed to severe environmental stressors of either a physical or psychological nature, they decompensate and exhibit an underlying psychotic or mood disorder. This is, perhaps, best documented in the case of increased incidence of psychoses among recent immigrants (Coid et al., 2008; Zolkowska, Canto-Graae, & McNeil, 2001).

As a core psychology competency, the medical psychologist must gather a substantial knowledge of the vast array of psychological signs and symptoms secondary to substances of abuse. In the second author's treatment facility, all patients are interviewed for SUDs because comorbidity is a local norm. In many communities with inpatient or outpatient health-care capability, especially in communities where substance addiction and *substance dependence* is prevalent, addicted patients tend to present initially at their local emergency room or to their primary-care provider (PCP).

Dependence on alcohol, tobacco, and drugs are considered to be chronic medical illnesses with long-term complications like hepatitis C (McLellan, Lewis, O'Brien, & Kleber, 2000). Prescribing medical psychologists working in an integrated general medical setting are truly on the front lines of substance abuse treatment and prevention, and require a dynamic, working knowledge of SUDs which interfaces with other specialties to promote a crucible in which the fields of general medicine, behavioral and family medicine, psychopharmacology, and medical psychology are seamlessly melded.

In general, psychoactive substances exert such powerful effects on the central nervous system that their users may experience profound changes in their thoughts, emotions, and behaviors. In consequence to this, cognitive, emotional, and behavioral syndromes associated with drug use are ubiquitous and include depression, euphoria, anxiety, paranoia, hallucinations, and psychomotor agitation. Intoxication and withdrawal reactions may precipitate a cascade of physical effects and potentially life-threatening conditions. Due to the profound effects of SUDs on the clinical presentation, substance abuse should be considered a diagnosis of exclusion on every working differential diagnosis.

Table 7.5 Differential Diagnosing and Prevention of Side Effects With Psychotropic Medication

Provoked Symptom	Possible Drug Involvement	Diagnostic Differentiators/Prophylaxis/Treatment
Cardiac		Cardiac clearance (EKG).
1. Torsades de pointes	1. Phenothiazines & TCAs.	1. & 2. Screen for history of ischemic heart disease, myocardial infarction, arrhythmias, hypokalemia, hypomagnesia (eating disorders).
2. Palpitations/arrhythmias	2. Amphetamines/methylphenidates, TCAs.	
3. Hypertension	3. Amphetamines/methylphenidates, MAOI.	3. Take blood pressure at baseline and periodically thereafter.
4. Orthostatic hypotension	4. TCAs, neuroleptics.	4. Discontinue if hypotension is pronounced or if patient is elderly.
Movement Disorders		Neurological Exam
1. Tardive dyskinesia	1. Neuroleptics.	1. Discontinue meds and/or prescribe anticholinergics. Consider clozapine.
2. Dyskinesia	2. Cocaine.	2. Drug testing/cocaine detoxification.
3. Akathisia	3. Neuroleptics, SSRIs.	3. Reduce dose or discontinue meds. Consider adding diphenhydramine, mirtazapine, or propranolol.
Anxiety		TSH hyperthyroidism; treatment of hypothyroidism with thyroxin can cause anxiety.
1. Panic, anxiety	1. Amphetamines.	1. Switch amphetamine for guanfacine or atomoxetine in treatment of ADHD.
Depression/mania		Family history of MDD/BPD
1. Depression	1. Benzodiazepines, alcohol.	1. Discontinue benzos, detoxify alcohol.
2. Mania	2. Nearly all antidepressants have potential to induce mania in bipolar patients.	2. Consider lamotrigine.
Rash		Screen for similar reaction to any medications.
1. Stevens-Johnson Syndrome	1. Lamotrigine, carbamazepine, valproic acid, chlorpromazine.	1. Stop meds immediately at slightest indication of rash. Refer to emergency medicine, as needed.

Category	Drugs	Recommendations
Psychoses 1. Prescription drugs 2. Drugs of abuse	1. Amphetamine, Parkinson's treatments, anticholinergic compounds, steroids. 2. Cannabinoids, LSD, mescaline, cocaine, amphetamines, phencyclidine, various designer drugs.	Thorough medical/drug history is essential. Lab screen in case of drugs of abuse. 1. Discontinue medication until psychosis resolved. Switch to alternative meds, or rechallenge at lower dose, when appropriate. 2. Support, reassurance during psychosis. Substance abuse counseling after episode.
Cognitive dysfunction 1. Cognitive blunting 2. Memory 3. Dementia	1. Lithium, carbamazepine, topiramate, valproate. 2. Benzos, marijuana, alcohol. 3. TCAs, alcohol.	Screen drug interactions that raise serum levels. Adjust drug to population age. 1. Switch to lamotrigine or oxcarbazepine. 2. Avoid benzos in elderly/student population. Drug counseling for abuse. 3. Switch from TCAs to SSRI for elderly. Screen for Korsakoff's.
G.I./urinary 1. Loss of appetite 2. Overeating (metabolic syndrome) 3. Sexual dysfunction	1. Amphetamine, bupropion, venlafaxine, alcohol. 2. Olanzapine, risperidone, mirtazapine, quetiapine, gabapentin, lithium. 3. SSRIs/SNRIs.	Screen for problematic eating or sexual dysfunction before prescribing. 1. Dietary changes or medication switching; alcoholism treatment. 2. Screen for diabetes/prediabetes. Take baseline weight, and make periodic checks. 3. Switch to bupropion.
Toxicity syndromes 1. Serotonin syndrome 2. Neuroleptic malignancy syndrome	1. MAOIs SSRIs, SNRIs, TCAs, and many more. 2. Haloperidol, phenothiazines; abrupt withdraw from Parkinson's treatment (dopaminergics).	Screen for syndromes by presenting symptoms and drug history. 1. Increase pulse, dilated pupils, hyperthermia, myoclonus, mental confusion. 2. Fever, muscle rigidity, autonomic instability, elevated CPK, leukocytosis.

Source: Muse (2010).

Every drug, illicit or legal, has side effects, and nearly all the psychotropic agents can produce unwanted emotional, cognitive, behavioral, and medical symptoms. Table 7.5 lists several symptoms associated with iatrogenic drug side effects as well as symptoms associated with drugs of abuse. These potentially confounding associations must be weighed in making an accurate differential diagnosis.

The *DSM-IV-TR* (American Psychiatric Association, 2000) describes broad diagnostic categories of *substance-related disorders (SRD)* that include: (1) disorders (SUDs) that are caused by substances taken by individuals with intent to alter mood or behavior, (2) disorders that are caused by unintentional use of a substance, and (3) medication side effects. SUDs include (1) abuse and (2) dependence, whereas substance-induced disorders (SIDs), through intentional or unintentional use, include (1) intoxication, (2) withdrawal, (3) delirium, (4) dementia, (5) sexual dysfunction, (6) amnesia, (7) psychosis, (8) mood, (9) anxiety, and (10) sleep disorders.

The differential diagnosis of SUDs include many of the general elements of a psychological evaluation, but with particular focus on ruling-in and ruling-out elements of SUDs and SIDs. Such a focus emphasizes early urine toxicological screening, safety evaluation to determine which level of medical care is required (inpatient, detoxification, or outpatient) and collaboration with the PCP. Also part of standard SUDs evaluation is a review of current medical and psychosocial signs and symptoms, the ordering of general lab panels to cover liver, kidney, electrolytes, and hemocytes, as well as more specific tests, such as vitamins B_1, B_{12}, and folate acid levels in alcoholism. A review of the patient's substance-use history is essential in this process, as is the presence of comorbid medical conditions and/or comorbid psychiatric and SUD/SID, any history of suicidal/homicidal ideation, and/or premorbid/comorbid physical disability and cognitive impairment. Family history, including SUDs in the family and current family support or lack thereof, are essential social factors that compose the psychobiosocial assessment of the medical psychologist.

In some settings, the potential for an SUD/SID to color any clinical presentation is so great, especially in an acute presentation, that the differential diagnostic process might be presumptively and appropriately weighted toward a SUD/SID early in the assessment process; other Axis I and Axis II possibilities can be deferred for later reevaluation. In the authors' experience, it can be very difficult to separate symptoms of chronic intoxication and withdrawal from those of preexisting Axis I or Axis II pathological conditions.

The ability to identify key psychological, physiological, cognitive, and behavioral signs and symptoms of overdose, withdrawal, delirium, dementia, or psychosis associated with various drug types can provide a good starting point for the working differential diagnosis. A case in point is *Korsakoff syndrome*. For the discerning clinician working in the emergency room setting, a patient brought in with anterograde amnesia and persistent delusions might be interviewed with a family member present. Although all possible etiologies of the symptoms are explored (head trauma, schizophrenia, brief psychotic episode due to extreme stress exposure, history of mood disorder, toxic food/chemical ingestion, iatrogenic drug reaction, and substance abuse), the right questions will likely elicit the clues needed for a more discriminating evaluation. A history of alcoholism would raise the possibility of acute alcohol poisoning, head trauma, or vitamin B_1 deficiency. Ruling out the first two possibilities, and confirming the third with the proper lab test, confirms a diagnosis of Korsakoff.

In the emergency setting, drug overdose and complicated withdrawal can be medical emergencies with potentially life-threatening consequences and safety is, therefore, the first priority in any SUD/SID assessment. Once the direct, transient substance-related symptoms are assessed, however, the evaluator needs to pursue chronic, pernicious secondary symptoms of SUDs, which include not only the physically based pathologies such as *Wernicke-Korsakoff syndrome*, but also such *sociopsychological* symptoms as depression, low self-esteem, poor social skills, divorce, and poor parenting skills, as well as vocational/economic problems.

SUD/SIDs are commonly first seen in emergency departments, and often only the medical emergency is addressed. Nonetheless, psychological dysfunction, behavior, and personality factors, mental illness, and a broad range of overlapping signs and symptoms are associated with the use of psychoactive substances (Huggins, 1990; Little, 2001), and a full spectrum biopsychosocial evaluation can guide for follow-up treatment beyond the initial ER visit. Despite recent studies that demonstrate a slight decline in adolescent drug and alcohol use, adolescent substance abuse remains a primary medical concern, especially in the emergency department (Solhkhah, 2003). Solhkhah documents the growing presentation of so-called club drugs like ecstasy (3,4-methylenedioxymethamphetamine/MDMA), *ketamine, and gamma hydroxybutyrate (GHB),* along with ever-present alcohol, cocaine, and heroin. Complicating the differential diagnosis in ERs is the high incidence of adolescents presenting with SUDs and comorbid psychiatric disorders.

Beyond recreational drugs, one must also be alert for steroid abuse and other esoteric uses of dietary substances.[7] Muzina (2008), for example, discusses a 20-year-old male who was referred by his primary-care physician and psychotherapist for medical management of his mood swings, anxiety, and general confusion. This young man reported unremitting sadness for more than a year, leaving him feeling dead inside. Muzina documented that the young man's use of steroids and supplements significantly complicated the clinical picture and the general differential diagnosis. Another case in point, Capwell (1995) reported an ephedrine-induced mania from a herbal diet supplement that contained *Ma-huang*.

Researchers continue to suggest the critical need for, and complexity of, informed and accurate differential diagnoses for an increasingly recognized comorbid SUD/SID population. Kinzie and Friedman (2004) review the complicating clinical challenges of finding the appropriate psychopharmacology interventions for various cultural refugee and asylum-seeker patients who present with culturally varied manifestations and descriptions of PTSD, major depression, perceptual distortion/psychosis, and schizophrenia, intermixed with alcohol dependence (Kinzie & Friedman, 2004). Hjorthoj, Fohlmann, and Nordentoft, (2009) found cannabis use to be prevalent among people with schizophrenia spectrum disorders, and Kaiser, Lohrer, Morgan, and Hambrecht (2005) documented the early signs of psychosis in patients who suffered from both drug dependence and schizophrenia. Korkeila et al. (2005) have presented research that points out that those vulnerable to psychosis are more prone to lifetime alcohol abuse and SUD.

The seminal work of Siris (1990) reviewed overlapping diagnoses and treatment strategies for patients with dual diagnoses of schizophrenia and substance abuse, highlighting the role of neuroleptic medication, and the adjunctive roles of antiparkinsonian medications, tricyclic antidepressants, and benzodiazepines. Pharmacokinetic and pharmacodynamic interactions of psychotropic medications and substances

---

[7]Medical psychologist George Kapalka's (2010) *Nutritional and Herbal Therapy for Children and Adolescents: A Handbook for Mental Health Clinicians* is an excellent reference.

of abuse were also considered. Siris documents the strategic value of psychosocial interventions throughout schizophrenics' vulnerability life cycle, and the critical need for substance abuse treatment during all stages of the course of the disease.

In summary, to gain and maintain competence in the SUD/SID field, the medical psychologist must continually augment knowledge of the ever-changing substances available on the illicit drug market, and remain current in research on the biobehavioral effects of psychoactive drugs, genetic studies, neuropsychological aspects of SUD/SIDs, reward systems and addictive behavior, molecular mechanism of addictive substances, interactions between food and addiction, and the ever growing pharmacotherapy field. Medicine has a core competency in addiction medicine with all appropriate board-level examinations. As medical psychology continues to mature, it is hoped that more prescribing medical psychologists will opt to gain the additional certification in substance abuse from APA's College of Professional Psychology, and will make addiction medical psychology a subspecialty, prepared to attend to significant numbers of patients with SUDs.

THE VARIED PRESENTATIONS OF PSYCHOLOGICAL DISORDERS IN DIFFERENT POPULATIONS

Just as it is important that the medical psychologist consider medical disorders that present as psychological disorders, psychological disorders that often present in primary-care settings as medical problems, and the impact of drugs and other substances on the clinical presentation of our patients, prescribing medical psychologists must consider the manner in which our patients' culture, gender, age, and ethnicity influence their experience and communication of mental illness.

Consider the example of a young mother who brings her seven-year-old son to a clinic, at the behest of his teacher, to request medication for Attention Deficit–Hyperactivity Disorder (ADHD). The patient's mother may describe her son's behaviors as hyperactive, distracted, inattentive, fidgety, disruptive, and so forth. In fact, ADHD may very well be the proper diagnosis, but are there other possibilities that can account for the symptoms presented by this patient's mother? As psychologists, we know that children, owing to their developmental immaturity, are relatively more behaviorally expressive than verbally. Often, the behaviors displayed by young children communicate relative comfort or discomfort, without clear indications about the precise nature of their personal experience.

In fact, if we were to consider this young patient's symptoms at face value and without further exploration, many diagnostic possibilities come to mind including: Attention Deficit–Hyperactivity Disorder, adjustment disorders, oppositional defiant disorder, anxiety disorders, childhood depression, bipolar spectrum disorders, Tourette's syndrome, pervasive developmental disorders, auditory processing disorders, posttraumatic stress disorder, the influence of medications, and even heavy metal poisoning. Until we conduct a thorough psychological assessment of this child's behavioral, environmental, and medical history, none of the aforementioned can be completely ruled out. The gathering of a thorough history is the first step in ruling in or ruling out any number of possibilities during the first diagnostic interview.

During the first diagnostic interview, the medical psychologist will likely learn about the patient's birth and early developmental milestones, the structure of his family, his home environment, the parents' involvement in his school activities, the presence or absence of childhood trauma, and changes in the patient's behavior

across environmental settings such as home, school, and play. Such a thorough interview is intended to provide the practitioner sufficient information to explain symptoms in terms of one or more simultaneous, overlapping, or sequential patterns. In
the example offered, our patient may indeed have a single syndrome like Attention
Deficit–Hyperactivity Disorder. On the other hand, we may learn through the interview process that our patient actually has a learning disorder in the context of a
chaotic home environment to which he is learning to adapt emotionally by avoiding
responsibility, while manipulating the emotions of authority figures in order to mitigate his anxiety. Clearly, the effectiveness of the treatment plan, whether it includes
psychotherapy, medication, or both, will depend on an expert differential diagnosis
(Muse, Brown, & Cothran-Ross, 2011).

A sound approach to differential diagnosis is indispensable, regardless of the age
group at issue, though the facts and characteristics of various age groups may differ.
Some elderly patients must confront challenges similar to those of younger patients,
while simultaneously confronting developmental challenges completely different
from anything that they have encountered before. On the one hand, elder patients
may appear more frail and vulnerable and may experience themselves as increasingly more dependent, as when they were very much younger. Nonetheless, elders
have the benefit of experience and, in many cases, the often-overlooked advantage
of wisdom.

Charged with the pivotal task of developing an accurate diagnosis, medical psychologists must apply their trusted systematic diagnostic tools to develop a reasoned
and informed explanation for their elderly patients' behaviors while recognizing the
many inherent resources inevitably associated with long life. "Due to accumulation
of losses and distress this wisdom can be hidden away for a while, but should be
uncovered in psychotherapy to help the client in better coping with the conditions
of old age" (Munk, 2010). However, all too often the misunderstood behaviors of
elders are the subject of prejudice, particularly when such behaviors are interpreted
through the eyes of less experienced professionals who may too quickly dismiss wisdom as inconvenient, senile ranting. Such a professional error can have devastating
consequences for the patient and the patient's family, particularly when it leads to
a misdiagnosis and unnecessary and ineffective treatment or outright mistreatment.
The elderly Spanish patient comes to mind who often repeated "El pan no es pan, y
el vino ya no es vino" (bread is not bread and wine is no longer wine). Such repetitive speech might easily be diagnosed as tangential, if not delusional. However, this
90-year-old gentleman was referring to the way life had changed during his lifetime.
Even the bread and the wine, staples of his Spanish culture, had changed, just as he
had, to nearly unrecognizable forms during the century he had experienced them.

It is commonly understood that dementia leads to or exacerbates depression;
however, emerging research points to the possibility of depression leading to cognitive deficits. Many individuals with depression present to primary care clinics with
complaints of memory loss, which may be associated with symptoms of depression,
and many elderly patients with mild cognitive impairment associated with the early
stages of Alzheimer's disease may present with the very same initial complaints. In
fact, some of these patients may be moderately depressed with no dementia. Others
may be describing their early experience of a progressive dementing disease, and still
others may be experiencing the simultaneous symptoms of mild depression with mild
cognitive impairment.

The art and science of differential diagnosis continue to develop, and more objective tools are being sought to support and improve the objectivity and clarity of the

diagnostic process. McCaffrey, Duff, and Solomon (2000) for example, conducted a study to cross-validate and extend the hypothesis that olfactory dysfunction could discriminate between groups of patients with Alzheimer's disease and those with major depression. They concluded that olfactory assessment adds to the diagnostic utility in the differential diagnosis of Alzheimer's disease versus major depression in elderly patients. More recently, Murray (2010) has suggested that the inclusion of *discourse sampling* and analyses (with a focus on *informativeness*) into comprehensive assessment protocols may lead to more accurate discrimination of depression and early Alzheimer's disease in the elderly. Kornhuber et al. (2009) have explored the use of brain imaging studies to support definitive differential diagnosis.

Like age, gender differences are significant. Across the lifespan, age and gender often intersect in important ways. For example, according to the World Health Organization (WHO, 2002) adolescent girls have a much higher prevalence of depression, suicidal ideation, suicide attempts, and eating disorders than adolescent boys. On the other hand, boys appear to have more anger problems, high-risk behaviors, and completed suicides than girls. The WHO reported that symptoms experienced by girls are often more inwardly directed than those of boys.

In adulthood, women are reported to experience greater distress than men, given a similar level of symptoms. In fact, according to the WHO (2002), "depressive disorders account for close to 41.9% of the disability from neuropsychiatric disorders among women compared to 29.3% among men." Part of this difference may be due to the tendency of women to more often experience distress, but it also may reflect women's greater propensity to seek professional consultation. Nonetheless, in the report entitled "Gender and Mental Health," the WHO (2002) reported that once men recognize they have a problem, they are as likely as women to use mental-health services. In contrast to women, men were more likely than women to report alcohol abuse and to be diagnosed with antisocial personality disorder (WHO, 2011).

The female reproductive cycle, menopause, and other biological factors, combined with pressure from multiple roles, gender discrimination, and associated poverty, hunger, malnutrition, overwork, domestic violence, and sexual abuse, may account for women's higher incidence of poor mental health (WHO, 2011). Likewise, male biology and sociocultural expectations for men contribute to a more outwardly directed response to stress and distress.

When the medical psychologist's knowledge of gender differences is an integrated component of a thorough clinical evaluation, the patient benefits. Such discriminative discernment notwithstanding, improperly applied statistics, isolated from the whole picture, may fuel a bias that compromises clinical goals. The WHO (2011), for example, reports that female gender is a significant predictor of being prescribed mood-altering psychotropic drugs. This phenomenon begs the question of whether there is a bona fide need for more pharmacotherapy with this gender, or whether the greater symptom disclosure by women is part of an untoward decision to medicate, or whether women's advice-seeking behavior renders them more vulnerable to current treatment fashions.

Socio-cultural and ethnic factors are also crucial considerations for practicing medical psychologists. Accuracy of diagnosis and efficacy of treatment depend on recognition of cultural variation in symptomatology of mental illness (Geltman & Chang, 2004). Caribbean Latinos have been observed to present in outpatient settings with a higher-than-expected incidence of hallucinations; yet, little is known about this phenomenon and whether it reflects psychotic illness. The first author of this chapter has observed that among his Mexican and Mexican-American patients, hallucinations appear to be a normal, uncomplicated, and time-limited part of the grieving process. The risk is that such hallucinations will be reinterpreted or misinterpreted to the patient as pathology or disorder by the culturally insensitive health-care provider.

In African-American and Caucasian populations presenting with symptoms of psychotic mania, African Americans were more likely to describe hallucinations than their Caucasian counterparts and more likely to be misdiagnosed with schizophrenia (Strakowski, McElroy, Keck, & West, 1996). Whaley (2004) reported that the prevalence of diagnoses of paranoid schizophrenia is particularly striking among African-American inpatients, and that prevalence studies of inpatient samples have found paranoid schizophrenia to be the most frequent diagnosis given to African Americans. Whaley suggests that the cultural bias of clinicians who attribute characteristics of violence to African Americans contributes to the disproportionate prevalence of the diagnosis of paranoid schizophrenia in that population.

To date, no single tool has been designed to measure the multitude of patient variables that significantly contribute to any given person's mental health. An appreciation of this fact and the ability to employ critical thinking are the cornerstone of differential diagnosing.

PSYCHOLOGICAL TESTING, PHYSICAL AND LABORATORY ASSESSMENT, AND MEDICATION RESPONSE AS VEHICLES FOR CLARIFYING DIAGNOSTIC DILEMMAS

Critical thinking and the diagnostic interview, as indispensable as they are to the differential diagnosis, do not stand alone in the clinician's toolbox. Physical examination, psychological testing, laboratory assessment, and medication response may suggest to the medical psychologist new diagnostic possibilities, confirm or rule-out hypotheses, or help to uncover underlying contributions to pathology.

Ideally, the examining psychologist will establish a working relationship with each patient, one that engenders a collaborative alliance by respecting and drawing on the patient's insights and perception of the source of the suffering. Unfortunately, this level of participation from patients is not always possible. Due to apprehensiveness, lack of insight, perceptual distortion, disability, or deception, even the most seasoned clinician may be misled during the initial examination. Mild cognitive impairment or disordered personality traits, for example, may not present as the patient's chief complaint, but may, nonetheless, have a significant impact on the presenting complaint. In such cases, the use of psychological tests to gather standardized, objective measures of symptom complexes and underlying dynamics, which are subsequently interpreted within the context of the patient's history, can be decisive in generating the best differential diagnosis.

A vast range of psychological tests exist from which to choose. Variations in reliability, administration time, interpretation ease, and clinician familiarity with a particular test are common considerations when selecting a test to use with a particular patient. When selecting a test for an individual with a physical or sensory impairment, accommodations must often be made to ensure accessibility to the patient and validity of the results. These accommodations may address testing environment, scheduled breaks, test administration procedures, test format (audio vs. written), and other adaptations such as those pertaining to language and cultural differences (Artman & Daniels, 2010). In the event that a particular psychological test cannot be made adequately accessible without compromising the validity of the results, alternative means of assessment must be identified. Prior to administering any test, the clinician must take every reasonable measure to ensure adequacy of the testing environment and test materials. Frequently used instruments such as the MMPI-II, Wechsler intelligence scales, and Wechsler Memory Scale (Kaufman & Lichtenberg, 2006) may be widely employed, and the appropriate test or combination of tests selected for any given individual will depend on the referral question and the diagnoses under consideration.

Consider the case of a 23-year-old male, married with two young children, who presented with a primary complaint of anger outbursts, irritability, and depressed mood. The patient reported completing the ninth grade of high school with a history marked by poor academic achievement and behavioral disruptions, primarily regarding truancy and classroom behavior. The patient also reported an ongoing struggle to maintain employment, growing frustration with his inability to provide for his family, feelings of worthlessness, hypersomnia, and decreased appetite.

Such a presentation may suggest multiple diagnostic possibilities, including depressive disorders, impulse-control disorders, bipolar disorders, substance-abuse disorders, and others. Without further exploration, this patient might be prematurely diagnosed, leaving the office with a diagnostic label and a prescription for medication to help stabilize his mood and behavior. On the other hand, appropriate questioning of this not-atypical patient revealed a complete absence of past psychological testing in school or as an adult. Testing was ordered to acquire a measure of his intellectual functioning and it was discovered that the patient's IQ was below average and a very likely contributor to his continued frustration in new work environments, despite his desire to excel. It was also concluded that a similar history of academic frustration years earlier may have contributed to his disruptive behavior in school and the formation of a set of expectations and associated emotional responses that continued to influence his thoughts, feelings, and behaviors. The administration of psychological testing in this patient's case led to a more comprehensive and targeted treatment plan, and averted the otherwise fairly high probability of medication to treat what might have appeared to be a mood disorder with behavioral dyscontrol. The patient was better treated with problem-solving approaches destined to achieve a better fit between his abilities and his vocational placement, and to aid the patient in adjusting goals and expectations to ensure success rather than failure.

When cognitive impairment is first discovered later in the life of a patient, a careful evaluation of the patient's cognitive performance over time is recommended in order to rule out or refer for evaluation of acute organic changes or progressive neurological diseases that might account for the deterioration. Psychological tests can be instrumental in gauging current deficits, and interviewing the patient and family members can aid in gathering developmental material that will help to place current deficits in a broader perspective.

The range of scales measured by objective and projective personality tests allows for a finer differentiation within and across Axis I and Axis II diagnoses. The usefulness of all scales contained within the various tests of personality is beyond the scope of this chapter. Continued research supports the utility of the Restructured Clinical Scales of the MMPI-II in detecting the presence or absence of a comorbid personality disorder with an Axis I diagnosis (Kamphuis, Arbisi, Ben-Porath, & McNulty,

2008) and the use of the validity scales is indicated to differentiate between valid medical impairments and exaggeration of somatic complaints (Greiffenstein, 2010). Similarly, the Millon Clinical Multiaxial Inventory-III (MCMI-III) has proved useful in identifying and differentiating Axis II personality disorders, whereas more subtle differentiations between dissociative identity disorder, borderline personality disorder, and psychosis have been shown using the Rorschach protocol. Such a differentiation can be difficult in an initial interview due to similarities between self-image, affect presentation, high rates of self-harm, traumatic histories, and stress response (Brand, Armstrong, Loewnstein, & McNary, 2009).

Consider the patient who presented with a history of dysthymic disorder and a long history of ineffective decision making. He was prescribed sertraline and reported no adverse side effects during the first month of use. The patient, however, experienced significant anxiety at a standard dose, and in a timeframe normally associated with clinical improvement. The patient self-discontinued the medication. He was then administered the MCMI-III, and the test results suggested that the depression was a long-standing characteristic of the patient's personality. Given the depressive personality trait as an important piece of the diagnostic puzzle, the patient's growing anxiety response as depression lifted is more readily understandable when the depression is appreciated as a defense/coping mechanism. This case illustrates that psychological test results can be a very valuable piece of the diagnostic process and are worthy of the same consideration given to the physical examination. The difficulty in insurance reimbursement for psychometrics, however, is a patent example of the continued lack of parity between physical and mental accessibility to diagnostic workup.

Physical examination, including a neurological exam, is integrated with the clinical interview and psychological testing by the prescribing medical psychologist in the formulation of differential diagnoses. The physical examination may be available in patient's records or it can be accomplished quickly as an integrated part of the initial diagnostic interview. The value of incorporating the physical exam in the medical psychologist's decision making cannot be overemphasized, for it may (a) yield no abnormal physical findings and help the examiner to focus on possible psychological factors contributing to the presenting problems; (b) yield remarkable physical findings, which require additional consideration as possible contributing factors to the patient's presenting problem; (c) yield remarkable physical finding seemingly unrelated to the presenting problem, but warranting referral to the patient's primary-care practitioner for further evaluation; and/or (d) identify an urgent or emergent physical illness requiring immediate life-saving action.

Medical psychologists are not expected to perform a full physical examination as might be performed by a physician. In fact, it is uncommon for psychiatrists to perform such a comprehensive examination in routine clinical practice. However, medical psychologists are expected to observe the patient's general appearance and to collect, whenever possible, vital signs such as blood pressure, pulse, respiratory rate, height, and weight. During the initial interview, the condition of the patient's exposed skin can easily be observed for dryness, dehydration, rashes, edema, or other abnormalities, and a verbal review of systems (ROS) can yield rich decision-making data.

A brief neurological examination is readily accomplished during the initial diagnostic interview and includes evaluation of a patient's speech for slurring, aphasias, word-finding difficulties, and perseveration. Examination of the patient's body movement is simple, unobtrusive, and essential to detect or rule-out weakness, clumsiness, ataxia, facial asymmetry, asymmetry of movements, choreiform movements, abnormal gait, tremor, motor stereotypy, or other abnormalities of movement. A patient's eyes should be briefly examined to ensure that there is no nystagmus, that the eyes move equally and fully in all directions, and that the pupils are equal and reactive. Along with this information, basic urine and blood screens can be ordered to further rule out biological conditions and to establish current baseline measurements against which to make future comparisons.

When the physical examination is combined with information regarding the patient's current health status and a comprehensive behavioral and medical history, the medical psychologist may formulate reasonable hypotheses regarding psychological or medical factors contributing to presenting problems. Armed with this information the clinician may formulate a diagnosis or decide to order specific medical or psychological tests to help clarify examination findings or initial clinical hypotheses. A referral or consult with the patient's primary-care practitioner may be indicated, according to the findings.

Occasionally, the physical examination findings during the initial diagnostic interview or follow-up visit may require immediate medical intervention. Consider the 350-pound, *diaphoretic*, *tachypnic*, 37-year-old male who presented to the first author's office for a follow-up, reporting no problems since the last appointment except for significant chest tightness for the past several hours. In that case, the medical psychologist and primary care physician agreed that immediate hospital care was the proper next step.

Under nonemergent conditions the medical psychologist usually has the option to select from among the many laboratory tests available to clinicians today. However, it is neither practical nor reasonable to order laboratory tests covering every organ system in order to be sure that nothing has been missed in the assessment process. How, then, does the medical psychologist decide which laboratory tests to order?

Consider the example of a 27-year-old female patient who presents for an initial interview with complaints of irritability, social isolation, anxiety in public places, hypersomnolence, chronic fatigue, and general body aches. During the course of your diagnostic interview you observe no behavioral abnormalities and no neurological abnormalities, but you do notice that her arms and upper chest are decorated with tattoos. Upon inquiry, the patient describes a history of intravenous heroin use during the past 2 years of incarceration from which she was recently released. The patient reports, also, that she obtained her tattoos early during her incarceration. The patient reports that needle sharing was a common prison practice, whether for tattooing or injecting drugs. At the completion of the interview, you are confident that the patient is suffering from depression, but you suspect that her intravenous drug use and prison tattooing have placed her at risk for hepatitis C, which may also be contributing to her symptoms of body aches and chronic fatigue. In fact, the suspicion that she has hepatitis C and her recent release from prison may be significant contributors to her depression. It would seem reasonable to order a liver panel and to consult with the patient's primary care practitioner. In a different patient with similar psychological complaints, but no history of intravenous drug use, tattooing, or prison history, a liver panel might not be warranted.

Consider also the 45-year-old businessman who presents to the prescribing medical psychologist with complaints of gradual onset of personal disorganization, in contrast to his normal high level of organizational skills. The patient reported that he has experienced frustration, increasing fatigue and depression, and has noticed significant weight gain during the previous year. The patient appears to be somewhat bewildered insofar as he cannot identify any problems in his life other than the presenting symptoms and his frustration over recent work deficiencies. He expresses concern that his performance at work seems to be deteriorating. Upon physical examination, the patient's skin feels cold, but not particularly dry, considering the local climate. No other obvious pathological neurological signs are observed and vital signs are normal. Although there may be psychological explanations for each of the symptoms presented by the patient, one fairly common endocrine problem may account for all of the symptoms: hypothyroidism. Hypothyroidism may be associated with an enlarged thyroid that may or may not be visible or palpable in some cases. A thyroid panel here would seem to be a reasonable and simple test to be ordered by the medical psychologist.

Similarly, tests for specific endogenous and exogenous substances may be warranted when patients present with mania-like symptoms. Hyperthyroidism may produce behaviors like those of mania in some patients. Medication for the treatment of chronic obstructive pulmonary disease and asthma, including *albuterol* and *theophylline*, may mimic mania in some individuals. Active cocaine use has frequently been associated with behaviors similar to mania. Any of these possibilities may be addressed through the use of medical laboratory testing. In short, laboratory tests are ordered for patients during the diagnostic workup or in preparation for pharmacotherapy in three stages: (1) general function tests that are absent from the patients file such as liver, kidney, electrolyte, and blood chemistry might be routinely ordered to screen for hidden conditions; (2) specific tests that might shed light on particular symptoms such as thyroid panel for fatigue or agitation are ordered to aid in differential diagnosing as needed; and (3) tests that are relevant to medications being prescribed, such as serum levels of lithium and valproic acid, are ordered as part of medication monitoring.

As indicated earlier, a patient's response to any drug, whether abused or taken as prescribed, yields important information that must not be overlooked. The patient's unexpected response to any prescribed medication may suggest other clinical possibilities worthy of consideration. Perhaps the dose is too strong or too weak. Perhaps the patient is a *poor metabolizer*, *ultrametabolizer,* allergic or otherwise sensitive to the medication. Perhaps the diagnosis is incorrect. The possibilities are many, in large part due to the fact that the symptoms of various mental conditions, though often thought of as belonging to one disorder or another, frequently overlap.

PSYCHOPHARMACOLOGICAL IMPLICATIONS FOR MENTAL DISORDERS WITH OVERLAPPING SYMPTOMATOLOGY

Since the publication of the first edition of the *DSM* (*Diagnostic and Statistical Manual of Mental Disorders*) in 1952, psychiatrists, psychologists, and almost all health-care providers have proceeded to cluster psychiatric symptoms into discrete disorders. Since that time, the *DSM* has been revised five times to add, remove, or change the identified mental disorders (Nobleza & Carlat, 2011). The number of disorders has increased throughout the revisions of the text, as have the philosophical bases for the manual (from a psychodynamic to medical model). To this day, there is much disagreement among health-care providers regarding psychiatric diagnoses and their corresponding symptom criteria (e.g., the prevalence of early-onset bipolar disorder).

It is important to remember that the *DSM* is a manual designed to be used as a guideline for diagnosing and treating mental disorders. The diagnoses have come about after many decades of observations by providers that mental-health symptoms often cluster into cohesive groups. That being said, there are also innumerable cases of patients who have symptoms that cross over two or more distinct diagnoses, or whose symptoms do not meet criteria for any one disorder (e.g., symptoms of mixed anxiety and depression).

The lack of organization or possible overlap of presenting symptoms in a patient does not have to impede the medical psychologist's treatment protocol. By contrast, having a patient with a clear mental-health disorder may not simplify treatment of that disorder. For example, even if a patient meets criteria for bipolar disorder, that patient may be interested in addressing only the most debilitating and acute symptoms or may desire to target symptoms not considered important to the psychologist. Therefore, a frank and informative discussion with the patient regarding such issues is advised.[8] With informed consent and agreement, patient and practitioner can move forward more confidently, having begun the therapeutic relationship on the basis of mutual respect and participation in the treatment process.

With regard to patients who present with debilitating symptoms that cut across diagnostic categories and who require treatment of several different sets of symptoms, it is crucial for the prescribing medical psychologist to ensure that the medications selected to treat one set of symptoms do not impact other symptoms in such a manner as to leave the patient worse off than before treatment began. Consider the case of children who present with comorbid ADHD and bipolar disorder (Papolos & Papolos, 2006). The quandary for the prescribing psychologist is to safely treat the hyperactivity and inattention of the first disorder without exacerbating rage and mania associated with the second disorder. A particular knowledge of the neurochemical etiology of the symptoms in question is essential under these circumstances. It is generally agreed by medical providers that the rage and mania of bipolar disorder are the result of excessive dopaminergic activity and, considering that most psychostimulants are dopamine agonists, careful monitoring is advised when using such agents for the treatment of patients with comorbid bipolar disorder and ADHD. (Diehl & Gershon, 2004; Joyce et al., 1995; Swerdlow & Koob, 1987). In some cases, first-line ADHD agents for such patients could deregulate the patient's mood. Under such circumstances, the selection of an alternative ADHD treatment such as a glutamate agonist (e.g. modafinil), or an alpha-2_A agonist (e.g. clonidine, guanfacine) may be safer and better tolerated. Alternatively, if stimulant medication has been used by the bipolar patient without any change in anger, rage, or mania, one might reconsider the diagnosis of bipolar disorder. Although response to medication is never taken as a single source for ruling in or ruling out a diagnosis, it is, nonetheless, information worth considering when periodically reviewing a patient's diagnosis. Diagnoses, after all, are not static, definitive pronouncements but, rather, working hypotheses.

As a second example, consider the patient who presents with schizophrenia and depression. Again, knowledge of the neurotransmitters involved in the origin of these symptoms is crucial. In addition to its involvement with mania and rage, excessive

---

[8]One of the pillars of medical psychology is its insistence on incorporating the patient, to the degree that the patient is available, into all aspects of treatment. This model of care specifically repudiates unilateral decision making on the part of the professional, and avoids patronizing, authoritarian, and coercive/manipulative management. This orientation is an integral part of the ethics of prescribing as practiced by medical psychologists and is subsumed under the tenets of informed consent (see Chapter 10).

dopamine activity is thought to be involved in the production of hallucinations and other psychotic symptoms. Following this line of reasoning, it would be generally contraindicated for the medical psychologist to prescribe bupropion as a first-line antidepressant for the depressed patient with comorbid schizophrenia, because that particular agent is a dopamine reuptake inhibitor that acts to increase brain dopamine levels and could, consequently, exacerbate psychotic symptoms.

Although many medications prescribed to treat a target set of symptoms may produce unacceptable exacerbation of other symptoms or other undesirable side effects, there are many cases in which the prescribing medical psychologist and the patient may conclude that the unwanted side effects of a particular medication are an acceptable and perhaps unavoidable cost. At times, the benefits outweigh the cost of side effects, and may even be welcome, as in the case of SSRI-induced delayed orgasm in a depressed male with premature ejaculation dysfunction.

On the other hand, certain pharmacologic agents' mechanism of action (MOA) may prove to have multiple symptom relief applications. For example, when ADHD and unipolar depression occur together with no other symptoms to contraindicate the use of a dopamine reuptake inhibitor, the medical psychologist may consider using bupropion as the drug of choice given its FDA approval for use in the treatment of both disorders. In this case, the increased dopamine activity associated with this drug could be efficacious for treating both the inattention/hyperactivity and the depression. Granted, this one medication may not ultimately address all the patient's symptoms, but it would be a very logical beginning strategy.

As another example of the use of one agent to treat overlapping symptoms from two disorders, consider the patient presenting with major depression and generalized anxiety. Although these are considered two discrete disorders in the *DSM*, they both often respond well to agents that increase serotonin and norepinephrine levels in the brain. Venlafaxine is just such an agent. This is a medication that is often preferred by patients because it is less often associated with weight gain and reduced libido relative to serotonin-only agents. Additionally, it may improve focus and concentration in many cases and act as an activator in depression with vegetative symptoms.

Although it may not be possible to address all overlapping symptoms with one medication, it is preferable that the prescribing medical psychologist utilize the fewest medications at the lowest dose to achieve therapeutic goals. This practice avoids polypharmacy and reduces the possibility of side effects, drug interactions, and cost, all of which may become impediments to full patient compliance; and the cultivation of compliance through a thoughtful, collaborative approach is extremely important for ethical and effective patient care.

When one is treating patients who have overlapping psychological symptoms, it is imperative to be aware of the presence of atypical symptom presentation, because this may be an indication of an underlying confounding condition or subject variable. As previously mentioned at the beginning of this chapter, there is a specific protocol to follow during the diagnostic process to assess for the presence of organicity. Additionally, when working with a multidisordered patient, race, gender, age, medical history, and drug use history (both prescription and non-) are important considerations.

It is also important to be aware that some patients may have paradoxical reactions to medications, because this, too, can be an indication of an underlying medical condition, such as *polymorphism* in the CYP450 enzyme system. To reiterate, a thorough family history can often glean whether such a reaction is consistent among family members, or whether there are particular hereditary medical conditions to consider. Finally, given the challenge of working with a patient who has overlapping symptoms, it is fundamental to work with the patient to establish reasonable expectations and treatment goals.

KNOWLEDGE OF DUAL DIAGNOSIS AND COMORBID CONDITIONS

Dual diagnoses and *comorbid conditions* present another layer of complication for the diagnosing clinician. Symptoms rarely present in neat packages awaiting a single, quickly identified label. More often, the patient's presentation is a complicated blend of psychological symptoms, environmental stressors, medical disorders, substance use, iatrogenic effects of medications and other factors. The lack of succinct differential diagnosing clouds treatment options, as does the oversimplification of symptoms with a single, inadequate diagnosis.

When conducting the intake evaluation of a new patient, presented histories of multiple diagnoses must be assessed carefully. It is neither likely that all diagnoses are correct nor that each time a new diagnosis replaces a previous one it represents the full remission of the prior and emergence of a new disorder. When looking into a lengthy history, consider how these multiple diagnoses can inform your diagnosis. Don't simply add to the list. Multiple diagnoses may represent the patient's symptom progression over time, or they may simply point to inadequate or inappropriate diagnoses, with consequent inadequate treatment, resulting in the patient's growing frustration with therapies and increasing resistance to treatment.

When mental-health disorders are comorbid with medical disorders, they can adversely influence prognosis. Accurate diagnosis of comorbid psychiatric diagnoses will allow for the modification of treatment goals to reflect the difficult road ahead. In such cases, rather than the single goal of complete symptom remission, it may sometimes be more efficacious to focus initially upon a select set of a patient's priority symptoms. Such an approach increases the probability of attaining near-term therapeutic goals, thereby motivating greater treatment compliance and reinforcing a more durable therapeutic relationship.

Any number of mental, emotional, and behavioral diagnoses can co-occur, however, a few diagnostic pairs have been observed to co-occur at significantly higher rates. Although the following examples do not provide an exhaustive list of these diagnoses, they are presented to illustrate both the relationship between diagnoses and the importance of appropriate diagnosing for effective treatment planning.

Comorbidity of anxiety disorders and major depressive disorder (MDD) is quite common, occurring in up to 60% of patients with MDD (Cameron, 2007). Rates vary across anxiety disorders. For example, of individuals diagnosed with generalized anxiety disorder (GAD) more than 50% also meet criteria for MDD; and of those diagnosed with social anxiety disorder, over 30% meet criteria for MDD (Aina & Susman, 2006). A clear differentiation between the symptoms of depression and anxiety in a single patient is difficult because there is significant overlap in the diagnostic criteria of MDD and GAD, specifically symptoms of sleep disturbance, difficulty concentrating, restlessness, and fatigue. Factors that favor the MDD diagnosis include symptoms such as anergic hopelessness, feeling as if one just can't go on, anhedonia, and early morning awakenings, whereas problems such as initial insomnia, worry, or fears, and specific behaviors such as avoidance or phobias point to anxiety (Aina & Susman, 2006). Anxiety tends to precede depression, with a median age of onset of 11 years for anxiety and 30 years for mood disorders (Cameron, 2007).

Individuals diagnosed with comorbid anxiety and MDD tend to have poorer prognoses than those with one diagnosis alone, including increased symptom severity, poorer compliance with treatment, more significant functional impairment, increased complications due to medical disorders, and higher risk for suicide (Cameron, 2007). In patients that present with medical disorders, such as heart disease, diabetes, HIV/AIDS, and pulmonary disease or disorders, close observation is advised for the potential of poorer medical and behavioral health treatment outcomes, including increased mortality, decreased compliance with medical care, and increased functional impairment (Aina & Susman, 2006).

In order to avoid overmedication, practitioners treating those with significant medical disorders must be cognizant of potential medication side effects and the possible iatrogenic effects of medications that the patient is currently prescribed. Cognitive behavioral therapy (CBT) is the nonpharmacological treatment approach most commonly used to treat anxiety and depressive disorders, although other psychosocial therapies have not been adequately tested to afford a comparison of effectiveness of CBT over those options;[9] additional options to improve symptoms might include exercise and support groups.

The diagnosis of depression in individuals with Alzheimer's-type dementia was introduced earlier in this chapter.[10] The identification of depressive symptoms can be complicated by the patient's impaired ability to articulate feelings of sadness and hopelessness due to cognitive deficits. The presence of MDD in individuals with Alzheimer's disease is associated with more severe apathy, delusions, anxiety, pathological crying, irritability, deficits in activities of daily living, impairments in social functioning, and parkinsonism than in those individuals that were not diagnosed with comorbid depression (Starkstein, Jorge, Mizrahi, & Robinson, 2005). Causality, however, is not known and while depression may worsen the prognosis for individuals with Alzheimer's, the reverse may also be true.

When an individual is diagnosed with schizophrenia and a co-occurring substance abuse disorder, which is the case in about 50% of individuals with schizophrenia, the road ahead may look grim. Such patients present an increased risk for poor treatment response, psychiatric hospitalization, homelessness, incarceration, infections secondary to drug abuse (such as hepatitis C and HIV/AIDS), violence, and lack of social support due to family strain. Despite these inherent complications with this particular dual diagnosis, research suggests that the long-term outcome for individuals referred to appropriate forms of treatment offers hope of significant improvement. Drake et al. (2006) reported that, 3 years after the initiation of treatment, such patients did not show significant improvement; however, at the 10-year follow-up, it was observed that substantial gains in the patients' quality of life had been achieved. An important consideration in this study was that, prior to engaging in treatment,

---

[9]See Chapter 2 for a discussion of the need for a greater range of therapies in studies of comparative effectiveness.

[10]See also Chapter 4, Table 4.1, for an extensive review of disease-modifying strategies for Alzheimer's.

patients identified their treatment goals. These treatment goals not only guided therapy but were used to determine improvement.

An integrated treatment program for dually diagnosed individuals that presents a consistent and clear message and one that addresses medication treatment, substance abuse counseling, and psychosocial support, is central to continued stability (Green, Drake, Brunette, & Noordsy, 2007). Substance use should be addressed directly with patients in the initial interview in a nonjudgmental way that encourages open communication about use. Such individuals often face numerous obstacles to their recovery, but if their co-occurring disorders are identified and addressed with consistent, integrated support, their chances for recovery are greatly improved. The provider needs to be alert for signs of substance abuse with all patients, even with those patients who initially indicate that they are substance free; changes in behavior or treatment compliance may signal emergence of new substance use or a recurrence of past use. Here, a periodic drug screening, with patient informed consent, may bolster the goal of optimal management of potential dual diagnoses.

Chronic depressions, such as *double depression* (dysthymic disorder with superimposed episodes of MDD) and recurrent MDD can exemplify the complex nature of dual versus single diagnoses. In a study by Klein (2004) a significant familial aggregation was found for those diagnosed with chronic forms of depression (i.e., double depression and chronic MDD) that was not found for episodic MDD. These forms of chronic depression are often associated with more functional impairment. The prognosis, however, for individuals diagnosed with dysthymic disorder is complicated by more than the presence or absence of an episode of MDD, which occurs at some time for the majority of patients diagnosed with dysthymic disorder. Comorbid anxiety, cluster C personality traits (obsessive-compulsive, avoidant, dependent), chronic stress and depressive personality traits were found to be associated with significantly lower recovery rates (Hayden & Klein, 2001).

Diagnoses must not be oversimplified to the detriment of the patient. Sometimes a single diagnosis is not the best answer and an acknowledgment of the interaction of two diagnoses will lead to better explanation of the cause, treatment options, and outcome. Improper or hasty diagnosing can lead to ineffective treatment of symptoms without targeting the cause; such an inadequate diagnostic workup may lead to untoward complications, relapse, and a reduction in compliance as well as truncated prognosis for the patient's chances for remission.

IATROGENIC EFFECTS OF MEDICATION VERSUS PRIMARY SYMPTOMS OF DISEASE PROGRESSION

As discussed, dual diagnoses and comorbid conditions are common and very important considerations in the diagnostic process. The causes of such conditions are often beyond our control. Sometimes, however, comorbid and/or dual diagnoses may be caused by prescribed treatments and, thus, may be preventable. Knowledge of iatrogenic effects of medication versus primary symptoms of disease or disease progression can be crucial, not only in the treatment of our patients, but also in the prevention of iatrogenic harm and the avoidance of unnecessary complications or discomfort to the patient. Such harm may bring symptoms that were heretofore nonexistent, such as agitation, akathisia, and drug dependence.

Broadly speaking, *iatrogenesis* may be caused by acts of omission and acts of commission and almost always are caused by a combination of the two. Some of the most serious acts of omission occur during the process of a differential diagnosis. Whether novice or veteran, clinicians can become overly reliant on the previous diagnoses reported by their patients or by other clinical practitioners in their patient's history. Such overreliance can result in the omission of important elements of a comprehensive evaluation, which would otherwise promote correct diagnoses, and a subsequent act of commission by prescribing the wrong treatment based on the incorrect diagnosis. Consider the following excerpt abstract published by Bury and Bostwick (2010).

This report presents a patient incorrectly diagnosed first with parasitic infestation and then with primary delusional parasitosis (DP). Neither diagnosis was correct. As she traveled from doctor to doctor, however, the primary DP label gained credibility via repetition, with her ongoing symptoms seen as proof of its truth.

Patient history is valuable for what it adds to the diagnostic process, but, it is not a shortcut. Omissions in the diagnostic process, whatever the reason, can result in errors of commission and unintended iatrogenic consequences. Likewise, failure to consider patient medication sensitivities, *drug–drug interactions*, drug side-effect profiles, potential for abuse, idiosyncratic medication contraindications, and drug effect–illness symptom overlap, can lead to secondary errors of commission.

An example of the latter is found in the case of an 85-year-old female patient who was admitted to hospital subsequent to a motor vehicle accident. In addition to treatment for a fractured spine with concomitant pain, this patient was prescribed and administered risperidone to reduce agitation that had been reported by emergency department staff. Upon administration of the risperidone, the patient responded with less agitation and progressed well. Prior to her discharge and after a period of relative calm, hospital staff observed an increase in unusual motor activity and emotional irritability and concluded that the patient's agitation had returned. Risperidone was discontinued and quetiapine, another atypical antipsychotic medication, was prescribed. The patient was discharged to the care of her primary-care physician and psychiatrist who observed that the patient, once again, became less agitated over time. The psychiatrist attributed this period of calm to the quetiapine. Quetiapine, thereafter, became a permanent part of the patient's treatment that no other practitioner challenged for months. Over time, as the physical pain resolved, the patient became increasingly irritable. The patient's spouse and primary-care physician requested a consultation by a medical psychologist who diagnosed *iatrogenic neuroleptic akathisia*. Quetiapine was discontinued and other medications added to address the akathisia, which improved during the ensuing 9 months, but it never resolved.

The patient's initial calm had been erroneously attributed to the therapeutic effect of risperidone, without apparent consideration of other possibilities. The reemergence of discomfort after a period of healing was actually iatrogenic akathisia that had been misinterpreted as a failure of the risperidone, rather than as a result of risperidone. When the second round of apparent agitation ceased with the replacement of risperidone by quetiapine, the decision to prescribe quetiapine was viewed as a good choice. As the patient began physical therapy, her growing discomfort was interpreted as a consequence of physical therapy–induced pain, not quetiapine-induced *akathisia*, which remained in the patient's treatment plan as a sedating agent and sleep aid. All the while, antipsychotic medication maintained incessant discomfort during the waking hours as the patient became increasingly depressed and suicidal.

Medical psychologists are familiar with the risk of extrapyramidal side effects of neuroleptic medications. It is important for the prescribing medical psychologist to understand primary conditions that may result in similar motor disturbance.[11] People with schizophrenia may later develop neuromuscular illnesses such as multiple sclerosis or amyotrophic lateral sclerosis. They may suffer head injury or develop other upper motor neuron lesions as a result of spinal cord injury, hypoxic encephalopathy, and so forth. The medical psychologist prescribing neuroleptic medication must take care to consider all possibilities and make appropriate referrals. One mistake can lead to another. Although it may be based on an act of omission, prescribing the wrong medication is a serious act of commission that can have significant undesirable consequences. Absent a thorough consideration of context, pathology-based akathisia is often seen as a neuroleptic side effect rather than a primary symptom of a disease process. On the other hand, iatrogenic akathisia can look like agitation, mania, hyperactivity, anxiety, and many other conditions.

In elderly patients, distinguishing between depression, dementia, delirium, and anxiety can be a daunting challenge, but, once again, a systematic approach allows the prescribing medical psychologist to monitor the development of symptoms and treatment outcomes. As a rule of thumb, avoid polypharmacy in the elderly. Prescribing multiple medications, especially all at once, may make it very difficult for the patient to tolerate the treatment and for the prescriber to determine which medications are producing observed effects. If the clinician cannot effectively monitor outcomes, both safety and efficacy are compromised.

Consider the 94-year-old female resident of an assisted living center who had been homebound and bedridden since she was 90 years of age. She reported that she had been prescribed gabapentin for pain and had been taking it for approximately 4 years. After she became depressed, she was prescribed antidepressants, which had consistently failed to provide relief. The patient reported that she did not believe that the gabapentin was helping much either, but no one had questioned its use since it was first prescribed. The patient was advised to check with her primary-care practitioner regarding the advisability of discontinuing the medication. On discontinuation of gabapentin, the patient's depression promptly lifted and she resumed an active schedule. A practical awareness that gender and age assumptions may mask the adverse effects of some drugs, even when patients point out their concerns, and that some drugs can mimic or trigger mental illness is pivotal to proper medication management, especially when more than one psychotropic is prescribed.

Not only psychotropic medication can mimic mental illness. Elliott (2009) provides a short list of common medications that can mimic anxiety including codeine (for pain relief), calcium channel blockers (for high blood pressure), angiotensin converting enzyme (ACE) inhibitors (for high blood pressure), statins (for high cholesterol), and benzodiazepines (for treating anxiety). Each of these drugs can cause dizziness; several can cause nausea; some can cause flushing, headache, or other symptoms often associated with anxiety.

In summary, differential diagnosing is what psychologists do best. The history of clinical psychology was founded on the construction of the Army Alpha and Beta test (Gregory, 2010), which provided much-needed diagnosing during World War I; this tradition continues today, with psychological testing and measurement pertaining almost exclusively to the science and practice of psychology. Prescribing

---

[11]See Chapter 4, Tables 4.3 and 4.4.

medical psychologists apply psychometrics, and further augment their competency in diagnostics by including physical examination, laboratory testing, and pharmacological results. No matter what the technique used in the diagnostic armamentarium, however, the development of patient rapport, a collaborative effort with other providers, and an appreciation for the continual need for reassessment as each case progresses in treatment is the cornerstone for integrating diagnosis with treatment.

CHAPTER 7 KEY TERMS

Addiction medicine: A medical specialty that focuses on addictive disease, both psychiatric and medical, with specialized study and training in both the prevention and treatment of such disease. This integrative specialty often crosses over into other areas, since various aspects of addiction fall within the fields of public health, psychology, social work, psychiatry, and internal medicine, among others. With the American Society of Addiction Medicine (ASAM), there are two primary routes to specialization: (1) psychiatric pathway and (2) other fields of medicine.

Akathisia (iatrogenic neuroleptic): The unintended development of akathisia secondary to the prescription of neuroleptic medications such as haloperidol, quetiapine, etc.

Albuterol: A drug that is a fast-acting bronchodilator prescribed for the treatment or prevention of breathing difficulties, bronchospasms, and chest tightness from lung diseases such as asthma or chronic obstructive pulmonary disease (COPD).

Baseline EKG: An electrocardiogram that is used to screen for cardiovascular disease before initiating treatment. It also serves as a point of comparison for later EKG repeats.

College of Professional Psychology: The American Psychological Association (APA) Practice Organization's College of Professional Psychology, among other things, offers a mechanism for psychologists who are licensed health service providers to identify clearly to third-party payers and other consumers of psychological services (a) that they have earned credentials in the treatment of persons for alcohol and other psychoactive substance use disorders; and (b) that pharmacologically trained medical psychologists have completed postdoctoral psychopharmacology training programs and have taken the Psychopharmacology Examination for Psychologists (PEP).

Comorbid conditions: A term that describes the co-occurrence of medical and psychiatric diagnoses within a patient, such may occur when a patient has two psychiatric disorders such as major depression and schizophrenia or when a patient has a psychiatric disorder and medical condition, such as generalized anxiety disorder and heart disease.

Comprehensive metabolic panel: A blood test that measures a patient's sugar (glucose) level, electrolyte and fluid balance, kidney function, and liver function.

Consultation-liaison psychiatry: A branch of psychiatry that specializes in the interface of medicine and psychiatry in the hospital or medical setting.

Dementia with Lewy bodies: Dementia with the presence of Lewy bodies. The dementia is characterized by cognitive decline in alertness and attention as well as recurrent visual hallucinations and parkinsonian motor symptoms.

Denial of blindness: A type of anosognosia (unawareness or denial of a neurological deficit) usually seen in recent brain trauma victims and includes a denial of disability; in this case, physiological blindness.

Denial of hemiparesis: A type of anosogonosia seen in brain trauma victims; in this case, the denial of weakness on one side of their body.

Diaphoretic: A state of excessive sweating, which may indicate the presence of an underlying medical condition or a side-effect of medications.

Discourse sampling: A term referring to processes utilized to gather information regarding human discourse, specifically the manner in which humans share information through conversation or text.

Drug–drug interactions: A drug–drug interaction (DDI) occurs when the effectiveness or toxicity of a drug is altered by the administration of another drug or substance that is administered for medical purposes. Unintentional drug–drug interactions are errors that are often preventable.

Double depression: A term used to describe the co-occurrence of major depression and dysthymic disorder.

Dual diagnosis: A term used to refer to the co-occurrence of both a psychiatric disorder and substance-related disorder.

Factitious disorders: The intentional and pathological production or feigning of physical or psychological signs or symptoms to assume the sick role.

Gamma hydroxybutyrate (GHB): A central nervous system depressant that has been used in a medical setting to treat conditions such as insomnia, clinical depression, narcolepsy, and alcoholism. GHB was first researched extensively in the 1960s. It is produced naturally by the body in small amounts, but its physiological function is unclear. GHB is frequently abused for recreational purposes.

Graves disease: An autoimmune disorder that leads to overactivity of the thyroid gland (hyperthyroidism).

Iatrogenesis: The unintended adverse effects that arise as a result of medical treatment; for example, increased suicidal thoughts brought on by antidepressant medication treatment; the development of tardive dyskinesia or akathisia from the prescription of neuroleptic medications, and so on.

Informativeness: A term used to describe the extent to which sampled human discourse produces accurate or correct information units during structured discourse tasks.

Ketamine: As a hydrochloride salt, ketamine is a noncompetitive NMDA receptor antagonist that binds to the neurotransmitter glutamate, blocks the receptor, and mediates the analgesic (reduction of pain). Since it can induce dissociative states, ketamine's effects are seen in analgesia, anesthesia, hallucinations, elevated blood pressure, bronchodilation, and reduced depression. Ketamine is also commonly abused as a recreational drug.

Korsakoff syndrome (KS): A neurological disorder caused by the lack of thiamine (vitamin B_1) in the brain with six major symptoms: Anterograde amnesia, retrograde amnesia, confabulation, meager content in conversation, lack of insight, and apathy. In Wernicke-Korsakoff Syndrome, Wernicke's encephalopathy represents the "acute" phase of the disorder and Korsakoff's amnesic syndrome represents the "chronic" phase.

Mental status examination: A structured method of observing and describing a patient's current state of mind, under the domains of appearance, attitude, behavior, mood and affect, speech, thought process, thought content, perception, cognition, insight and judgment.

Ma-huang: Ephedra sinica, a species of ephedra (Chinese ma huang), contains the alkaloids ephedrine and pseudoephedrine, which are nonselective sympathomimetic agents with both alpha- and beta-adrenergic activities that stimulate the central nervous system causing bronchodilation and vasoconstriction.

Nosology: A branch of medicine that deals with classification of diseases.

Phenylketonuria (PKU): A rare condition in which a baby is born without the ability to properly break down the amino acid phenylalanine.

Polymorphism: In genetics and biochemistry polymorphism refers to the occurrence of two or more clearly different phenotypes in the same population of a species. With respect to drug metabolism, relevant examples in pharmacology include such phenotypes as poor metabolizers, extensive metabolizers, intermediate metabolizers, and ultra-rapid metabolizers.

Polypharmacy: The administration of multiple medications in excess of what is necessary to treat the underlying disorder, increasing the risk for adverse effects.

Presumptive clues: Within the process of differentiating between organic and psychological etiologies of psychiatric symptoms, this type of clue is a symptom or event, which would lead the clinician to the assumption that the origin of the disorder is organic.

Poor metabolizer (PM): In reference to drugs metabolized by a particular cytochrome P450 enzyme, persons who metabolize such drugs slower than others. Note that a person can be a PM of one drug, and an extensive metabolizer of another.

Psychosomatic medicine: A scientific and clinical specialty that integrates multiple clinical disciplines in the diagnosis and treatment of patients with complex medical conditions and psychological/psychiatric disorders.

Reduplicative paramnesia: A rare delusional misidentification disorder usually attributable to traumatic brain injury (specifically, damage to the right cerebral hemisphere and to both frontal lobes) in which the individual believes that a place or location has been duplicated, existing in two or more places simultaneously, or that it has been "relocated" to another site.

Review of systems (ROS): As a part of the physical examination and health history, an ROS is the patient's subjective report of the presence or absence of common symptoms related to each major body system.

Sociopsychological: Refers to the scientific study of the ways in which human psychological variables (thoughts, feelings, and behaviors) are influenced by the actual, imagined, or implied presence of others in their social and cultural context.

Somatization: The tendency, in the absence of an organic etiology, to experience and communicate somatic distress in response to psychosocial stress, to attribute this distress to physical illness or disease, and to seek medical help for these symptoms.

Somatoform disorder: A group of disorders that are characterized by physical symptoms that suggest physical illness or injury, but which cannot be explained fully by a general medical condition, direct effect of a substance, or attribution to another mental disorder.

Substance abuse (SA): Substance abuse, also known as drug abuse, refers to a maladaptive pattern of use of a substance, whose pattern of use is not considered to constitute dependence, but which does not exclude dependence. Substance abuse is a form of substance-related disorder.

Substance dependence (SD): A condition characterized by persistent use of alcohol or other drugs despite problems related to use of the substance. Compulsive and repetitive use may result in tolerance to the effect of the drug and may also result in withdrawal symptoms when use is reduced or stopped. A substance dependence diagnosis may be associated with evidence of tolerance or withdrawal and may be assigned with or without evidence of physiological dependence. SD and SA are considered SUDs.

Substance-related disorders (SRD): An umbrella term to describe any of the mental disorders associated with excessive use of or exposure to psychoactive substances, including drugs of abuse, medications, and toxins. The group is divided into substance use disorders and substance-induced disorders.

Substance-induced disorders (SID): A subgroup of substance-related disorders comprising a variety of behavioral or psychological anomalies resulting from ingestion of or exposure to a drug of abuse, medication, or toxin.

Substance use disorders (SUD): A subgroup of substance-related disorders in which psychoactive substance use or abuse repeatedly results in significantly adverse consequences. The group comprises substance abuse and substance dependence. Substance use disorders refer to a characteristic pattern of continued pathological use of any medication or toxin that results in adverse consequences and could lead to substance abuse, dependence, or addiction.

Tachypnic: A state of rapid respiration that leads to a build-up of carbon dioxide in an individual and may result in fainting, also known as hyperventilation.

Teratogenic risk: A term used to describe the relative probability that exposure to a particular substance might adversely impact the normal development of a fetus or embryo.

Theophylline: A xanthine derivative bronchodilator that has a direct effect on the smooth muscles of the bronchi and blood vessels in the respiratory tract. This class of drugs does not work as rapidly as beta-adrenergic agonist drugs.

Ultrametabolizer: In reference to drugs metabolized by a particular cytochrome P450 enzyme, persons who metabolize such drugs much more extensively than others.

Wernicke-Korsakoff syndrome (WKS): A combined manifestation of two eponymous disorders, Korsakoff's syndrome and Wernicke's encephalopathy. Wernicke-Korsakoff syndrome (also called wet brain, Korsakoff's psychosis, alcoholic encephalopathy, Wernicke's disease, and encephalopathy) is a manifestation of thiamine (vitamin B_1) deficiency, or beriberi, and is usually secondary to alcohol abuse. It is characterized by (Wernicke's encephalopathy) confusion, nystagmus, ophthalmoplegia, anisocoria, ataxia, sluggish pupillary reflexes, coma, and death if untreated and (Korsakoff's psychosis) anterograde and retrograde amnesia, confabulation, and hallucinations.

Chapter 7 Questions

1. When administering neuroleptic medications, especially to children, Native Americans, obese adults, elders, or patients with diabetes, it is important to order the following laboratory test:
   a. Thyroid stimulating hormone level (TSH)
   b. Comprehensive metabolic panel (CMP)
   c. Electrocardiogram (EKG)
   d. Sedimentation Rate (Sed Rate)
   e. Complete Blood Count (CBC)

2. Catalina, Macias, and de Cos (2008) found that the most frequent symptoms associated with _____ were inconsistent response to treatment, worsening of the symptoms when faced with the prospect of a discharge plan, disappearance of the symptoms just after being admitted, and intense relationships with other patients or staff during the hospitalization.
   a. Somatoform pain disorder
   b. Dependent personality disorder
   c. Factitious disorder
   d. Borderline personality disorder
   e. Conversion reaction

3. Van Dijke et al. (2010) found an inverse correlation with _____ and borderline personality disorder (BPD) along a continuum of affect dysregulation.
   a. Obsessive compulsive disorder
   b. Bipolar disorder
   c. Major depressive disorder
   d. Somatoform disorder (SoD)
   e. Malingering

4. Patients with medically unexplained symptoms may be subject to unnecessary diagnostic investigations, polypharmacy, and polysurgery, which, together, may place them at high risk of
   a. Iatrogenic disease.
   b. Alcohol dependence.
   c. Major depressive disorder.
   d. Anxiety disorders.
   e. Opioid dependence.

5. A patient's response to a prescribed medication is _____
   a. A practical approach to ruling in or ruling out a diagnosis.
   b. Not very useful when evaluating affective disorders or anxiety disorders.
   c. Essential information to diagnosis of Attention–Deficit Hyperactivity Disorder.

    d. Information worth considering when periodically reviewing a patient's diagnosis.

    e. Irrelevant to the diagnostic process as medication is not prescribed until the correct diagnosis is determined.

6. According to the World Health Organization (WHO) (2011), _____ is a significant predictor of being prescribed mood-altering psychotropic drugs.

    a. Ethnicity

    b. Age

    c. Past suicidal ideation

    d. Male gender

    e. Female gender

7. Whaley (2004) reported that the prevalence of diagnoses of paranoid schizophrenia is particularly striking among _____.

    a. Mexican Americans.

    b. Hispanic Americans.

    c. American Indians.

    d. African Americans.

    e. Irish Americans.

8. According to the World Health Organization (WHO, 2002), boys seem to have more _____ than girls.

    a. Depression

    b. Alcohol abuse

    c. Suicidal ideation

    d. Suicide attempts

    e. Completed suicides

9. A patient cannot identify any problems in his life, but reports frustration over recent work deficiencies and concern that his performance at work seems to be deteriorating. Upon physical examination, the patient's skin feels cold, but not particularly dry, considering the local climate. No other obvious pathoneurological signs are observed and vital signs are normal. A _____ is a logical laboratory test to order before prescribing medications.

    a. TSH

    b. Toxicology screen

    c. Hematocrit

    d. Liver panel

    e. All of the above

10. With respect to visual hallucinations, an organic origin is more likely the case when such hallucinations occur_____.

    a. In the absence of physical symptoms.

    b. While under the influence of an hallucinogenic drug.

    c. In the absence of a head injury.

    d. In the absence of psychological symptoms.

    e. All of the above

    Answers: (1) b, (2) c, (3) d, (4) a, (5) d, (6) e, (7) d, (8) e, (9) a, and (10) d.

REFERENCES

Abbey, S. E. (2005). Somatization and somatoform disorders. In J. L. Levenson (Ed.), *Textbook of psychosomatic pedicine* (pp. 271–279). Arlington, VA: American Psychiatric Publishing.

Aina, Y., & Susman, J. (2006). Understanding comorbidity with depression and anxiety disorders. *Journal of the American Osteopathic Association, 106,* S9–S14.

American Psychiatric Association. (1994). *Diagnostic and statistical manual of mental health disorders* (4th ed.). Washington, DC: Author.

American Psychiatric Association. (2000). *Diagnostic and statistical manual of mental disorders* (4th ed., text rev.). Washington, DC: Author.

Artman, L., & Daniels, J. (2010). Disability and psychotherapy practice: Cultural competence and practical tips. *Professional Psychology: Research and Practice, 41*(5), 442–448.

Bózzola, F. C., Gorelick, P. B., & Freels, S. (1992). Personality changes in Alzheimer's disease. *Archives of Neurology, 49*(3), 297–300.

Brand, B., Armstrong, J., Loewnstein, R., & McNary, S. (2009). Personality differences on the Rorschach of dissociative identity disorder, borderline personality disorder, and psychotic inpatients. *Psychological Trauma: Theory, Research, Practice, and Policy, 1*(3), 188–205.

Bury, J. E., & Bostwick, J. M. (2010). Iatrogenic delusional parasitosis: A case of physician-patient folie a deux. *General Hospital Psychiatry, 32*(2), 210–212.

Byrne, G. J., & Pachana, N. A. (2010). Anxiety and depression in the elderly: Do we know anymore? *Current Opinion in Psychiatry, 23*(6), 504–509.

Cameron, O. (2007). Understanding comorbid depression and anxiety. *Psychiatric Times, 24*(14).

Capwell, R. R. (1995). Ephedrine-induced mania from an herbal diet supplement. *The American Journal of Psychiatry, 152*(4).

Catalina, M. L., de Ugarte, L., & Moreno, C. (2009). Factitious disorder with psychological symptoms: Is confrontation useful? *Actas Españolas de Psiquiatría, 37*(1), 57–59.

Catalina, M. L., Macias, V. G., & de Cos, A. (2008). Prevalence of factitious disorder with psychological symptoms in hospitalized patients. *Actas Españolas de Psiquiatría, 36*(6), 345–349.

CDC. (2009, July 17). Morbidity and mortality weekly report. *Centers for Disease Control and Prevention.*

Chuang, L. (2009, October 29). Mental disorders secondary to general medical conditions. *eMedicine.* Retrieved January 28, 2011 from http://emedicine.medscape.com/article/294131-overview

Clay, R. (2000). Earning certification in substance abuse: Psychologists find APA certification helps their substance abuse patients, and their practices. *APA Monitor, 31,* 36.

Coid, J., Kirkbride, J., Barker, D., Cowden, F., Stamps, R., Yang, M., & Jones, P. (2008). Raised incidence rates of all psychoses among migrant groups: Findings from the east London First Episode Psychosis Study. *Archives of General Psychiatry, 65,* 1250–1258.

Diehl, D. D., & Gershon, S. (2004). The role of dopamine in mood disorders. *Comprehensive Psychiatry, 33*(2), 115–120.

Drake, R., McHugo, G., Xie, H., Fox, M., Packard, J., & Helmstetter, B. (2006). Ten-year recovery outcomes for clients with co-occurring schizophrenia and substance use disorders. *Schizophrenia Bulletin, 31*(3), 464–473.

Elliott, C. (2009). When anxiety isn't anxiety. *Psych Central.* Retrieved January 28, 2011 from http://blogs.psychcentral.com/anxiety/2009/05/when-anxiety-isnt-anxiety

Galanter, M., & Kleber, H. D. (Eds.). (2008). *The American psychiatric publishing textbook of substance treatment,* 4th ed. Arlington, VA: American Psychiatric Association.

Geltman, D., & Chang, G. (2004). Hallucinations in Latino psychiatric outpatients: A preliminary investigation. *General Hospital Psychiatry, 26*(2), 153–157.

Green, A., Drake, R., Brunette, M. & Noordsy, D. (2007). Schizophrenia and co-occurring substance use disorder. *American Journal of Psychiatry, 164*(3), 402–408.

Green-Hernandez, C., Singleton, J. K., & Aronzon, D. Z. (2001). *Primary care pediatrics.* Philadelphia, PA: Lippincott, Williams & Wilkins.

Gregory, R. (2010). *Psychological testing: History, principles and applications.* Canada: Pearson Education.

Greiffenstein, M. (2010). The MMPI-2 symptom validity scale (fbs) not influenced by medical impairment: A large sleep center investigation. *Assessment, 17*(2), 269–277.

Hayden, E., & Klein, D. (2001). Outcome of dysthymic disorder at 5-year follow-up: The effect of familial psychopathology, early adversity, personality, comorbidity, and chronic stress. *American Journal of Psychiatry, 158*(11), 1864–1870.

Hjorthot, C., Fohlmann, A., & Nordentoft, M. (2009). Treatment of cannabis use disorders in people with schizophrenia spectrum disorders—A systematic review. *Addictive Behaviors, 34*(6-7), 520–525.

Huggins, N. (1990). Psychiatric and psychological consequences of substance abuse. In W. D. Lerner & M. A. Barr (Eds.), (1990). *Handbook of hospital based substance abuse treatment* (pp. 85–111). Elmsford, NY: Pergamon Press.

Joyce, P. R., Fergusson, D. M., Woollard, G., Abbott, R. M., Horwood, L. J., & Upton, J. (1995). Urinary catecholamines and plasma hormones predict mood state in rapid cycling bipolar affective disorder. *Journal of Affective Disorders, 33*(4), 233–243.

Julien, R. (2011). To intend or not to intend, that is the question: Sedatives, behavior, amnesia and intent. *American Society for the Advancement of Pharmacotherapy,* APA Division 55. Washington, DC: Midwinter Conference.

Kaiser, R., Lohrer, F., Morgan, V., & Hambrecht, M. (2005). Changes in the pattern of substance abuse after the onset of psychosis. *Australian and New Zealand Journal of Psychiatry, 39*(6), 467–472.

Kamphuis, J., Arbisi, P., Ben-Porath, Y. & McNulty, J. (2008). Detecting comorbid axis-II status among inpatients using the MMPI-2 restructured clinical scales. *European Journal of Psychological Assessment, 24,* 157–164.

Kapalka, G. M. (2010). *Nutritional and herbal therapies for children and adolescents: A handbook for mental health clinicians.* San Diego, CA: Elsevier Science.

Kaufman, A., & Lichtenberger, E. (2006). *Assessing adolescent and adult intelligence* (3rd ed.). Hoboken, NJ: Wiley.

Kinzie, J. D., & Friedman, M. J. (2004). Psychopharmacology for refugee and asylum-seeker patients. In J. P. Wilson & B. Drooek (Eds.), *Broken spirits: The treatment of traumatized asylum seekers, refugees, war and torture victims* (pp. 580–600). New York, NY: Brunner-Routledge.

Kirmayer, L. J., & Young, A. (1998). Culture and somatization: Clinical, epidemiological and ethnographic perspectives. *Psychosomatic Medicine, 60,* 420–430.

Klein, K., Shankman, S., Lewinsohn, P., Rohde, P., & Seeley, J. (2004). Family study of chronic depression in a community sample of young adults. *American Journal of Psychiatry, 161*(4), 646–653.

Korkeila, J. A., Svirskis, T., Heinimaa, M., Ristkari, T., Huffunen, J., Ilonen, T., . . . & Salokangas, R. K. R. (2005). Substance abuse and related diagnoses in early psychosis. *Comprehensive Psychiatry, 46*(6), 447–452.

Kornhuber, J., Schmidtke, K., Frölich, L., Perneczky, R., et al. (2009). Early and differential diagnosis of dementia and mild cognitive impairment: Design and cohort baseline characteristics of the German Dementia Competence Network. *Dementia and Geriatric Cognitive Disorders, 27*(5), 404–417.

Leo, R., & Ahrens, K. (1998). Visual hallucinations in mild dementia: A rare occurrence of Lhermitte's Hallucinosis. *Psychosomatics, 40,* 360–363.

Levenson, J. L. (2005). Psychiatric assessment and consultation. In R. J. Shaw & D. R. DeMaso (Eds.), *Textbook of psychosomatic medicine* (p. 4). Arlington, VA: American Psychiatric Publishing.

Lipowski, Z. J. (1988). Somatization: The concept and its clinical application. *American Journal of Psychiatry, 145,* 1358–1368.

Little, J. (2001). Treatment of dually diagnosed clients. *Journal of Psychoactive Drugs, 33*(1), 27–31.

Madhusoodanan, S., Danan, D., & Moise, D. (2007). Psychiatric manifestations of brain tumors: Diagnostic implications. *Expert Review of Neurotherapeutics, 7*(4), 343–349.

McCaffrey, R. J., Duff, K., & Solomon, G. S. (2000). Olfactory dysfunction discriminates probable Alzheimer's dementia from major depression: A cross-validation and extension. *Journal of Neuropsychiatry & Clinical Neurosciences, 12*(1), 29.

McLellan, A. T., Lewis, D. C., O'Brien, C. P., & Kleber, H. D. (2000). Drug dependence, a chronic medical illness implications for treatment, insurance, and outcomes evaluation. *Journal of American Medicine Association, 284*(13), 1689–1695.

Miller, N. S. (1991). *Comprehensive handbook of drug and alcohol addiction.* New York, NY: Marcel Dekker.

Miller, N. S., & Kipnis, S. S. (2006). *Detoxification and substance abuse treatment: A treatment improvement protocol (TIP) 45.* Rockville, MD: U.S. Department of Health and Human Services.

Merriam-Webster. (2010). *Dictionary and thesaurus.* Retrieved January 9, 2012 from http://www.mirriam-webster.com

Morrison, J. (1997). *When psychological problems mask medical disorders: A guide for psychotherapists.* New York, NY: Guilford Press.

Munk, K. P. (2010). New aspects of late life depression. *Nordic Psychology, 62*(2), 1.

Murray, L. L. (2010). Distinguishing clinical depression from early Alzheimer's disease in elderly people: Can narrative analysis help? *Aphasiology, 24*(6–8), 928–939.

Muse, M. (2010). *Clinical psychopharmacology for non-mental health prescribers.* Rockville, MD: Mensana Publications.

Muse, M., Brown, S., & Cothran-Ross, T. (2011). Psychology, psychopharmacology, and pediatrics: When to treat and when to refer. In G. Kapalka (Ed.), *Pediatricians and pharmacologically trained psychologists* (pp. 3–16). New York, NY: Springer.

Muse, M., & McGrath, R. (2010). Training comparison among three professions prescribing psychoactive medications: Psychiatric nurse practitioners, physicians, and pharmacologically-trained psychologists. *Journal of Clinical Psychology, 66,* 1–8.

Muzina, D. J. (2008). Depression and anxiety: Distinguishing unipolar and bipolar disorders. *Annals of Clinical Psychiatry, 20*(Suppl. 4), S19–S23.

Niesink, R. J. M., Jaspers, R. M. A., Kornet, L. M. W., & van Ree, J. M. (1999). *Drugs of abuse and addiction: Neurobehavioral toxicology.* Washington, DC: CRC Press.

Nobleza, D., & Carlat, D. (2011). DSM-5: A guide to coming changes. *The Carlat Psychiatric Report, 9,* 1–6.

Ouimette, P., & Brown, P. J. (2003). *Trauma and substance abuse: Causes, consequences, and treatment of comorbid disorder.* Washington, DC: American Psychological Association.

Papolos, D., & Papolos, J. (2006). *The bipolar child: The definitive and reassuring guide to childhood's most misunderstood disorder* (3rd ed.). New York: Broadway Books.

Siris, S. G. (1990). Pharmacological treatment of substance-abusing schizophrenic patients. *Schizophrenia Bulletin, 16*(1), 111–112.

Solhkhah, R. (2003). The psychotic child. *Child and Adolescent Psychiatric Clinics of North America, 12*(4), 693–722.

Starkstein, S., Jorge, R., Mizrahi, R., & Robinson, R. (2005). The construct of minor and major depression in Alzheimer's disease. *American Journal of Psychiatry, 162*(11), 2086–2093.

Strakowski, S. M., McElroy, S. L., Keck, P. E., & West, S. A. (1996). Racial influence on diagnosis in psychotic mania. *Journal of Affective Disorders, 39*(2), 157–162.

Swerdlow N. R., & Koob, G. F. (1987). Dopamine, schizophrenia, mania, and depression: Toward a unified hypothesis of cortico-striatopallido-thalamic function. *Behavioral and Brain Sciences, 10,* 197–208.

Taylor, R. (2007). *Psychological masquerade: Distinguishing psychological from organic disorders* (3rd edition). New York, NY: Springer Publishing.

Van Dijke, A., Ford, J. D., van der Hart, O., van Son, M., van der Jeijden, P., & Buhrin, M. (2010). Affect dysregulation in borderline personality disorder and somatoform disorder: differentiating under- and over-regulation. *Journal of Personality Disorder, 24*(3), 296–311.

Van Reekum, R., Stuss, D. T., & Ostrander, L. (2005). Apathy: Why care? *Journal of Neuropsychiatry and Clinical Neuroscience, 17,* 7–19.

Whaley, A. L. (2004). Paranoia in African-American men receiving inpatient psychiatric treatment. *Journal of the American Academy of Psychiatry Law, 32,* 282–290.

World Health Organization. (2002). Gender and mental health. *Gender and health.* Retrieved on January 31, 2011 from http://whqlibdoc.who.int/gender/2002/a85573.pdf

World Health Organization. (2011). Gender disparities and mental health: The facts. *Gender and Women's Mental Health.* Retrieved on January 31, 2011.

Zolkowska, K., Cantor-Graae, E., & McNeil, T. (2001). Increased rates of psychosis among immigrants to Sweden: Is migration a risk factor for psychosis? *Psychological Medicine, 31,* 669–678.

Chapter 8

PHARMACOLOGY

Randall Tackett

Pharmacology is the basic science of how drugs interact in the body to produce both their therapeutic and toxic effects. Pharmacology incorporates knowledge from a multitude of disciplines, which include biochemistry, physiology, pathophysiology, medicinal chemistry, pharmaceutics, and toxicology. *Medicinal chemistry* describes the chemical interaction between the structure of the drug and the molecular receptors. Because specific chemical structures interact with molecular receptor structures, often both the therapeutic and toxic effects of drugs can be predicted based on their chemical structures. This is referred to as *structure activity relationships*. *Pharmaceutics* describes the relationships between the dosage forms of drugs, their disposition in the body, and the clinical response observed.

Psychopharmacology focuses specifically on drugs that interact within the central nervous system (CNS) to produce their therapeutic actions. It is important to note that drugs used to treat CNS disorders must reach the CNS and the brain by passing through peripheral sites. The drugs will be metabolized and excreted by the liver and kidneys. Thus, although the main therapeutic effect that is seen is through an interaction in the brain, there are several peripheral sites where drugs can and will interact, resulting in clinically significant drug interactions and/or side effects.

In evaluating drug actions, pharmacology considers the effects of a drug from a *pharmacodynamic* and *pharmacokinetic* aspect. Pharmacodynamics describes the interaction of the drug molecule with the tissues that results in the therapeutic or toxic effect of the drug. Pharmacokinetics addresses the distribution of the drug throughout the body and describes the *absorption*, *distribution*, *metabolism*, and *excretion* (ADME) of the drug. Pharmacokinetic parameters are related to the onset and the duration of the drug.

PHARMACODYNAMICS

Drug/Receptor Interactions

Drugs produce their actions by chemically interacting with other molecules. A drug can interact chemically with another chemical. For example, antacids neutralize stomach acid through a simple chemical interaction. However, most drugs, as well as neurotransmitters and hormones, produce their actions by binding to specific proteins. A drug can bind to an enzyme, neutralizing the effect of the enzyme, such as the case with phenelzine that binds to monoamine oxidase and neutralizes the enzyme. However, most drugs produce their action by binding to receptors as indicated by the following:

Drug + Receptor ➔ Drug-Receptor Complex

Drug binding is dictated by specific structural requirements of the receptor that match with that of the drug. The rate at which the drug binds to the receptor is referred to as the *association constant*, whereas the rate at which the drug releases from the receptor or deactivates the receptor is known as the *dissociation constant* and represents how tightly a drug binds to the receptor as well as how long the receptor will be affected.

Drugs exist as *enantiomers*, which are optical *isomers* that are mirror images of each other and are defined by the direction in which the isomer rotates polarized light. Isomers that rotate light clockwise are described as the (+) or *d-isomer* (dextrorotary). If the isomer rotates light in the opposite direction, it is referred to as the (–) or *l-isomer* (levorotary). Most drugs are available as the *racemic mixture* consisting of equal amounts of the d- and l-isomers. However, only one of the isomers is biologically active. Advances in technology have made it feasible to isolate the biologically active isomer, and these have become available therapeutically as evidenced by d-amphetamine and escitalopram, which are commercially available isomers.

There are a number of receptor types that account for drug actions. Perhaps one of the simplest types of receptors is the *ion channel*. Ion channel receptors exist as *ligand gated*, *voltage gated*, and *second messenger* regulated receptors. The net effect of activation of these receptors is an increased permeability of a specific ion or hydrophilic molecule across the membrane. Ion channels tend to be structurally similar in that they are tubelike channels that pass through the cell membrane. Benzodiazepines represent a class of drugs that bind to ion channel receptors.

The most frequently encountered receptor type is the *G protein-coupled receptors*.[1] All the G protein-coupled receptors consist of a single polypeptide chain that has seven transmembrane regions. The receptors are exposed on the extracellular site of the cell membrane but the transmembrane regions have intracellular components connected to G-proteins that participate in intracellular signaling mechanisms. When a drug binds to the extracellular component of the G protein-coupled receptor site, this results in activation of an *effector protein* such as adenylyl cyclase or phospholipase C. These effector proteins then activate intracellular second messengers that serve as signaling molecules intracellularly. The most common second messengers are cyclic AMP (cAMP) and cyclic GMP (cGMP). Phospholipase C is another frequently encountered second messenger that has been shown to have a prominent role in the regulation of intracellular calcium. Diacylglycerol (DAG) and inositol-1-4, 5-triposphosphate (IP_3) are also recognized second messenger molecules that can activate protein kinase C to produce the cellular response observed after receptor activation.

A number of G proteins have been identified, each with unique properties. G_s is a stimulatory protein that has been shown to activate calcium channels and adenylyl cyclase. G_i is an inhibitory G protein that inhibits potassium channels and inhibits adenylyl cyclase. G_o inhibits calcium channels and G_q activates phospholipase C. Of the G protein-coupled receptors, the best characterized is the β-adrenergic receptor. These G proteins serve an important means of amplifying a signal initiated by a few drug or transmitter molecules that bind to the receptor.

Intracellular *transcription factors* represent another type of receptor known as *intracellular receptors*. Activation of this type of receptor requires that the drug is lipophilic so that it can enter the cell to interact with the receptor. Binding of the

---

[1]See Chapter 3, Figure 3.3.

drug to a transcription factor results in activating or inhibiting RNA transcription, which dictates the response seen. Steroids produce their actions by binding to intracellular receptors.

A final class of receptors is the *enzymatic transmembrane receptors*, which possess enzymatic cytosolic domains. Drugs bind to an extracellular receptor site, which then activates an intracellular enzyme. Of this class of receptors, the largest group is associated with tyrosine kinase. When a drug binds to the extracellular site, tyrosine kinase located at the cytoplasmic tail of the receptor is activated, and it can then initiate a number of intracellular signaling mechanisms. Insulin represents a drug that acts through this receptor type.

Drug receptor binding is dictated by the orientation of the specific amino acids in the receptor proteins and the chemical geometry or structure of the drug. The fluid nature of the cell membrane in which the receptor exists allows for conformational changes to occur when a drug binds to the receptor. Receptors exist in either an activated or resting state. If a drug binds to and activates the receptor, it is referred to as an *agonist*. If the drug inactivates or inhibits the receptor, it is considered an *antagonist*. In some cases, a drug may bind to a portion of the enzyme or receptor molecule that is not considered the active site. This is referred to as *allosteric binding* and can result in either enhancement or inhibition of the receptor's actions.

If a drug binds to the receptor and completely activates the receptors, it is referred to as a *full agonist*. A full agonist will have a high affinity for the receptor, and, in high enough concentrations, should activate all the existing receptors. A *partial agonist* is a drug that activates the receptors but the effect is less than maximal even though all the receptors are bound. Some drugs may be classified as *inverse agonists* because they have a higher affinity for receptors that are in the resting state than those in the active state.

The propensity for a drug to bind to a receptor is referred to as its *affinity*. Most drug binding interactions are the results of *electrostatic binding,* which is reversible. However, a few drugs may bind covalently to a receptor. *Covalent binding* interactions are considered essentially irreversible.

Dose response curves are used to quantify drug receptor binding as a function of dose. There are basically two types of dose response curves. *Graded dose response curves* are presented as semilogarithmic plots of the effect of drug receptor binding versus the dose of the drug. These sigmoidal plots demonstrate the efficacy and the potency of a drug. The *potency* of a drug is a relative description of where the drug's dose response curve is positioned compared to other drugs. Potency between different drugs is often expressed by comparing their $ED_{50}s$, which is the *effective dose* at which 50% of the maximal response is observed. The lower the ED_{50}, the greater the potency of the drug. It is important to note that potency has minimal clinical significance. A more potent drug will produce an effect at a lower dose, but that does not imply superiority. A low-potency drug may be just as effective in achieving the desired therapeutic effect but simply requires a larger dose to do so. The only disadvantage one would have with a lower-potency drug would be if the amount of drug necessary to produce a therapeutic response would be difficult to administer. *Efficacy*, on the other hand, describes the ability of a drug to bind to a receptor and produce an effect and is demonstrated by the maximal effect, referred to as the E_{max}, or the dose at which the maximal effect occurs. The ED_{10} represents the dose at which 10% of the response occurs and is often used as the estimation of the threshold dose. Note in Figure 8.1 that the second dose response curve is very steep. Drugs with steep dose response curves are of particular concern because small changes in

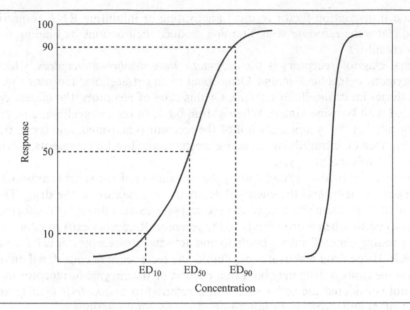

Figure 8.1   Graded Dose Response Curve

dose can result in a large effect. Thus, toxicity can occur quickly and often at doses very similar to those needed to produce the therapeutic actions.

Quantal dose response curves express the percentage of a population that responds to a particular dose. Compared to a graded dose response curve, a quantal dose response evaluates whether a response occurred or did not occur at a given dose. These curves can be used to determine the median effective and median toxic doses. If the frequency of response is plotted on a quantal dose response curve, a bell-shaped curve results. In a normally distributed population, it is anticipated that 95% of the population will respond within 2 standard deviations of the mean. Those individuals that fall on the far left of the mean dose would be considered hypersensitive, whereas those to the far right of the mean would be patients that are resistant to the drug, as shown in Figure 8.2.

Figure 8.3 shows several graded dose response curves. Curve A depicts a dose response curve of an agonist. If the dose response curve shifts to the left, it is indicative of an increase in potency, whereas a shift to the right represents a decrease in potency. In the presence of a *competitive antagonist*, the dose response curve will be shifted to the right as shown by Curve B. This indicates that a greater dose of the agonist is necessary to produce the same effect in the presence of the reversible antagonist. This is typical of most competitive binding interactions. Curve C demonstrates the effects of an interaction with a noncompetitive antagonist. Note that the curve is shifted further to the right, but also the maximal effect is reduced. This is due to the receptors being irreversibly bound by the covalent antagonist.

Physiological antagonism represents another drug interaction that occurs in some cases but does not require an interaction at the same receptor site. In physiological antagonism, two agonists offset each other by activating different receptor sites. For example, during an anaphylactic reaction, histamine is released and can cause severe bronchoconstriction by activating histamine receptors. Epinephrine is administered to antagonize the severe bronchoconstriction by activating beta receptors in the lungs to produce bronchodilation.

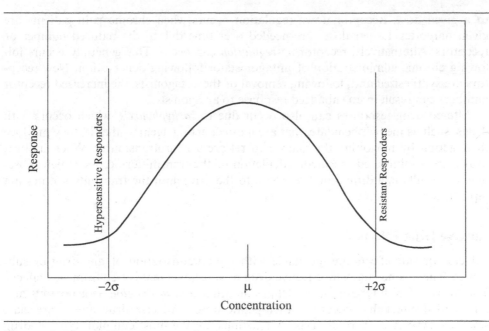

Figure 8.2   Quantal Dose Response Curve

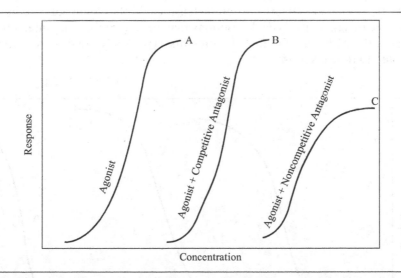

Figure 8.3   Graded Dose Curve With Sole Agonist, and With Agonist/Antagonist Interactions

Receptor Regulation

Receptors are dynamic entities and can change in the presence of drugs or neurotransmitters. These changes can occur over a matter of minutes or, in many cases, over a much longer period of time such as days or weeks. A reduction in receptors is referred to as *down-regulation* and often occurs when the receptors are exposed to agonists. The reduction in receptor number is demonstrated as a reduced response to a given dose. Receptor down-regulation occurs when chronic pain patients are given narcotics. Larger doses are needed over time due to the reduced number of receptors. Alternatively, receptor *up-regulation* can occur. This generally occurs following chronic administration of antagonists or following denervation. New receptors are synthesized and, following removal of the antagonists, the increased receptor numbers can result in an enhanced response to an agonist.

Altered drug responses can also occur due to *tachyphylaxis,* which occurs with drugs, such as methylphenidate, that are indirect acting agents—that is, they produce their action by provoking the neuron to release a neurotransmitter. When indirect drugs are administered repeatedly, depletion of the transmitter occurs, which subsequently results in a diminished response to the drug until the transmitter stores are replenished.

Adverse Drug Effects

Adverse or side effects are inevitable with the administration of any drug or substance. There is no clinically effective drug or substance that is free from side effects. The World Health Organization defines an *adverse drug reaction* as a noxious and unintended effect that occurs at therapeutic doses. Adverse drug effects are classified as Type A or Type B. Type A reactions are the most common type of drug reactions and are the most predictable. These reactions are dose dependent and are exaggerated extensions of the pharmacological action of the drug. For example, excessive sedation that may occur with the use of a benzodiazepine or excessive bradycardia with use of a beta blocker (to treat, for example, posttraumatic stress disorder) represent side effects that are extensions of the therapeutic actions. With psychotropic drugs, many Type A reactions may be due to the drug interacting with receptors in the periphery. Figure 8.4 represents Type A adverse drug reactions, typically related to dose response.

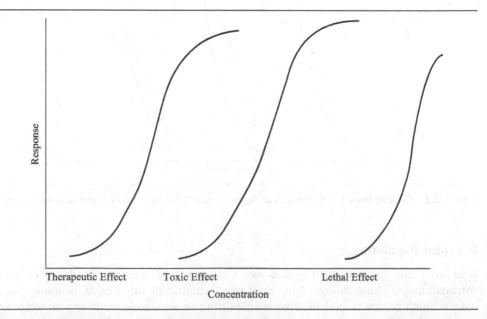

Figure 8.4   Type A Adverse Drug Reaction

Type B reactions are much more unpredictable and are often referred to as idiosyncratic reactions. Type B reactions generally are immunological or allergic in nature and can occur at any dose and following any route of administration (Edwards & Aronson, 2000). Adverse drug reactions are more common in the very young and the elderly. In the elderly, adverse reactions are more common because of age-related changes in physiology, the presence of comorbid disease states, and concomitant administration of several drugs. Women are also reported to have higher rates of adverse drug reactions than males.

PHARMACOKINETICS

Pharmacokinetics describes the disposition of drugs in the body, beginning with administration to excretion, and provides a foundation for determining the duration and intensity of the drug effect. Additionally, pharmacokinetics provides us with a basis for how often a drug needs to be dosed.

Absorption

For a drug to be effective, it must reach the site of action after administration. *Bioavailability (F)* represents the fraction of the administered drug that reaches the systemic circulation and ultimately reaches the site of action. For example, if a drug has a bioavailability of 65% and is administered as a 10 mg dose, this means that 6.5 mg of the drug reaches the circulation. Obviously, a drug that is administered IV will have a bioavailability of 100% because the drug would be administered directly into the systemic circulation. Absorption of a drug is dependent on a number of factors such as the chemical properties of the drug, the site where the drug is administered, and what specific membrane barriers are present that must be crossed in order for the drug to reach the ultimate site of action. All these factors can affect a drug's bioavailability. Most drugs are administered orally, taking advantage of the large absorptive area of the gastrointestinal tract. This route is convenient for most patients and is particularly helpful if multiple doses or chronic drug administration is required. However, a major disadvantage is the exposure of the drug to the high acidic environment of the stomach, which can destroy the active ingredient. Additionally, the drug may be irritating to the GI tract, resulting in nausea, vomiting, or even GI bleeding. Enteric coated drugs have been developed to protect the drug from the acid in the GI tract and/or to reduce irritation of the GI tract by the drug. Drugs that are *lipophilic*, such as most psychotropic drugs, tend to cross most membranes easily and, thus, are more easily absorbed. *Hydrophilic* drugs, alternatively, have a more difficult time being absorbed across the GI tract unless there are specific drug-transport mechanisms present.

Most drugs are absorbed in the small intestine where the intestinal microvilli provide a large absorptive surface area. Once the drug is absorbed across the intestinal epithelium, the drug enters the *portal circulation* and is carried to the liver (see Figure 8.5). With some drugs, the initial pass through the liver results in extensive metabolism of the drug, which may significantly reduce the amount of drug that can reach the site of action. This is referred to as *first pass metabolism*. If a drug undergoes significant first pass metabolism, this usually requires a longer time to reach therapeutic levels. In some cases, the first pass metabolism may be so extensive that it precludes administering the drug orally. Oral administration is the only route in which a drug is subject to first pass metabolism.

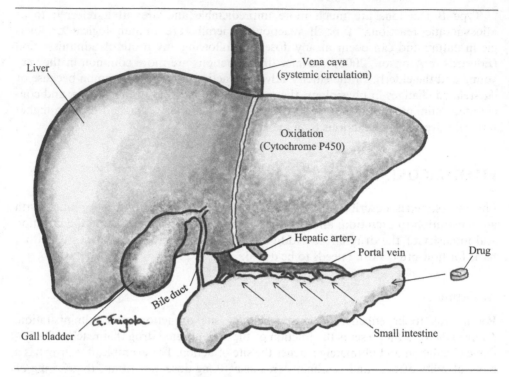

Figure 8.5   First Pass Drug Metabolism

Intravenous administration has a bioavailability of 100%, in part because first pass metabolism is circumvented, because the drug is administered directly into the systemic circulation; it also results in the most rapid onset of action. There is a greater risk with this route of administration since it is more invasive and the effects occur so quickly. Sublingual or buccal administration takes advantage of direct administration of the drug to a well vascularized mucous membrane. Additionally, this has provided a convenient mechanism to bypass the portal circulation and first pass metabolism. Onset of action is usually very rapid. Transdermal administration is useful for drugs that are highly lipophilic and allow drug absorption through a gel or a patch application. The lipophilic nature of the drug facilitates diffusion across the skin and subcutaneous tissues where it can enter systemic circulation. The onset of transdermally administered drugs is usually delayed, but this route of administration can provide a prolonged administration of a drug over several hours or days, avoiding sharp increases in plasma concentrations as exhibited by oral or *parenteral administration*.

Distribution

Distribution of a drug throughout the body is primarily achieved by the systemic circulation following absorption. Distribution into the various tissues is often dependent on the blood flow to those tissues. As such, disease states that may affect blood flow (i.e., cardiovascular disease, renal disease) may affect the distribution of the drug.

Volume of distribution (Vd) is a calculated pharmacokinetic parameter that describes the fluid volume that would be required to contain the amount of drug during steady state. *Steady state* is achieved when the peak and trough plasma concentrations of the drug are relatively constant. Generally, it requires four to five half-lives for a drug to reach steady state.

If a drug is hydrophilic, it tends to be contained primarily within the vascular compartment, so its volume of distribution is low. Highly lipophilic drugs are widely distributed in the body's various tissues and membranes, so the volume of distribution of these drugs generally greatly exceeds the blood volume. In general, drugs that have a higher volume of distribution require larger initial doses to obtain a therapeutic plasma level. Additionally, the volume of distribution in women is greater than that in men due to the larger amount of lipid tissue in women. Also, the volume of distribution can be affected by a change in the body mass or composition. Elderly patients often demonstrate a decrease in skeletal muscle mass, which could decrease the volume of distribution. Conversely, the increase in mass in obese patients could increase the volume of distribution.

Another important determinant of drug distribution is *plasma protein binding*. Several drugs may reversibly bind to plasma proteins, specifically *albumin* or *alpha-1 glycoprotein*. Albumin is the most prominent plasma protein and thus accounts for the majority of drug binding. If a drug is bound to plasma protein, the protein bound drug complex is simply too large for the drug to leave the vascular compartment. Unbound or free drug, however, can leave the vascular compartment to interact with the tissue receptors or undergo metabolism and/or excretion. Drugs that are highly protein bound (i.e., >90%) can be subject to drug interactions. If another highly protein bound drug is administered concomitantly, competition for the protein binding sites can result in an increase in the free drug concentration of one of the drugs, which may result in toxicity. Additionally, in some disease states involving the liver or kidneys there may be a reduction in plasma proteins (*hypoalbunemia*), which reduces the protein binding sites and increases the free drug concentrations of a highly protein bound drug, resulting in toxicity.

Metabolism

Termination of a drug's action is often accomplished through the metabolism of the drug. In general, drug metabolism changes the drug molecule so that its pharmacological actions are terminated and the drug becomes more water-soluble. The increase in water solubility facilitates excretion of the drug by the kidneys. However, some drugs can become pharmacologically activated through metabolism and their pharmacological actions increase. A drug, such as codeine, that is activated by metabolism is referred to as a *prodrug*. It is also not uncommon for the metabolic process to produce active *metabolites*. These active metabolites can be toxic, especially if they accumulate. This is the case with acetaminophen. In other instances, the metabolites may be active and extend the therapeutic actions of the drug, as is the case with some selective serotonin reuptake inhibitors such as fluoxetine.

The liver is usually identified as the major organ involved in metabolism. However, several other organs such as the GI tract, skin, kidneys, lungs, and even the blood can contribute to the metabolism of a drug. For example, monoamine oxidase is present in the intestinal mucosa, the kidneys, and the lungs, and can metabolize *sympathomimetic drugs*. Acetylcholinesterase is present in the blood and can metabolize many cholinergic drugs.

In the liver, the *hepatocytes* contain the specific enzymes that are located intracellularly on the endoplasmic reticulum. The primary enzymes involved in the metabolism of most drugs belong to the *cytochrome P450* class, which includes several *isozymes* (Nebert & Russell, 2002; Nelson et al., 1996; Frye, 2004). Drugs may be metabolized by a specific isozyme or in some cases there may be a major pathway involving one isozyme and then another minor pathway involving another isozyme. Even though there are a number of isozymes of the cytochrome P450 system, the CYP3A4 isozyme is involved in the metabolism of the most drugs. CYP2D6 represents another isozyme involved with the metabolism of a number of drugs but not to the same degree as CYP3A4. Other isozymes identified in drug metabolism to a lesser extent include CYP2C, CYP1A2, and CYP2E1.

Figure 8.6 presents the proportion of drugs metabolized by the different CYP450 enzymes (Wrighton, 1992), and the percentage of different CYP450 enzymes present in the liver (Pain et al., 2006; Shimada et al., 1994).

There are two phases of reactions in drug metabolism. In Phase I, the drug binds to the cytochrome P450 enzyme and then undergoes *hydroxylation, oxidation, hydrolysis,* or *reduction*. The net effect of these interactions is to produce a reactive site on the drug molecule. This can be done by either removing a chemical group from the drug molecule or inserting a reactive chemical entity onto the drug molecule. This site will be important in the Phase II reactions. The formation of these reactive sites accounts for some of the toxic effects of some metabolites. Table 8.1 lists the psychotropic drugs that are substrates for various CYP450 isozymes.

In Phase II reactions, a large chemical group is added to the molecule in a process referred to as *conjugation*. This is accomplished using *transferases*. During these reactions, glucuronic acid, sulfuric acid, acetic acid, or some other chemical group is attached to the reactive site on the drug molecule that was created during the Phase I reactions. These conjugation reactions result in a metabolite that has a different structure from the parent compound. Thus, virtually all products of conjugation have reduced pharmacological activity since the molecule is chemically altered and does not fit the receptor. These reactions may also be named according to the chemical group added, for example, *glucuronidation, acetylation, sulfation.* Additionally,

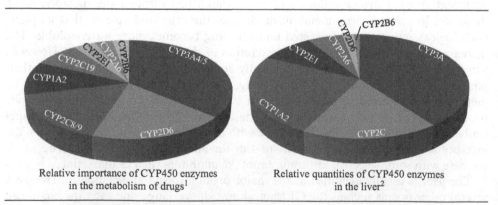

Relative importance of CYP450 enzymes
in the metabolism of drugs[1]

Relative quantities of CYP450 enzymes
in the liver[2]

Figure 8.6   Relative Importance of CYP450 Enzymes
[1]As reported in Wrighton and Stevens (1992).
[2]As reported in Paine et al. (2006) and Shimada, Yamazaki, Mimura, Inui, and Guengerich (1994).
Adapted from Borges (2008).

Table 8.1   Cytochrome P450 Enzymes and Respective Substrates

	CYP3A4	CYP2D6	CYP1A2	CYP2C9
S	Alprazolam	Amitriptyline	Amitriptyline	Amitriptyline
U	Aripiprazole	Aripiprazole	Caffeine	Imipramine
B	Buspirone	Desipramine	Clomipramine	Phenytoin
S	Citalopram	Fluoxetine	Clozapine	
T	Clomipramine	Haloperidol	Imipramine	
R	Diazepam	Imipramine	Olanzapine	
A	Escitalopram	Metoprolol		
T	Flunitrazepam	Paroxetine		
E	Fluoxetine	Perphenazine		
	Haloperidol	Propranolol		
	Imipramine	Risperidol		
	Midazolam	Risperidone		
	Norfluoxetine	Thioridazine		
	Risperidone	Venlafaxine		
	Sertraline			
	Triazolam			
	Venlafaxine			
	Ziprasidone			

the conjugation reactions increase the polarity of the drug, which renders the drug more water soluble (hydrophilic), increasing its ability to be excreted by the kidneys.

Phase II metabolism occurs in multiple organs (e.g., liver, kidneys, lungs, spleen, intestines), although it is principally accomplished in the liver. Once the conjugation reaction has occurred, the metabolite is transported to the small intestine via the bile. The metabolite is then absorbed across the intestinal villi where it enters the systemic circulation and is carried to the kidneys, to be filtered across the glomerulus and excreted. Nonetheless, some drugs may undergo *enterohepatic recirculation*, a process in which the conjugated drug is converted back to the parent compound by enzymes in the small intestine. With enterohepatic recirculation the drug regains its pharmacological activity and can be carried to the active sites in the body via the vena cava or through absorption from the small intestine to the systemic circulation. Enterohepatic circulation, as seen in Figure 8.7, can concentrate the potency of the drug and can also increase the duration of the original effect.

Drug metabolism enzymes can be influenced by the drugs that undergo metabolism. Several drugs are known to bind to the cytochrome P450 enzymes resulting in their inhibition. This can result in a decrease in the rate of metabolism of the drug or another concomitantly administered drug. The drug can accumulate and become toxic. However, in the presence of an inhibitor, a prodrug may not be activated and an inadequate therapeutic response may occur, because the prodrug relies on metabolism for its activation.

Drug metabolism enzymes can also be induced by some drugs such as anticonvulsants. Induction results in an increased synthesis and/or activity of the enzymes. This results in an acceleration of the metabolism of drugs. This can decrease the therapeutic response of the inducing drug or of concomitantly administered drugs. Generally, inducers result in a decreased therapeutic response. One consequence of induction is that an inducing drug can induce its own metabolism, resulting in the

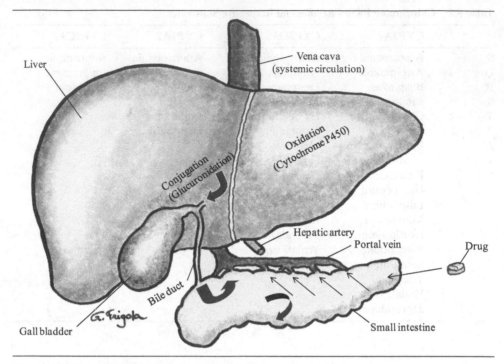

Figure 8.7   Enterohepatic Drug Metabolism
Note: Drug is absorbed through the portal vein, conjugated in the liver, and returned to the small intestine through the bile duct, where it is enzymatically converted to the original drug and reabsorbed into the liver where it is concentrated or is absorbed from the small intestine into the systemic circulation.

need for larger doses over time. A list of some drugs that can act as *inducers* and *inhibitors* are shown in Table 8.2.

Although the majority of drugs undergo metabolism, there are a few drugs that are not subject to liver metabolism but, rather, are eliminated unchanged through the kidneys. Lithium, an element with no metabolic value, is an important example of such a drug. Lithium is excreted through the kidneys and, therefore, changes in renal function can have significant clinical implications; decreased renal function can result in toxic accumulation of lithium.

Excretion

Most drugs are excreted from the body through the kidneys. As described earlier, lipophilic drugs, due to their chemical nature, have minimal water solubility, and must be made more hydrophilic by metabolism. Some excretion of a drug will occur through the fecal route because most orally administered drugs are incompletely absorbed. The bioavailability of orally administered drugs is not 100%. The unabsorbed portion of the drug will pass through GI tract and be excreted unchanged.

The kidneys receive approximately 25% of the total systemic blood flow. This allows for very good filtration of the blood. As the blood is filtered through the glomerulus, only unbound, free drug can pass across the glomerular membrane unless there is renal damage. Therefore, the main factors that affect renal excretion of a drug are the *glomerular filtration rate*, the renal blood flow, and the protein

Table 8.2   CYP 450 Inhibitors and Inducers

	CYP3A4	CYP2D6	CYP1A2	CYP2C9
Inhibitors	Cimetidine Erythromycin Ketaconazole Grapefruit juice Omeprazole	Fluoxetine Paroxetine Haloperidol	Cimetidine Fluvoxamine Erythromycin	Cimetidine Disulfiram
Inducers	Carbamazepine Phenobarbital Modafinil St. John's Wort	Carbamazepine	Smoking Carbamazepine Modafinil Charred grilled meat	Carbamazepine St. John's Wort

binding of the drug. If any of these factors change, there can be a significant alteration in the renal excretion of a drug. As one ages, we typically see a reduction in renal function and this can result in the accumulation of a drug. This is one of the main reasons that drug dosages are frequently reduced in the elderly. With some drugs, it is important to adjust the dosage based on the glomerular filtration rate, and *creatinine clearance* is calculated to provide an estimate of the glomerular filtration rate.

In addition to the kidney and liver, *P-glycoprotein*, a transporter protein, has been demonstrated to have an important role in excretion as well as movement of some drugs across membranes. In the small intestine, P-glycoprotein usually transports drug molecules out of the intestinal cells into the lumen where the drug can be eliminated. Inhibition of P-glycoprotein, for example, with grapefruit juice, can have important consequences by allowing a drug to accumulate to toxic levels in the body. P-glycoproteins may be subject to *polymorphisms* as discussed later in this chapter.

Regardless of whether a drug is metabolized or simply excreted, drugs are eventually eliminated from the body. Most drugs are eliminated through *first-order kinetics* in which the rate of elimination is proportional to the concentration in the plasma. The plasma concentration of the drug will decrease exponentially over time, and the decrease will be constant. Regardless of the concentration, the amount of drug will decrease by 50% over each half-life of the drug.

A few drugs (e.g., phenytoin and ethanol) do not undergo first-order elimination kinetics. Instead, they follow *zero-order kinetics* in which the rate of elimination is constant regardless of the concentration in the plasma. Rather than exponentially, the rate of elimination is linear. Zero-order kinetics occur with drugs that saturate their elimination mechanisms.

Pharmacokinetic Parameters

Half-life is a useful parameter for estimating the duration of action of a drug and can be used to determine dosing intervals. Half-life is defined as the time required to reduce the plasma concentration by one-half. For example, if a dose of a drug produces a plasma concentration of 10 mg, the half-life would be the amount of time required for the plasma concentration to decrease to 5 mg. The metabolism, excretion, and the volume of distribution of the drug affect half-life. The half-life of a drug may be increased in individuals that are obese (increased distribution), who have cardiac, renal, and/or liver disease (decreased clearance) or who have reduced cytochrome P450 enzyme action (decreased metabolism). Alternatively, the half-life of a drug may be decreased as a result of aging (decreased distribution) or secondary to cytochrome P450 induction (increased metabolism).

Area under the curve (AUC) is determined by integrating the plasma concentration of a drug over time. This parameter is important in providing an estimate of bioavailability. As discussed earlier, bioavailability of drugs given intravenously is 100%. The bioavailability of a drug given by a different route of administration can be calculated using the following equation:

$$\text{Bioavailability (F)} = AUC_{\text{(route of administration)}} / AUC_{\text{(IV)}}$$

Parenthetically, as discussed later, generic drugs must demonstrate that their AUC is equivalent to that of the brand drug in order to gain FDA approval.

Clearance represents the rate of elimination of a drug from the plasma. This is not the same as excretion. Drugs may be cleared from the plasma and enter tissue but still remain in the body. Excretion refers to elimination of the drug from the body. Clearance is dependent on the chemical properties of the drug, the efficiency of the organs at extracting the drug from the plasma, and the blood flow to the organ, which determines the rate of delivery of the drug to the target site. Clearance can be greatly affected by disease states, especially those diseases involving the cardiovascular, hepatic, and renal systems.

When a drug is administered multiple times, steady state occurs when the rate of administration equals the rate of elimination. In general, steady state is achieved in 4–5 half-lives. At steady state, the minimum plasma concentration (C_{min}) and the maximum plasma concentration (C_{max}) are relatively constant. Ideally, the plasma concentration between C_{max} and C_{min} represents the *therapeutic window* for the drug. Once dosing stops, it generally takes 4–5 half-lives to eliminate the drug from the plasma.

PHARMACOGENOMICS

The genetic make-up of an individual dictates how that individual will respond to drugs. *Pharmacogenomics* represents the characterization of these genetic components and their clinical and therapeutic implications. Genetic differences in drug metabolism and response has long been recognized. For example, the historical literature has described fast and slow metabolizers of several drugs. There is renewed interest in this area with the hope that by determining a patient's metabolic profile, it will be possible to optimize therapy by choosing the correct drug, dose, and dosage interval (Evans & McLeod, 2003).

Pharmacogenetic differences can impact both the pharmacokinetics and the pharmacodynamics of a drug. These differences remain stable throughout the individual's lifetime. The clinical relevance of a particular polymorphism is dependent on a number of factors, such as whether the enzyme system involved represents a major or minor metabolic pathway, whether there are active metabolites, and the steepness of the dose response.

Polymorphisms often segregate patients into poor metabolizers or extensive or ultrarapid metabolizers. *Poor metabolizers* often demonstrate exaggerated drug responses such as prolonged drug effects and toxicity due to the accumulation of the drug. In the case of prodrugs, poor metabolizers will have a diminished therapeutic response because there will be a delay in the formation of the active component of the drug or, in some cases, insufficient active drug produced. Ultrarapid or *extensive metabolizers* frequently experience subtherapeutic drug levels and subsequent therapeutic failure due to their rapid metabolism. If given a prodrug, toxicity can occur due to the rapid formation of the active component. With significant polymorphism, inhibition or induction of the enzymes can result in greatly exaggerated responses.

Several polymorphisms have been identified with psychotropic drugs. Many of these have been related to a polymorphism of CYP2D6 (Mrazek, 2006; Wall, Oldenkamp, & Swintak, 2010). For example, increased extrapyramidal symptoms have been observed in patients that are poor metabolizers of haloperidol. In addition to polymorphisms identified with metabolic enzymes, polymorphisms of receptors and P-glycoprotein have also been described.

DRUG DEVELOPMENT

Currently, the Food and Drug Administration (FDA) must approve all drugs sold in the United States as being safe and effective. This has not always been the case. In 1906, the Pure Food and Drug Act resulted in the creation of the FDA, which was then charged with assuring that drugs met established standards for quality and purity. The Food, Drug and Cosmetic Act that was passed in 1938 required that a drug manufacturer provide proof of a drug's safety and purity. Subsequently, the Food, Drug and Cosmetic Act was amended in 1962 to required proof of efficacy and safety for all new drugs approved. This amendment also provided important and needed guidelines about clinical testing and the reporting of adverse drug events (Lipsky & Martin, 2001).

Today, pharmaceutical companies must demonstrate various qualities of the drug through extensive testing. Before administration into human subjects, extensive preclinical testing is conducted. During this preclinical phase of drug development, a thorough description of the drug's chemical structure and properties, its receptor binding profile, and toxicity is undertaken. The initial characterization is done using *in vitro* testing as well as extensive testing of the drug's pharmacology and toxicology in at least three animal species, with at least some of the tests being conducted in a nonrodent animal. These studies provide important information concerning the absorption, distribution, metabolism, and excretion of the drug in the animal models.

Additionally, the *mechanism of action* is defined. Using *in vitro* binding studies defines which receptors the drug will interact with at therapeutic concentrations. These studies can also provide insight into potential toxic effects by determining which receptors are bound at high drug concentrations. The administration of the candidate drug *in vivo* is important in characterizing what effects the drug will have on the various systems of the intact organism. For example, an antidepressant is designed to have a therapeutic effect primarily in the central nervous system. However, since it is given orally, it can and will interact with peripheral sites such as the heart or peripheral autonomic nervous system, which may explain some of its side effects.

These preclinical studies provide important information regarding the metabolic profile of the drug—that is, whether there are active or toxic metabolites formed and, if so, how their actions could contribute to the overall pharmacological actions of the drug. Also, by determining the metabolic pathways, important information is gained about potential sites of drug interactions by determining which specific enzymes are involved in the metabolism of the drug.

Prior to administering the drug to humans, the toxicology of the drug is characterized. Animal studies will have previously determined the dose of drug at which no effect occurs (no-effect dose), the minimum lethal dose, and the median lethal dose. The effects of the drug on specific organ systems are also determined. Although all organ systems are usually evaluated, we are particularly interested in a drug's effects on the liver, kidneys, cardiovascular, and hematological systems. In most cases, the drug is administered to normal animals as well as animal that fit models of the disease for which the drug is being tested.

Although many of the preclinical studies are relatively short in duration (a few hours to a few months), longer studies that may last several months or a year may be initiated, especially in the case where a drug would be given for a long period of time. Additionally, preclinical studies will be done in which the drug is administered to pregnant animals to determine if there are any teratogenic or mutagenic effects of the drug. *Teratogenic effects* are those that may result in birth defects due to changes in somatic tissues as seen with several psychotropic drugs such as lithium, valproic acid, benzodiazepines, and selective serotonin reuptake inhibitors. *Mutagenic effects* are those effects in which the genetic material is altered and can result in inheritable abnormalities. Mutagenic effects are usually evaluated using the *Ames test*, which is an *in vitro* test. Drugs are also tested for their carcinogenic potential.

The overall purpose of the preclinical studies is to provide sufficient evidence to the FDA demonstrating that the drug is reasonably safe for administration to humans. All the preclinical studies are compiled, analyzed, and submitted to the FDA as an *Investigational New Drug Application,* which is referred to as an IND. In addition to the preclinical pharmacology and toxicology studies, the IND also provides information concerning the proposed *clinical trials* as well as the demonstration that the manufacturer can consistently produce the drug in its proposed dosage form. Once the IND is submitted to the FDA, the FDA reviews and evaluates the information. The IND is reviewed on three general levels: chemical, pharmacology/toxicology, and medical. The chemical review basically evaluates the stability of the proposed drug molecule as well as the ability of the drug manufacturer to consistently manufacture or produce the drug. The pharmacology/toxicology review focuses on the safety of the drug as demonstrated by preclinical animal/*in vitro* studies. The medical review determines whether the proposed clinical trial protocols are adequately designed and powered sufficiently to gain meaningful data. The medical review also determines whether any of the clinical trial participants would be exposed to any undue risks.

When its review is completed, if the FDA approves, the IND clinical trials can then begin. In some cases, the FDA may request additional preclinical studies be done prior to approval or, conversely, the FDA can disapprove the drug. Once the IND is approved, the drug can be tested in humans. However, it is common that additional *in vitro* and long-term animal studies are done to gain more information about the drug while the human clinical studies are initiated. Additional animal or *in vitro* studies are often conducted as new information arises during clinical trials.

After approval of the IND, the proposed drug undergoes three phases of clinical trials. *Phase I trials* represent the first administration of the drug into humans and are designed to establish the safety of the drug as well as how well the drug will be tolerated in humans. These studies are relatively small, usually involving between 20 and 100 subjects. The subjects chosen for Phase I studies are healthy individuals and it is not uncommon for these studies to be unblinded. The main goal of Phase I studies is to determine the absorption, distribution, metabolism, and excretion of the drug. Generally, subjects are started on a dose of the drug that is not expected to have an effect and the dose can be increased to determine the maximal tolerated dose of the drug. During the Phase I studies, side effects are particularly noted as well as pharmacokinetic parameters in humans. This information will be particularly useful in the designing of Phase II and III clinical trials. Thus, the primary objectives of Phase I clinical trials are to establish safety, pharmacokinetic parameters, and the toxicity of the drug. It is estimated that more than 50% of proposed drugs do not make it past Phase I.

Phase II trials represent the first instance when the drug is administered to patients with the disease that the drug is intended to treat. The primary objectives of Phase II studies are to further define the efficacy and safety of the drug when treating the indicated disease. Phase II studies are larger than Phase I studies, often evaluating several hundred patients. Thus, the studies have more power to detect side effects that may be encountered when the drug is marketed. Moreover, Phase II studies build on the data obtained during the initial Phase I studies by further defining the dose response relationships. During this phase of clinical trials, single blind studies are often done with the test drug compared to either placebo and/or another drug. Assuming demonstrated efficacy as well as no safety concerns, the results of Phase II studies provide important direction for conduction of *Phase III trials*.

The largest, most complex clinical trials are conducted in Phase III. It is in this stage of drug development that the randomized, double blind, controlled trials are done. Several hundred to several thousand patients at multiple clinical sites are employed. The trials can last for several months or even years, depending on the proposed use of the drug. The FDA requires the studies to have specific predetermined primary and secondary endpoints. Generally, the FDA requires a minimum of two randomized controlled trials for a drug to obtain approval.

Upon completion of the Phase III trials, the drug manufacturer files a *New Drug Application (NDA)*. The NDA includes the information in the IND, the results of the clinical trials done in Phases I, II, and III, as well as any new additional *in vitro* or animal studies. The format for all NDAs is outlined explicitly in the Code of Federal Regulations and undergoes reviews that specifically evaluate the drug from the perspectives of chemistry, *biopharmaceutics*, pharmacology, statistics, and medical; in addition, antibiotic drugs will undergo a microbiology review. NDAs are reviewed internally but may also utilize external advisory committees. Once an NDA is reviewed, the FDA either deems the application approved, not approved, or approvable. An approved NDA allows the marketing of the drug for the approved indication using the approved dosage range. If an NDA is not approved or is ruled approvable, the FDA provides the drug manufacturer with the specific deficiencies that resulted in the drug not being approved. In general, if an NDA is deemed not approved, there are major deficiencies, and significant additional studies will be required. Under such prospects, not-approved drugs are usually dropped from further development. An approvable NDA usually only requires a few additional studies or a supporting data.

Once approved by the FDA, a drug can be marketed only for the indication, the population, and in the dose that it was approved. The approved drug may be prescribed by providers for other indications, populations, and/or dosages than approved. This is referred to as *off-label use* and is based on the prescriber's clinical judgment. Off-label use is common in children because many drugs, in the past, were never approved for use in children because this population was not frequently included in clinical trials during drug approval. It is important to remember that since safety and efficacy have not been established for off-label use, the prescriber uses the drug off-label at his or her own liability risk.

After approval, additional clinical studies are often conducted. These are *Phase IV Trials* or postmarketing studies. These studies have become particularly important for monitoring the safety of the drug by detecting rare side effects or for detecting drug interactions. Because of the relatively small number of subjects involved in the Phase I to III clinical studies, it is unlikely that rare side effects (e.g., those that occur in 1 out of 10,000 patients or more) will be detected. Furthermore, Phase IV studies may also evaluate potential drug interactions that may arise when the drug becomes marketed in the real world. The overall drug approval process and timeline is shown in Figure 8.8.

After a drug is marketed, it is also important to monitor the safety of the drug because more patients are exposed in very diverse conditions (i.e., comorbid disease states, concomitant drug administration). It is important to remember that drug safety is dynamic. Just because a drug is approved by the FDA as being safe and effective, this does not guarantee that the drug will retain these attributes throughout the life of the drug. It is the duty of drug manufacturers to continually monitor the safety of the drug postapproval, and to update the prescribing information as soon as new safety information becomes available (Friedman et al., 1999; Lurie & Sasich, 1999).

The science of monitoring drug safety is referred to as *pharmacovigilance*. The FDA requires drug companies to monitor, assess, and report adverse events of their products. To facilitate the reporting of adverse events, the FDA established the MEDWATCH *program* in 1993. Medical psychologists and other providers, as well as patients, are encouraged to report adverse events of drugs to the FDA. The minimal information required to report an adverse event through the MEDWATCH program is a patient, a drug, the particular side effect and an identifiable reporter. However, as much information as possible should be provided. It is not necessary to prove causation in order to report the adverse event. A copy of the MEDWATCH form is shown in Figure 8.9.

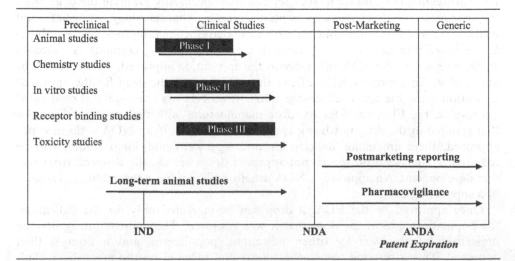

Figure 8.8   Drug Evolution: From Clinical Trials to Generic Availability

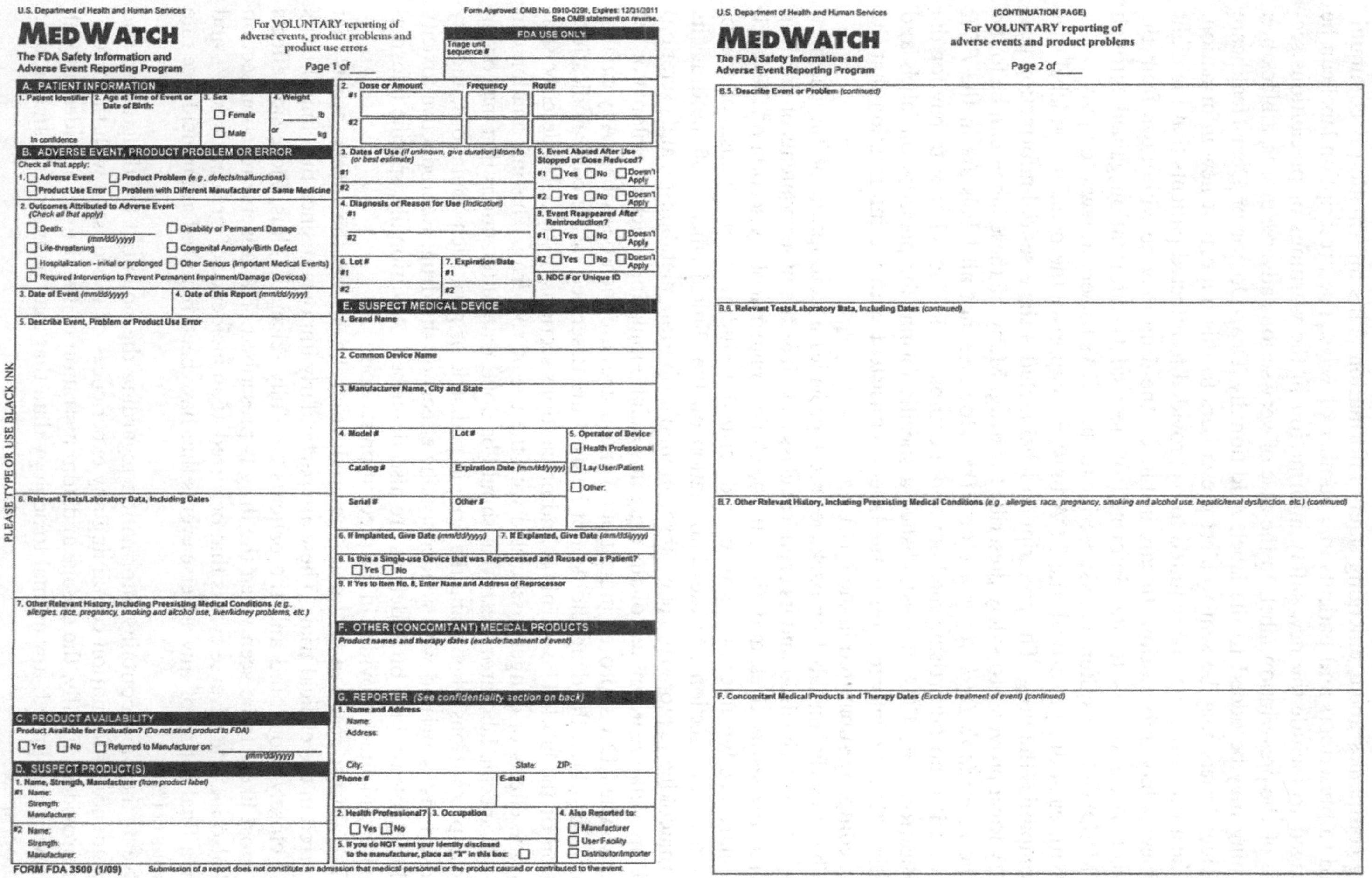

Figure 8.9 MEDWATCH Form

The information gained from the MEDWATCH program is collected in the FDA's *Adverse Events Reporting System (AERS)* database and used to alert the FDA and drug companies about emerging safety information. This information is communicated to prescribers and patients in a number of ways. The prescription label can be changed to include the new safety information in the warnings or precautions sections of the prescription label. In the case of very serious adverse events, a black box warning may be added to the label. Additionally, Dear-Doctor or Dear-Healthcare Provider letters may be sent to alert prescribers to this important new information. Medication guides may be required to be provided to affected patients that highlight the new safety information. In rare instances, the drug may be withdrawn from the market. An easy way to stay informed of new safety information gained through the MEDWATCH system is to subscribe to the FDA's listserv at www.fda.gov

With each drug approval, the FDA must also approve the prescription label that accompanies the drug. The prescription label includes the essential information necessary for a provider to safely prescribe the drug. Many of these labels can be found in the *Physician's Desk Reference* or *PDR*. However, not all labels are in the *PDR* because it is an advertising medium and a company may not choose to pay for the publication. The FDA has established a specific format for prescription labels and requires that the information in the label is consistent with the information that the drug company submitted in the NDA.

The prescription label or package insert provides a description of the chemical description of the drug and its chemical class as well as the other contents of the drug such as *excipients*, dyes, and fillers. In the clinical pharmacology section of the label, the pharmacodynamics of the drug are described, including the mechanism of action. Moreover, this section provides information on the clinical efficacy of the drug, its pharmacokinetic properties (e.g., absorption, distribution, metabolism, and excretion) and any data regarding use of the drug in special populations such as children or the elderly. The FDA approved indication(s) and usages are then described. Any circumstances in which the drug should not be used are described in the contraindications section of the label. The warnings and precautions sections of the label describe serious side effects or dangers associated with the use of the drug. This information can include specific laboratory tests that should be done, drug interactions that may occur, special precautions when using the drug in pediatric or geriatric populations, and any precautions associated with gender-specific effects of the drug. Reproductive toxicity and the potential for birth defects are also described. Additionally, specific information for patients is provided in the precaution section.

The adverse reaction section of the product label describes the adverse events that occurred in the clinical trials. These are particularly important since the clinical trials were closely monitored and the patients carefully selected. Thus, those side effects are most likely to be seen when the drug is prescribed. The adverse reaction section will also include adverse events that occurred at an incidence of greater than 1%, and then a final listing of any adverse events that have been reported at an incidence rate less than 1%.

Next, the label contains information regarding the potential for drug abuse and dependence. Information containing any experiences of overdosage with the drug is also provided. Finally, the dosage and administration of the drug is provided, as well as how it is supplied, any animal toxicology data that may be pertinent, and product photographs.

The FDA has recognized that the old label format was complex and very difficult for prescribers to find answers to specific questions. The package insert was written for prescribers, and not for patients. In assessing the usefulness of the label, the FDA also recognized that the approval date of the drug was not included in the information or whether there were any recent changes to the label. As a result, the FDA recently instituted a new label format that contains a highlight section that provides an overview of the risks and benefits of the drug. A contents section is also provided that presents an easy-to-use reference to more detailed safety and efficacy information. The highlighted section provides an abbreviated summary of the most clinically relevant information needed by the prescriber.

Although every package insert contains a contraindication, warnings, and precautions section, some drugs may require an additional type of warning known as a *black box warning*. The black box warning represents the most serious warning that a drug can have. The warning is placed at the top of the label in a bold black box so that it is prominently displayed. This warning is generally reserved for problems that may lead to serious injury or death with the use of the medication and must be approved by the FDA. In some cases, all drugs in a particular class receive a black box warning. This is referred to as a class warning; the risk of increased suicidal ideation associated with antidepressants is an example.

Generic Drugs

Generic drugs came into existence as a major remedy to offset rising health-care costs. Prior to 1984, generic drugs went through the same efficacy and safety evaluation process as brand-name prescription drugs. Since this was expensive with regard to cost and time, very few generic drugs were prescribed. The availability of generic drugs is dependent on when the patent of the brand-name drug expires. Most patents in the United States are applied for just prior to the initiation of animal testing and protect the brand drug for 20 years. However, in 1984, the Hatch-Waxman Act was passed that provided an abbreviated FDA approval process for generic drugs by allowing generic drug companies to rely on the safety and efficacy studies that were done when the drug was a brand-name drug. It additionally allowed generic drug companies to initiate product development before the brand name company's patent expired.

Generic manufacturers apply for generic drug approval by submitting an abbreviated new drug application referred to as an ANDA. Since a generic drug contains identical amounts of the active drug as the brand-name, has the same indications, dosage form, and route of administration, a generic company only needs to demonstrate that its active ingredient is *bioequivalent* to the *reference listed drug (RLD)*. The reference listed drug is the standard drug to which all generics are compared and is usually the name brand drug. The purpose of the RLD is to minimize variations between generic drug products elaborated and manufactured by different companies. A generic drug company must also demonstrate that it can consistently produce the drug product within the necessary manufacturing specifications. Compared to the approval process for the brand name drug, which usually requires between 10 and 14 years, the generic drug approval process is usually only 2 to 4 years (Hornecker, 2009).

A key requirement of generic drugs is the demonstration that the drug is bioequivalent. A drug that is deemed to be bioequivalent to the brand product means that the bioavailability of the drugs in the body does not differ significantly. Typically, this is determined by giving a single oral dose of the generic drug to 24 to 36 healthy adults and then determining two absorption parameters: area under the curve (AUC) and the maximal concentration (C_{max}). The generic drug must demonstrate that the 90% confidence intervals for these parameters must fall within 80% to 125% of that of the branded drug in order for the generic to be considered bioequivalent. This requirement was an FDA regulatory decision that was based on the concept that most drugs with the same active ingredient would not have clinically significant differences in blood levels and, thus, therapeutic effects would presumably be equivalent (Chen et al., 2001; Kesselheim et al., 2008). There is debate, however, about whether all drugs that are bioequivalent are also therapeutically equivalent because bioequivalence is based on pharmacokinetic parameters whereas therapeutic equivalence is dependent on pharmacodynamics parameters such as efficacy and toxicity. Therapeutic equivalence is not directly tested but is assumed based on the bioequivalency testing.

The issue of therapeutic equivalence versus bioequivalence is of most concern with drugs that have a *narrow therapeutic index*. The FDA defines a narrow therapeutic index drug as one that has less than a twofold difference in the median lethal dose and the median effective dose or less than a twofold difference in the minimum toxic concentration and the minimum effective blood concentration. Additionally, these drugs would require careful titration and monitoring in order to be used safely. Drugs that meet these criteria include digoxin, lithium, phenytoin, theophylline, and warfarin. In addition to the FDA, several other health-care organizations have also included antiarrhythmics, anticonvulsants, and immunosuppressants. Thus, with these drugs, prescribers often request brand drugs in order to minimize variability. Nevertheless, one should be vigilant concerning adverse effects when one is shifting from brand to generic or vice versa. Because of differences in appearances between brand and among generics, patients are often less likely to note a misfilled prescription if it occurs.

Over-the-Counter (OTC) Drugs or Nonprescription Drugs

Almost every drug sold OTC was initially approved as a prescription drug and sold as such for several years until its safety was well established. Several of the OTC products are simply lower dosages of the prescription medications. OTC drugs are considered to have considerable safety margins and are believed to be able to be used without the supervision of a prescriber. This does not mean that OTC medications are without side effects or drug interactions. In fact, both side effects and drug interactions have been well documented.

Supplements

Dietary supplements include vitamins, herbs, minerals, and botanicals. Although the FDA oversees the safety and health claims made of dietary supplements, the efficacy and safety of these substances are not evaluated with the same scrutiny as drugs. The FDA can restrict or halt the sale of these substances if it can demonstrate the substances are unsafe. Supplements cannot make claims of treating any particular disease.

Scheduled Drugs

The Controlled Substances Act identifies and classifies drugs according to their potential for abuse. *Controlled drugs* are classified by the Drug Enforcement Administration (DEA) and a current list of drugs in each class is available on the DEA's web site.

Table 8.3   DEA Scheduled Drugs

Schedule	Examples
I	Marijuana, LSD, Ecstasy (MDMA), Peyote, Heroin
II	Cocaine, Fentanyl, Methadone, Lisdexamfetamine, Dextroamphetamine, Methylphenidate, Morphine
III	Anabolic steroids, Marinol, Buprenorphine, Hydrocodone
IV	Benzodiazepines
V	Promethazine

There are five classes or schedules. Schedule I drugs are defined as those drugs that have no approved medical use and have a high potential for abuse that can lead to severe psychological or physical dependence. Schedule II drugs have a high abuse potential but have an approved medical use. Schedules III, IV, and V all have medical uses but they also carry the potential for abuse and dependence in decreasing order. Because of the high level of abuse of controlled substances, there is a greater accountability of their use. Examples of *scheduled drugs* are noted in Table 8.3.

CHAPTER 8 KEY TERMS

Absorption: The passage of the drug into the circulatory system.

Acetylation: A reaction that introduces an acetyl functional group into an organic compound.

Adverse drug reaction: Injurious reaction to medication given at a normal indicated dose.

AERS (Adverse Events Reporting System): The Adverse Event Reporting System (AERS) is a computerized information database designed to support the FDA's post-marketing safety surveillance program for all approved drug and therapeutic biologic products.

Affinity: The tendency of a neural transmitter or drug to form strong or weak chemical bonds with a receptor.

Agonist: A drug that activates the receptor when it binds to it.

Albumin: Serum albumin is the most abundant protein in the blood; one of its functions is to transport certain substances like hormones and drugs.

Alpha-1 glycoprotein: A plasma protein, like albumin, which may act to transport drugs.

Allosteric binding: Binding outside of the receptor site, which affects the receptor through secondary processes.

Ames test: A biological assay that detects certain chemicals that affect DNA and may have mutagenic potential.

Antagonist: A drug that inhibits or inactivates the receptor when it binds to the receptor; an antagonist does not cause the opposite effect of an agonist, but merely attenuates the agonist's effect (see *Inverse agonist*).

AUC (Area under the curve): The area under the plot of serum concentration of a drug against the time after drug administration.

Association constant: A mathematical description of the affinity of a ligand for a receptor protein at equilibrium.

Bioavailability (F): The percent or fraction of an administered drug that reaches the systemic circulation.

Bioequivalent: Two pharmaceutical products are bioequivalent if their bioavailabilities after administration are similar.

Biopharmaceutics: The study of a drug's chemical properties in relation to onset, duration, and intensity of drug action at specified dosage.

Black box warning: Highlighted information in a drug insert that indicates a significant risk of serious or life-threatening adverse effect.

Clearance: The rate at which a drug is removed from the body; clearance is defined as the rate of drug elimination divided by the plasma concentration of the drug.

Clinical trial: A clinical trial is a research study to answer specific questions about vaccines or new therapies or new ways of using known treatments. Clinical trials (also called medical research and research studies) are used to determine whether new drugs or treatments are both safe and effective. Trials are in four phases: Phase I tests a new drug or treatment in a small group; Phase II expands the study to a larger group of people; Phase III expands the study to an even larger group of people; and Phase IV takes place after the drug or treatment has been licensed and marketed. (See *Phase I, II, III,* and *IV trials.*)

Competitive antagonist: A substance, such as a drug, that binds to a receptor, thereby occupying it, without activating the receptor.

Conjugation: Phase II metabolism consists of conjugation, which adds molecular weight to carboxyl, hydroxyl, amino, and sulfhydryl groups, and usually renders the molecule inert.

Controlled drug: A controlled (scheduled) drug is one whose use and distribution is tightly controlled because of its abuse potential or risk.

Covalent binding: Covalent binding is based on the binding of enzymes and proteins by covalent or irreversible bonds.

Creatinine clearance: The creatinine clearance test compares the level of creatinine in urine with the creatinine level in the blood.

Cytochrome P450 (CYP450): An extensive family of enzymes located primarily in the liver that metabolizes drugs.

D-isomer: An asymmetric stereoisomer whose carbon atom rotates plane-polarized light clockwise (to the right).

Dissociation constant: An equilibrium constant that measures the propensity of a ligand to separate (dissociate) reversibly from a receptor.

Distribution: Describes the reversible transfer of drug from one location to another within the body.

Dose response curve: Defines the relationship between dose and response to the agent. The response can be therapeutic or it can detail side effects.

Down-regulation: Through RNA transcription, an adaptive decrease in the number of surface receptors, rendering the cell less sensitive to neural transmitters, hormones, or drugs.

Effective dose: (see *Potency*). The dose needed to effect a response.

ED50 (Effective dose): The dose that produces 50% of the maximum response.

Effector protein: An intermediate or go-between protein that is activated by postsynaptic binding with the G protein-coupled receptor site and which subsequently binds to and activates an intracellular secondary messenger.

Efficacy (E_{Max}): Refers to the capacity to produce an effect. E_{Max} refers to the maximum response achievable from a drug. It is not so much dose related as it is effect related.

Electrostatic binding: The temporary, weak binding of ligand to protein complexes through oppositely charged molecules.

Enantiomer: Chiral ("hand" in Greek) molecule that is one of two stereoisomers that are mirror images of each other; that is, they are nonsuperimposable, like the left and right hand.

Enterohepatic recirculation: Conjugated drugs that enter the intestines by way of the bile duct and are deconjugated in the small intestine and subsequently introduced back into systemic circulation as active metabolites.

Enzymatic transmembrane receptor: One of three transmembrane cell-surface receptors, this class of receptor is linked to enzymes within the cell such as protein kinases.

Excipient: An inert substance added to a drug as a carrier for the active ingredients of the medication.

Excretion: The process or act of expelling waste products from the body.

Extensive metabolizer: A person whose CYP450 enzyme(s) is/are particularly effective in metabolizing certain drugs. The extensive metabolizer may be identified through drug reaction testing, which uses genetic testing to predict how a particular person will respond to various drugs by checking for genes that code for specific CYP450 liver enzymes.

First-order kinetics: The rate of elimination is proportional to the amount of drug in the body.

First pass metabolism: The initial degradation of a drug in the liver and intestines before its remaining active ingredients are introduced into systemic circulation.

Full agonist: Compounds that exhibit full efficacy in receptor binding and activation.

Generic drug: A drug product that is comparable to a brand/reference listed drug in dosage form, strength, route of administration, quality and performance characteristics, and intended use.

Glomerular filtration rate: The volume of liquid filtered from the glomerular capillaries into Bowman's capsule per unit of time.

Glucuronidation: A part of Phase II metabolism in which the addition of glucuronic acid to a substrate through conjugation renders it inert.

G protein-coupled receptor: Seven-transmembrane α-helix structured receptors that are activated by agonists on the postsynaptic membrane and trigger intracellular signal transduction pathways that result in changes in cellular response.

Graded dose response curve: Plots the degree of a given response against the concentration of the drug.

Half-life: The time it takes for the blood plasma concentration of a substance at steady-state to be reduced by half.

Hepatocytes: The chief functional cells of the liver, involved in metabolic, endocrine, and secretory activities.

Hydrolysis: A reaction in which water is added to a molecule.

Hydroxylation: A reaction, catalyzed by enzymes, which incorporates a hydroxyl group into an organic compound.

Hydrophilic: Hydrophilic molecules are typically charge-polarized and capable of hydrogen bonding; it is this nature that makes them attracted to, and often dissolved by, water.

Hypoalbunemia: Abnormally low levels of serum albumin.

IND (Investigational New Drug Application): After successful preclinical drug trials, the IND is the mechanism by which a drug formally progresses to clinical trials in human subjects.

Inducer: A substance that speeds up the drug's enzymatic metabolism. The drug itself may self-induce greater metabolic action, or such a reaction might be caused through an interaction with other inducing substances.

Inhibitor: A substance that slows down the metabolism of a drug.

Intracellular receptor: A receptor within the cell that is activated by an effector protein, secondary messenger, or transcription factor and serves as a link in intracellular signaling mechanisms.

Inverse agonist: A substance that binds to a receptor and induces a response opposite to that of an agonist.

Ion channel: Pores, formed by proteins embedded in the cell membrane, that control the flow of ions down their electrochemical gradient.

Isomers: Compounds that are formed of the same elements and in the same proportions but in different configurations (structural arrangements).

Isozymes: Enzymes of different structure but which catalyze the same reaction.

Ligand gated: An ion channel-linked receptor that is opened or closed in response to the binding of a chemical messenger such as a neurotransmitter or drug.

Lipophilic: Literally, fat loving, refers to molecules that are attracted to, and dissolvable in, fat, lipids, oils and nonpolar medium. Lipophilic substances are repelled by water.

L-isomer: Left-handed isomer of a chiral molecule.

Mechanism of action: In pharmacodynamics, the biochemical interaction by which a pharmacologic agent produces its effect on the organism; usually, this includes identifying the specific receptor target that a drug binds to and the effect of such binding on the cell's functioning.

Medicinal chemistry: The application of biochemical research in the design and synthesis of pharmaceuticals.

MEDWATCH: The Food and Drug Administration's program for reporting serious reactions, product quality problems, therapeutic nonequivalence/failure, and product use errors with human medical products, such as drugs and medical devices.

Metabolism: Two related chemical reactions that sustain life within organisms: (1) Catabolism breaks down organic matter, whereas (2) anabolism uses the energy of catabolism to construct components of cells.

Metabolite: Metabolites are the products of enzyme-catalyzed reactions that occur naturally within cells; drug metabolites may be inactive or partially active or activated (prodrugs) through metabolism.

Mutagenic effects: Influences that change reproductive genes, producing mutations in subsequent generations.

Narrow therapeutic index: FDA definition: (1) a drug with less than a twofold difference between median lethal and median effective dose, or (2) a drug with less than a twofold difference between minimum toxic and minimum effective concentrations in the blood, and (3) the safe and effective use of the drug product requires careful titration and patient monitoring.

NDA (New Drug Application): The process by which a drug manufacturer formally applies to the FDA for the right to market and sell a pharmaceutical product in the United States.

Off-label use: The prescribing of a drug for uses, dosages, ages, or populations other than those approved by the FDA.

Oxidation: The loss of electrons, or an increase in oxidation state in an atom, molecule, or ion. The CYP450 enzymes work largely by catalyzing the oxidation of the drug by inserting on atom of O_2 into the substrate.

Parenteral administration: Introduction of a substance other than by mouth or rectum.

Partial agonist: A drug that possesses affinity for a receptor, but unlike a full agonist, will elicit only a small degree of the pharmacological effect, even if a high proportion of receptors are occupied by the compound.

P-glycoprotein: A cell membrane associated protein that is found throughout the body but is responsible for transporting many drugs from the intestine into the circulatory system.

Pharmaceutics: The process or science of developing a chemical entity into a safe and effective medicine.

Pharmacodynamic: The effect of drugs on living organisms, including mechanism of action and the result of such action.

Pharmacogenomics: The study of the influence of genetic variation on drug response.

Pharmacokinetics: The effect of the body on the drug, measured by the rate at which the substrate is absorbed, distributed, metabolized, and eliminated.

Pharmacology: The study of chemicals' (drugs and poisons) effects on the body's functioning.

Pharmacovigilance: The detection, assessment, and prevention of adverse side effects.

Phase I trials: Initial studies to determine the metabolism and pharmacologic actions of drugs in humans, the side effects associated with increasing doses, and to gain early evidence of effectiveness; done in healthy participants and/or patients.

Phase II trials: Controlled clinical studies conducted to evaluate the effectiveness of the drug for a particular indication or indications in patients with the disease or condition under study and to determine the common short-term side effects and risks.

Phase III trials: Expanded controlled and uncontrolled trials after preliminary evidence suggesting effectiveness of the drug has been obtained; they are intended to gather additional information to evaluate the overall benefit-risk relationship of the drug and provide an adequate basis for prescriber labeling.

Phase IV trials: Postmarketing studies to delineate additional information, including the drug's risks, benefits, and optimal use.

Physiological antagonism: A substance that mimics the effects of a ligand antagonist without binding to the receptor associated with the effect. This may occur when two drugs have opposing actions in the body and cancel one another out.

Plasma protein binding: Many drugs bind to blood proteins and are carried through the systemic circulation without being free to react with receptors while they are bound to the transport protein. Only unbound or free agents exert a pharmacologic effect at the target site.

Polymorphism: The existence of different genotypes and phenotypes in a population of a species. In pharmacology, polymorphisms showing allelic variations are associated with differences in CYP450-mediated metabolic reactions.

Poor metabolizer: A person who metabolizes a drug slower or less completely than others.

Portal circulation: Refers to the circulation of blood from the small intestine to the liver, via the portal vein.

Potency: The dose needed to produce an effect. A more potent drug will produce an effect at a lower dose.

Prodrug: A substance that is a precursor to a drug and is administered in its inactive form, which requires metabolism to be converted to the active drug.

Psychopharmacology: The research (experimental psychopharmacology) and application (clinical psychopharmacology) of drugs that induce changes in emotion, cognition and behavior.

Quantal dose response curve: Generally a bell-shaped curve that expresses the percentage of a population that responds to a particular dose.

Racemic mixture: A stereoisomeric mixture with equal amounts of left- and right-handed enantiomers of a chiral molecule.

Reduction: The gain of electrons or a decrease in oxidation state in an atom, molecule, or ion.

RLD (reference listed drug): An approved drug product to which new generic versions are compared to show that they are bioequivalent.

Scheduled drug: A controlled (scheduled) drug is one whose use and distribution is tightly controlled because of its abuse potential or risk. Controlled drugs are rated in the order of their abuse risk and placed in Schedules by the federal Drug Enforcement Administration (DEA). The drugs with the highest abuse potential are placed in Schedule I, and those with the lowest abuse potential are in Schedule V.

Second messenger: Molecules that relay signals from receptors on the cell surface to target molecules inside the cell.

Steady state: Steady state is achieved when the rates of drug administration and drug elimination are equal.

Structure activity relationship (SAR): The relationship between the chemical or three-dimensional structure of a drug molecule and its biological effect on the organism.

Sulfation: A phase II enzyme reaction. This conjugation process transfers a sulfonate anion to a drug molecule.

Sympathomimetic drug: Substances that mimic the effects of the sympathetic nervous system.

Tachyphylaxis: Diminished response to a substance because of previous exposure to the same substance; in pharmacology this results in diminished response to repeatedly administered drugs.

Teratogenic effect: The effect of a substance that is able to disturb normal growth and development of an embryo or fetus.

Therapeutic window: The range of a drug's dosing or its serum concentration at which a therapeutic effect is achieved without toxicity occurring.

Transcription factor: An array of proteins that act as receptor/agonist by binding to specific DNA sequences, thereby controlling the flow of genetic information from DNA to mRNA.

Transferase: An enzyme that catalyzes the transfer of a functional group from one molecule to another.

Up-regulation: An increase in the number of receptors on the surface of cells, making the cell more sensitive to ligands.

Voltage gated: Access of ions to and from the interior of a cell is activated by changes in electrical potential difference near the ion channel.

Volume of distribution (Vd): The volume of body fluid in which a compound is apparently distributed. It may consist of plasma or tissue fluid.

Zero-order kinetics: The rate of elimination of a drug over time is constant and unaffected by the level of drug concentration.

Chapter 8 Questions

1. Chronic administration of an antagonist would be expected to produce
   a. Tachyphylaxis.
   b. Receptor down-regulation.
   c. Receptor up-regulation.
   d. Bioequivalence.
2. Drug A is administered to a patient and produces an increase in blood pressure by 10 mmHg. Drug B is administered to the patient and produces an increase

in blood pressure, also by 10 mmHg. When the two drugs are combined, an increase in blood pressure of 40 mmHg. occurs. This is an example of

a. Pharmacological antagonism.

b. Additivity.

c. Potentiation

d. Synergism.

3. The science of collecting, evaluating, and analyzing adverse drug events is referred to as

a. Pharmaceutics.

b. Pharmacovigilance.

c. Medicinal chemistry.

d. Pharmacokinetics.

4. Compared to the brand drugs, the FDA requires generic drugs to be

a. Bioequivalent.

b. Biotherapeutic.

c. Both bioequivalent and biotherapeutic.

d. Either bioequivalent or biotherapeutic.

5. Which of the following is responsible for metabolizing the largest number of drugs?

a. Albumin

b. CYP3A4

c. CYP1A2

d. P-glycoprotein

6. In the presence of a competitive antagonist, the dose response curve of the agonist

a. Is not affected.

b. Would be reduced in maximal response.

c. Would be shifted to the right.

d. Would be shifted to the left.

7. Alprazolam is metabolized by CYP3A4. If a person took their dose of alprazolam with grapefruit juice, you would anticipate:

a. An increased metabolism of alprazolam.

b. A decreased metabolism of alprazolam.

c. Grapefruit juice should not affect the metabolism.

d. An induction of the enzymes.

8. The amount of drug that enters the systemic circulation is referred to as:

a. Bioavailability.

b. Half-life.

c. Polymorphism.

d. Steady state.

9. Which of the following provides information about the variation in sensitivity to a drug within the population studied?

a. Graded dose-response curves

b. Quantal dose-response curve

c. Therapeutic index

d. Half-life

10. Which form of a drug would most readily cross biological membranes?

a. Un-ionized

b. Ionized

c. Glucuronidated

d. Protein bound

11. Hepatic dysfunction would have which effect on a prodrug?

a. Increased effect

b. Decreased effect

c. Prodrugs are unaffected by hepatic activity

d. None of the above.

12. Addiction and abuse would be the most likely in which class of drugs?

a. Schedule I

b. Schedule II

c. Schedule III

d. Schedule IV

13. Which of the following is true about drug protein binding?

a. Binding of the drug to the protein is usually reversible.

b. Only free drug can produce pharmacological effects.

c. Only free drug can undergo metabolism by the liver.

d. All of the above.

14. High tissue binding would be associated with a:

a. High volume of distribution.

b. Low volume of distribution.

c. None of the above.

d. All of the above.

15. A drug with the following characteristics would reach steady state the quickest:

a. Long half-life

b. Small volume of distribution

c. Short half-life

d. Large volume of distribution

Answers: (1) c, (2), d, (3) b, (4) a, (5) b, (6) c, (7) b, (8) a, (9) b, (10) a, (11) b, (12) a, (13) d, (14) a, and (15) c.

REFERENCES

Borges, S. (2008). *Impact of CYP450 genetic testing on the clinical use of SSRI.* Silver Spring, MD: FDA, Office of Clinical Pharmacology Center for Drug Evaluation and Research.

Chen, M., Shah, V., Patnaik, R., Adams, W., Hussain, A., Conner, D., . . . & Williams, R. (2001). Bioavailability and bioequivalence: An FDA regulatory overview. *Pharmaceutical Research, 18*, 1645–1650.

Edwards, I., & Aronson, J. (2000). Adverse drug reactions: Definitions, diagnosis and management. *Lancet, 356*, 1255–1259.

Evans, W., & McLeod, H. (2003). Pharmacogenetics—drug disposition, drug targets and side effects. *New England Journal of Medicine, 34,* 538–549.

Friedman, M., Woodcock, J., Lumpkin, M., Shuren, J., Hass, A., & Thompson, L. (1999). The safety of newly approved medicines: Do recent market removals mean there is a problem? *Journal of the American Medical Association, 281,* 1728–1734.

Frye, R. (2004). Probing the world of cytochrome P450 enzymes. *Molecular Interventions, 4,* 157–162.

Hornecker, J. (2009). Generic drugs: History, approval process and current challenges. *US Pharmacist, 34,* 26–30.

Kesselheim, A., Misono, A., Lee, J., Stedman, M., Brookhart, A., Choudhry, N., & Shrank, W. Clinical equivalence of generic and brand-name drugs used in cardiovascular disease: A systematic review and metanalysis. *Journal of the American Medical Association, 300,* 2514–2526.

Lurie, P., & Sasich, L. (1999). Safety of FDA approved drugs. *Journal of the American Medical Association, 282,* 2297.

Lipsky, M., & Sharp, L. (2001). From idea to market: The drug approval process. *Journal of the American Board Family Practice, 14,* 362–367.

Mrazek, D. (2006). Psychiatric pharmacogenomics. *Focus, 4,* 339–343.

Nebert, D., & Russell, D. (2002). Clinical importance of the cytochromes P450. *Lancet, 360,* 1155–1162.

Nelson, D., Koymans, L., Kamataki, T., Stegeman, J., Feyereisen, R., Waxman, D., . . . & Nebert, D. (1996). P450 superfamily: Update on new sequences, gene mapping, accession numbers and nomenclature. *Pharmacogenetics, 6,* 1–42.

Paine, M., Hart, H., Ludington, S., Haining, R., Rettie, A., & Zeldin, D. (2006). The human intestinal cytochrome P450 "pie." *Drug Metabolism and Disposition, 34,* 880–886.

Shimada, T., Yamazaki, H., Mimura, M., Inui, Y., & Guengerich, F. (1994). Interindividual variations in human liver cytochrome P-450 enzymes involved in the oxidation of drugs, carcinogens and toxic chemicals: Studies with liver microsomes of 30 Japanese and 30 Caucasians. *Journal of Pharmacology and Experimental Therapeutics, 270,* 414–423.

Wall, C., Oldenkamp, C., & Swintak, C. (2010). Safety and efficacy pharmacogenomics in pediatric psychopharmacology. *Primary Psychiatry, 17,* 53–58.

Wrighton, S. A., & Stevens, J. C. (1992). The human hepatic cytochromes P450 involved in drug metabolism. *Critical Reviews in Toxicology, 22*(1), 1–21.

Chapter 9 ————————————————————————————

THE PRACTICE OF CLINICAL PSYCHOPHARMACOLOGY

William J. Burns

Lenore Walker

Jose A. Rey

This chapter is designed to address the knowledge and skills that are needed to carry out the practice of clinical psychopharmacology by psychologists trained in the integration of psychotherapeutic and pharmacotherapeutic modalities of treatment. Necessarily, psychologists who take responsibility for a combination of psychological and psychopharmacological treatments are called on to be well informed in evidence-based practice in both clinical psychology and clinical psychopharmacology (Burns, Rey, & Burns, 2008). The chapter is organized into five main sections, each describing key aspects of the clinical care offered by prescribing medical psychologists to their patients: (1) evaluation, (2) treatment initiation, (3) treatment monitoring, (4) considerations of special populations, which encompasses gender and age differences as well as the integration of pharmacotherapy with the treatment of substance abuse disorders and the integration of cultural issues into psychopharmacology, and (5) a review of general classes of psychotropics as well as a review of specific drugs within each class.

EVALUATION

The evaluation of signs and symptoms of psychopathology precedes and provides direction to treatment planning. The proper formulation of a plan for pharmacotherapy relies on the medical psychologist's knowledge of the three major principles of pharmacology: *Pharmacodynamics, pharmacokinetics, and pharmacotherapeutics.* Pharmacodynamics is the process by which drugs influence cell physiology (typically the receptors) to achieve a desired result. Pharmacokinetics is the process by which the body absorbs the drug into the bloodstream, distributes it to its site of action, metabolizes it, and excretes it. Pharmacotherapeutics is the desired or intended effect or reason that the drug is administered to a particular patient at a given time (also called the indication or usage of the drug). Pharmacotherapeutic usage of drugs depends, in turn, on knowledge of pharmacodynamics (what the drug will do to the body) and pharmacokinetics (how well the body will be able to metabolize the drug). The two essential skills necessary for the evaluation of patients and treatment planning are a knowledge of indications and contraindications, as well as knowledge of the factors involved in the selection of medication.

INDICATIONS AND CONTRAINDICATIONS

The Food and Drug Administration (FDA) approves drugs only for a specific use after research trials have provided evidence that a given drug is appropriately indicated for the treatment of a given illness and type of patient. When the FDA publishes the approved indication(s) for the use of a specific drug, it often includes some *contraindications* and specifies situations that make the use of a specific medication inadvisable. Typically, the source of medication contraindications in psychopharmacology is related to negative side effects and/or outcomes related to drug–drug, drug–physiology, or drug–food interactions. When contraindications have been reported by the FDA for a specific drug, it becomes the responsibility of the skilled clinician, in collaboration with the patient, to decide whether the benefits outweigh the risks when a decision is made to administer such a drug. When a clinician decides to prescribe a drug for a condition that has not been FDA approved, the usage is called off-label, and may be justified if the need outweighs the contraindications. However, this places the prescriber at risk for various medicolegal issues. Table 9.1 provides a sample list of psychotropic medications with the conditions for which they are FDA approved (indications). The issue of contraindications will be discussed further in the third section of this chapter under the title: "Monitoring the Course of Treatment." In that section, Table 9.3 is introduced to list major contraindications for psychotropic drugs.

SELECTION FACTORS

Practitioners of clinical psychopharmacology are faced with a complex array of factors, which must be considered in order to select a medication most appropriate for each patient under their care, because there may be a wide range of drugs that have been indicated by the FDA for the same condition. For example, as of January 1, 2011, the FDA has approved 20 different antidepressants from which a clinician may select in order to treat depression. From such an array of choices, a clinician's decision must be based on the following:

1.   Diagnosis must be the first step in the clinical process before treatment of any kind can begin, because the prescriber must know what is being treated. A good example of the type of diagnostic precision that is required is the issue of the distinction between major depression and bipolar disorder in which the patient's current episode is that of depression. If the clinician were to treat such a patient with antidepressants alone under the diagnostic assumption of a unipolar depression, and the patient were in fact bipolar, it might cause the patient to switch to a manic episode or lead to a rapid cycling pattern. A clinician must know the treatment of choice that best fits the diagnosis that has been assigned to his or her patient on the basis of the signs and symptoms which have thoroughly been evaluated.

2.   Clinicians must choose those symptoms that are to be the target of their treatment, those symptoms that are the most basic aspects of the diagnosis, and those symptoms that the prescribing medical psychologist has contracted with their patient to target. Target symptoms should be behavioral, objective, and measurable so that they can be assessed repeatedly over time to establish the effectiveness of the treatment, thus being easily identified by both the prescriber and patient. The clinician must include those symptoms that will offer the clearest indicators of treatment

Table 9.1 Drug Indications, Dosage Ranges, Side Effects, Routes of Administration, FDA Approval for Children, and Pregnancy Risk

Antidepressant	Brand Name	Usual Dosage Range	Sedation	Other Uses and (Side Effects)	Routes of Administration	Child Approved	Pregnancy Category*
I Antidepressants:							
MAO inhibitors (FwO)				Significant Drug/Food interactions,			
Phenelzine	Nardil	45–90 mg/d	+++	Atypical depression (SE: Orthostatic hypotension, HTN CRISIS)	Oral	No	C
Tranylcypromine	Parnate	20–40 mg/d	+	MDD (SE HTN CRISIS, Orthostatic hypotension, edema, tachycardia, HA, insomnia)	Oral	No	C
Selegiline	Eldepryl EMSAM	5–10 mg/d (oral for PD) 6–12 mg/d (transdermal for MDD)	+	MDD, Parkinson's disease (5–10 mg/d) (SE: HA, insomnia, dizziness, nausea)	Oral Transdermal	No	C
Tricyclic compounds (FwO)							
Amitriptyline	Elavil	25–300 mg/d	++++	Depression (SE: See Footnote)	Oral	12+	Not formally assigned C / D?
Doxepin	Adapin/ Sinequan/ Silenor	25–300 mg/d	++++	Most sedating TCA Silenor is FDA-approved for insomnia	Oral, Topical	12+	C
Imipramine	Tofranil	25–300 mg/d	+++	Enuresis in children	Oral	12+	Not formally assigned D?
Trimipramine	Surmontil	25–300 mg/d	+++		Oral	No	C

Side effects (SE) are placed in parenthesis. See Table 9.3 for major contraindications.

(continued)

Table 9.1 (Continued)

Antidepressant	Brand Name	Usual Dosage Range	Sedation	Other Uses and Side Effects/ Comments	Routes of Administration	Child Approved	Pregnancy Category*
Nortriptyline	Pamelor/ Aventyl	25–200 mg/d	+++		Oral	No	D
Desipramine	Norpramin	25–300 mg/d	++		Oral	12+	C
Protriptyline	Vivactil	10–60 mg/d	++		Oral	12+	Not formally assigned
Clomipramine	Anafranil	25–250 mg/d	++++	FDA approved for OCD only	Oral	10+	C
Tetracyclic compounds (FwO)							
Amoxapine	Asendin	25–600 mg/d	+++	(SE: Possible EPS)	Oral	16+	C
Maprotiline	Ludiomil	25–225 mg/d	+++	(SE: Possible Seizures)	Oral	No	B
SSRIs				(SE: Take all SSRIs w/ food Class effects: Sexual Dys., Insomnia, Anxiety, GI discomfort)			
Fluoxetine	Prozac Serafem Prozac Weekly	10–80 mg/d 10–80 mg/d 90 mg/d (weekly*)	–/+	Approved for MDD, OCD, bulimia, PMDD, panic and in combination with Olanzapine for bipolar depression/resistant depression	Oral	8+ for MDD 7+ for OCD	C
Sertraline	Zoloft	25–200 mg/d	–/+	OCD, Panic, PTSD, PMDD, & social anxiety	Oral	6+ for OCD only	C
Paroxetine	Paxil (hcl) Pexeva (mesylate)	10–60 mg/d	+	Approved for GAD, OCD, PMDD, PTSD, Pain, & Social Anxiety	Oral	No	D

Fluvoxamine	Luvox	100–300 mg/d	+	OCD, social anxiety; unlabeled uses: MDD, anxiety in children, PTSD & panic	Oral	8+ for OCD only	C
Citalopram	Celexa	10–40 mg/d	+	Depression (SE: insomnia, nausea, xerostomia, diaphoresis QT-prolongation >40mg/d)	Oral	No	C
Escitalopram	Lexapro	10–40 mg/d	+	MDD, GAD SE: HA, insomnia, nausea, sexual dys.	Oral	12+ for MDD	C
Others							
Trazodone	Desyrel/Oleptro	50–600 mg/d	+++	(SE: Orthostasis, sedation, priapism)	Oral	No	C
Nefazodone	Serzone* brand removed from U.S. market	100–600 mg/d	+-	(SE: Sedation, orthostasis, hepatotoxicity risk)	Oral	No	C
Vilazodone	Viibryd	10–40 mg/d	-/+	(SE: Similar to SSRI profile: e.g., GI disturbances & insomnia) *Also a 5HT-1a partial agonist*	Oral	No	C
Bupropion	Wellbutrin IR/SR/XL Zyban/ Budeprion/ Aplenzin	100–450 mg/d	–	(SE: Used for smoking cessation and Social Anxiety Disorder HA, insomnia, nausea, constipation, dry mouth, dermatological seizures)	Oral	No	C
Venlafaxine	Effexor I Effexor XR	25–375 mg/d 37.5–225 mg/d	+	(SE: Approved for GAD, social anxiety, and Panic Disorder HA, sedation, BP changes at high doses HTN risk, insomnia, nervousness, dizziness, xerostomia, anorexia, constipation, weakness, diaphoresis)	Oral	No	C

(continued)

Table 9.1 (Continued)

Antidepressant	Brand Name	Usual Dosage Range	Sedation	Other Uses and Side Effects/ Comments	Routes of Administration	Child Approved	Pregnancy Category*
Desvenlafaxine	Pristiq	50–400 mg/d	+	Approved for MDD only (SE: HA, sedation, GI distress, BP changes at high doses insomnia, nervousness, dizziness, xerostomia, anorexia, constipation, weakness, diaphoresis)	Oral	No	C
Mirtazapine	Remeron	15–45 mg/d	+ + +	(SE: sedation, weight gain, dizziness, dry mouth, inc. abnormal LFTs,† 2%)	Oral	No	C
Duloxetine	Cymbalta	20–60 mg/d	+	MDD, GAD, chronic pain, fibromyalgia SE: HA, dizziness, insomnia, fatigue, xerostomia, constipation, GI distress	Oral	No	C

*FDA Pregnancy Categories

A   Controlled studies in pregnant women fail to demonstrate a risk to the fetus in the first trimester with no evidence of risk in later trimesters. The possibility of fetal harm appears remote.

B   Either animal-reproduction studies have not demonstrated a fetal risk, but there are no controlled studies in pregnant women, or animal-reproduction studies have shown an adverse effect (other than a decrease in fertility) that was not confirmed in controlled studies in women in the first trimester, and there is no evidence of a risk in later trimesters.

C   Either studies in animals have revealed adverse effects on the fetus (teratogenic or embryocidal effects or other) and there are no controlled studies in women, or studies in women and animals are not available. Drugs should be given only if the potential benefits justify the potential risk to the fetus.

D   There is positive evidence of human fetal risk, but the benefits from use in pregnant women may be acceptable despite the risk, (e.g. if the drug is needed in a life-threatening situation or for a serious disease for which safer drugs cannot be used or are ineffective.)

X   Studies in animals or human beings have demonstrated fetal abnormalities or there is evidence of fetal risk based on human experience, or both, and the risk of the drug in pregnant women clearly outweighs any possible benefits. The drug is contraindicated in women who are or may become pregnant.

† LFTs: Liver Function Tests

Key Abbreviations:

FwO = **possibly Fatal with Overdose**
TCA = **Tricyclic/Tetracyclic Antidepressant (most are SNRIs either stronger at serotonin or norepinephrine reuptake)**
SSRI = **Selective Serotonin Reuptake Inhibitor**
MAOI = **Monoamine Oxidase Inhibitor**
SNRI = **Serotonin-Norepinephrine Reuptake Inhibitor**
GI = **Gastrointestinal distress (generally nausea/vomiting/diarrhea)**
HA = **Headache**
OCD = **Obsessive Compulsive Disorder**
MDD = **Major Depressive Disorder**

Adverse Events for Antidepressants Summarized:

MAOIs: Orthostasis, dizziness, anticholinergic SEs, sedation, inc. risk of hypertensive crisis (dietary restrictions), sexual dysfunction, hepatic complications, and insomnia

TCAs: Anticholinergic effects (dry mouth, blurred vision, dec. memory, urinary retention, constipation, confusion), sedation, orthostatic hypotension, cardiac conduction abnormalities (arrhythmias), sexual dysfunction, behavioral disturbances (activation, psychosis), lower seizure threshold, headache, GI disturbances, rash, hepatic, blood dyscrasias, weight gain. *All TCAs are very lethal in overdose.*

SSRIs: Headache, nausea/vomiting, diarrhea, sexual dysfunction, insomnia, nervousness, anxiety, akathisia
Serotonin Syndrome and discontinuation syndromes.

(continued)

Table 9.1 (Continued)

II. Anxiolytics

Benzodiazepine (C-IV) (Side Effects: see footnotes)	Brand	Usual Dosage Range	Approx. Equivalent	FDA Approved Uses	Routes of Administration	Child Approved	Pregnancy Category
Long-Acting							
Chlordiazepoxide	Librium	15–100 mg/d (200 mg)	10	Anxiety Disorder, Acute Alcohol Withdrawal, Preoperative Apprehension	Oral, IM, IV	No	D
Diazepam	Valium	2–60 mg/d	5	Anxiety Disorder, Alcohol Withdrawal, Muscle Relaxant, Preprocedural Sedation, and Amnesia	Oral, IM, IV, Rectal	Infancy+	D
Clonazepam	Klonopin	1.5–10 mg/d (20 mg)	0.25	Panic Disorder; Seizure disorders (Lennox-Gastaut syndrome; akinetic; myoclonic)	Oral	No	D
Clorazepate	Tranxene	7.5–60 mg/d	7.5	GAD, Alcohol Withdrawal	Oral	No	Not formally assigned
Flurazepam	Dalmane	15–30 mg/d	15	Insomnia	Oral	15+	X
Shorter-Acting							
Alprazolam	Xanax	0.75–4 mg/d (8 mg)	0.5	GAD, Panic Disorder, Anxiety Associated with Depression	Oral	No	D
Lorazepam	Ativan	2–6 mg/d (10 mg)	1	Anxiety Disorder, Anxiety Associated with Depression	Oral, IV, IM	No	D
Oxazepam	Serax	30–120 mg/d	15	Anxiety Disorder, Alcohol Withdrawal	Oral	No	D
Temazepam	Restoril	15–30 mg/d	15	Insomnia	Oral	No	X
Triazolam	Halcion	0.125–0.5 mg/d	0.125	Insomnia	Oral	No	X
Quazepam	Doral	7.5–15 mg/d	7.5	Insomnia	Oral	No	X
Estazolam	Prosom	1–2 mg/d	1	Insomnia	Oral	No	X

Common side effects of the benzodiazepines: drowsiness, sedation, ataxia, dizziness, anterograde amnesia, decreased concentration, rare-paradoxical excitation, disinhibition. *All benzodiazepines will cause physical dependence at normal and regular doses within 2 weeks to 2 months. Factors contributing to dependence: high potency agents (alprazolam, lorazepam, clonazepam, and triazolam), length of treatment, higher doses, and dependent personality traits.*

Other Anxiolytics	Brand	Usual Dosage Range	Other Uses and Side Effects	Routes of Administration	Child Approved	Pregnancy Category
Buspirone	BuSpar	15–60 mg/d	GAD Nonaddicting	Oral	No	B
Diphenhydramine	Benadryl	25–200 mg/d	Insomnia, (SE: sedation, anticholinergic)	Oral, IM, IV	2 +	B
Hydroxyzine	Vistaril	50–400 mg/d	Anxiety Disorder, Preop Sedation (SE: sedation, mild anticholinergic)	Oral, IM	6 +	C
Meprobamate (C-IV) (muscle relaxant)	Miltown (USA Brand Name Discontinued)	400–1600 mg/d	**Anxiety Disorder, (SE: Potential dependence/ addiction** **Related to Carisoprodol Soma, now a C-IV in the U.S.A.**	**Oral**	No	D
Sedative-Hypnotics (C-II-IV)						
Zolpidem (C-IV)	Ambien	5–10 mg/HS	For insomnia only	Oral	No	C
Zaleplon (C-IV)	Sonata	5–20 mg/HS	For insomnia only	Oral	No	C
Eszopeclone (C-IV)	Lunesta	1–3 mg/HS	For insomnia only	Oral	No	C
Doxepin	Silenor	3–6 mg/HS	For insomnia	Oral	No	C
Ramelteon	Rozerem	8 mg/HS	For insomnia only	Oral	No	C
Phenobarbital (C-II-IV)	Luminal	30–120 mg/HS	Sedative (SE: fatal in OD)	Oral, IM, IV, subcutaneous	Infants	D
Secobarbital	Seconal	6–200 mg/d	For insomnia & sedation	Oral	Infants	D

C-I-II-III & IV = Drug Enforcement Administration (DEA) control code (U.S. Dept. of Justice Prescription Drug Monitoring Programs (PDMP)).

(continued)

Table 9.1 (Continued)

Generic Category Phenothiazines (FwO)	Brand	Dosage Range	Sedation	EPS	Indications and Special Side Effects	Routes of Administration	Child Approved	Pregnancy
III. Antipsychotics								
Chlorpromazine	Thorazine	50–2000 mg/d	+++	+++	Psychosis, Mania (SE: EPS)	Oral, IM, IV	6 months+	C
Thioridazine	Mellaril	50–800 mg/d	++++	++	Schizophrenia (SE: Pigmentary retinopathy, QT changes, sedation, very anticholinergic)	Oral	No	C
Mesoridazine	Serentil	50–400 mg/d	+++	++	Schizophrenia	Oral, IM	No	C
Perphenazine	Trilafon	8–64 mg/d	++	+++	Schizophrenia	Oral	No	C
Prochlorperazine	Compazine	10–40 mg/d	++	+++	Also used for N&V	Oral, IM	12+	C
Trifluoperazine	Stelazine	2–80 mg/d	++	+++	Approved for Schizophrenia and Anxiety	Oral	6+	C
Fluphenazine	Prolixin	2–40 mg/d	+	++++	Schizophrenia (SE: High EPS)	Oral, IM, LAI	No	C
Other								
Thiothixene	Navane	5–60 mg/d	++	+++	Schizophrenia	Oral	No	C
Haloperidol	Haldol (Depot)	1–100 mg/d (50–450 mg/ month)	+	++++	Schizophrenia, Tourette's, severe behavior problems in children (SE: High EPS)	Oral, IM, LAI	3+	C
Loxapine*	Loxitane	20–250 mg/d	++	++	Psychotic Disorder Metabolite=amoxapine	Oral	No	C
Molindone*	Moban	15–225 mg/d	++	++	Schizophrenia and weight loss *No longer available in United States*	Oral	3+	C

Atypical Aps

Generic	Brand	Dose			Indication / SE	Route	Peds	Preg
Clozapine	Clozaril	75–900 mg/d	++++	–/+	Schizophrenia (SE: Low EPS, agranulocytosis, seizures, anticholinergic, orthostasis, weight gain)	Oral	No	B
Risperidone	Risperdal (Consta Inj.)	1–16 mg/d (25–50 mg/ 2 wks)	–/+	+*	Schizophrenia and Acute Mania or Mixed Episode Bipolar I Disorder, Aggression with Autistic Disorder (SE: Dose-related EPS, orthostatic hypotension, inc. PRL)	Oral, IM, LAI	5+ autism 10+ bipolar 13+ Schizophrenia	C
Olanzapine	Zyprexa (Zydis & Inj.)	5–20 mg/d	+++	+	FDA approved for adult, adolescent, and child Schizophrenia, Bipolar I Mania, (SE: Low EPS, weight gain, sedation, anticholinergic)	Oral, IM, LAI	No	C
Quetiapine	Seroquel	200–800 mg/d	+++	–/+	Schizophrenia, acute manic or depressive episodes of bipolar (SE: Low EPS, **sedation**, orthostatic hypotension)	Oral	No	C
Ziprasidone	Geodon	40–160 mg/d	+	+	Schizophrenia, Approved for mania (SE: Low EPS, GI distress, QT changes, low weight gain)	Oral, IM	No	C
Aripiprazole	Abilify	10–30 mg/d	–/+	+	Schizophrenia, Bipolar, Autistic disorder (SE: Low EPS, N&V, HA, insomnia, agitation, low weight gain)	Oral, IM	6+ autism 10+ Bip. 13+ Schiz.	C
Paliperidone	Invega	3–12 mg/d	–/+	+	Schizophrenia, **Schizoaffective** disorder (SE: dose-related EPS, low weight gain)	Oral, IM, LAI	12+	C

(continued)

Table 9.1 (Continued)

Generic Category Phenothiazines (FwO)	Brand	Dosage Range	Sedation	EPS	Indications and Special Side Effects	Routes of Administration	Child Approved	Pregnancy
Iloperidone	Fanapt	2–24 mg/d	+	+	Schizophrenia (SE: Low EPS, low wt. gain, QT changes)	Oral	No	C
Asenapine	Saphris	5–20 mg/d SL	++	+	Schizophrenia, Acute mania (SE: Low EPS, low weight gain Approved for bipolar)	Sublingual	No	C
Lurasidone	Latuda	40–80 mg/d	+	+	Schizophrenia (SE: Low EPS, low metabolic syndrome) Approved for bipolar disorder	Oral	No	B

Side effects of antipsychotics summarized:

Histamine receptor blockade: sedation, weight gain, potentiation of other CNS depressants

Muscarinic receptor blockade: (anticholinergic)-urinary retention, cognition and memory effects (confusion), sinus tachycardia, dry mouth, blurred vision, and constipation

Alpha-1 adrenergic receptor blockade: orthostatic hypotension, reflex tachycardia, and potentiation of antihypertensives

Dopamine D_2 receptor blockade: (also reason for antipsychotic effect), EPS side effects (dystonias, akathisias, pseudoparkinsonism, tardive dyskinesia), prolactin elevation (galactorrhea, amenorrhea, gynecomastia)

Other: sexual dysfunction 25%–60% (highest w/Mellaril), Neuroleptic Malignant Syndrome—rare, seizures, impaired thermoregulation (including with low pot.), behavioral changes, ophthalmic (lens opacities, retinitis pigmentosis, exacerbation of glaucoma, photophobia), hematological (clozapine), hepatic, increases in QT intervals (arrhythmias: highest with Mellaril/Serentil and Geodon)

Anti-EPS/ Antiparkinsonian Agents	Brand Name	Usual Dosage Range	Uses and Side Effects	Routes of Administration	Approved for Children	Pregnancy Category
Antimuscarinics						
Benztropine	Cogentin	1–8 mg/d	Approved for treatment of EPS. (SE: tachycardia, confusion, disorientation, memory loss, GI symptoms)	Oral, IM, IV	>3	C
Trihexyphenidyl	Artane	2–15 mg/d	Treatment of drug-induced EPS (SE: tachycardia, confusion, dry skin, GI symptoms, blurred vision)	Oral	No	C

Antihistamines

Diphenhydramine	Benadryl	50–400 mg/d	Treatment of drug-induced EPS (SE: mild sedation, anticholinergic)	Oral, IM, IV	2+	B
Dopamine Agonists						
Amantadine	Symmetrel	100–400 mg/d	Antibiotic and treatment of EPS	Oral	No	C

Mood Stabilizer	Brand Name	Usual Dosage Range	Plasma Levels	Uses, Side Effects, and Signs of Toxicity	Route of Administration	Approved for Children as Mood Stabilizer	Pregnancy Category

IV. Mood Stabilizers

Mood Stabilizer	Brand Name	Usual Dosage Range	Plasma Levels	Uses, Side Effects, and Signs of Toxicity	Route of Administration	Approved for Children as Mood Stabilizer	Pregnancy Category
Lithium	Eskalith	300–2400 mg/d	0.8–1.2 mEg/L (acute episode) 0.4–1.0 mEg/L (maintenance)	Bipolar and mania (SE: GI dist, sedation, tremor, headache, polyuria, dipsia and phagia, weight gain, leukocytosis, rash, memory impairment, decreased attention and libido) TOX signs: tremors, slurred speech, ataxia, rigidity, seizures, sedation, BP changes, delirium, arrhythmia, coma	Oral	12+	D
Carbamazepine	Equetro (Tegretol)	400–1600 mg/d	4–12 mu grams/ml	Bipolar I acute mania and mixed episodes. (SE: GI dist., dizziness, drowsiness, inc. LFT, ataxia, diplopia, blurred vision, aplastic anemia, rash, weight gain, SIADH)** TOX signs: cardiac changes, seizures, GI dist, delirium, sedation, coma	Oral	No	D

**SIADH: Syndrome or Inappropriate Antidiuretic Hormone

(continued)

Table 9.1 (Continued)

Mood Stabilizer	Brand Name	Usual Dosage Range	Plasma Levels	Uses, Side Effects, and Signs of Toxicity	Route of Administration	Approved for Children as Mood Stabilizer	Pregnancy Category
Valproic acid	Stavzor Depakene Depakote	250–3000 mg/d	5–120 mu grams/ml	Mania Associated with Bipolar Disorder (SE: GI dist., dizziness, drowsiness, inc. LFTs, ataxia, alopecia) TOX. Signs: mental status changes, including sedation, gait dist., slurred speech.	Oral, IV, Sprinkles	No	D
Lamotrigine	Lamictal	25–400 mg/d	—	Bipolar I (SE: rash, cog. Impairment, Stevens Johnson Syn.)	Oral	No	C

V. Psychostimulants/Agents for ADHD

Generic	Brand Names	Dose Range	Uses and Side Effects	Routes of Administration	Approved for Children	Pregnancy Category
Dextroamphetamine and amphetamine (C-II) (mixed salts)	Adderall Adderall XR	5–40 mg/d 5–30 mg/d	ADHD XR available (SE: reduced appetite, insomnia, headache, GI pain, xerostemia, irritability)	Oral	3+	C
Dextroamphetamine (C-II)	Dexedrine Dexedrine Spansule (ER)	2.5–40 mg/d	ADHD (SE: reduced appetite, insomnia, headache, inc. BP, GI distress xerostomia, irritability)	Oral (tablet/liquid)	3+	C
Methampetamine (C-II)	Desoxyn	5–30 mg/d	Approved for ADHD (Crank, Crystal Meth = MDMA – 3,4-methylenedioxy-methamphetamine can be made from the OTC pseudoephedrine)	Oral	6+	C

Drug	Brand	Dose	Route	Indication / Side Effects	Age	Cat.
Methylphenidate[‡] (C-II)	Ritalin/Concerta Daytrana	5–60 mg/d	Oral, Transdermal	ADHD, (SE: insomnia, nausea, appetite decrease, tics, headache, GI pain, irritability)	6+	C
Dex-methylphenidate (C-II)	Focalin Focalin XR	5–20 mg/d peds 5–30 mg/d adult	Oral	ADHD, (SE: paradoxical aggravation of symptoms, insomnia, nausea, decreased appetite, decreased tics, headache, GI pain, irritability)	6+	C
Lisdexamfetamine (C-II)	Vyvanse	20–70 mg/d	Oral	ADHD, Dextroamphetamine with reported lower abuse potential. (SE: decreased appetite, insomnia, headache, GI pain, xerostomia, irritability)	6+	C
Atomoxetine U.S.A. Box Warning: May cause suicidal ideation	Strattera	18–100 mg/d	Oral	ADHD, Not a controlled substance (SE: inc. BP, HR, HA, insomnia, GI pain, nausea, xerostomia, decreased appetite, cough)	6+	C
Clonidine	Catapres (TTS) Kapvay (ER)	0.1–4 mg/d	Oral, Transdermal (7d) Oral	(SE: fatigue, sedation, depression, hypotension, bradycardia)	6+	C
Guanfacine	Tenex Intuniv (ER)	1–4 mg/d	Oral	(SE: fatigue, sedation, depression, hypotension, bradycardia, HA)	6+	B

Possible uses include: weight loss, narcolepsy/somnolence, pain, ADD/ADHD

[‡]All are abusable and can cause physical dependence

C-I-II-III & IV = Drug Enforcement Administration (DEA) control code (U.S. Dept. of Justice Prescription Drug Monitoring Programs [PDMP]

XR or ER = extended release formulation; SR = sustained release formulation efficacy so that they can decide whether to maintain treatment, increase dose, switch to another medication, or add an augmenting agent. For instance, a patient who is being treated for depression with an antidepressant medication can be monitored for improvements in sleep, appetite, activity levels, and other symptoms. These symptoms can be measured using self-report type measures or clinician-administered instruments.

3. A patient's past history of a diagnosis similar to the current diagnosis and a history of successful treatment with that diagnosis would justify the choice to prescribe the previously successful agent as a first choice for the current episode. For instance, if a patient had been diagnosed with unipolar depression previously, and had a good response to venlafaxine, then it would be reasonable to start treatment for the current episode with venlafaxine.

4. Clinicians need to sift through the family history of their patients for clues about the treatments that have worked best for other family members. For instance, a mother who had benefited from treatment with lithium to manage bipolar disorder may predict successful treatment of a daughter's bipolar disorder with lithium as well.

5. Demographics such as age, gender, ethnicity, and body mass are important to consider when selecting medications. These factors may predict response to a medication, determine dosing level and rate, and inform differences in metabolic enzyme activity.

6. Assessment of comorbid medical conditions allows a clinician to estimate the impact of the selected medication on other coexisting conditions as well as the target symptoms of the primary condition. For example, a clinician should be concerned about treating a patient who suffers from glucose intolerance with a second-generation antipsychotic (e.g., quetiapine, olanzapine) due to the increased risk of producing a metabolic syndrome.

7. An existing medication regimen raises the issue of potential *drug–drug interaction. Cytochrome P450 enzyme* substrate or inhibitor matches have the potential to significantly increase the blood level of medications with such matches. For instance, a patient who is taking Coumadin (warfarin) can trigger enhanced effect and bleeding by simultaneously taking selective serotonin reuptake inhibitors (SSRI), tricyclic antidepressants (TCA), *ginkgo biloba,* or *St. John's wort.* Table 9.2 shows the interactions in which drugs share common cytochrome P450 metabolizing enzymes with other medications.[1]

Potential for drug–food interaction also exists. For example, the consumption of foods that have high tyramine content such as certain cheeses, raisins, bananas, chocolate, or yogurt may affect the pharmacokinetics and pharmacodynamics of MAOIs and can potentially lead to hypertensive crisis.

APPROACHES TO THE INITIAL PHASE OF TREATMENT: APPOINTMENT SCHEDULING

For most pharmacologically trained psychologists who obtain privileges to prescribe, it is assumed that a recommendation to patients for treatment of a mental disorder will include both psychological and psychopharmacological components.

---

[1]Also see Chapter 8, Tables 8.1 & 8.2.

Table 9.2   Metabolism and CYP450 Drug Interactions for Psychiatric Medications

| | Medications Used in Depression | | |
Drug	How Metabolized	Induces	Inhibits
Bupropion	**2B6**	None	**2D6**
Citalopram	**2C19**, 2D6, **3A4**	None	1A2, 2B6, 2C19, 2D6
Duloxetine	1A2, **2D6**	None	**2D6**
Escitalopram	**2C19**, 2D6, **3A4**	None	2D6
Fluoxetine	2C9, 2C19, **2D6, 3A4**	None	1A2, **2B6**, 2C8/9, 2C19, **2D6**, 3A4
Fluvoxamine	1A2, **2D6**	None	**1A2, 2B6**, 2C8/9, **2C19**, 2D6, **3A4**
Mirtazapine	1A2, **2D6, 3A4**	None	1A2, 3A4
Nefazodone	**2D6, 3A4**	None	1A2, 2C8/9, 2D6, **3A4**
Paroxetine	**2D6**	None	1A2, **2B6**, 2C8/9, 2C19, **2D6**, 3A4
Sertraline	**2B6, 2C8/9**, 2C19, 2D6, **3A4**	None	**2B6, 2C9, 2C19**, 2D6, **3A4** (dosages >200mg)
St. John's Wort	**3A4**	**3A4**	None
Trazodone	2D6, **3A4**	None	2D6
Venlafaxine	2C8/9, 2C19, **2D6, 3A4**	None	2B6, 2D6, 3A4
Tricyclic Antidepressants			
Amitriptyline	**2D6**, 3A4, 2C19, 2C9, 2B6, 1A2	None	1A2, 2C9, 2C19, 2D6, 2E1
Amoxapine	**2D6**	None	None
Clomipramine	**2D6, 2C19, 1A2**, 3A4	None	**2D6**
Desipramine	**2D6**,1A2	None	**2D6, 2A6, 2B6, 3A4**, 2E1
Doxepine	**2D6**, 3A4, 1A2	None	None
Imipramine	**2D6, 2C19**, 3A4, 2B6, 1A2	None	**2D6**, 1A2, 2C19, 2E1
Maprotiline	**2D6**	None	None

(continued)

Table 9.2 (Continued)

Drug	How Metabolized	Induces	Inhibits
	Medications Used in Depression		
Nortriptyline	**2D6**, 3A4, 2C9, 1A2	None	2D6, 2E1
Protriptyline	**2D6**	None	None
Trimipramine	**2D6, 3A4, 2C19**	None	None

Drug	How Metabolized	Induces	Inhibits
	Medications Used in ADHD		
Amphetamine(s)	**2D6**	None	None
Atomoxetine	2C19, **2D6**	None	None
Methylphenidate(s)	**2D6**	None	None
Modafinil	3A4	None	Mild 2C19, 2D6

Drug	How Metabolized	Induces	Inhibits
	Medications Used for EPS		
Benztropine	2D6	None	None
Bromocriptine	**3A4**	None	**3A4**
Diphenhydramine	None	None	2D6
Trihexyphenidyl	None	None	None

Medications Used in Psychosis

Drug	How Metabolized	Inducers	Inhibits
Atypical Antipsychotics			
Aripiprazole	**2D6, 3A4**	None	None
Clozapine	**1A2**, 2C19, **2D6, 3A4**	None	2C8/9, 2D6, 3A4
Iloperidone	**2D6**, 3A4	None	2D6
Olanzapine	**1A2**, 2D6	None	1A2, 2C8/9, 2C19, 2D6, 3A4
Quetiapine	2D6, **3A4**	None	None
Paliperidone	**2D6, 3A4**	None	None
Risperidone	**2D6**, 3A4	None	2D6
Ziprasidone	1A2, 3A4 (*primarily via aldehyde oxidase*)	None	2D6, 3A4
Asenapine	**1A2**, UGT1A‡	None	2D6
Typical Antipsychotics			
Chlorpromazine	**2D6**, 1A2, 3A4	None	**2D6**, 2E1
Fluphenazine	**2D6**	None	1A2, 2C9, 2D6, 2E1
Haloperidol	**2D6**, 1A2, 3A4	None	**2D6**
Perphenazine	**2D6**, 1A2, 2C9, 2C19, 3A4	None	1A2, 2C19
Thioridazine	**2D6**, 2C19	None	**2D6**, 1A2, 2C9, 2E1
Thiothixane	1A2	None	2D6

Medications Used in Anxiety and Insomnia

Drug	How Metabolized	Induces	Inhibits
Alprazolam	**3A4**	None	None
Buspirone	2D6, **3A4**	None	None
Chlordiazepoxide	**3A4**	None	None

UGT1A‡, a glucuronosyltransferase isozyme, metabolizes through conjugation and subsequent elimination.

(continued)

Table 9.2 (Continued)

Drug	How Metabolized	Induces	Inhibits
Clonazepam	1A2, **3A4**	None	None
Diazepam	2B6, 2C9, **2C19**, **3A4**	None	None
Eszopeclone	3A4	None	None
Hydroxyzine	None	None	2D6
Lorazepam	Almost none	None	None
Quazepam	3A4	None	None
Temazepam	2B6, 2C8/9, 2C19, 3A4	None	None
Triazolam	**3A4**	None	2C8, 2C9
Zaleplon	3A4, *(primarily via aldehyde oxidase)*	None	None
Zolpidem	1A2, 2C8/9, 2C19, 2D6, **3A4**	None	None

	Medications Used in Bipolar Disorder		
Drug	How Metabolized	Induces	Inhibits
Carbamazepine	2C8/9, **3A4**	**1A2, 2B6, 2C8/9, 2C19, 3A4** (autoinducer)	None
Lamotrigine	Minimal CYP, glucuronidation	None	None
Lithium	No CYP involvement	None	None
Valproic acid/derivatives	2A6, 2C9, 2C19	2A6	2C8/9, 2C19, 2D6

Note: (Bold type refers to major enzymes implicated in each drug's metabolism.)
Source: Lacy, Armstrong, Goldman, and Lance (2007).

If the medical psychologist is providing psychotherapy, then session frequency will be dictated by the contracted frequency for psychotherapy sessions. In the case of weekly appointments designed to use a combination of psychotherapy and psychopharmacology, the clinician can monitor the effect of medication on a weekly basis. During the acute phase of treatment, at least monthly drug monitoring would be recommended. During the maintenance phase, the frequency of monitoring visits can be every 3 to 6 months, if the patient is stable and free of adverse reactions. In such a monitoring session the clinician should assess the following parameters:

1. Progress in the improvement of the psychological condition based on psychological and pharmacological treatment.
2. Complaints (signs and symptoms) regarding adverse drug reactions, failure to improve, or worsening of the patient's condition.
3. Signs or symptoms of interactions with other medications or other physical or psychological factors that could be affecting progress.
4. Laboratory testing of blood levels of any drugs that raise risks of toxicity, especially those with a narrow therapeutic window.
5. Routine examination of blood pressure, heart rate, and weight to monitor for changes from previous baseline.

ROUTES OF ADMINISTRATION

Pharmacologically trained psychologists must be versed in the available routes, which may be used for administration of medication (oral, lingual, sublingual, rectal, intravascular, intramuscular, subcutaneous, transdermal, inhalation, intranasal, *intrathecal,* and topical), as well as the differential responses that patients show to each of these routes. Because there are no current formulations of psychotropic medications for subcutaneous, inhalation, intranasal, or intrathecal routes, these will not be discussed here.

The choice of a route is most often determined by the chemical properties of the drug (e.g., hydrophilic versus hydrophobic) and by therapeutic needs (e.g., rapid onset; maximizing amount of medication reaching receptors in the brain).

Enteral routes are in the gastrointestinal tract. Parenteral routes are outside the alimentary tract and, therefore, are useful for drugs that are poorly absorbed or unstable in the GI tract. The parenteral routes may be used for unconscious patients and those cases requiring rapid onset of drug effect. Table 9.1 presents available psychotropic medications and the formulations using routes of administration for each.

Oral Administration

When drugs are given by mouth (per ora), they are absorbed into systemic circulation at the level of the stomach, the duodenum, or the intestine. Before they enter general circulation, orally ingested drugs enter the portal circulation of the liver where *first-pass metabolism* limits their efficacy. This first-pass metabolism is the reason that oral doses must be higher than intravenous doses, which enter the bloodstream without going through the liver. It is also the reason that patients with liver disease will have a more difficult time metabolizing drugs that are given orally (Mycek, Harvey,

Champe, Fisher. & Cooper, 2000). In patients with liver disease/dysfunction, the first pass of the drug through the liver may not remove as much of the drug from circulation as would a healthy liver. Therefore, the oral dose of that drug would need to be adjusted downward for a patient with liver disease/dysfunction, in order to avoid undesirably higher blood concentrations of the drug. A subcategory of the oral route is lingual administration, used primarily with patients who have difficulty swallowing pills or have tendencies to cheek medication. When lingual drugs (such as Risperdal M-tabs or Fazaclo, a lingual formulation of Clozapine) are placed on the tongue, they disintegrate rapidly and follow the same GI tract metabolism as tablets or liquid administration.

Sublingual Administration

When certain drugs are put under the tongue, they diffuse into the capillary network and enter the systemic circulation directly. Because this route bypasses the GI tract and liver, first-pass metabolism does not limit their efficacy.

Rectal Administration

When drugs are administered rectally, 50% of their content bypasses portal circulation, which minimizes the effect of first-pass metabolism. This route avoids vomiting and the destruction of the drug by intestinal enzymes or low pH in the stomach.

Intravascular Administration

To avoid first-pass metabolism, intravenous injection is the route of choice. IV (venous) or IA (arterial) allow for rapid onset of action and maximum control over circulating levels of the drug. Although rare, the risk of infection must be avoided with this route, and rate of infusion must be carefully controlled to avoid delivery that is too rapid or highly concentrated.

Intramuscular Administration

Intramuscular administration (IM) route can involve either an aqueous solution for the drug in order to obtain rapid absorption, or a depot preparation, wherein the drug is suspended in a nonaqueous solution such as ethylene glycol or peanut oil in order to provide slow absorption. Examples of IM psychotropics include Risperdal Consta and haloperidol decanoate.

Transdermal Administration

This route is used to apply drugs directly to the skin in order to achieve systemic effects, typically by means of a transdermal patch. An example of a transdermal patch is the MAO-1 inhibitor Selegiline (EMSAM) which was FDA approved in 2006 for use as an antidepressant.

Topical Administration

This route is used when localized effect of the drug is desired. An example of topical application is the use of steroid cream for the treatment of rashes.

DOSING OF MEDICATIONS

Prescribing medical psychologists must have a detailed knowledge of the recommended doses for each medication they are licensed or credentialed to prescribe. Such knowledge must include not only the initial dose and the maximum dose that are recommended, but also the half-life and adverse effects, as well as patient factors that must be considered in dose adjustment (weight, gender, ethnicity, age, and concurrent medical condition). Some examples of the recommended dosage ranges for common psychoactive medications are offered in Table 9.1.

DOSAGE ADJUSTMENT

Monitoring a patient's progress by using the selected target symptoms as reference is the only objective way to assess the need for any changes in the course of treatment. Based on the assessment of changes in target symptoms, a prescriber has several options including *titration,* switching, and discontinuation.

Titration

If the patient demonstrates no change or only partial improvement in the target symptoms, an option for the prescriber is to increase the dose of the medication until the patient reacts in one of the following ways (Green, 1995, pp. 39–40):

1. Adequate symptom control is established.
2. The upper limit of the maximum FDA approved range is reached or risk-benefit analysis provides justification to exceed that range.
3. Adverse drug effects that preclude further increase begin to occur.
4. A plateau is reached wherein no more improvement or worsening occur.

The benefit of using titration to adjust dosage is that the cost/benefit ratio of improvement versus adverse drug effects is maximized.

Switching

A second option is to replace an ineffective or intolerable medication with a new one. There are several methods for accomplishing the switching process, including stopping one drug and starting another at the equivalent dose or stopping one drug and starting another at a reduced dose and then titrating upward. Cross-titration, also called cross-taper, is the process in which a clinician adds one medication to a patient's *medication regimen,* gradually increases the dosage while the dosage of the original medication is gradually reduced and finally discontinued or kept at a minimal therapeutic dose. Such *cross-tapering* provides a relatively safe and cautious method for substituting one medication for another. An example of decision making in which cross-tapering is needed is the switch from one SSRI to another, in order to obtain a more favorable side effect profile. Switching can occur due to a patient's inability to tolerate the original drug or if, after an adequate time and dose, the original drug has not produced any benefit. There is the special case of switching between non-MAOI and MAOI antidepressants, in which there must be a discontinuation of one with a washout period before the other is started.

Discontinuation

Medications that are not associated with improvement over baseline or that are associated with adverse side effects that outweigh any improvement should be discontinued. Such discontinuation, however, must be carried out in a fashion that will not trigger adverse drug effects from the sudden withdrawal. Frequently, it is required that the discontinuation be accomplished through a process of successive approximation to cessation of usage of the medication.

The antidepressants (SSRIs, SNRIs, TCAs, and MAOIs), as well as antipsychotics and anxiolytics, are capable of causing a discontinuation syndrome following any sudden interruption, dosage reduction, or cessation of usage. The effects are typically brief and mild, but they may be distressing for some patients. Reported symptoms of such withdrawal reactions include: problems with balance (vertigo, dizziness, weakness), GI tract disturbances (nausea, emesis, diarrhea, cramping), nervous system reactions (headache, malaise, agitation, irritability, nervousness, sleep disturbance, confusion, parasthesias), flulike symptoms, and psychiatric reactions (anxiety, depression, or general return of former mental disturbance). Estimates of the frequency with which patients have reported such symptoms following discontinuation range from 20% to 80%. These reactions were originally called the SSRI discontinuation syndrome,[2] due to the first reports in the 1990s by patients who had discontinued using fluvoxamine (Luvox) and paroxetine (Paxil). SSRIs with the shortest half-life, such as fluvoxamine and paroxetine, and those with inactive metabolites, such as sertraline (Zoloft), are thought to have a higher risk for such a reaction, whereas fluoxetine (Prozac), because of its exceptionally long half-life (4–6 days), is thought to be at lower risk for causing SSRI discontinuation syndrome (Finkel, Clark, & Cubedu, 2009). Discontinuation syndrome can be avoided when clinicians appropriately taper the reduction in dosage. Such tapering should include a drop of no more than 25% of the dosage every 3 to 7 days (Stern, Herman, & Slavin, 1998).

There is some controversy over the naming of the syndrome. As noted, in order to avoid a public reaction over the notion of dependence, the syndrome was contrived as discontinuation syndrome rather than withdrawal or dependence syndrome. However, the symptoms immediately following abrupt cessation of the dosage would seem to indicate a physical withdrawal. The greatest concern would be that the discontinuation of an antidepressant could be premature, and that the symptoms of the anxiety or depression that led to starting the treatment could return. Therefore, therapist and patient need to consider whether the symptoms represent discontinuation syndrome or a return of the original symptoms.

MONITORING AND MANAGEMENT DURING THE COURSE OF TREATMENT

The prescribing medical psychologist needs to be aware of major contraindications for specific medications in order to avoid drug reactions in their patients. Table 9.3 presents a list of the reported contraindications for psychotropics in current use. Side

---

[2]It is interesting to note that manufacturers of the SSRIs fought to have dependency symptoms associated with their drugs termed *discontinuation syndrome* rather than *withdrawal symptoms*, and more recently have used terms such as *symptoms on stopping* (SoS) (Healy, 2009).

Table 9.3 Medication Contraindication and Warnings

Drug Category and Name	Contraindications and Warnings
MAO Inhibitors Phenelzine Tranylcypromine Isocarboxazide Selegiline	1. Contraindicated for patients with hypersensitivity or cross-sensitivity to MAOI. 2. Contraindicated for use with other MAOI, TCAs, SSRIs, SNRIs, CNS depressants, cyclobenzaprine, dextromethorphan, ethanol, meperidine, buproprion, or buspirone. 3. Contraindicated, due to risk potential for hypertensive crisis, for use with foods containing tyramine, tryptophan, or dopamine, for example, cheese, yeast products, pickled herring, alcoholic beverages (especially red wine), liver, aged meats. 4. Contraindicated for patients with congestive heart failure, pheochromocytoma, abnormal liver function tests or history of hepatic disease, renal disease or severe renal impairment. 5. Contraindicated with concurrent use of sympathomimetics (including amphetamines, cocaine, dopamine, epinephrine, methylphenidate, norepinephrine, or phenylephrine) and related compounds (methyldopa, levodopa, phenylalanine, tryptophan, or tyrosine), as well as ophthalmic alpha 2-agonists, may result in hypertensive reaction. 6. Contraindicated with concurrent use of CNS depressants, and sufficient amount of time must be given for clearance of serotonergic agents and their active metabolites before initiation of phenelzine. At least 2 weeks should elapse between the discontinuation of phenelzine and serotonergic agent initiation. **Warnings/precautions:** Increased risk of suicidal thinking and behavior in children, adolescents, and young adults (18–24) with MDD and other psychiatric disorders. May worsen psychosis or risk a shift to mania. Monitor patients with diabetes for increased sensitization to insulin. Use with caution in patients with glaucoma or seizures.
Tricyclic Antidepressants Amitriptyline Amoxapine Clomipramine Desipramine Doxepin Imipramine Maprotiline Nortriptyline Protriptyline Trimipramine	1. Contraindicated for patients with hypersensitivity and cross-sensitivity to TCAs. 2. Contraindicated for use with MAO inhibitors within the past 14 days. 3. Contraindicated during the acute recovery phase following myocardial infarction. 4. Contraindicated for concurrent use of cisapride. **Warnings/precautions:** Increased risk of suicidal thinking and behavior in children, adolescents, and young adults (18–24) with MDD and other psychiatric disorders. TCAs are fatal on overdose. May worsen psychosis or risk shift to mania in patients with bipolar disorder. Obtain CBC and monitor for infection since TCAs may cause bone marrow suppression. May affect blood sugar control in diabetes. Discontinue prior to surgery. Avoid use with patients predisposed to seizures due to previous seizures, brain damage, alcoholism, or use of other drugs that lower seizure threshold. Avoid use with other anticholinergics or neuroleptics during hot weather, which increases the risk of hyperpyrexia. May increase the risks associated with the use of electroconvulsive therapy. Avoid use in elderly patients with hepatic and renal dysfunction. Avoid abrupt discontinuance in patients receiving high doses for prolonged periods. TCAs may cause hyponatremia and/or syndrome of inappropriate antidiuretic hormone hypersecretion (SIADH); volume depletion and diuretics may increase the risk.

(continued)

Table 9.3 (Continued)

Drug Category and Name	Contraindications and Warnings
SSRI Antidepressants	
Citalopram	1. Contraindicated for patients with hypersensitivity or cross-sensitivity to any components of these formulations. 2. Contraindicated in patients using MAO inhibitors or within 2 weeks of discontinuation of use of MAO inhibitors. 3. Contraindicated with concomitant use with pimozide. **Warnings/precautions:** Increased risk of suicidal thinking and behavior in children, adolescents, and young adults (18–24) with MDD and other psychiatric disorders. Increased risk of prolonged QT interval when prescribed over 40 mg per day. May worsen psychosis or risk shift to mania. Risk of serotonin syndrome or neuroleptic malignant syndrome when used alone or with serotonergic or antidopaminergic agents. Use with caution in patients with renal or hepatic dysfunction. Use caution with concomitant use with aspirin, NSAID, warfarin, or other drugs that affect coagulation because the risk of bleeding may be potentiated. SSRIs may cause hyponatremia/SIADH; volume depletion and diuretics may increase the risk.
Escitalopram	1. Contraindicated for patients with hypersensitivity or cross-sensitivity to any components of these formulations. 2. Contraindicated in patients using MAO inhibitors or within 2 weeks of discontinuation of use of MAO inhibitors. 3. Contraindicated with concomitant use with pimozide. **Warnings/precautions:** Increased risk of suicidal thinking and behavior in children, adolescents, and young adults (18–24) with MDD and other psychiatric disorders. May worsen psychosis or risk shift to mania. Risk of serotonin syndrome or neuroleptic malignant syndrome when used alone or with serotonergic or antidopaminergic agents. Use with caution in patients with renal or hepatic dysfunction. SSRIs may cause hyponatremia/SIADH; volume depletion and diuretics may increase the risk. Use with caution in patients predisposed to seizures or who have had previous seizures, brain damage, alcoholism, or use of other drugs which lower seizure threshold. Use caution with concomitant use with aspirin, NSAID, warfarin, or other drugs that affect coagulation because the risk of bleeding may be potentiated. May increase risks associated with electroconvulsive therapy.

Fluoxetine

1. Contraindicated for patients with hypersensitivity or cross-sensitivity to any components of these formulations.
2. Contraindicated in patients using MAO inhibitors or within 2 weeks of discontinuation of use of MAO inhibitors.
3. Contraindicated with concomitant use with pimozide or thioridazine.
4. Treatment with MAO inhibitors or thioridazine should not be initiated until 5 weeks after the discontinuation of fluoxetine.

Warnings/precautions: Increased risk of suicidal thinking and behavior in children, adolescents, and young adults (18–24) with MDD and other psychiatric disorders. May worsen psychosis or risk shift to mania.

Risk of serotonin syndrome or neuroleptic malignant syndrome when used alone or with serotonergic or antidopaminergic agents. Fluoxetine use has been associated with the occurrence of significant rash and allergic events including vasculitis, lupus-like syndrome, laryngospasm, anaphylactoid reactions, and pulmonary inflammatory reactions. Use with caution in patients with renal or hepatic dysfunction. SSRIs may cause hyponatremia/SIADH; volume depletion and diuretics may increase the risk. Use with caution in patients predisposed to seizures or who have had previous seizures, brain damage, alcoholism, or use of other drugs that lower seizure threshold. Use caution with concomitant use with aspirin, NSAID, warfarin, or other drugs that affect coagulation because the risk of bleeding may be potentiated. May increase risks associated with electroconvulsive therapy. Use caution with history of myocardial infarction or unstable heart disease. May alter glycemic control in patients with diabetes. May exacerbate sexual dysfunction.

Fluvoxamine

1. Contraindicated for patients with hypersensitivity or cross-sensitivity to any components of these formulations.
2. Contraindicated in patients using MAO inhibitors or within 2 weeks of discontinuation of use of MAO inhibitors.
3. Contraindicated with concomitant use with pimozide, thioridazine, tizanidine, and alosetron.

Warnings/precautions: Increased risk of suicidal thinking and behavior in children, adolescents, and young adults (18–24) with MDD and other psychiatric disorders. May worsen psychosis or risk shift to mania.

Risk of serotonin syndrome or neuroleptic malignant syndrome when used alone or with serotonergic or antidopaminergic agents. Use with caution in patients with renal or hepatic dysfunction. SSRIs may cause hyponatremia/SIADH; volume depletion and diuretics may increase the risk. Use with caution in patients predisposed to seizures or who have had previous seizures, brain damage, alcoholism, or use of other drugs that lower seizure threshold. Use caution with concomitant use with aspirin, NSAID, warfarin, or other drugs that affect coagulation because the risk of bleeding may be potentiated.

Paroxetine

1. Contraindicated for patients with hypersensitivity or cross-sensitivity to any components of these formulations.
2. Contraindicated in patients using MAO inhibitors or within 2 weeks of discontinuation of use of MAO inhibitors.
3. Contraindicated with concomitant use with pimozide and thioridazine.
4. Contraindicated during pregnancy.

(continued)

Table 9.3 (Continued)

Drug Category and Name	Contraindications and Warnings
	Warnings/precautions: Increased risk of suicidal thinking and behavior in children, adolescents, and young adults (18–24) with MDD and other psychiatric disorders. May worsen psychosis or risk shift to mania. Risk of serotonin syndrome or neuroleptic malignant syndrome when used alone or with serotonergic or antidopaminergic agents. Use with caution (dose reduction is recommended) in patients with renal or hepatic dysfunction. SSRIs may cause hyponatremia/SIADH; volume depletion and diuretics may increase the risk. Use caution with concomitant use with aspirin, NSAID, warfarin, or other drugs that affect coagulation because the risk of bleeding may be potentiated. Use with caution in patients predisposed to seizures or who have had previous seizures, brain damage, alcoholism, or use of other drugs that lower seizure threshold. May exacerbate sexual dysfunction. Use caution with narrow-angle glaucoma. May increase risks associated with electroconvulsive therapy.
Sertraline	1. Contraindicated for patients with hypersensitivity or cross-sensitivity to any components of these formulations.
	2. Contraindicated in patients using MAO inhibitors or within 2 weeks of discontinuation of use of MAO inhibitors.
	3. Contraindicated with concomitant use with pimozide and with disulfiram.
	Warnings/precautions: Increased risk of suicidal thinking and behavior in children, adolescents, and young adults (18–24) with MDD and other psychiatric disorders. May worsen psychosis or risk shift to mania. Risk of serotonin syndrome or neuroleptic malignant syndrome when used alone or with serotonergic or antidopaminergic agents. Use with caution (dose reduction is recommended) in patients with renal or hepatic dysfunction. SSRIs may cause hyponatremia/SIADH; volume depletion and diuretics may increase the risk. Use caution with concomitant use with aspirin, NSAID, warfarin, or other drugs that affect coagulation because the risk of bleeding may be potentiated. Use with caution in patients predisposed to seizures or who have had previous seizures, brain damage, alcoholism, or use of other drugs that lower seizure threshold. May exacerbate sexual dysfunction. May increase risks associated with electroconvulsive therapy. Sertraline acts as a mild uricosuric, so use with caution in patients at risk of uric acid nephropathy.
Dopamine Reuptake Blockers	1. Contraindicated for patients with hypersensitivity or cross-sensitivity to bupropion or for use with other dosage uses of bupropion, for example, Zyban.
Bupropion	2. Contraindicated in patients with seizure disorders.
	3. Contraindicated in patients with a history of anorexia/bulimia.
	4. Contraindicated for use with MAO inhibitor within 14 days of discontinuation of the MAOI.
	5. Contraindicated for use with patients undergoing abrupt discontinuation of ethanol or sedatives (including benzodiazepines).

Warnings/precautions: Increased risk of suicidal thinking and behavior in children, adolescents, and young adults (18–24) with MDD and other psychiatric disorders. May worsen psychosis or risk a shift to mania. The risk of seizures is dose dependent and is increased in patients with a history of seizures, anorexia/bulimia/head trauma, CNS tumor, severe hepatic cirrhosis, abrupt discontinuation of sedative-hypnotics or ethanol, and medications that lower seizure threshold. May cause CNS stimulation, restlessness, anxiety, insomnia, or anorexia. May increase risks associated with electroconvulsive therapy. Discontinue prior to elective surgery. May cause weight gain. Use with caution in patients with all types of cardiovascular disease. Use with caution in patients with renal and hepatic disease.

Serotonin/Norepinephrine Reuptake Inhibitors

Duloxetine

1. Contraindicated for patients with hypersensitivity or cross-sensitivity to SNRIs.
2. Contraindicated for use with MAO inhibitors.
3. Contraindicated for use with patients with uncontrolled narrow-angle glaucoma.
4. Contraindicated for use with patients with hepatic impairment or severe renal impairment.

Warnings/precautions: Increased risk of suicidal thinking and behavior in children, adolescents, and young adults (18–24) with MDD and other psychiatric disorders. May worsen psychosis or risk a shift to mania. Use caution for patients with diabetes, seizure disorders, brain damage, or alcoholism. Risk of serotonin syndrome or neuroleptic malignant syndrome when used alone or with serotonergic or antidopaminergic agents. Use with caution (dose reduction is recommended) in patients with renal or hepatic dysfunction. Use caution with concomitant use with aspirin, NSAID, warfarin, or other drugs that affect coagulation because the risk of bleeding may be potentiated. Modest increase in serum glucose and hemoglobin A1C have been observed in some diabetic patients receiving Duloxetine therapy for diabetic peripheral neuropathy. May cause increased urinary resistance. Avoid use with patients with substantial ethanol intake, evidence of chronic liver disease, or hepatic impairment. May cause hyponatremia/SIADH; volume depletion and diuretics may increase the risk.

Desvenlafaxine
Venlafaxine

1. Contraindicated for patients with hypersensitivity or cross-sensitivity to venlafaxine.
2. Contraindicated for use with MAO inhibitors. Venlafaxine should not be initiated within 14 days of the discontinuation of an MAOI and an MAOI should not be initiated within 7 days of the discontinuation of venlafaxine.

(continued)

Table 9.3   (Continued)

Drug Category and Name	Contraindications and Warnings
	Warnings/precautions: Increased risk of suicidal thinking and behavior in children, adolescents, and young adults (18–24) with MDD and other psychiatric disorders. May worsen psychosis or risk a shift to mania. Risk of serotonin syndrome or neuroleptic malignant syndrome when used alone or with serotonergic or antidopaminergic agents. Use with caution (dose reduction is recommended) in patients with renal or hepatic dysfunction. Use caution with concomitant use with aspirin, NSAID, warfarin, or other drugs that affect coagulation because the risk of bleeding may be potentiated. Use caution in patients with recent history of myocardial infarction, unstable heart disease, or hypothyroidism. Control preexisting hypertension before initiating venlafaxine. May cause hyponatremia/SIADH; volume depletion and diuretics may increase the risk. May increase risks associated with electroconvulsive therapy or a history of seizures. Use caution with narrow-angle glaucoma.
Serotonin Receptor Antagonists	
Nefazodone Trazodone	1. Contraindicated for patients with hypersensitivity or cross-sensitivity to Trazodone or Nefazodone.
	Warnings/precautions: Increased risk of suicidal thinking and behavior in children, adolescents, and young adults (18–24) with MDD and other psychiatric disorders. May worsen psychosis or risk a shift to mania. Priapism, including cases resulting in permanent dysfunction, has occurred with the use of Trazodone. Use caution in patients during acute recovery phase of myocardial infarction and patients with a history of cardiovascular disease (including a previous MI, stroke, tachycardia, or conduction abnormalities). Use caution for concurrent use with MAOI. Due to sedation caused by trazodone, caution should be used with CNS depressants and ethanol. Use with caution for patients with seizure disorders, brain damage, alcoholism, or use of drugs that lower seizure threshold or for use with patients with hepatic impairment or renal dysfunction.
Noradrenergic Antagonist	
Mirtazapine	1. Contraindicated for patients with hypersensitivity or cross-sensitivity to Mirtazapine. 2. Contraindicated for use with MAO inhibitors. Mirtazapine should not be initiated within 14 days of the discontinuation of an MAOI.
	Warnings/precautions: Increased risk of suicidal thinking and behavior in children, adolescents, and young adults (18–24) with MDD and other psychiatric disorders. May worsen psychosis or risk a shift to mania. Discontinue immediately if signs and symptoms of neutropenia/agranulocytosis appear. Sedative effects may be additive with other CNS depressants and ethanol. May increase appetite and stimulate weight gain. Use with caution for patients with seizure disorders, brain damage, alcoholism, or use of drugs that lower seizure threshold.

Benzodiazepines

Alprazolam

1. Contraindicated for patients with hypersensitivity or cross-sensitivity to other benzodiazepines.
2. Contraindicated in patients with acute narrow-angle glaucoma.
3. Contraindicated for use with ketoconazole or itraconazole.
4. Contraindicated during pregnancy.

Warnings/precautions: Rebound or withdrawal symptoms, including seizures, may occur 18 hours to 3 days following abrupt discontinuation or large decreases in dose or prolonged treatment. Use with caution in renal impairment or predisposition to urate nephropathy. Use with caution with the elderly or debilitated patients and patients with hepatic disease including alcoholics, renal impairment, or obese patients. Causes dose-related CNS depression, which may impair physical and mental capabilities including anterograde amnesia. May potentiate the effects of sedatives and ethanol. Benzodiazepines have been associated with falls and traumatic injury, especially in the elderly. Use with caution with patients with respiratory disease or gag reflex. Use with caution with patients with suicide risk or with patients at risk for shift to mania. Paradoxical reactions including hyperactivity and aggressiveness have been reported with benzodiazepines. Fatal on overdose.

Chlordiazepoxide

1. Contraindicated for patients with hypersensitivity or cross-sensitivity to other benzodiazepines.
2. Contraindicated in patients with acute narrow-angle glaucoma.
3. Contraindicated during pregnancy.

Warnings/precautions: Use with caution with the elderly or debilitated patients and patients with hepatic disease including alcoholics, renal impairment. Use with caution with patients with respiratory disease, gag reflex, or porphyria. Avoid parenteral administration in comatose or shock patients. Causes dose-related CNS depression, which may impair physical and mental capabilities including anterograde amnesia. May potentiate the effects of sedatives and ethanol. Benzodiazepines have been associated with falls and traumatic injury, especially in the elderly. Caution with patients with a history of drug dependence. Benzodiazepines have been associated with dependence and acute withdrawal symptoms on discontinuation or reduction in dose, including seizures and anterograde amnesia. Paradoxical reactions including hyperactivity and aggressiveness have been reported with benzodiazepines. Fatal on overdose.

(continued)

Table 9.3 (Continued)

Drug Category and Name	Contraindications and Warnings
Clonazepam	1. Contraindicated for patients with hypersensitivity or cross-sensitivity to other benzodiazepines. 2. Contraindicated in patients with acute narrow-angle glaucoma. 3. Contraindicated during pregnancy. 4. Contraindicated in patients with significant liver disease. **Warnings/precautions:** Use with caution in depressed patients due to risk of suicide. Use with caution with the elderly or debilitated patients and patients with hepatic disease including alcoholics, renal impairment. Use with caution with patients with respiratory disease or gag reflex. Monitor CBC and liver function tests. Caution with patients with a history of drug dependence. Benzodiazepines have been associated with dependence and acute withdrawal symptoms on discontinuation or reduction in dose including seizures and anterograde amnesia. Paradoxical reactions including hyperactivity and aggressiveness have been reported with benzodiazepines. Causes dose-related CNS depression, which may impair physical and mental capabilities including anterograde amnesia. May potentiate the effects of sedatives and ethanol. Benzodiazepines have been associated with falls and traumatic injury, especially in the elderly.
Diazepam Lorazepam Oxazepam	1. Contraindicated for patients with hypersensitivity or cross-sensitivity to other Benzodiazepines. 2. Contraindicated in patients with acute narrow-angle glaucoma. 3. Contraindicated in patients with severe hepatic insufficiency. 4. Contraindicated in patients with myasthenia gravis. 5. Contraindicated in patients with severe respiratory insufficiency. 6. Contraindicated in patients with sleep apnea syndrome. 7. Contraindicated during pregnancy. **Warnings/precautions:** Withdrawal has been associated with an increase in the seizure frequency. Use with caution with the elderly or debilitated patients, obese patients, patients with hepatic disease including alcoholics or renal impairment. Use with caution with patients with respiratory disease or gag reflex. Acute hypotension, muscle, apnea, and cardiac arrest have occurred with parenteral administration. Acute effects may be more prevalent in patients receiving concurrent barbiturates, narcotics, or ethanol. Avoid intra-arterial injection or extravasation of the parenteral formulation. Causes dose-related CNS depression resulting in sedation, dizziness, confusion, or ataxia, which may impair physical or mental capabilities. Benzodiazepines have been associated with falls and traumatic injury, especially in the elderly. Use with caution in depressed patients due to risk of suicide. Use with caution with patients with a history of dependence. Benzodiazepines have been associated with dependence and acute withdrawal symptoms on discontinuation or reduction in dose, including seizures and anterograde amnesia.

Estazolam
Flurazepam
Quazepam
Temazepam
Triazolam

1. Contraindicated for patients with hypersensitivity or cross-sensitivity to other benzodiazepines.
2. Contraindicated during pregnancy.

Warnings/precautions: Congenital malformations have been noted in a case report following maternal use during the first trimester of pregnancy and also with the use of similar agents. Patients using this class of drugs are encouraged to enroll themselves in the AED Pregnancy registry (1-888-233-2334; www.aedpregnancyregistry.org). Use with caution in depressed patients due to risk of suicide. Use with caution with the elderly or debilitated patients, patients with hepatic disease including alcoholics, renal impairment. Use with caution with patients with respiratory disease, gag reflex, or sleep apnea. Causes dose-related CNS depression resulting in sedation, dizziness, confusion, or ataxia, which may impair physical or mental capabilities. Use with caution in patients receiving other CNS depressants or psychoactive agents. Effects of other sedative drugs or ethanol may be potentiated. Benzodiazepines have been associated with falls and traumatic injury, especially in the elderly. Use caution in patients with depression, especially if suicidal risk is present. Benzodiazepines have been associated with dependence and acute withdrawal symptoms on discontinuation or reduction in dose, including seizures and anterograde amnesia. Paradoxical reactions including hyperactivity and aggressiveness have been reported with benzodiazepines.

Other Anxiolytics

Buspirone

1. Contraindicated for patients with hypersensitivity or cross-sensitivity to buspirone.
2. Not recommended for use with patients with hepatic impairment or renal dysfunction.
3. Use with MAOI may result in hypertensive reaction.
4. Does not prevent or treat withdrawal from benzodiazepines.
5. Restlessness syndrome has been reported in a small number of patients.
6. Buspirone does not exhibit cross-tolerance with benzodiazepines or other sedative/hypnotic agents, therefore if substituting Buspirone for any of these agents gradually withdraw the drugs prior to initiating buspirone.

Diphenhydramine

1. Contraindicated for patients with hypersensitivity or cross-sensitivity to diphenhydramine.
2. Contraindicated for patients with bronchial asthma or while breastfeeding.

Warnings/precautions: Causes sedation, so caution must be taken when driving or operating machinery. Sedative effects of CNS depressants or ethanol are potentiated, especially in the elderly. Antihistamines may cause excitation, especially in young children. Use with caution in patients with angle-closure glaucoma, pyloroduodenal obstruction (including stenotic peptic ulcer), urinary tract obstruction (including bladder neck obstruction and symptomatic prostatic hyperplasia), asthma, hyperthyroidism, increased intraocular pressure, and cardiovascular disease (including hypertension and tachycardia). Avoid use in patients sensitive to soy protein, peanuts, or phenylalanine.

(continued)

Table 9.3 (Continued)

Drug Category and Name	Contraindications and Warnings
Hydroxyzine	1. Contraindicated for patients with hypersensitivity or cross-sensitivity to hydroxyzine. 2. Subcutaneous, IV, and intra-arterial administrations are contraindicated due to tissue damage. 3. Contraindicated during early pregnancy. **Warnings/precautions:** Causes sedation, so caution must be taken when driving machinery. Potentiates the effects of CNS depressants or ethanol. Use with caution for patients with narrow-angle glaucoma, prostatic hyperplasia, bladder neck obstruction, asthma, or COPD.
Meprobamate	1. Contraindicated for patients with hypersensitivity or cross-sensitivity to meprobamate. 2. Contraindicated for use with geriatric patients because it is a highly addictive and sedating anxiolytic. Those using it for long periods may become addicted and need to be withdrawn slowly. 3. Contraindicated during pregnancy.
Sedative-Hypnotics	
Eszopiclone	No contraindications listed by manufacturer. **Warnings/precautions:** Use with caution in patients with depression or a history of drug dependence. Abrupt withdrawal may lead to withdrawal symptoms. Use with caution in patients receiving other CNS depressants or psychoactive medications. Hypnotic sedatives have been associated with abnormal thinking and behavior changes including decreased inhibition, aggression, bizarre behavior, agitation, hallucinations, amnesia, and depersonalization. These behaviors may occur unpredictably and may indicate previously unrecognized psychiatric disorders. This drug may impair physical and mental abilities. It has been associated with anaphylaxis as well as angioedema. There is a risk for hazardous sleep-related activities such as sleep driving, cooking, eating food, and making phone calls while asleep. Use with caution in patients with respiratory compromise or hepatic dysfunction. Because the onset of action is so rapid, administration should be given as the patient is getting into bed.
Phenobarbital Secobarbital	1. Contraindicated for patients with hypersensitivity or cross-sensitivity to phenobarbital. 2. Contraindicated in patients with hepatic impairment, dyspnea, airway obstruction, or porphyria. 3. Contraindicated in patients with addiction, since potential for drug dependency exists. 4. Contraindicated for intra-arterial or subcutaneous administration. 5. Contraindicated for patients with a history of sedative/hypnotic addiction. 6. Contraindicated for patients with nephritic disease. 7. Contraindicated during pregnancy.

Warnings/precautions: Cardiac defects and hemorrhagic diseases have been reported in newborn infants of mothers who were taking phenobarbital during pregnancy. Withdrawal symptoms have been noted in the infant following delivery. Potential for drug dependency exists; abrupt cessation may precipitate withdrawal, including status epilepticus in epileptic patents. Do not administer to patients in acute pain. Use caution in elderly, debilitated, renal or hepatic dysfunction, or pediatric patients. May cause paradoxical responses including agitation and hyperactivity, particularly in acute pain and pediatric patients. Use caution in patients with depression or suicidal tendencies or patients with a history of drug abuse. Tolerance, psychological and physical dependence, may occur with prolonged use. May cause CNS depression, which may impair physical and mental abilities. Effects with other sedative drugs or ethanol may be potentiated. May cause respiratory depression or hypotension especially when administered IV. Use with caution in hemodynamically unstable (hypovolemic shock, CHF), or patients with respiratory disease. Not recommended as a sedative in the elderly. Use has been associated with cognitive deficits in children.

Zaleplon
Zolpidem

1. Contraindicated for patients with hypersensitivity or cross-sensitivity to similar compounds.

Warnings/precautions: Use with caution in patients with suicidal risks or with a history of drug dependence. Hypnotic sedatives have been associated with abnormal thinking and behavior changes including decreased inhibition, aggression, bizarre behavior, agitation, hallucinations, amnesia, and depersonalization. These behaviors may occur unpredictably and may indicate previously unrecognized psychiatric disorders. This drug may impair physical and mental abilities. Causes sedation, so caution must be taken when driving machinery. Effects with other sedative drugs or ethanol may be potentiated. Amnesia can occur. Use with caution in patients receiving other CNS depressants or psychoactive medications. It has been associated with anaphylaxis as well as angioedema. There is a risk for hazardous sleep-related activities such as sleep driving, cooking, eating food, and making phone calls while asleep. Use with caution in elderly patients with respiratory compromise or hepatic dysfunction. Because the onset of action is so rapid, administration should be given as the patient is getting into bed. Use zolpidem with caution in patients with myasthenia gravis and sleep apnea.

Typical Antipsychotics

Chlorpromazine
Fluphenazine
Loxapine
Mesoridazine
Molindone

1. Contraindicated in patients with hypersensitivity or cross-sensitivity to dopamine antagonists (especially phenothiazines).
2. Contraindicated for patients with severe central nervous system depression or coma.
3. Fluphenazine is contraindicated for patients with brain damage, blood dyscrasias, or hepatic disease.
4. Thiothixene is contraindicated for patients with blood dyscrasias and circulatory collapse.
5. Thrifluoperazine is contraindicated for patients with blood dyscrasias, severe hepatic disease, and bone marrow suppression.

(continued)

Table 9.3 (Continued)

Drug Category and Name	Contraindications and Warnings
Perphenazine Thiothixene Trifluoperazine	**Warnings/precautions:** Elderly patients' dementia-related psychosis treated with antipsychotics are at risk for death (due to heart failure or pneumonia). Use with caution in patients with Parkinson's disease, hemodynamic instability, predisposition to seizures, subcortical brain damage, severe cardiac, hepatic, renal, or respiratory disease. Esophageal dismotility, aspiration, and increased prolactin levels have occurred. Antiemetic effects may mask temperature regulation or toxicity. Cardiac conduction alterations and life-threatening arrhythmias have occurred. Avoid use with patients with preexisting low **WBC** or history of drug-induced leuko/neutropenia or agranulocytosis since typical antipsychotics can cause fatal leukopenia, neutropenia, and agranulocytosis. Use with caution in patients at risk for hypotension (which may occur with parenteral administration). Extrapyramidal symptoms frequently occur.
Haloperidol	1. Contraindicated in patients with hypersensitivity or cross-sensitivity to dopamine antagonists. 2. Contraindicated for patients with severe central nervous system depression or coma. 3. Contraindicated for Parkinson's disease.
	Warnings/precautions: Elderly patients with dementia-related psychosis are at risk of death (due to heart failure or pneumonia) when treated with dopamine antagonists. Maximum dosage ranges should not be exceeded due to risk of altering cardiac function or producing prolonged QT interval. Avoid use with patients with pre-existing low WBC or history of drug-induced leuko/ neutropenia or agranulocytosis.
Thioridazine	1. Contraindicated in patients with hypersensitivity or cross-sensitivity to dopamine antagonists (especially phenothiazines). 2. Contraindicated for patients with severe central nervous system depression or coma. 3. Contraindicated for patients with severe hyper-hypotensive heart disease. 4. Contraindicated to be used in combination with other drugs that are known to prolong the QT interval, and in patients with congenital long QT syndrome or a history of cardiac arrhythmias.
	Warnings/precautions: Thioridazine has dose-related effects on ventricular repolarization leading to QT prolongation, a potentially life-threatening event. Therefore, it should be reserved with patients with schizophrenia who have failed to respond to adequate levels of other antipsychotic drugs. Use with caution in patients with orthostatic hypotension. Elderly patients' dementia-related psychosis treated with antipsychotics are at risk for death. Use with caution in patients with Parkinson's disease, hemodynamic instability, predisposition to seizures, subcortical brain damage, severe cardiac, hepatic, renal, or respiratory disease. Esophageal dismotility, aspiration, and increased prolactin levels have occurred. Antiemetic effects may mask temperature regulation or toxicity. Avoid use with patients with preexisting low WBC or history of drug-induced leuko/neutropenia or agranulocytosis.

Atypical Antipsychotics

Clozapine

1. Contraindicated in patients with hypersensitivity or cross-sensitivity to atypical antipsychotics.
2. Contraindicated in patients with a history of agranulocytosis, granulocytopenia, or bone marrow suppression.
3. Contraindicated in patients with uncontrolled epilepsy, severe CNS depression or coma, paralytic ileus, or myeloproliferative disorders.

Warnings/precautions: In elderly patients with dementia-related psychosis (risk of death). In patients with WBC <3,500 cells/mm^3 due to risk of agranulocytosis (life threatening). In patients with a history of seizures, head trauma, brain damage, alcoholism, or concurrent use of drugs that lower the seizure threshold. It has been associated with benign self-limiting fever (<100.4 F within the first 3 weeks), with severe febrile reactions including neuroleptic malignant syndrome. In patients with deep vein thrombosis, myocarditis, pericarditis, pericardial effusion, cardiomyopathy, and heart failure. May cause anticholinergic effects. Use caution with patients with urinary retention, benign prostatic hyperplasia, narrow angle glaucoma, xerostomia, visual problems, constipation, or bowel obstruction. May cause hyperglycemia, ketoacidosis, hyperosmolar coma, or death. Use caution in patients with hepatic or renal disease, cardiovascular or pulmonary disease, or hypotension. May cause tachycardia. There is a suicide risk for patients with psychosis or bipolar disorders. Medication should not be stopped abruptly. Significant weight gain has been observed.

Aripiprazole
Asenapine

1. Contraindicated in patients with hypersensitivity or cross-sensitivity to atypical antipsychotics.

Warnings/precautions: Increased risk of suicidal thinking and behavior in children, adolescents, and young adults (18–24) with MDD and other psychiatric disorders. In elderly patients with dementia-related psychosis (risk of death). Caution should be used in cases of preexisting low WBC or a history of drug-related leuko-/neutropenia. For use with patients with Parkinson's disease. For use with patients with disposition to seizures and severe cardiac disease. Caution for patients with diabetes and other disorders of glucose regulation for risk of developing hyperglycemia. May cause EPS.

Iloperidone
Paliperidone
Risperidone

1. Contraindicated for patients with hypersensitivity or cross-sensitivity to illoperidone, paliperidone, or risperidone or any component of that formulation.
2. Warning/precaution: Elderly patients with dementia-related psychosis (risk of death). Use with caution with iloperidone in disorders with CNS depression, predisposition to seizures, hepatic impairment, esophageal dysmotility, and aspiration or risk of aspiration pneumonia (Alzheimer's disease). With paliperidone and risperidone caution should be used in cases of preexisting low WBC or a history of drug related leuko/neutropenia. Iloperidone and risperidone may alter cardiac conduction and prolong the QT interval or arrhythmia or when used in combination with other drugs that cause cardiac problems. Paliperidone and risperidone may cause EPS, suicidal effects and increased prolactin levels.

(continued)

Table 9.3 (Continued)

Drug Category and Name	Contraindications and Warnings
Ziprasidone	1. It is contraindicated for patients with hypersensitivity or cross-sensitivity to ziprasidone. 2. Contraindicated for patients with a history of prolonged QT, congenital long QT syndrome, recent myocardial infarction, heart failure, concurrent use of other QT-prolonging agents (including arsenic, trioxide, chlorpromazine, class 1a antiarrhythmics, class 3 antiarrhythmics). 3. Warnings/precautions: Elderly patients with dementia-related psychosis (risk of death). Caution should be used in cases of preexisting low WBC or a history of drug related leuko/neutropenia. May cause EPS. Use with caution in disorders with CNS depression, predisposition to seizures, hepatic impairment, esophageal dysmotility, and aspiration or risk of aspiration pneumonia. Caution in the case of patients at high risk for suicide who have psychotic illness or bipolar disorder.
Olanzapine	1. Contraindicated for patients with hypersensitivity or cross-sensitivity to olanzapine. **Warnings/precautions:** Elderly patients with dementia-related psychosis (risk of death). Caution should be used in cases of pre-existing low WBC or a history of drug-related leuko/neutropenia. Caution in the case of patients at high risk for suicide who have psychotic illness or bipolar disorder. Use with caution in disorders with CNS depression, predisposition to seizures, hepatic impairment, esophageal dysmotility and aspiration, or risk of aspiration pneumonia. Caution patients regarding driving and operating machinery. Patients with ischemic heart disease, prior myocardial infarction, hemodynamic instability, or any history of cardiac disease may be at risk for orthostatic hypotension or arrhythmia. Patients with decreased gastrointestinal motility, urinary retention, BPH, xerostomia, or narrow-angle glaucoma are at risk for anticholinergic effects. Olanzapine may be associated with neuroleptic malignant syndrome. Caution for patients with diabetes and other disorders of glucose regulation for risk of developing hyperglycemia.
Quetiapine	1. Contraindicated for patients with hypersensitivity or cross-sensitivity to quetiapine. **Warnings/precautions:** Increased risk of suicidal thinking and behavior in children, adolescents, and young adults (18–24) with MDD and other psychiatric disorders. Increased risk of arrhythmias when combined with other antipsychotic medication. Elderly patients with dementia-related psychosis (risk of death). Caution should be used in cases of preexisting low WBC or a history of drug-related leuko/neutropenia. Caution for patients with diabetes and other disorders of glucose regulation for risk of developing hyperglycemia. Patients with decreased gastrointestinal motility, urinary retention, BPH, xerostomia, or narrow-angle glaucoma are at risk for anticholinergic effects. Caution in patients with a history of seizures. May cause a decrease in thyroxine, elevations in liver enzymes, cholesterol, and triglyceride levels, and hyperprolactinemia in patients with breast cancer.

Anti-EPS / Anti-Parkinsonian Agents

Amantadine
Trihexyphenidyl

1. Contraindicated for patients with hypersensitivity or cross-sensitivity to amantadine.

Warnings/precautions: May cause CNS depression, which may impair mental and physical abilities. May cause suicidal thinking. Use caution with patients with liver disease, a history of dermatitis, uncontrolled psychosis, severe neurosis, seizures, or those receiving CNS stimulants. Use reduced dose in renal disease. Abrupt discontinuation may cause agitation, anxiety, delirium, delusions, depression, hallucinations, paranoia, Parkinsonian crisis, slurred speech, or stupor. Use with caution with patients with peripheral edema or orthostatic hypertension. Dopamine antagonists have been associated with compulsive behaviors (e.g., gambling, hypersexuality, and binge eating).

Benztropine

1. Contraindicated for patients with hypersensitivity or cross-sensitivity to benztropine.
2. Contraindicated for pyloric or duodenal obstruction, stenosing, peptic ulcers.
3. Contraindicated in bladder neck obstruction, achalasia, and myasthenia gravis.

Warnings/precautions: Use with caution in hot weather during exercise due to anhydrosis and hypothermia particularly in the elderly, alcoholics, patients with CNS disease, and those with prolonged outdoor exposure in hot weather. Caution in elderly patients with atherosclerosis. Caution in patients with tachycardia, cardiac arrhythmia, hypertension, hypotension, glaucoma, prostatic hyperplasia, especially the elderly who tend toward urinary retention, liver, or kidney disorders, or obstructive diseases of the GI tract. May cause weakness and inability to move. May be associated with confusion or hallucinations or CNS depression.

Diphenhydramine

See above in Anxiolytics

Mood Stabilizers

Carbamazepine

1. Contraindicated in patients hypersensitive to carbamazepine, tricyclic antidepressants, or any components of these formulations.
2. Contraindicated in bone marrow depression.
3. Contraindicated with or within 14 days of MAO inhibitor use.
4. Contraindicated for concurrent use of nefazodone.
5. Contraindicated during pregnancy.

(continued)

Table 9.3 (Continued)

Drug Category and Name	Contraindications and Warnings
	Warnings/precautions: Potentially fatal blood cell abnormalities have been reported. Increased risk for suicidal behaviors and thoughts. Use with caution in patients with cardiac damage, ECG abnormalities, or hepatic or renal disease. Potentially serious or fatal multiorgan sensitivity reactions. Dizziness and drowsiness may interfere with operating machinery. Effects with other sedative drugs or ethanol may be potentiated. Severe dermatologic reactions including toxic epidermal necrolysis and Stevens-Johnson syndrome have resulted in fatalities. It is important to screen for the genetic susceptibility genotype (HALA-B 1502 allele) in Asian patients. To avoid dermatologic complications, patients with positive results should not be started on Carbamazepine. Elderly patients may have an increased risk of SIADH-like syndrome.
Lamotrigine	1. Contraindicated for patients with hypersensitivity or cross-sensitivity to lamotrigine.
	Warnings/precautions: Severe and potentially life-threatening skin rashes requiring hospitalization have been reported. Risk may be increased by co-administration with valproic acid at higher than recommended starting doses and rapid dose titration. Increased risk for suicidal behaviors and thoughts. Acute multiorgan failure and hematologic effects (e.g. neutropenia and leukopenia, thrombocytopenia, pancytopenia, anemia, aplasticanemia, and pure red cell aplasia) have been reported. Use caution in patients with impaired renal, hepatic, or cardiac function. Avoid abrupt cessation. May cause CNS depression, which may impair physical or mental abilities. Binds to melanin and may accumulate in the eye or other melanin-rich tissues.
	1. Contraindicated for patients with hypersensitivity or cross-sensitivity to lithium. 2. Avoid use in patients with severe cardiovascular disease. 3. Contraindicated with patients with severe debilitation, dehydration, or sodium depletion. 4. Contraindicated for use during pregnancy.
Lithium	**Warnings/precautions:** Lithium toxicity is closely related to serum levels and can occur at therapeutic doses. Serum level determinations are required to monitor therapy. Use with caution in patients with thyroid disease, mild to moderate renal impairment, or mild to moderate cardiovascular disease. Use with caution in patients receiving medications that alter sodium excretion (e.g., diuretics, ACE inhibitors, NSAIDs), or in patients with significant fluid loss. Chronic therapy results in diminished concentrating ability (usually reversible when lithium is discontinued). Use with caution in patients with risk of suicide. Neuroleptic malignancy syndrome-like syndrome has been reported in patients receiving concurrent treatment with neuroleptics medications. Lithium may affect alertness for driving a car. The effect of neuromuscular blocking agents may be prolonged with concomitant use with lithium. Higher serum concentrations may be required and tolerated during manic episodes, but the tolerance decreases when symptoms subside. Salt and fluid intake must be monitored and managed during therapy.

Valproic acid

1. Contraindicated with hypersensitivity to valproic acid derivatives or any component of the formulation.
2. Contraindicated in hepatic disease or significant hepatic impairment.
3. Contraindicated in patients with urea cycle disorders.
4. Contraindicated for use during pregnancy.

Warnings/Precautions: Hepatic failure resulting in fatalities has occurred in patients (children less than 2 years of age are at considerable risk). Use with caution in patients with organic brain disease, mental retardation with severe seizure disorders, congenital metabolic disorders, and patients on multiple anticonvulsants. Monitor patients closely and discontinue immediately with signs and symptoms of hepatotoxicity (e.g., malaise, weakness, facial edema, anorexia, jaundice, and vomiting). Cases of life-threatening pancreatitis occurring at the start of therapy or after years of use have been reported in adults and children. Symptoms of abdominal pain, nausea, vomiting, or anorexia should be regarded as warnings to discontinue therapy. Potential for teratogenic effects such as neurotube defects (spina bifida). May cause severe thrombocytopenia, inhibition of platelet aggregation, and bleeding. Tremors may indicate overdose. Use with caution in patients using other anticonvulsants. Valproic acid has been associated with dermatologic and hematologic changes such as eosinophilia, neutropenia, or thrombocytopenia. Hyperammonemia and encephalopathy, sometimes fatal, have been reported and may be present with normal transaminase levels. Ammonia levels should be measures in patients who develop unexplained lethargy and vomiting or changes in mental status or in patients who present with hypothermia. Evaluate possible urea cycle disorder before initiating therapy. Use with caution in patients with risk of suicide such as bipolar patients. May cause CNS depression, which may impair physical or mental abilities and may potentiate the effects of other sedative drugs.

Psychostimulants

Atomoxetine

1. Contraindicated for patients with hypersensitivity or cross-sensitivity to atomoxetine.
2. Contraindicated for use with or within 14 days of MAO inhibitor use.
3. Contraindicated for use with patients with narrow-angle glaucoma.

Warnings/precautions: Increased risk of suicidal ideation in pediatric patients. Use caution with patients with hepatic or renal disease. May cause urinary retention or hesitancy or bladder outlet obstruction. Priapism has been associated with use. Orthostasis can occur in patients predisposed to hypotension, changes in heart rate or blood pressure. CNS stimulants have been associated with serious cardiovascular events including sudden death with preexisting structural cardiac abnormalities, stroke, and myocardial infarction. Avoid use in patients with heart rhythm abnormalities. May increase heart rate or blood pressure. Allergic reactions may occur (including angioneurotic edema, urticaria, and rash). Growth should be monitored during treatment. Height and weight gain may be reduced during the first 9 to 12 months of treatment, but should recover by 3 years of therapy.

(continued)

Table 9.3 (Continued)

Drug Category and Name	Contraindications and Warnings
Lisdexamfetamine Dextroamphetamine Dextroamphetamine and amphetamine	1. Contraindicated for patients with hypersensitivity or cross-sensitivity or idiosyncratic reaction sympathomimetic amines. 2. Contraindicated in advanced arteriosclerosis, symptomatic cardiovascular disease, or moderate to severe hypertension. 3. Contraindicated in patients with hyperthyroidism, glaucoma, agitated states, or a history of drug abuse. 4. Contraindicated for concurrent use or within 2 weeks of use of MAOI. **Warnings/precautions:** Use has been associated with serious cardiovascular events, including sudden death in patients with preexisting structural cardiac abnormalities or other serious heart problems. Avoid use in patients with heart arrhythmia problems or coronary artery disease. Use caution in patients with psychiatric or seizure disorders. Amphetamines may exacerbate symptoms of behavior or thought disorder in psychotic patients or unmask tics in patients with Tourette's syndrome. Potential for drug dependency exists, especially in prolonged use. Avoid use in patients with a history of ethanol or drug abuse. Abrupt discontinuation may result in symptoms of withdrawal. Appetite suppression and slow growth rate may occur. Treatment interruption may be necessary for children who are not growing or gaining weight.
Methylphenidate Dexmethylphenidate	1. Contraindicated for patients with hypersensitivity or cross-sensitivity to methylphenidate. 2. Contraindicated in patients with marked anxiety, tension, and agitation. 3. Contraindicated in patients with glaucoma. 4. Contraindicated during or within 14 days following MAOI therapy. 5. Contraindicated when there is a family history or diagnosis of Tourette's syndrome or tics. **Warnings/precautions:** CNS stimulant use has been associated with serious cardiovascular events including sudden death in patients with preexisting structural cardiac abnormalities or serious heart problems. Use with caution in patients with hypertension, cardiac arrhythmia, hyperthyroidism, or increased heart rate. Use with caution in patients with bipolar disorder. May exacerbate symptoms of behavior and thought disorder in psychotic patients. Use caution in patients with seizure disorders and patients with a history of ethanol or drug abuse. Potential for drug dependency exists. Avoid abrupt discontinuation. Visual disturbances have been reported. Should not be used in patients with esophageal motility disorder or preexisting severe gastrointestinal narrowing (history of peritonitis, cystic fibrosis, chronic intestinal pseudo-obstruction, or Meckel's diverticulum). Metadate CD and Metadate ER contain sucrose and lactose, respectively. Avoid administration in hereditary galactose intolerance, Lapp lactase deficiency, or glucose-galactose malabsorption. Transdermal administration may cause allergic contact sensitization characterized by intense local reactions (edema and papules).

effects, unexpected adverse drug reactions, toxicities, and the use of medications with special populations such as women of child-bearing age are some of the factors that have been taken into consideration in determining the contraindication of a drug, and for the use of particular drugs for a specific type of patient.

SIDE EFFECTS, ADVERSE DRUG REACTIONS, DRUG TOXICITY, AND OVERDOSE

The term *side effects* refers to expected reactions to normal doses of a drug. The term *adverse drug reactions* (ADRs) refers to unexpected effects of a drug that is given at a normal therapeutic dose. And the term *drug toxicity* refers to the undesirable effects of a drug seen at higher-than-normal doses, or normal doses that create toxic effects due to irregularities in the patient's physiology.

Practitioners must be aware of methods to best manage expected side effects, unexpected adverse drug reactions, and drug toxicities, including those that occur during overdose. They must be cognizant of the indications in their patients of any physical reactions that call for referral for appropriate medical specialties—for example, acute allergic reactions, glucose intolerance, or hypertensive crisis. Therapeutic monitoring of patients for adverse reactions to drugs should include the following areas of knowledge:

1. Knowledge of the oral doses at which each drug is likely to be toxic, for all medications prescribed and over-the counter (OTC) taken by a patient.
2. Physiological and behavioral toxicity indications for each of these drugs.
3. Methods for monitoring and managing drug levels, including laboratory test results and interpretation of these results.

Side Effects of Medications

All medications have the possibility of side effects, even when blood concentration levels are within normal range. The expected side effects for each drug approved by FDA, when given within the recommended therapeutic dose range, are listed in the package insert. The toxic reactions are listed as overdose/toxicology, and the unexpected adverse reactions caused by interactions with other medications are listed as drug interactions. Notwithstanding individual patient variations, certain effects tend to be common within drug categories. For instance:

1. Anticholinergic side effects of some antipsychotics and antidepressants are known to increase heart rate, temperature, and pupil size with a decrease in bowel sounds and sweating.
2. Tricyclic antidepressants may cause cardiovascular side effects, such as orthostatic hypotension, tachycardia, and ECG changes.
3. CNS depressants and tranquilizers such as barbiturates and benzodiazepines tend to cause lethargy, shallow breathing, and weak, irregular, slow, or fast pulse.
4. Stimulants and hallucinogens, such as amphetamines, ecstasy, cocaine, and LSD cause symptoms of hyperactivity, agitation, sweating, tremor, dilated pupils, and auditory or visual hallucinations.

Adverse Drug Reaction (ADR) Symptomology

Symptoms of unexpected adverse drug reactions vary depending on the specific type of drug that has been taken; but, in general, they are similar to the symptomology observed with expected side effects. Adverse drug reactions may occur with both prescription and *over-the-counter* medications, and are often due to variations in patient metabolic processes created by immunological sensitivities, organ dysfunction, aging, or illness.

Drug Toxicity

Drugs are chemical substances that alter the body's normal chemistry. Most, if not all drugs, have a negative effect on the body, in addition to the positive or desired effect for which they are intended. Nonetheless, it is possible that the blood concentration levels of a particular medication or herbal supplement may rise to an excessive level that could become toxic. Toxic levels may occur when the dosage is too high, when other drugs have depleted or inhibited the CYP450 enzymes needed for metabolism, or when a dysfunctional liver or kidney is not able to remove the drug properly from the bloodstream. In other words, a person with drug toxicity has accumulated an excessive concentration of a medication in their bloodstream. The negative effects of medication become more pronounced as the blood concentration of that medication increases. At toxic levels the adverse drug effects can be severe and debilitating.

Drug–Drug Interactions

Some drug interactions are due to the system of cytochrome P450 enzymes that is used to clear drugs predominantly from the intestines and liver. Drugs may increase or decrease the activity of CYP isozymes either by inducing the biosynthesis of an isozyme (induction) or by inhibiting the activity of the CYP isozyme (inhibition). This is a major source of adverse drug reaction because changes in CYP enzyme activity may affect the metabolism and clearance of some drugs. For example, if one drug inhibits the CYP-mediated metabolism of another drug, the second drug may accumulate within the body to toxic levels. Such drug interactions may necessitate dosage adjustments or argue for choosing drugs that do not interact with the CYP system. Such drug interactions are especially important to take into account when using drugs of vital importance to the patient, drugs with significant side effects, and drugs with a narrow dosing range. An example is phenytoin (Dilantin), which induces CYP1A2, 2C9, 2C19, and 3A4. Substrates for 3A4 may be drugs with critical doses like carbamazepine, whose blood *plasma concentration* may decrease because of enzyme induction caused by phenytoin. Table 9.2 shows interactions with other medications that share common cytochrome P450 metabolizing enzymes.

Some psychotropic drugs may have very small therapeutic windows (e.g., lithium) and yet are regarded as treatment of choice for a given diagnosis (i.e., bipolar disorder). In the case of such a drug, one must carefully weigh the risk-benefit ratio. In lithium treatment of bipolar disorder, the concurrent use of caffeine may decrease the serum concentration of lithium by increasing the urinary elimination of the drug. Furthermore, the concurrent use of ACE inhibitors may increase the serum concentration of lithium to neurotoxic levels (Hulisz & Jakab, 2007).

Other Interactions

Some nondrug substances, such as foods and naturally grown supplements, are known to induce or inhibit CYP enzyme activity. Bioactive compounds found in grapefruit juice have been found to inhibit CYP3A4-mediated metabolism of some medications and, therefore, lead to increased bioavailability and risk of overdose on medications such as benzodiazepines and antihistamines. Due to this risk, grapefruit juice consumption should be limited or, if possible, avoided by patients taking certain drugs. St. John's wort induces CYP3A4 and is an inhibitor of 1A1, 1B1, 2D6, and 3A4. Tobacco smoking induces CYP1A2, whose substrates are clozapine, olanzapine, and fluvoxamine. Smoking, which is three times as high among schizophrenic patients as the general population (George & Vessicchio, 2001), may require increasing certain antipsychotic doses to obtain effective results. If a smoking-cessation program is implemented and causes a reduction or cessation of smoking, the dose of drugs like clozapine will need to be decreased because the reduction of enzymatic activity will cause the drug level in the blood to rise.

Therapeutic Index

The ratio of the lethal dose to the therapeutic dose is called the *therapeutic index*. Drugs with a narrow therapeutic index are more risky to use due to the lethal dose being close to the therapeutic dose and anything that increases the blood levels of the drug can easily produce a toxic reaction. Conversely, drugs with a wide therapeutic index are safer. Related to the therapeutic index, but more difficult to establish is the therapeutic window, which is the range of blood levels within which a beneficial effect is known to occur.

Management of Drug Side Effects

Prevention of all side effects may be an unreasonable goal. However, minimizing untoward side effects can be accomplished by using caution when increasing dosage, switching to different medications and discontinuing medications. Patients need to be educated about accidental interactions of their medication with other prescriptive medications, substances of abuse, OTC drugs, and foods. For instance, patients who are prescribed CNS depressants need to be educated about the simultaneous ingestion of other nonprescriptive CNS depressants such as alcohol. Prescribing medical psychologists must interview patients frequently about the possible interactive substances in their daily lives. Initial interviews should include a visual inspection of all prescribed and OTC medications. In the case of patients who take multiple medications for a variety of medical disorders, the prescribing medical psychologist should require them to bring all their medications, including OTC drugs, for inspection and recording in their records. This is particularly true for geriatric patients. Such cautious regulation, education, and monitoring by the clinician will reduce the risk of untoward side effects and provide for enhanced awareness and reporting on the part of the patient.

Collaborative Management of Adverse Drug Reactions

Collaboration and consultation is a best practice standard between medical psychologists and physicians. Just as it is incumbent upon medical providers to consult with psychologists and other mental-health professionals concerning emotional, cognitive and behavioral symptoms beyond their expertise, the medical psychologist consults with his medical colleagues on health concerns that impact on the management of mental-health conditions. It is a given that medical psychologists engage in coordination of care with appropriate medical specialists. For instance, when the risk of adverse drug reactions is due to comorbid disease states or pregnancy risk, appropriate physician specialists should be consulted. In the case of diseases that cause renal or hepatic insufficiency that alters drug metabolism, consultation with a nephrologist or liver specialist would be recommended.

FDA provides guidance on the drug insert with prescription medications to guide dosing for patients with impaired renal function based on estimation of the glomerular filtration rate, which, in turn, is based on lab measures of creatinine. In the case of genetic factors that may cause abnormal drug metabolism during either phase I oxidation or phase II conjugation, as well as inherited abnormal alleles of cytochrome P-450 that may alter drug metabolism, consultation with a geneticist is recommended. Drug toxicity may be a concern for a pregnant woman with a life-threatening depression that requires psychotropics with known risk of teratogenicity; such a case might be closely coordinated between gynecologist/obstetrician and psychologist.

Referral to hospital may be required when patients present to a clinician with life-threatening conditions such as anaphylactic (allergic) response to medication or food, respiratory or heart failure, loss of consciousness, seizure, or other medical emergencies. These are not likely to occur when the patient is in the medical psychologist's office. Yet, if the patient or concerned other is reporting these reactions, usually by phone, the obvious response should be referral to an emergency room.

Management of Overdose

Overdose can be a medical emergency in which basic life support (BLS) procedures become necessary. In the state of Louisiana, medical psychologists are required to maintain their BLS certification. Regardless of whether a medical psychologist is BLS certified, the first step should be to call 911 and to keep the patient comfortable until emergency medical service (EMS) arrives. Patients should be supine with head turned to the side and feet elevated and provided with a body cover to retain warmth until emergency help arrives. Initial intervention for overdose should focus on stabilization of the patient's airway, breathing rate and circulatory system (ABC). When EMS arrives, they may determine that ventilation is required if there are long apnea spells, or blood gases show hypoxia. If the patient goes into hypovolemic, vasodilatory, or cardiogenic shock—in which blood pressure drops so low that cells, tissues, and organs can be damaged due to lack of oxygenated blood—brain, kidneys, liver, or heart may cease to function. If untreated, shock may be fatal.

Drug toxicity may include drug lethality. For those cases in which toxicity raises the risk of lethality, for example, overdose of tricyclic antidepressant or benzodiazepine drugs, immediate action is required by the medical psychologist, and may consist of facilitating BLS intervention by alerting EMS, with subsequent hospital emergency room referral.

Drug toxicity is not always provoked by drug overdose, but it may result from interplay of multiple drugs. More than one third (36%) of all drugs are metabolized by the CYP450 enzyme 3A4/5. And 19% are metabolized by 2D6. The monitoring of CYP-inducing and/or -inhibiting drug interactions in the practice of a prescribing medical psychologist is complicated by the multiple directions from which an interaction may be produced. Drug–drug interactions may be due to a psychotropic interacting with another psychotropic, a psychotropic inducing or inhibiting a non-psychotropic (e.g., an SSRI such as paroxetine inhibiting an antiemetic such as promethazine), or a nonpsychotropic inducing or inhibiting a psychotropic. If one of two drugs inhibits the CYP-mediated metabolism of another drug, the second drug may accumulate within the body to toxic levels. And, in turn, if one of two drugs induces the CYP-mediated metabolism of another drug, the second drug may fail to accumulate within the body the concentration sufficient to produce a therapeutic effect.[3] If the clinical decision is made to prescribe a psychotropic with drug–drug interaction potential, the prescribing medical psychologist may need to adjust the dosage to lower the risk of adverse drug reactions.

RELAPSE PREVENTION, MAINTENANCE, AND PROPHYLAXIS

Pharmacotherapy parallels the phase of psychosocial treatment and, indeed, is intertwined. The recovery from depression, for example, depends on environmental events and relapse may reoccur when a toxic environment is reencountered or recalled. It has been proposed that there are three phases to the treatment of severe mental-health disorders; such treatment phases refer to the application of psychotherapy as well as pharmacotherapy. For example, the treatment of depression with antidepressant medications ideally follows a sequence through the acute, continuation, and maintenance phases (Reimherr, Amsterdam, Quitkin, Rosenbaum, Fava, Zajecka, et al., 1998).

1. Acute Therapy. During the first 8 to 12 weeks, the treating psychologist starts with a low dose and slowly increases the dosage to reach a therapeutic range. Regular monitoring for side effects and assessment of desired effects should be a part of this acute phase.

2. Continuation Therapy. During the 5 to 6 months following the disappearance of the acute symptoms the prescriber continues to administer the medication in order to continue the regulation of the disorder.

3. Maintenance Therapy. Maintenance therapy is a form of treatment in which psychopharmacological medication is prescribed for a patient who is at risk for reoccurrence of symptoms even after a period of remission. Such continuation of treatment during a period of remission is assumed to be an effective form of relapse prevention. A good example of such maintenance therapy is the case of a patient who has had several repeated episodes of major depression and is likely to suffer recurrence. Antidepressants of a similar type and in dosages comparable to those used during the acute phase are usually recommended to prevent recurrence.

Practitioners must be skilled in strategies for ensuring treatment *adherence*, preventing recurrence of symptoms, and maintaining gains in the process of treatment.

---

[3]A different variation on drug interaction occurs with prodrugs, such as codeine, which require metabolism by CYP450 enzymes to become active. In the case of codeine, for example, CYP3A4 anabolism is required to convert inert codeine into narcodeine, and CYP2D6 to convert codeine into morphine. Grapefruit, a significant CYP3A4 inhibitor, can substantially reduce the effectiveness of codeine.

Relapse and Recurrence

In pharmacotherapy, relapse is defined as a return to the same episode of illness after an initial response in the acute or continuation phase of treatment. Recurrence is defined as the evolution of a new episode of illness after recovery from the previous episode and during the maintenance phase of treatment.

Relapse prevention (RP) methods need to be applied as a part of treatment for mental disorders such as anxiety, depression, bipolar disorder, and schizophrenia. In the practice of cognitive-behavioral therapy, relapse prevention of depressive disorder may be applied by using a technique called coaching near the termination phase of treatment. Patients are coached in the recognition of the signs of relapse and offered practice in taking steps to prevent relapse from occurring. Periodic checkup telephone calls or office visits are very helpful in preventing relapse. The use of periodic checkups following termination allows the therapist to aid patients in the recognition and acceptance of the signs of relapse, and to make suggestions about prevention or remediation.

In their practice of prescribing medical psychology, clinicians need to train patients to recognize prodromal symptoms that could predict relapse or recurrence and to contact the prescriber for evaluation and possible adjustments in the treatment protocol. Similar to the practice of psychotherapists, medical psychologists need to help their patients to be realistic about the efficacy of treatment, and to understand that changing environmental contingencies may introduce risks for relapse. Patients are taught to recognize the warning signs of relapse, such as a return of depressive symptoms, manic symptoms, or prodromal psychotic symptoms. Some therapists model for their patients how to act as if they were a therapist, and to imitate, through role-play, how to talk themselves into contacting their therapist when faced with the warning signs of relapse. Patients are taught to conceptualize the feelings of relapse proclivity and when to decide that they need outside intervention in order to prevent relapse.

Prophylaxis

Preventive medical treatment of disease and preventive psychological treatment are both forms of *prophylaxis*. In clinical practice, preventive medicine and preventive psychology often take the form of OTC medications, dietary supplements, and self-help psychology skills. Prophylactic prescriptive medication is employed in the use of anticonvulsant medication following brain surgery, despite the lack of any seizure activity. Because the risk-benefit ratio is very high in this case, the use of antiseizure medication is justified as a preventive measure. An example of the use of psychopharmacological treatment for prophylactic reasons would be the administration of diphenhydramine along with haloperidol to prevent dystonia.

Maintenance of Treatment Goals

During the final course of treatment, and after symptoms have remitted, a medical psychologist may decide to continue the use of medications that will help a patient to remain symptom free when there is a risk of the recurrence of previous symptomology. An example of such a maintenance strategy is the prescription of lithium to a patient who is at risk for a manic episode due to a past history of manic episodes.

Ensuring Treatment Adherence

A patient's verbal agreement to carry out a prescribed regimen of treatment may not be a guarantee that the treatment steps will be carried out. The nonadherence rate for short-term medication prescription not being filled is 30%–35%, and stopping medication after several days is 20%–25% of those who filled the prescription, with 70%–80% who do not finish a 10-day course of the medication. Nonadherence for long-term use is 50% and 70% for lifestyle suggestions (e.g., dietary habits) (Nockowitz, 1998). Signs of nonadherence include missing scheduled appointments, having leftover medications observed during pill counts, or failure to achieve the desired effects of treatment despite close monitoring and expected effectiveness of the interventions. Intervention for nonadherence should target the reason for the nonadherence. Rather than use intrusive methods such as assessing side effects, pill counting, and serum drug levels, it is best to intervene with education and psychological methods. Education often helps to uncover false beliefs about the disorder under treatment. Psychological methods help to uncover psychosocial difficulties that interfere with adherence, and they lead to interventions that are suitable for the patient's recovery.

The Special Case of OTC Drugs and Supplements

The first step in monitoring of patient use of OTC drugs, dietary supplements, and medications begins during the initial interview. Patients are asked to bring all their prescription medication containers, OTC products, and dietary supplements to their first session. This may be the only method by which a clinician can use direct observation to confirm the product brands and daily dosages of these products. Subsequently, a history of past experiences with medications and supplements may be obtained, as well as a current and historical estimation of the use of recreational substances and any treatments for abuses of those substances. Drug-seeking behaviors and potential for abuse should also be assessed.

Aging and disease alter bodily distribution and elimination of OTC drugs in a manner similar to that of prescription medications. Reduction in metabolism and excretion, even in the healthy elderly person, can precipitate bad outcomes to *polypharmacy* and potentiate greater side effects with both prescription and OTC drugs. Because of their diminished physiological reserve and greater susceptibility to drug side effects, OTC stimulants, hypnotics, insomnia remedies, and pain pills can cause special problems for the elderly. For example, OTC drugs that contain caffeine (also coffee, tea, cola, and chocolate) can be a cause of disturbed sleep in the elderly. Because the stimulant action of caffeine lasts 12 to 20 hours after ingestion, older patients may experience diminished restfulness even when they do sleep, and they may have delayed sleep onset, lighter sleep, and increased morning drowsiness. Likewise, nicotine use can diminish sleep quality and may increase the risk of sleep apnea. Diphenhydramine (Benadryl, Nytol, or Sominex) is an OTC antihistamine that is commonly used as a sleeping pill. However, in the elderly, rather than producing actual sleep, this antihistamine may be more likely to produce sedation and aggravate preexisting cognitive loss (Gillin & Ancoli-Israel, 1998).

Another category of frequently used OTC drugs by the elderly is medication for pain (analgesic), fever (antipyrexia) and anti-inflammation. Nonsteroidal anti-inflammatory drugs (NSAIDs) include common OTC drugs such as aspirin, ibuprofen (Advil, Motrin), and indomethacin (Indocin). In the elderly, NSAIDs are of concern due to their capacity to raise blood pressure, reduce renal function, produce mental confusion, and cause gastropathy and hemorrhage (Avorn, 1998).

Dietary supplements that contain iron are often consumed by the elderly, although their normal diet may contain a sufficient amount of the daily requirement. An iron supplement could be counterproductive if it were to mask an underlying cause of anemia, such as early-stage colon cancer blood loss in which anemia is a warning sign. Most of the vitamin and mineral supplementations may be unproductive in their use to counteract the onset of heart disease and cancer. Epidemiological studies are much more supportive of the effectiveness of a diet rich in fruits and vegetables in preventing heart disease and cancer (Avorn, 1998). In fact, vitamin and mineral supplements can actually be counterproductive in the elderly if they are used instead of fruits and vegetables.

The extract of an ancient tree, ginkgo biloba, has been widely used as an herbal supplement to treat vascular insufficiency, impaired mental performance, tinnitus, deafness, diabetic retinopathy, impotence, premenstrual syndrome, depression, and allergies. The leaf extract has been observed during drug-trial research to produce gastrointestinal discomfort, headache, and dizziness (Murray, 1995).

St. John's wort is the extract of the flower of a perennial shrub that has been used as an antidepressant, antiviral, antibiotic, and psychotropic herbal supplement. Adverse reactions to St. John's wort have included photosensitivity, skin disease, and gastric upset. Individuals who have taken St. John's wort are counseled to avoid exposure to strong sunlight and ultraviolet light because of the risk of photosensitivity. Similar to patients who are taking MAO inhibitors, patients on St. John's wort are counseled to avoid foods with significant tyramine content and drugs such as L-dopa and 5-hydroxytryptophan (dopamine and serotonin) (Murray, 1995).

OTC drugs interact with medications in a manner similar to drug–drug interactions between prescription medications. A good example of such an OTC drug that is at high risk for interaction with certain medications is the OTC antacid, histamine H_2 antagonist, cimetidine (Tagamet), which is used to treat duodenal ulcers and gastroesophageal reflux. Cimetidine is a powerful inhibitor of cytochrome P450 liver enzymes 2D6, 3A4, and 1A2 (Martinez et al., 1999). In one study, cimetidine was shown to increase the half-life of imipramine (Tofranil) from 10.8 to 22.7 hours (Wells, Pieper, & Self, 1986). Imipramine is affected by cytochrome P450 enzyme 2D6, and depends heavily on this enzyme for its metabolism. In another study cimetidine was found to increase serum paroxetine (Paxil) levels by 50% (Greb et al., 1989). Other histamine subtype 2 (H_2) receptor blockers such as ranitidine (Zantac) do not pose the same problems (Cozza, Armstrong, & Oesterheld, 2003).

Dietary supplements and herbal remedies may also interact unfavorably with medications. St. John's wort induces CYP450 enzyme 3A4, and consequently places oral contraceptives at risk for failure, and vitamin C is known to increase or prolong oral contraceptive activity (Cozza, Armstrong, & Oesterheld, 2003). St. John's wort is a potent inducer of P-glycoprotein transporters that are present on the villus tips of enterocytes in the jejunum (the primary site of absorption of oral drugs) to transport hydrophobic substances across the cell into the gut and urine and out of the brain. St. John's wort has been found to increase P-glycoprotein levels in the intestine by one and one-half times. When St. John's wort is administered with digoxin (Lanoxin), an antiarrhythmic, the plasma concentration of digoxin is reduced (Cozza, Armstrong, & Osterheld, 2003).

Corticosteroids, which are Phase II metabolism inducers metabolized partly by CYP450 3A4 enzymes, have been found to reduce salicylic acid (aspirin) levels when given simultaneously. Phenobarbital and phenytoin (Dilantin), which are inducers of 3A4, have been found to decrease transplant survival and to necessitate higher doses of prednisone to maintain efficacy (Wassner et al., 1977). Caffeine depends primarily on the cytochrome P450 enzyme 1A2 for oxidative clearance and is often inhibited in its metabolism to cause patient jitters, which clinicians may misinterpret as side effects of prescribed medications. For instance, in a study by Jeppesen, Loft, and Poulsen (1996) it was found that the selective serotonin reuptake inhibitor, fluvoxamine (Luvox), when coadministered with caffeine, increases the half-life of caffeine from 5 to 31 hours.

SPECIAL POPULATIONS OF PATIENTS

Pregnant women, elderly patients, disabled patients, children, substance abusers, and the culturally diverse may all present special issues for the prescribing medical psychologist. Each of these special populations of patients may present with needs and issues that are specific to their life status. For example, during pregnancy the blood supply for the fetus carries to the fetal brain any medications taken by the mother. Research trials carried out by the FDA have indicated special categories of risk for these unborn children.

FDA PREGNANCY RISK CATEGORIES

These categories indicate the potential of a systemically absorbed drug causing birth defects. The difference between categories is based on the reliability of documentation and the risk-benefit ratio as listed in the following:

Category A: Controlled studies of women show no evidence of risk.

Category B: No controlled studies have been carried out.

Category C: Studies in animals have shown evidence of teratogenicity, but no studies have been done in women to confirm teratogenicity. Drugs should be given only if the potential benefits justify the potential risk to the fetus.

Category D: There is evidence of human fetal risk, but the benefits from use in pregnant women may be acceptable despite the risk, for example, if the drug is needed in a life-threatening situation or for a serious disease for which safer drugs cannot be used or are ineffective.

Category X: Studies in animals or humans have demonstrated fetal abnormalities or there is evidence of fetal risk based on human experience or both, and the risk of the use of the drug in pregnant women clearly outweighs any benefit. The drug is contraindicated in women who are or may become pregnant.

Examples of psychotropic medications that are known to be teratogens include several of the benzodiazepines. Examples of those with considerable risk of causing birth defects include anticonvulsants and lithium (see Table 9.1, as well as Chapter 5, Table 5.3).

THE ELDERLY

Since the early 1900s in the United States, the proportion of the population over 65 has tripled from 4% to 12%, and the cohort of elderly over 85 years of age is the fastest growing cohort in the country (Lebowitz, Pearson, & Cohen, 1998). Approximately 80% of elderly over 65 have at least one chronic illness. These facts place an ever-increasing burden on medical psychologists to treat the mental disorders of the elderly within the context of their overall health. Arthritis, high blood pressure, diabetes, heart disease, and dementia frequently coexist with depressive reactions in the elderly. In addition, medical conditions of the elderly, such as thyroid disorders, electrolyte imbalances, delirium, and hypertension, can present in the context of psychological disorders. Psychological stress can be the trigger for the appearance of physical illness or the occasion for an increase in functional disability of a current medical condition.

Clinicians who prescribe psychotropic medications for the elderly can more readily avoid complications such as ADRs and overdose in this population by attending to the following three critical issues:

1. From among the wide range of intervention methods that are available to treat emotional problems, the prescribing medical psychologist must be aware of those methods that are most appropriate for the elderly. For example, in most cases, the decision to use a benzodiazepine to treat anxiety and depression in the elderly may not be appropriate because of the confusion and sedation that can impact cognitive functioning.

2. Since aging is known to change receptor-site sensitivity, the prescribing medical psychologist must be acutely aware of the recommended dosages of psychotropic medication that are most appropriate for each age range. For example, although the recommended adult initial dosage for fluoxetine (Prozac) is 20 mg, the recommended initial dosage for elderly is 10 mg (Lacy, Armstrong, Goldman, & Lance, 2007). Despite the fact that an unintended overdose of an SSRI may not be life threatening, the side effects of overdose may be temporarily disabling for an elderly person.

3. Since aging is known to reduce the efficiency with which the GI tract and liver metabolize ingested drugs, drugs are distributed less efficiently throughout the bodies of the elderly. Therefore, a medical psychologist who prescribes drugs for oral transmission needs to assess each patient for renal impairment or digestive disorders, in addition to general compensation for age. For example, the prescription of lithium to an elderly patient with declining glomerular filtration rate (GFR) could lead to a dangerous build-up of lithium in the plasma.

A prime example of a cohort of patients who are at risk for organ deterioration morbidity is that of nursing-home patients. Although they represent only 5% of the entire elderly population, there are between one and two million elderly patients in nursing homes in the United States (Mitchell, Teno, Miller, & Mor, 2005). The population of the elderly in nursing homes is mostly over 85 years in age and female, with moderate to high levels of disability. Most of these residents have a diagnosable mental disorder. Primary conditions found in these patients are dementia, behavioral problems, and depression. Notwithstanding the failure of primary care providers to often diagnose depressive conditions in these patients, they are often treated with antipsychotics to manage behavior problems and agitation.

Consequently, excessive use of antipsychotics may occur in nursing homes (Lebowitz, Pearson, & Cohen, 1998), and federal regulations are now in place to manage the use of neuroleptics and sedative hypnotics with nursing home patients (Royner, Edelman, Cox, & Schmuely, 1992).

The very old (85+) nursing home patient presents special challenges for prescribing medical psychologists. They are very likely to have more than one physical illness in addition to a mental disorder. They are very likely to be taking multiple medications without the sufficient understanding of the effects of these medications that would allow them to participate fully in their own health care. Age-related alterations in brain function cause reduced awareness and sensitivity to medications; and altered distribution and excretion of drugs produced by aging and disease, as well as widespread polypharmacy, combine to lower the threshold of toxicity in these very old patients (Lebowitz et al., 1998). Therefore, prescribing medical psychologists should add to the list of medications of these patients with great caution. If psychotherapy is not an option, and medication appears to be the treatment of choice, the prescriber should choose those medications with the lowest risk of adding to the problems that these patients already carry. For example, if anxiety is to be treated, the prescribing psychologist may want to choose a low-risk drug such as buspirone (BuSpar) rather than a benzodiazepine. For sleeping problems, rather than use a hypnotic such as zolpidem (Ambien), which is a GABA-a receptor agonist and prone to affect cognitive function, the first attempt to resolve insomnia might best be behavior management of sleeping.

CHILDREN

The special needs of the pediatric population offer a challenge to clinicians inasmuch as modification of adult norms is usually in order for the use of medication with these children. A child is not a small adult. Children differ from adults in their dynamic response to a given plasma concentration of some drugs. For example, in children, higher doses of some drugs can be achieved with lower toxicity (e.g., tricyclic antidepressants) because the liver function of the young tends to be more vigorous. Also, in children it has been found that lower plasma levels with some drugs are required to achieve a desired therapeutic effect (e.g., haloperidol). Similar to adults, however, and regardless of the age of a child, the distribution and elimination of the drug will depend on the interaction between the chemical properties of the drug and the patient's own physiology (which is altered by development and disease). The course of normal development in the child increases volume of distribution and body weight in a linear fashion. Consequently, the initial loading dose of a prescribed drug for a child must be modified to achieve a given plasma concentration by factoring in weight (Green, 1995).

Research findings indicate that higher concentrations of alpha-1-acid glycoprotein are found in children compared to adults, and that this increases the protein binding of some psychotropic drugs, such as haloperidol, which in turn results in reduced free-drug concentrations. Age-related changes in drug distribution due to the child's small body size or increased drug binding may shorten a drug's half-life. The smaller the child, the smaller the volume of distribution and the shorter the half-life of the drug. The half-life of imipramine, for example, has been found to be shorter in 5- to 12-year-olds (11–42 hours) than in 13- to 16-year-olds (14–89 hours). The caveat for the prescriber occurs with drugs that have narrow therapeutic windows, for which adjustments need to be made by increasing the frequency of dosing intervals in order to remain within the therapeutic window (because of the drug's shortened half-life). And this caveat remains true despite adequate drug elimination, because volume of distribution alterations can be expected to influence drug half-life independent of drug clearance (Green, 1995).

For the treatment of mental disorders in children, psychotherapy should always be considered as treatment of choice, since most children seen in clinics and private practice do not need medication, and the long term effects of psychoactive medications on the maturation and development of children and adolescents have not been well researched. The list of psychoactive drugs that has received FDA approval for children is brief and often limited to older children. Dosing regimens and side effects of unapproved medications for children are largely unknown, and the off-label use of such drugs should be done only for exceptional cases and for reasons that justify their use (Green, 1995).

PATIENTS WITH DISABILITY

Patients with congenital intellectual disability (mental retardation) are often at risk for misunderstanding the purpose of medications prescribed for them or the regimen required for their use. Consequently, these patients often take better advantage of treatments that include the collaboration of a relative or significant other who is not disabled. Such informants as parents, spouse, siblings, friends, neighbors, or social workers should be included in the diagnostic phase, as well as the treatment phase of appointments with such patients. An increased amount of time per session with intellectually disabled patients may be needed in order to sort out those environmental contingencies that may aid or hinder the *compliance* of disabled patients with a prescribed regimen of treatment. Disabled patients frequently show evidence of failure to give informed consent appropriately and may need a legal guardian to consent for them. Problems that develop with intellectually disabled patients often take the form of compliance failures (e.g.,, not taking the drugs at all, not taking the proper dose, not following the prescribed timing for taking the drugs, or taking too much medication at once or over a period of time). Tactics that may be used by clinicians to overcome these compliance failures include:

1. Offering both patient and informant written as well as oral instructions about the treatment regimen in plain and simple language.
2. Frequent follow-up and checkups using both office visits and telephone checkups to determine the quality of adherence.
3. Requesting that the informant keep a diary of daily regimen adherence and nonadherence that can be used at the next formal session.
4. Behavioral compliance interventions for patient and informant as part of their therapy sessions.
5. Consider routes other than oral administration, such as IM depot in the cases where drugs are available for that route of delivery.

In addition to adherence failure, these patients frequently present with inability to properly report adverse drug reactions (ADRs) or behavioral manifestations of progress. Again, clinicians need to rely on informants, as well as laboratory tests to help determine success or failure of medication treatment.

Patients with acquired cognitive disability, such as Alzheimer's dementia or other forms of degenerative brain disease, often present in earlier stages with memory disability rather than intellectual disability. This finding may also be true of patients with traumatic brain injury, brain tumors, cranial infections, toxic-metabolic conditions, epilepsy, and heart or lung disease. Cognitive disability in these patients may range as widely as intellectual, memory, attention, language, motor, personality, and executive disorders. Each of these disabling domains brings with it special challenges for the prescription of psychotropic medications. Most of these patients are in need of some type of intervention, whether that be psychotherapy, psychopharmacological treatment, or rehabilitation. Not only do their disabilities in each of the forementioned domains make it difficult for them to be compliant with prescribed regimens of treatment, but psychotropic medications will often be found to interact with the drugs prescribed for them by their neurologist, internist, cardiologist, pulmonologist, or other physicians.

Patients with physical disabilities such as cerebral palsy, quadriplegia, amputated limbs, blindness, deafness, heart or lung disease, liver or kidney disease, or any chronic illness often require specific modifications and considerations (similar to those with elderly and other disabled patients) in their psychopharmacological treatment.

DUAL DIAGNOSIS PATIENTS

Many of the recreational substances are addictive (e.g., alcohol, tobacco, heroin, marijuana, amphetamines), and thereby make it very difficult for consumers to cease their use of these substances. Consequently, the treatment of substance abuse most often must focus on the motivation to enter treatment and the uncovering of the behaviors that maintain craving, drug seeking, and relapse.

The most frequently abused substance in the United States is alcohol. It is rapidly absorbed as a very small molecule and has a brief half-life. It inhibits excitatory neurotransmitters and increases the release of serotonin and the binding of GABA to receptors. It causes a decline in the consolidation of new memories (which may be escalated to the point of blackout when ingested with benzodiazepines) and a decrease in motor control. Most often, alcohol abuse is a comorbid condition that is present, simultaneously, with mental disorders, especially with depression, bipolar disorder, and psychosis. In many patients, it may be an attempt to self-medicate and to find relief from the negative experiences of severe emotional symptoms. Some psychiatric patients with comorbid alcoholism come to outpatient therapy sessions in a state of intoxication. It is important that clinicians recognize the signs of intoxication (mental confusion, motor discoordination, slurred speech, and disinhibition) and calmly address the issue of the intoxication and the underlying alcoholism as a comorbid disorder that complicates the treatment of their primary disorder.

An example of a well-designed model for the treatment of alcoholism (that is adaptable to other types of substance abuse and mental disorders) is that of Marlatt and colleagues (Larimer, Palmer, & Marlatt 1999). They hypothesize two types of causes of relapse for alcoholism: immediate determinants and covert antecedents. For alcoholism, the immediate determinants are high-risk environments, personal coping abilities, personal expectancies for outcome, and the *abstinence-violation effect*. Covert

408 The Practice of Clinical Psychopharmacology

antecedents for alcoholism are personal cravings, urges, and lifestyle. Relapse prevention techniques, including booster sessions, maintenance therapy, prophylactic medication, and extended periods of approximation to termination are all good methods for sustaining remission after treatment for substance abuse. Following remission and termination of formal treatment sessions, such patients should be frequently monitored through the use of randomly scheduled telephone calls to the patient and to their trusted informants. Check-up sessions should be scheduled for face-to-face meetings in the clinician's office, where random drug screen could be carried out. Any signs of tendency to relapse should be a signal to schedule booster sessions or the restarting of formal therapy sessions.

Outpatient intervention may be effective for people with mild alcohol problems, but referral to a specialized treatment center usually is required for patients who are alcohol dependent. During recovery, alcoholics pass through a series of somewhat predictable stages. Successful treatment involves helping the patient to move from one stage to the next with the greatest efficiency. Patients may recycle through these stages several times before attaining recovery completely. The first stage is marked by the change from a state of unawareness of the problem of alcoholism to awareness that drinking is problematic. The second stage involves a decision to stop drinking. The third stage is a trial and error process in which drinking is temporarily terminated with relapses after each attempt. In the fourth stage, a new nondrinking behavior pattern is attained with the help of relapse-prevention techniques. And the fifth stage involves a major relapse in which efforts to change are abandoned. These five stages typically repeat themselves until recovery is complete (Renner & Bierer, 1998).

During detoxification, benzodiazepines are the best drugs to cushion the withdrawal, because their side effects are minimal. Diazepam (Valium) is an example of a long-acting benzodiazepine that may be used. Lorazepam (Ativan) is a shorter-acting benzodiazepine that may be used for patients with liver disease, cognitive impairment, significant medical problems, or old age. The *cross-dependence* of alcohol and benzodiazepines is exploited in alcohol detoxification treatment, wherein the effects of alcohol are replaced by the effects of the benzodiazepine. Benzodiazepines have a longer half-life than alcohol, which allows them to be slowly tapered. The detoxification process is made smoother for the addict, thereby reducing the risk of withdrawal symptoms and side effects, which, in turn, reduces the risk of relapse (Nestler, Hyman, & Malenka, 2001).

For maintenance and long-term treatment, the opiate antagonist naltrexone (Depade, Vivitrol) may be used to reduce craving and relapse. However, naltrexone should not be used with patients who have hepatitis or liver failure. Disulfiram (Antabuse), which inhibits alcohol metabolism by blocking the enzyme acetaldehyde dehydrogenase, allows acetaldehyde to accumulate in the blood, producing nausea and vomiting when the patient drinks. It has not been shown, however, to be better than placebo in sustaining abstinence, and works best in stable, well-motivated patients (Renner & Bierer, 1998).

Relapse prevention and intervention methods may include various modes of psychological intervention, such as psychotherapy or behavior modification. Patients are often taught to identify high-risk situations and predictors of relapse, and then offered strategies to cope with minimal versus major relapse episodes. Maintaining frequent contact with a therapist who is available to intervene on a 24-hour basis may be critical for vulnerable patients. The Marlatt & Gordon (1985) model also includes intervention strategies that address the different types of causes, such as identifying the high-risk environments, enhancing coping skills, and managing the relapses.

Smoking Cessation

Patients addicted to nicotine may also require closely monitored therapeutic interventions in order to terminate smoking behavior. Special attention is required with smokers who also take psychotropic medication for *comorbid conditions*. Smoking tobacco (nicotine) may decrease serum concentration of 2D6 substrates and is an inducer of CYP1A2. Any drug that is metabolized by 1A2 may need to be used at higher doses in smokers. Conversely, when a patient stops smoking, drug toxicity may occur several weeks after the cessation as the enzyme levels falls accordingly. Drugs such as clozapine (Clozaril) and olanzapine (Zyprexa) may reach the point of toxicity when smoking is stopped. It is strongly recommended that prescribers monitor serum levels of such drugs during transition from smoking to nonsmoking. During the period that the patient on olanzapine is smoking, they may need higher doses to achieve the desired effect because smoking increases the clearance of olanzapine by as much as 40% (Cozza, Armstrong, & Oesterheld, 2003).

TOLERANCE, DEPENDENCE, AND SENSITIZATION AMONG DUAL DIAGNOSIS PATIENT

Terminology

Although *tolerance* refers to a decreased effect that develops with continued drug use, *cross-tolerance* is a decreased response to a drug from continued exposure to a similar drug. *Sensitization* (or inverse tolerance) refers to an increased effect after repeated administrations of a drug, and *cross-sensitization* refers to an increased effect of a drug from continued exposure to a similar drug. Physiological or physical *dependence* refers to the adverse physical signs and symptoms that result from the absence of a drug. Taken together, these adverse symptoms are called withdrawal symptoms.

Psychological dependence can occur concomitantly with physical dependence as well as with drugs that do not produce tolerance and physical dependence. Psychological dependence is the craving or emotional memory of the pleasure connected with drug taking. Drug addiction is the drug-seeking and drug-taking behavior that interferes with normal living and causes the addict to continue using the drug despite increasingly damaging consequences (Galanter & Wartenberg, 2005).

Another cross-reactivity that is important to mention in this context is the cross-dependence that is found in drugs that affect the same neuroreceptors in the nervous system. The prime example of cross-dependence is the case in which alcohol is ingested with benzodiazepines or barbiturates. The effect produced by such drug use is greatly intensified because each of these drugs alters GABA-a receptor conformation to increase the efficacy of the other. This synergistic cross-reactivity can be life threatening (Nestler, Hyman, & Malenka, 2001). Therefore, it is incumbent on prescribers of benzodiazepines to warn their patients about the risk.

Treatment

Treatment of the tolerance that has developed after repeated use of a drug depends on the characteristics of the drug. Some drugs, such as morphine, can be tolerated at very large doses when there has been a gradual increase of dosage over time. Tapering of dosage over time in order to withdraw the drug must be done slowly in order to avoid withdrawal symptoms, which, in the case of morphine, could be life threatening. A similar phenomenon can be seen with heroin addicts who have become tolerant to high doses of heroin as the relevant receptor sites downregulate in response to habitual use. After building this tolerance to ever-increasing doses over time, they may eventually come to methadone clinics for treatment. In order to mask the actual timing of dosage reduction, most methadone clinics put the daily dose of methadone in a solution such as Kool-Aid in order that addicts will not know whether the dose they have been given on a particular day has been cut from the day before.

Treatment of cross-tolerance may offer some challenges due to a mix-up about terminology. *Cross-tolerance* should not be confused with the term *cross-addiction*. *Cross-addiction* is meant to convey the notion that addiction to one mood-altering drug predisposes to addiction to all other mood-altering drugs. Although the term *cross-addiction* is used frequently in the education of alcoholics, there is a great deal of skepticism in the literature about this concept. The term *cross-tolerance* has a very different meaning. *Cross-tolerance* is defined as a decreased response to a drug (such as methamphetamine) due to previous exposure to a similar drug such as amphetamine or other stimulants. Cross-tolerance is often observed with antibiotics and analgesics. It may be observed in cigarette smokers who are less sensitive to the effects of caffeine since both drugs can affect nicotinic acetylcholine receptors. Because cross-tolerance is a form of tolerance, treatment can be carried out in a similar manner. Gradual tapering of dosage should be an initial strategy. If that strategy is not successful, a clinician may need to switch to another category of drug that will accomplish the same goal. For example, tolerance to a particular type of NSAID (such as ibuprofen) may require a switch to narcotic compounds for relief of pain, especially when cross-tolerance is encountered when a clinician has suggested switching to a different NSAID (such as aspirin).

ABUSE OF PRESCRIPTIVE MEDICATIONS

Abuse of narcotics, especially those used as painkillers, has been a common topic for news headlines and movie themes. These types of medication have a common effect: the relief from adverse stimulation. However, they have a common side effect: the potential for dependence and addiction. It is the combination of this effect and side effect that leads to their identification as drugs at risk for abuse.

Narcotics and painkillers are frequently abused by patients who were initially prescribed these medications legally to dampen their physical pain. When these patients become tolerant of the dosage that they have been prescribed they look for other sources of painkillers to increase their dosage, both legal and illegal. Their abuse of these drugs is not the pleasure seeking of a heroin addict, but it is relief from pain that drives them into dosages that escalate to the level of abuse.

Abuse of benzodiazepines has the same trajectory of development as abuse of narcotics. It generally begins with a legal prescription of a modest dosage of benzodiazepine in order to find relief from anxiety or depression. The rapid efficacy and low-side-effect profile of this medication makes it very attractive to patients who have struggled with the side effects and the latency period for efficacy typically found during the initiation of SSRIs. When SSRI drugs are co-prescribed with benzodiazepines for major depression, clinicians begin to taper the benzodiazepines downward as the SSRIs begin to have a therapeutic effect. At that moment, patients often express the desire to maintain their prescription of benzodiazepines and might insist that they do not want to be tapered off the benzodiazepines. It is at that point in treatment when some of these patients search for another prescriber who will refill their benzodiazepine prescription. Again, this type of abuse is not driven by the same motivation as that of a heroin addict or alcoholic but, rather, it is similar to the motivation of pain patients, which is the desire to remain symptom free without the hassle of bothersome side effects.

Stimulants are also abused, especially in the form of methamphetamine. The street form of methamphetamine is smoked and is illegally converted from pseudoephedrine (Contac, Dimetapp, Sudafed). Pseudoephedrine is an alpha-beta agonist that stimulates the alpha-adrenergic receptors of the respiratory mucosa causing vasoconstriction, and the beta-adrenergic receptors, causing bronchial relaxation (Finkel, Clark, & Cubeddu, 2009). Due to the illegal practice of making methamphetamine from pseudoephedrine, the pseudoephedrine products in pharmacy stores have been switched from an OTC drug to a behind-the-counter drug.

In cases of prescriptive medication abuse the first strategy of the prescribers should be preventative. Proper education of patients about the risks of taking these drugs will help patients to be vigilant for signs of tolerance and dependence that could lead to abuse. Diligent monitoring on the part of the clinician should also help to forestall some of the problems that tend to develop. Nevertheless, when the time comes for medication tapering to begin, the prescribing medical psychologist should firmly insist on the necessity for dosage reduction in order to avoid dependence, while educating the patient on the need for such a firm stance. When patients plead for one more month of full dosage, they may be largely unaware of the risk that they are taking. In this regard, there are two factors that can lead to dependence on benzodiazepines: the dosage and duration of use. The higher the dosage, the shorter the duration of treatment that will be needed to develop dependence. Still, even at therapeutic daily doses, clinically significant dependence may develop after only several weeks of treatment (Salzman, 1998). Gradual tapering should always be used as the method of reducing dosage, never abrupt termination. Withdrawal symptoms during abrupt or rapid dosage reduction can be painful and lead to resentment in the therapeutic relationship.

SENSITIVITY TOWARD CULTURALLY DIVERSE POPULATIONS

The most desirable outcome of pharmacotherapy and psychological treatment is the improvement of the quality of life. One method to help achieve this outcome is for the prescribing medical psychologist to involve the patient in decision making, especially in the process of medication selection. Quality of life is inextricably related to cultural norms and practices, and each individual patient's cultural leanings need to be assessed when prescribing. A person whose religious rules require fasting may not be able to take medication that must be taken with food during a period of fasting. For such a case, the prescriber would need to schedule a medication regimen that took the fasting into consideration. Religious beliefs also permeate the health activities of most ethnic minorities. It would be a mistake for the prescribing medical psychologist to presume that these patients could easily adjust to the notion that scientific knowledge must be preferred over religious beliefs in regard to their health.

Culturally appropriate educational techniques need to incorporate both religious and cultural values into a prescriptive regimen.

The language barrier that clinicians face with patients must be breached through the use of interpreters who are capable of accurately conveying the two-way communication between patient and clinician. The prescribing medical psychologist who works with immigrant populations and/or members of minority language groups will need to contract with a face-to-face or telephone interpretation service. For reasons that will not elude psychologists, the use of family members as interpreters, especially minors, should be avoided in the mental-health consultation. Since the population of Spanish speakers in the United States is 20% and increasing every day, it would be best that clinicians learn to speak and understand Spanish in order to serve these patients. Here, however, it is imperative that the Spanish spoken is of a proficient level, and it behooves the bilingual practitioner to become certified in medical interpretation to assure not only that proficiency in the second language is adequate, but also to ensure that the practicing bilingual prescriber is trained in proven methods of interpretation. In the meantime, consent forms and instructions for the use of medication need to be translated into all major secondary languages. In addition, it would be helpful to non-English speakers to have descriptions prepared in their language that explain different mental disorders and the medications used for their treatment. Nonetheless, some patients may not have sufficient formal education to read such instructions; in such cases a professional interpreter/translator should be available to read it to them and relay questions to the clinician. It is important to acknowledge that limited-English-speaking medical patients have the right to language interpretation during their visit. Precedence in this regard was first established as a provision within the Civil Rights Act of 1964, which required all federally funded hospitals to provide interpretation for non-English-speaking patients. It was more recently reinforced in 2003 by California Senate Bill 853, the Health Care Language Assistance Act, which mandates obligatory interpretation in a state where 40% of the population does not speak English in the home and 7 million self-identify with limited-English proficiency (Sundaram, 2009).

Patients seek treatment that corresponds with what they perceive as the cause of their illness (Zweber, 2002). Taking into account cultural influences, the prescribing medical psychologist should inquire first about the patient's own understanding of their illness, and secondly should inquire about any home remedies, herbs, or substances that might interact unfavorably with the psychopharmacological medications to be prescribed. Only after such an inquiry should the psychologist present his or her plan for treatment. After the prescriber is assured that the patient clearly understands the purpose and procedures to be employed, he or she should ask about the patient's agreement, disagreement, discomfort, or doubts about the treatment.

Patient complaints to primary-care providers about mental-health problems are often misunderstood by these providers due to the doctor's lack of familiarity with minority cultural traditions about mental disorders. For example, African-American patients who present with mania, depression, or alcohol-related symptoms are often misdiagnosed as having schizophrenia, because they have culturally shared beliefs that may be mistaken for delusions (Pi & Simpson, 2005). When the treating psychologist has any doubt about understanding the complaints of patients from a different culture, he or she should attempt to refer the patient to a clinician who is more knowledgeable in that culture, or to enlist the aid of family members who might better understand the communications of these patients. Each individual patient will come with his or her own beliefs, expectations, and cultural influences regarding his or her health problems and treatment. These cultural patterns will need to be assessed along with the patient's illnesses.

REVIEW OF PSYCHOACTIVE DRUGS

The eager student-initiate of prescribing medical psychology often focuses on assimilating the details of specific medications. While intimate familiarity with those medications that are available for prescribing to the mental health population is supremely important, we have left it for the last section of this chapter on clinical psychopharmacology because the principles enumerated in the first part of the chapter will endure through time and will form the foundation for the proper practice of psychopharmacology, while specific medications will come and go. In order to properly manage the drugs that we review below, it is imperative that the prescribing psychologist be competent in every single section covered in this book. Only then can specific knowledge of particular pharmaceuticals be balanced and integrated into the conscientious practice of clinical psychopharmacotherapy.

ANTIDEPRESSANTS

Psychopharmacology might well be traced to the origin of an offshoot of iminodibenzyl, which had been synthesized as early as 1889 (Byck, 1975). Chlorpromazine, a derivative of iminodibenzyl, was fortuitously discovered to have antipsychotic effects in the 1950s (Nelson, 2004) and, later in the same decade, imipramine, a tricyclic compound closely related to chlorpromazine, was found to have antidepressant qualities.[4] The tricyclic antidepressants (TCAs) share a common ancestry in their central three-ring molecular structure, but they are actually quite similar to other antidepressants in that they act as reuptake inhibitors. Although some tricyclics (amitriptyline, imipramine, and clomipramine) are primarily serotonin reuptake blockers, others work more at preventing norepinephrine reuptake (desipramine, nortriptyline, protriptyline). In fact, the majority of TCAs work on both reuptake transporters of serotonin and norepinephrine. Indeed, the problem with the TCAs is associated with their shotgun effect, in which they activate numerous pharmacodynamic mechanisms, including anticholinergic and antihistaminic effects, with their corresponding side effects (adverse cardiac reactions being most disturbing).

The attractiveness of second-generation antidepressants rests in their ability to selectively inhibit reuptake of either serotonin or serotonin and norepinephrine, without much involvement of muscarinic or histaminergic effects. The serotonin selective reuptake inhibitors, SSRIs (fluoxetine, sertraline, paroxetine, fluvoxamine, citalopram, escitalopram), and the serotonin norepinephrine reuptake inhibitors, SNRIs, (venlafaxine, duloxetine), and even the dopamine norepinephrine reuptake inhibitors, DNRIs (bupropion) all have exhibited the advantage of fewer side effects associated with anticholinergic and antihistaminic effects of the TCAs. Not too surprising, they have not demonstrated superiority among themselves in efficacious/

---

[4]A parallel discovery about the same time was that of iproniazid, a monoamine oxidase inhibitor (MAOI) antitubercular agent that was found to have antidepressant qualities in the 1950s (Crane, 1957).

effectiveness studies, nor are they demonstrably more therapeutic than their tricyclic counterparts.

Monoamine oxidase inhibitors, MAOIs, (phenelzine, isocarboxazid, tranylcypromine, selegiline) achieve an augmented presence of serotonin, epinephrine, and dopamine at the synapses through a different mechanism of action than the reuptake inhibitors, although the clinical result is felt to be the same. By retarding the degradation of monoamine within the neuron, MAOIs leave more active transmitters available for reintroduction into the synapses as a result of increased presence in the terminal end. Once again, efforts to show superiority of effect between MAOIs and other antidepressants have proved elusive. The MAOIs are, like the TCAs and the SSRIs, better defined by their side effects than by any singular therapeutic effect. The potential for life-threatening hyperserotonergic reactions with MAOIs is comparable to such a concern over *serotonin syndrome* for SSRIs and for anticholinergic effects with the TCAs.

Atypical antidepressants, such as the noradrenergic/specific serotonergic antidepressant (NaSSA) mirtazapine, which antagonizes 5-HT$_2$ and 5-HT$_3$, and trazodone, a highly selective serotonergic reuptake inhibitor with virtually no norepinephrine action, may be marketed as more selective, but their efficacy is no better than the other antidepressants, and their effectiveness may be less. Side effects of mirtazapine and trazodone include sedation, which stems from histaminergic affinity (antagonist) in the case of mirtazapine and α_1 adrenergic blockade in the case of trazodone.

Anxiolytic effects of reuptake inhibitor antidepressants have been demonstrated in clinical studies, and the FDA has approved several SSRIs and SNRIs for the treatment of various anxiety-related conditions, whereas the remaining reuptake inhibitors that have not been specifically approved for this purpose are frequently prescribed off-label as anxiolytics. Specifically (Chew, Hales, & Yudofsky, 2009): Citalopram (Celexa) is FDA approved for major depressive disorder (MDD), but it is used off-label for obsessive compulsive disorder (OCD), panic disorder, general anxiety disorder (GAD), social anxiety, and posttraumatic stress disorder (PTSD); escitalopram (Lexapro) is FDA indicated for MDD and GAD, but it is used for OCD, panic disorder, social anxiety, and PTSD; fluvoxamine (Luvox), approved for OCD and social anxiety disorder, was never approved for MDD, but it is used off-label for MDD, panic disorder, and PTSD; paroxetine (Paxil) completed the clinical studies necessary to be FDA approved for MDD, panic disorder, OCD, social anxiety disorder, GAD, and PTSD; fluoxetine (Prozac) is FDA approved for MDD and OCD, and it is used off label for panic disorder, GAD, social anxiety, and PTSD; (Zoloft) sertraline is indicated by the FDA for MDD, panic disorder, OCD, social anxiety disorder, and PTSD, but it is used off-label for the treatment of GAD; venlafaxine (Effexor) is FDA approved for the treatment of depression whereas Effexor XR is also approved for GAD, social phobia, and panic disorder; duloxetine (Cymbalta) is FDA indicated for MDD and GAD, but is used off-label for other anxiety disorders.

ANXIOLYTICS AND SLEEP AIDS

Apart from certain antidepressants and the occasional use of antihistamines (mirtazapine, diphenhydramine), psychopharmacotherapy relies on benzodiazepines and benzodiazepine-derived preparations for the treatment of anxiety and insomnia. Historically, anxiolytic effects and sedation/sleep were induced by the use of

Table 9.4   Benzodiazepines' Half-Lives

Drug	Elimination Half-Life
Alprazolam	6–12 hours
Chlordiazepoxide	5–30 hours
Clonazepam	18–50 hours
Clorazepate	36–100 hours
Diazepam	20–100 hours
Lorazepam	10–20 hours
Oxazepam	4–15 hours

phenobarbital in the first half of the twentieth century, but this practice was replaced with the safer benzodiazepines such as chlordiazepoxide and diazepam in the 60s and 70s; and in the 80s the use of new generation benzodiazepines sharply increased after alprazolam was shown to be effective in the treatment of panic (Sheehan et al., 1982). Around the same time that alprazolam was gaining acceptance for the treatment of anxiety, a parallel class of drugs, sometimes referred to as nonbenzodiazepine or benzodiazepine-like sedatives/hypnotics, was developed and shown to be effective for inducing sleep in the treatment of insomnia.

Benzodiazepines (chlordiazepoxide, diazepam, alprazolam, lorazepam, clonazepam, oxazepam, and clorazepate) work by activating the GABA-a benzodiazepine receptor complex, which acts to hyperpolarize neurons through the influx of chloride ions via increased permeability of that ion's channel pore, resulting in suppressed neuron firing. Certain side effects are held in common by the benzodiazepines, such as increased teratogenic threat[5] and anterograde amnesia, but their therapeutic influence differs mainly along the lines of potency[6] and longevity of effect. Table 9.4 presents benzodiazepines' elimination half-lives. The length of coverage of the different benzodiazepines is therapeutically more relevant than their respective potency. Although the prescribing psychologist must be aware of dose ranges when switching from one benzodiazepine to another because there can be as much as a 20-fold difference in equivalence (Riss, Cloyd, Gates, & Collins, 2008), the half-life of a particular benzodiazepine may or may not fit its therapeutic use and may require clinical discernment in the moment of selection. For example, clonazepam is often prescribed for the patient who requires lengthy anxiolytic coverage throughout the day, while alprazolam, a relatively short-acting agent, is preferentially used for public-speaking anxiety.

Nearly all benzodiazepines are primarily metabolized by CYP450 3A4, which is inhibited by ingesting grapefruit at the time that the medication is taken, and can result in overdosing due to interaction. Among benzodiazepines, the exception to the 3A4 rule is lorazepam and oxazepam, which are not metabolized by CYP450, and may, therefore, by appropriate when an alternative path of metabolism (conjugation) is advisable when liver function is a concern.

[5]See Chapter 5, Table 5.2.
[6]See Table 9.1 for dose equivalence.

Benzodiazepines are generally approved for the treatment of anxiety of short duration. They are often, however, used off-label to treat phobias, GAD, PTSD, OCD, and social anxiety. There is evidence that the use of benzodiazepines not only engenders physical dependency, but confounds therapeutic progress by interfering with psychosocial management of a variety of anxiety disorders (see Chapter 2). Lorazepam (Ativan) is FDA approved for short-term relief of symptoms of anxiety, as is chlordiazepoxide (Librium), which is also approved for alcohol withdrawal. Clonazepam (Klonopin) is FDA indicated for the treatment of panic disorder; oxazepam (Serax) is approved for short-term anxiety relief and alcohol withdrawal, as is clorazepate. Diazepam (Valium) is indicated for short-term relief of symptoms of anxiety, seizure disorder, and skeletal-muscle spasm. Alprazolam (Xanax) is FDA approved for short-term relief of anxiety symptoms and for panic attacks.

Although devoid of the fused benzene ring/diazepine ring that characterizes the molecular structure of the benzodiazepines, the benzodiazepine-like sedative hypnotics, nonetheless, act on the GABA receptor complex and provide for a reduction in neuronal firing. The drugs that comprise this class of hypnotics, zolpidem (Ambien), zaleplon (Sonata), and zopiclone/eszopiclone (Imovane/Lunesta), are especially sedating and have very short half-lives (1.5–2.4; 1.0–2.5; 5–6 hours, respectively), which makes them ideal for a night's sleep without morning residual hangover. Rebound insomnia, which is associated with benzodiazepines, does not appear to be a problem with the discontinuation of benzodiazepine-like hypnotics, and there is some evidence that REM sleep is less disturbed than with benzodiazepines (Jovanovic & Dreyfus, 1983). This class of drug also induces little respiratory depression, which is important for patients with sleep apnea and other respiratory-related conditions; in addition, the benzodiazepine-like hypnotics appear to be as habit forming as the benzodiazepines.

ANTIPSYCHOTICS

The explanation of antipsychotic medication effectiveness in addressing positive symptoms of schizophrenia and other psychotic sequelae is based on the *dopamine receptor antagonist hypothesis* in which it is assumed that agents that reduce the prevalence of dopamine help reduce symptomatology associated with psychosis. Both conventional and the newer atypical antipsychotics are hypothesized to work by blocking or antagonizing the action of dopamine at the receptor level. In addition to treating schizophrenia, antipsychotic medication has been used to treat delusions; hallucinations; disorganized thinking; and bizarre, agitated behavior found in other disorders such as major depressive disorder, bipolar disorder, and dementia-related psychosis. The use of such agents for impulse control, especially combative behavior among the adolescent population, is more controversial.

The discovery of the first conventional antipsychotic is shrouded, as are many such discoveries, in a heavy blanket of serendipity. Chlorpromazine, a compound originally produced in the effort to synthesize an antimalarial agent during World War II, owes its psychoactive discovery to the clinical appreciation of the substrate's ability to calm agitation. The sedating and antipsychotic qualities of chlorpromazine were recognized as chemical lobotomy by its advocate, Henri Laborit, who introduced the clinical use of chlorpromazine to his postwar psychiatric colleagues at the Val-de-Grace military hospital in Paris (Wilkaitis, Mulvihill, & Nasrllah, 2009). The first generation, or so-called classic, antipsychotics, which include chlorpromazine, fluphenazine, haloperidol, loxapine, thiothixene, pimozide, perphenazine, thioridazine, and trifluoperazine, proved to be highly effective in severe cases of psychosis. They also, unfortunately, proved to be toxic, and extrapyramidal side effects[7] as well as neuroleptic malignancy syndrome, seizure, and cardiac arrhythmias were unsettling consequences of their mechanisms of action.

Chlorpromazine (Thorazine) is approved by the FDA for the treatment of psychotic disorders, including schizophrenia, schizoaffective disorder, acute mania, and depression with psychotic features. Fluphenazine (Prolixin) is indicated by the FDA for the treatment of psychotic disorders, including schizophrenia, schizoaffective disorder, and drug-induced psychosis, and has been used off-label in conjugation with mood stabilizers to initially stabilize acute mania. Haloperidol (Haldol) is approved for use with psychotic disorders, Tourette's syndrome, and in children with explosive behavior. Thioridazine (Mellaril) is approved for use with psychotic disorders, acute mania, and, like haloperidol, in children with explosive behavior. Loxapine (Loxitane), thiothixene (Navane), perphenazine (Trilafon), and trifluoperazine (Stelazine) are approved for use with psychotic conditions, and have been used off-label with mood stabilizers for acute treatment of mania. Pimozide (Orap), an agent with a close molecular structure to haloperidol, has never been approved for the treatment of psychotic symptoms, and is rarely used off-label for this purpose. Rather, it is approved by the FDA for the treatment of Tourette's, and is almost exclusively used to this end.

Second generation antipsychotics (clozapine, risperidone, quetiapine, olanzapine, ziprasidone, paliperidone, and aripiprazole) are commonly referred to as atypical antipsychotics to distinguish them from the typical D_2 antagonism of conventional neuroleptics, although the newer atypicals continue to block D_2. Indeed, atypicals affect multiple mechanisms of action including D_2 antagonism and serotonin 5-HT_{2A} antagonism, and are purported to treat negative signs associated with psychosis as well as the more classic positive symptoms because of their relative preference, in comparison to conventional neuroleptics, for 5-HT_{2A} affinity. As discussed in Chapter 2, current analysis of clinical data puts in doubt the original claims that the atypical antipsychotics are more effective than conventional antipsychotics at treating positive or negative symptoms of schizophrenia. In addition, although their potential for provoking tardive dyskinesia appears less than the conventional antipsychotics, they are not free from this pernicious side effect. Moreover, the atypicals also contribute side effects that have come to be more associated with them than with the original antipsychotics, such as agranulocytosis, hyperprolactinemia, and metabolic syndrome (obesity/diabetes).

Clozapine (Clozaril) is the oldest of the second generation antipsychotics, but it got off to a slow start in the 1960s and 70s due to associated problems with agranulocytosis. It was initially used to good effect in Europe, but did not gain FDA approval until the late 1980s, and only then with restricted use. Clozapine is approved only for treatment-resistant schizophrenia that has not responded to conventional antipsychotics. It requires extensive laboratory monitoring,[8] but it has also proved to be the most effective of all antipsychotics in treating unresponsive psychotic disorders.[9] In 1994, risperidone (Risperdal) was approved as a new

---

[7]See Chapter 4, Table 4.4.
[8]See Chapter 6, Table 6.9.
[9]See Chapter 2, Table 2.2.

atypical antipsychotic for treatment of adult schizophrenia, with a greater than tenfold affinity for 5-HT$_{2A}$ over D$_2$. It proved to be well tolerated, although its high affinity for α_2 adrenergic receptors may contribute to orthostatic hypotension and tachycardia. Subsequent clinical trials have allowed risperidone to gain FDA approval for the treatment of schizophrenia in adolescents, acute manic and mixed episodes in adults and pediatric patients ages 10–17, and the treatment of irritability associated with autism. Quetiapine (Seroquel) was developed in the early 1980s along a molecular structure similar to clozapine, and it was approved by the FDA in 1997 with fewer restrictions since its safety profile was better. It, like all atypical antipsychotics, has a high affinity for 5-HT$_{2A}$ receptors, in addition to acting as a somewhat weaker antagonist at the D$_2$ receptor. However, it has an even greater affinity for histaminergic H$_1$ binding, which gives it a strong sedative effect. Quetiapine was originally approved for the treatment of schizophrenia, but it has more recently been granted indications for the treatment of depression and acute mania associated with bipolar disorder. It is also approved for maintenance treatment of bipolar disorder as an adjunct to lithium or valproic acid. In 1997, the FDA also approved olanzapine (Zyprexa), originally for the treatment of psychosis, but later extended its indications to include the treatment of bipolar disorder. Olanzapine has also been used off-label for treating several nonpsychotic conditions, among them anorexia nervosa. The most troubling side effect of olanzapine is weight gain, which may be an advantage with anorexia nervosa in which severe, delusional-like body distortion may be pharmacologically addressed while weight gain is potentiated by the same agent. Ziprasidone (Geodon) was initially approved in 2001 by the FDA for the treatment of schizophrenia and subsequently has obtained an additional indication for acute manic and mixed episodes in bipolar disorder. One concern, which delayed ziprasidone's approval, is the potential for prolonged QT interval (Crutchfield, 2005). The package insert contains warnings about the possibility of the dose-related prolongation, requiring avoiding its use with other drugs that are known to prolong the QT interval, and avoiding use in patients with congenital long QT syndrome or those with a history of cardiac arrhythmias. Paliperidone (Invega), similar to risperidone in structure, was approved for the treatment of schizophrenia in 2006 by the FDA. Finally, aripiprazole (Abilify) is an "atypical" atypical, inasmuch as it is not a true antagonist of D$_2$ and 5-HT receptors but, rather, is a partial agonist of D$_2$, and 5-HT$_{1A}$, as well as an antagonist of 5-HT$_{2A}$ (Jordan, et al., 2002). What this means as far as the *dopamine hypothesis* of schizophrenia is not very clear. Partial agonists may act, however, to reduce the activity of the affected receptor[10] when there is an overabundance of a transmitter by occupying the receptor and reducing access to a full agonist; this process with D$_2$ may lead to a "stabilizing effect" in receptor firing (Burris et al., 2002) and, following the dopamine hypothesis of schizophrenia, account for the therapeutic effect of aripiprazole with psychosis. Aripiprazole was initially gained FDA approval for the treatment of schizophrenia in adults, but subsequently was granted approval for the treatment of acute mania in bipolar disorder and more recently, in 2007 and 2008, was approved for the treatment of schizophrenia in adolescents, the treatment of manic and mixed episodes of bipolar disorder in adults and adolescents, and as an adjunctive to the treatment of MDD in adults.

---

[10]See Chapter 8.

MOOD STABILIZERS

Mood stabilizers consist of (1) lithium, (2) anticonvulsants (valproic acid, lamotrigine, carbamazepine, gabapentin, topiramate, oxcarbazepine), and (3) second-generation antipsychotics. Although some of the mood stabilizers share mechanism of actions, they are somewhat distinct to the extent in which one mechanism or another is thought to dominate. One might rightfully declare that the actual pharmacodynamic reason why these drugs address concerns of mood dysregulation in bipolar disorder is unknown, yet it is consensually believed that they all generally suppress overexcitatory processes in the brain.[11]

Lithium is speculated to work by causing immediate and long-term ("down-stream") inhibitory effects that include the inhibition of inositol monophosphatase,[12] the increase in glutamate reuptake from synapses, eventual gene expression resulting in general inhibition of cerebral activation, and, perhaps, neuroprotective effects (Kowatch, 2008). The anticonvulsants are generally believed to increase the inhibitory action of GABA, inhibit inositol transport, and/or reduce neuronal activity by restricting ion channel influx. Valproic acid (Depakote) is considered a "gamma-aminobutyric acid enhancing" (Goodwin & Jamison, 2007) mood stabilizer, while topiramate (Topamax) is thought to primarily increase GABA and inhibit glutamate receptor activation. Oxcarbazepine (Trileptal) and carbamazepine (Tegretol) are believed to increase limbic $GABA_B$ receptors while reducing GABA turnover and inhibiting calcium influx. Gabapentin (Neurontin) does not act as a GABA precursor, agonist, or antagonist (Fryre, 2004), but appears to increase the enzymatic action of glutamic acid decarboxylase, which converts glutamate to GABA; it may also increase enzymatic action to catabolized glutamate. Lamotrigine (Lamictal) does not affect GABA synthesis or deployment but, rather, acts to inhibit Na^+ influx presynaptically as well as to reduce the flow of Ca^{2+} and K^+ through voltage-sensitive channels, the result of which is to reduce glutamate activity. There is no consensus about how the atypical antipsychotics reduce agitation in bipolar mania, but the blockage of the excitatory transmitter dopamine might be assumed to be implicated.

The FDA approved lithium in 1970 for the treatment of acute mania, and later approved it for the prophylaxis of bipolar disorder. It is also indicated for the treatment of bipolar disorder in combination with olanzapine. Valproate was developed as an antiepileptic and gained FDA approval for this use in 1978. It was later approved for the treatment of mania in 1995. Carbamazepine and oxcarbazepine are not approved for use in bipolar disorder, but they are used for such off-label. They are largely considered alternatives to the first-line bipolar medications of lithium and valproate (American Psychiatric Association, 2002). Topiramate and gabapentin are FDA approved for the treatment of epilepsy, but are not FDA indicated for the treatment of mania or bipolar disorder, although they are used off-label much like carbamazepine and oxcarbazepine with conditions resistant to management by first-line

---

[11]How insightful was Ivan Pavlov's (1927) observations of "excitatory vs. inhibitory" regions of the brain and the balance among them as forming the basis to cerebral equilibrium!

[12]The *inositol depletion hypothesis* (Berridge, Downes, & Hanley,1982) proposes that lithium derives its effectiveness in treating mania by attenuating the phosphatidylinositol signal transduction pathway, which is accomplished through the inhibition of inositol monophosphatase, resulting in a depletion of inositol (Atack, 2000).

bipolar medications.[13] Lamotrigine was initially approved by the FDA for the treatment of epilepsy and was later approved for the treatment of acute mania associated with bipolar disorder. Clinical studies have shown lamotrigine to be useful in treating and preventing recurrence of bipolar-related depression and rapid cycling between depression and hypomania, and it is used off-label for this prophylactic goal (Chew et al., 2009).

The conventional antipsychotics chlorpromazine and thioridazine have FDA approval for the treatment of acute mania, whereas haloperidol is FDA approved for treating explosive behavior in children. Atypical antipsychotics indicated for treatment of acute mania and mixed episodes of bipolar disorder include ziprasidone, risperidone, and quetiapine. In addition, the FDA has approved risperidone for the treatment of irritability in autism, including aggression, self-injury, and temper tantrums. Quetiapine and olanzapine have been approved for the maintenance of bipolar disorder as adjuncts to lithium or divalproex (valproic acid), whereas Symbyax, a combined preparation of olanzapine and fluoxetine, is approved for the treatment of depressive episodes associated with bipolar disorder.

STIMULANTS

Stimulants or analeptics (amphetamine, methylphenidate) are used almost exclusively to treat Attention Deficit–Hyperactivity Disorder. Not all medications for the treatment of ADHD, however, are stimulants (e.g., guanfacine, bupropion).

Methylphenidate (Ritalin, Concerta) and amphetamine (Adderall) work respectively to increase dopamine singly or increase both dopamine and norepinephrine in synapses along the striatal-prefrontal trajectory (Taylor & Jentsch, 2000). This is achieved by an astounding number of ways, including the following (Muse, 2010): (a) amphetamine can bind to monoamine oxidase in the mitochondria and prevent the degradation of dopamine, leaving free dopamine in the nerve terminal; (b) amphetamine can interact with dopamine-containing synaptic vesicles, releasing free dopamine into the nerve terminal; (c) amphetamine can also bind to the presynaptic membrane of dopaminergic and noradrenergic neurons and induce the release of dopamine and norepinephrine from the nerve terminal; and (d) amphetamine can bind to the dopamine reuptake transporter (DAT) and to the norepinephrine transporter (NET), causing them to act in reverse and, respectively, transport free dopamine and norepinephrine out of the nerve terminal into the synaptic cleft. Methylphenidate, on the other hand, exerts its therapeutic effects (a) via blocking the reuptake of dopamine into nerve terminals, and (b) by stimulating the release of dopamine from nerve terminals, resulting in increased dopamine levels in the synapse.

Stimulant medications come in different packages or delivery systems which help to determine the rate, amount, and type of molecule to be released. Adderall is a racemic mix of amphetamine/dextroamphetamine salt that is available in immediate release tablets with an approximate duration of five hours and in extended release

---

[13]The clinical evidence for the use of the anticonvulsants in the treatment of bipolar disorder is equivocal, and a recent Cochrane review of topiramate found "insufficient evidence on which to base any recommendations regarding the use of topiramate in any phase of bipolar illness, either in monotherapy or as an adjunctive treatment" (Vasudev, Macritchie, Geddes, Watson, & Young, 2011).

capsules with coated beads that provide therapeutic coverage for about 8–10 hours. DextroStat and Dexedrine Spansules are isomeric dextroamphetamine preparations that are available in immediate as well as sustained release. Vyvanse, lisdexamfetamine, is a prodrug that requires metabolism to become active dexamphetamine, and extends its therapeutic effect for up to 12 hours. Ritalin, a methylphenidate, delivers the drug in immediate release, which lasts 2–5 hours, in sustained release, which gives 6–8 hours coverage but is delayed by 2–3 hours before reaching peak effects, and in a long-action capsule, which mixes immediate with sustained release methylphenidate to achieve fast onset and more sustained effect. Concerta uses a similar approach to Ritalin LA by delivering methylphenidate in two stages: immediate release and extended release. The Concerta capsule is coated with immediate release methylphenidate, and is further designed with an internal compartment that delays releasing the remainder drug as the compartment dissolves. Concerta is designed to provide fairly constant therapeutic effect over a period of 10–12 hours. Focalin XR, dexmethylphenidate extended release, is the d-isomer of racemic methylphenidate mix, and is delivered in a capsule that contains half immediate-release beads and half delay-release enteric-coated beads. Daytrana is a topical patch that delivers methylphenidate transdermally with action up to 12 hours.

Apart from stimulant medication, ADHD is treated with FDA approval by the reuptake inhibitors atomoxetine and bupropion, and the heretofore off-label antihypertensive drugs clonidine and guanfacine.[14] Atomoxetine (Strattera) is a norepinephrine reuptake inhibitor (NRI). Like other reuptake inhibitors, atomoxetine requires a 2- to 3-week break-in period before therapeutic benefit is observed. It provides, on the other hand, continuous coverage once a therapeutic level is achieved. Bupropion (Wellbutrin) is a dopamine norepinephrine reuptake inhibitor (DNRI) and, like atomoxetine, provides continuous coverage once the initial delayed therapeutic onset is overcome. Clonidine (Catapres) is an α_2 agonist, as is guanfacine (Tenex); the exact mechanism of action in the treatment of ADHD is unknown for the α_2 agonists.

There is ample evidence that stimulant medication is effective in mitigating ADHD in the short term. However, there is increasing evidence that its effectiveness diminishes substantially over the long term (Molina et al., 2008).[15] With ADHD, as with so many other disorders, diagnosis is paramount. If the provider follows only the descriptive criteria of the *DSM-IV*, it is too easy to falsely diagnosis ADHD when other alternative explanations may be more appropriate. This is where psychometrics make such a difference in determining if the symptoms stand out statistically from peers and warrant a diagnosis of disorder; attention deficit comes in many forms and degrees, and is age-related without necessarily being pathological. Distraction, impulsivity, and disorganization can equally well be the manifestation of adjustment reaction, anxiety or depression, developmental delay, or prodromal psychosis. Or, such symptoms can be a red herring for ineffectual parenting or family dysfunction. This is but one example of how the psychobiosocial approach can be so rewarding; not only can it differentially identify and treat conditions such as ADHD, but it can also identify misdiagnosis and offer alternative treatments beyond pure pharmacological approaches.

---

[14]FDA-approved extended release guanfacine and extended release clonidine as monotherapy or in conjunction with stimulants for ADHD in children in 2009 and 2010, respectively.
[15]See also Chapter 2's discussion of the MTA studies.

CHAPTER 9 KEY TERMS

Abstinence-violation effect: A person's sense of loss of control over his/her behavior that has an overwhelming and demoralizing effect. The guilt and perceived loss of control that a person feels whenever he or she slips and finds himself or herself returning to drug or alcohol use after an extended period of abstinence.

Adverse drug reactions: Drug-induced negative consequences that can be caused by an excessive dose, impaired metabolism or excretion of the drug (toxicity or overdose), undesirable effects of the chemical properties of the drug (side effects), depletion of metabolic enzymes by another drug (interaction), or an immune system hypersensitivity reaction (allergy).

Comorbid conditions: At least two simultaneous disorders affecting an individual at the same period of time.

Compliance: Treatment compliance is the patient's cooperation in carrying out the therapeutic contract with the therapist. Patients agree to comply with the instructions given by the therapist to carry out the steps of treatment.

Contraindications: All drugs have some undesirable or negative side effects to which patients must adjust, if they are to obtain the intended desirable effects of a drug. Some drugs should not be used for a particular indication, because they would be harmful or dangerous (absolute contraindications). Some drugs should be used with caution because they cause side effects or interactions (relative contraindications).

Cross-dependence: This is a form of cross-reactivity that is found in drugs that affect the same neuroreceptor, e.g., the cumulative CNS depressant effect of ingesting a combination of alcohol and benzodiazepines.

Cross-sensitization: The increased effect of a drug from continued exposure to a similar drug.

Cross-tapering: A type of medication adjustment in which a new medication is added to a patient's regimen, and its dose gradually increased, while the dosage of an original medication that was prescribed for the same clinical purpose is gradually reduced and finally discontinued.

Cross-tolerance: A decreased response to a drug from continued exposure to a similar drug.

Cytochrome P450 enzyme: These enzymes are needed in the catalytic metabolism of a drug in the GI tract or liver. They help to transform drug molecules by means of phase 1 metabolism to more-polar, water-soluble metabolites. This metabolic process inactivates the drug and allows it to be eliminated by the kidneys. Usage of drug substrates may deplete the number of a specific type of enzyme making it temporarily unavailable for use. Induction causes these enzymes to increase in number, and inhibition causes them to reduce in number.

Dependence: Psychological dependence is the craving or emotional memory of the pleasure connected with drug taking. Physical dependence refers to the adverse physical signs and symptoms which occur when the drug is absent or withdrawn.

Dopamine receptor antagonist hypothesis: Hypothesis that postulates that schizophrenia and other psychosis are due to excessive dopamine in certain pathways of the brain.

Drug–drug interaction: In pharmacodynamics, a drug interacts with other drugs at the receptor site, such that the drug with less affinity for a receptor may be displaced from its binding site by other drugs of greater affinity, which in turn decreases the pharmacodynamic effect (the action of the drug on the body) of the displaced drug. In pharmacokinetics, drugs that compete for, or inhibit one or more of the cytochrome P450 enzymes, can cause an increased plasma concentration of another drug that needs this specific enzyme for metabolism. Some drugs can also induce one of these enzymes and have the opposite effect, that is, increasing the pharmacokinetic (the action of the body on the drug) effect.

First-pass metabolism: Orally administered drugs enter the stomach, duodenum, and intestine for digestion and then drain through the venous system out of the intestines and into the liver before entering the vena cava of the heart to be circulated in the arterial bloodstream to tissues. This first pass through the liver metabolism extracts a great deal of the drug before it enters the tissue capillaries.

Gingko biloba: An herbal tree extract used to treat vascular insufficiency, impaired mental performance, tinnitus, deafness, diabetic neuropathy, impotence, premenstrual syndrome, depression, and allergies.

Inositol depletion hypothesis: Posits that lithium produces a lowering of myo-inositol in critical areas of the brain and the cascade effect is therapeutic in the treatment of bipolar disorder.

Intramuscular administration: An injection into muscular tissue may use an aqueous solution to increase the rate of absorption or a depot preparation wherein the drug is suspended in a nonaqueous solution such as peanut oil to slow down rate of absorption.

Intrathecal administration: The delivery of drugs into the cerebral spinal fluid.

Medication regimen: The instructions given to a patient in oral or written form that label the type of medication, the dosage, the time of day to administer the dosage, the frequency of the dosage, and the length of time that the regimen should be continued.

Neuroleptic malignancy syndrome: A life-threatening, idiosyncratic reaction to neuroleptic medication. The syndrome is characterized by fever, muscular rigidity, altered mental status, and autonomic dysfunction.

Over-the-counter (OTC) drugs: Medications that have been FDA approved for sale on an open counter in a store, in order that they may be purchased by customers without a prescription or consultation with a professional.

Pharmacodynamics: The actions of the drug on the body determine the group in which a drug is classified and makes up the components of the mechanism of action of the drug. The agonistic and antagonistic actions of drugs at the binding sites on the receptors.

Pharmacokinetics: The quantitative, time-dependent changes of both the plasma drug concentration and the total amount of drug in the body following the drug's administration. The movement of the drug through the body from the site of administration to the sites of drug action during absorption, metabolism, distribution, and elimination of the drug.

Pharmacotherapeutics: The application of the pharmacological principles of pharmacokinetics and pharmacodynamics to clinical practice.

Plasma concentration: The measurement of the amount of a drug that is present in the bloodstream at any given moment, usually in milligrams per deciliter or nanograms per milliliter.

Polypharmacy: Two meanings occur in the literature. The prescription of many drugs given at one time is the predominant meaning currently in use. Some authors use this term also to mean the excessive use of drugs, or even the overdose of a drug.

Prophylaxis: Preventative medical treatment of a disease or the medical agent used to prevent the disease. Also, preventative psychological treatment or the procedure used to prevent psychopathology.

Relapse prevention: Substance abusers or mental health patients who have recovered from their addiction or mental disorder are at risk for relapse (returning to their addiction or mental illness). In order to help these patients to prevent such relapse, therapists offer strategies whose purpose it is to prevent relapse from happening.

Sensitization: Sometimes called inverse tolerance, sensitization is an increased effect of a drug after repeated administrations.

Serotonin syndrome: Potentially life-threatening reaction to an overabundance of serotonin, the most severe symptoms include dangerous increase in heart rate and blood pressure, temperature above 41.1 °C (106.0 °F), metabolic acidosis, rhabdomyolisis, seizures, and renal failure.

St. John's wort: The herbal extract of the flower of a perennial shrub that is used as an antidepressant, antiviral, antibiotic, and psychotropic.

Therapeutic index: The ratio between the dosage of a drug that is effective in 50% of patients to the dosage that causes death in 50% of patients.

Titration: A procedure for the adjustment of the dosage of medication that is in use by a patient. The term was originally developed to describe a chemical laboratory procedure that has been applied to clinical practice, wherein it is the process of dosage adjustment in which the dosage of a medication is raised until the patient has adequate symptom control or has reached the upper limit of the maximum FDA approved range or severe ADRs appear or a plateau is reached where no improvements or worsening occurs.

Tolerance: The decreased drug effect that develops with the continued use of the drug.

Chapter 9 Questions

1. Which of the following refers to the indication or usage of the drug, approved by the FDA for a specific use after research trials have provided evidence that this drug is appropriately indicated for the treatment of a given illness and patient?
   a. Pharmacodynamics
   b. Pharmacokinetics
   c. Pharmacotherapeutics
   d. Pharmacogenetics
2. When a prescribing psychologist selects a medication that has not been FDA approved (off-label) for the age or the disorder presented by the patient, the psychologist may feel justified in making the selection when no other satisfactory drug is available to produce a needed effect, and
   a. The nonapproved drug has the same therapeutic target as a similar approved drug.
   b. The nonapproved drug has no black box warning against the usage as an off-label drug.

c. If the needed effect is known to be a primary effect of this drug.

d. If the need for the drug outweighs the contraindications.

3. Which of the following factors should be taken into consideration when selecting a psychopharmacological medication that is most appropriate for a patient under your care?

a. The treatment of choice that best fits the patient's diagnosis

b. The patient's comorbid medical conditions

c. The patient's existing medication regimen to avoid drug–drug interactions

d. All of the above.

4. Which of the following is the name of a procedure by which one medication is added to a patient's medication regimen and its dosage gradually increased, while the dosage of the original medication that was prescribed for the same clinical purpose is gradually reduced and finally discontinued?

a. Titration

b. Cross-tapering

c. Cross-dependence

d. Discontinuation

5. Intramuscular depot administration of an antipsychotic medication to a patient with a diagnosis of paranoid schizophrenia is selected by a prescribing medical psychologist in order to obtain which one of the following advantages in the care of a patient with psychosis?

a. To provide a slower absorption rate to last a longer time

b. To provide a faster absorption rate to get immediate effects

c. To avoid first-pass metabolism

d. To bypass the GI tract and liver

6. Which of the following medication categories is known to produce side effects that include increase in heart rate, temperature, and pupil size?

a. Opioids

b. CNS depressants

c. Anticholinergics

d. All of the above.

7. Which of the following events will have the highest likelihood of leading to drug toxicity?

a. The patient is prescribed a medication that requires a specific CYP450 enzyme for metabolism, and another medicine already in the patient's regimen has depleted that particular enzyme.

b. The patient is prescribed a medication that requires a higher dosage than has been given to attain any therapeutic effect.

c. The patient is prescribed a medication at a dosage that is too high for an initial dose, because the prescriber wrote in the amount of medication that should be taken after 2 weeks on the initial dose.

d. The patient is elderly and has been given an initial dosage that has been determined to be appropriate for a middle-aged adult.

8. Which of the following is an example of a drug–drug interaction that is frequently an accidental occurrence ?

a. Antipsychotic medication and alcohol

b. Benzodiazepines and alcohol

c. Anticonvulsants and phenobarbital

d. Antidepressants and anxiolytics

9. Which of the following is often the cause of relapse in individuals addicted to alcohol who are attempting to reach sobriety?

a. To enter the environment where drinking has occurred in the past

b. To allow themselves to think about the craving for alcohol

c. To enter a stressful environment that will trigger a need for anxiety relief

d. To nourish a sense of feeling sorry for themselves

10. The most commonly abused substances by the elderly are:

a. Wine and beer

b. Cocaine and nonsteroidal anti-inflammatory drugs

c. Whiskey and brandy

d. Marijuana and psychotropic medications

11. In general, what type of treatment should always be the first treatment of choice to be considered?

a. Medications specifically FDA approved for children

b. FDA-approved medications, but also safe off-label drugs

c. Any off-label drug that is needed as long as it is safe

d. Psychotherapy along with any medication

12. During detoxification for severe alcohol addiction, the medication treatment of choice for the first 24 to 48 hours is:

a. Haloperidol

b. Benzodiazepine

c. Prozac

d. Methadone

13. Of the following antidepressants, which class has the greatest diversity in mechanism of actions (affects the most receptors)?

a. SSRIs

b. TCAs

c. MAOIs

d. SNRIs

14. Mirtazapine is a

a. SSRI antidepressant.

b. NaSSA antidepressant.

c. Atypical antipsychotic.

d. New mood stabilizer.

15. First line treatment of GAD dictates beginning treatment with which of the following?

a. Olanzapine

b. Symbyax

c. Sertraline

d. Clonazepam

16. Which has proved least effective in the treatment of bipolar disorder?

    a. Gabapentin

    b. Lithium

    c. Lamotrigine

    d. Chlorpromazine

17. Which of the benzodiazepines is the shortest acting?

    a. Diazepam

    b. Lorazepam

    c. Alprazolam

    d. Clonazepam

18. How many mechanisms of action does amphetamine have in increasing dopamine and norepinephrine presence in the synapses?

    a. 2

    b. 4

    c. 6

    d. 8

Answers: (1) c, (2) d, (3) d, (4) b, (5) a, (6) c, (7) a, (8) b, (9) a, (10) d, (11) d, (12) b, (13) b, (14) b, (15) c, (16) a, (17) c, and (18) c

REFERENCES

American Psychiatric Association. (2002). Practice guideline for the treatment of patients with bipolar disorder. *American Journal of Psychiatry, 159*, 1–50.

Atack, J. (2000). Lithium, phosphatidylinositol signaling, and bipolar disorder: The role of inositol monophosphatase. In H. Manji, C. Bowden, & R. Belmaker (Eds.), *Bipolar medications: Mechanisms of action*. Washington, DC, American Psychiatric Press.

Avorn, J. (1998). Drug prescribing, drug taking, adverse reactions, and compliance in elderly patients. In C. Salzman (Ed.), *Clinical geriatric psychopharmacology*. Baltimore, MD: Williams & Wilkins.

Berridge, M., Downes, C., & Hanley, M. (1982). Lithium amplifies agonist-dependent phosphatidylinositol responses in brain and salivary glands. *Biochemistry Journal, 206*, 587–595.

Burns, W. J., Rey, J., & Burns, K. (2008). Psychopharmacology as practiced by psychologists. In M. Hersen & A. M. Gross (Eds.), *Handbook of clinical psychology, Vol. 1, Adults*. Hoboken, NJ: Wiley.

Burris, K., Molski, T., Xu, C., Ryan, E., Tottori, K., Kikuchi, T., . . . & Molinoff, P. (2002). Aripiprazole, a novel antipsychotic, is a high-affinity partial agonist at human dopamine D2 receptors. *Journal of Pharmacology, 302*, 381–389.

Byck, R. (1975). Drugs and the treatment of psychiatric disorders. In L. S. Gilman & A. Goodman (Eds.), *The pharmacological basis of therapeutics*. New York, NY: MacMillian.

Chew, R., Hales, R., & Yudofsky, S. (2009). *What your patients need to know about psychiatric medications*. Washington, DC: American Psychiatric Publishing.

Cozza, K. L., Armstrong, S. C., & Oesterheld, J. R. (2003). *Drug interaction principles for medical practice* (2nd ed.). Washington, DC: American Psychiatric Publishing.

Crane, G. E. (1957). Iproniazid (Marsalid) phosphate: A therapeutic agent for mental disorders. *Psychiatric Resarch Reports, 8*, 142–154.

Crutchfield, D. (2005). Ziprasidone: A new atypical antipsychotic. *Geriatric Times, 2,* 28–29.

Finkel, R., Clark, M. A., & Cubeddu, L. X. (2009). *Lippincott's illustrated reviews: Pharmacology.* Philadelphia, PA: Lippincott, Williams & Wilkins.

Frye, M. (2004). Gabapentin. In A. F. Schatzberg & C. B. Nemeroff (Eds.), *The American Psychiatric Publishing textbook of psychopharmacology* (pp. 607–614). Washington, DC: American Psychiatric Publishing.

Galanter, J. M., & Wartenberg, A. A. (2005). Pharmacology of chemical dependence and Addiction. In D. E. Golan, A. H. Tashian, Jr., E. J. Armstrong, J. M. Galanter, A. W. Armstrong, R. A. Aarnaout, & H. S. Rose, (Eds.), *Principles of pharmacology: The pathophysiological basis of drug therapy.* Philadelphia, PA: Lippincott, Williams & Wilkins.

Gillin, J. C., & Ancoli-Israel, S. (1998). The impact of age on sleep and sleep disorders. In C. Salzman (Ed.), *Clinical geriatric psychopharmacology.* Baltimore, MD: Williams & Wilkins.

George, T., & Vessicchio, J. (2001). Nicotine addiction and other psychiatric disorders. *Psychiatric Times, 18,* 39–42.

Goodwin, F., & Jamison, K. (2007). *Manic-depressive illness: Bipolar disorder and recurrent depression.* New York, NY: Oxford University Press.

Greb, W. H., Buscher, G., Dierdorf, H. D., Koster, F. E., Wolf, D., & Mellows, G. (1989). The effect of liver enzyme inhibition by cimetidine and enzyme induction by phenobarbitone on the pharmacokinetics of paroxetine. *Acta Psychiatrica Scandinavica, 80*(S350), 95–98.

Green, W. H. (1995). *Child and adolescent clinical psychopharmacology* (2nd ed.). Philadelphia, PA: Lippincott, Williams & Wilkins.

Healy, D. (2009). *Psychiatric drugs explained.* New York, NY: Elsevier.

Hulisz, D., & Jakab, J. (2007). Food-drug interactions: Which ones really matter? *U.S. Pharmacy, 32*(3), 93–98.

Jeppesen, U., Loft, S., Poulsen, H. E., & Brśen, K. (1996). A fluvoxamine-caffeine interaction study. *Pharmacogenetics, 6*(3), 213–222.

Jordan, S., et al. (2002). The antipsychotic aripiprazole is a potent, partial agonist at the human 5- HT_{1A} receptor. *European Journal of Pharmacology, 441,* 137–140.

Jovnovic, U., & Dreyfus, F. (1983). Poligraphical sleep recording in insomniac patients under zopiclone or nitrazepam. *Pharmacology, 27,* 136–145.

Kowatch, R. (2008). Mood stabilizers. In B. Geller. & M. Delbello (Eds.), *Treatment of bipolar disorder in children and adolescents.* New York, NY: Guilford Press.

Lacy, C. F., Armstrong, L. L., Goldman, M. P., & Lance, L. L. (2007). *Drug information handbook* (15th ed.). Hudson, OH: Lexicomp.

Larimer, M. E., Palmer, R. S., & Marlatt, G. A. (1999). Relapse prevention: An overview of Marlatt's cognitive-behavioral model. *Alcohol Research and Health, 23,*151–160.

Lebowitz, B. D., Pearson, J. L., & Cohen, G. D. (1998). Older Americans and their illnesses. In C. Salzman (Ed.), *Clinical geriatric psychopharmacology.* Baltimore, MD: Williams & Wilkin.

Marlatt, G. A., & Gordon, J. R. (Eds.). (1985). *Relapse prevention: Maintenance strategies in the treatment of addictive behaviors.* New York, NY: Guilford Press.

Martinez, C., Albet, C., Agundez, J. A., Herrero, E., Carillo, J. A., Marquez, M., . . . Ortiz, J. A. (1999). Comparative in vitro and in vivo inhibition of cytochrome P450 CYP1A2, CYP2D6, and CYP3A by H2-receptor antagonists. *Clinical Pharmacological Therapy, 65,* 369–376.

Mitchell, S., Teno, J., Miller, S., & Mor, V. (2005). A national study of the location of death for older persons with dementia. *Journal of the American Geriatric Society, 53,* 299–305.

Molina, B., Hinshaw, S., Swanson, J., Arnold, L., Vitiello, B., Jensen, P., . . . & MTA Cooperative Group. (2008). The MTA at 8 years: Prospective follow-up of children treated for combined-type ADHD in a multisite study. *Journal of the American Academy of Child & Adolescent Psychiatry, 48*, 484–500.

Murray, M. T. (1995). *The healing power of herbs.* Rocklin, CA: Prima Publishing.

Muse, M. (2010). *Psychopharmacology for the non-mental health prescriber.* Rockville, MD: Mensana Publications.

Mycek, M. J., Harvey, R. A., Champe, P. C., Fisher, B. D., & Cooper, M. (2000). *Lippincott's illustrated reviews Pharmacology.* Philadelphia, PA: Lippincott, Williams & Wilkins.

Nelson, C. (2004). Tricyclic and tetracyclic drugs. In A. F. Schatzberg & C. B. Nemeroff (Eds.), *The American Psychiatric Publishing textbook of psychopharmacology.* Washington, DC: American Psychiatric Publishing.

Nestler, E. J., Hyman, S. E., & Malenka, R. C. (2001). *Molecular neuropharmacology: A foundation for clinical neuroscience.* New York, NY: McGraw-Hill.

Nockowitz, R. (1998). Enhancing patient compliance with treatment recommendations. In T. A. Stern, J. B. Herman, & P. L. Slavin (Eds.), *The MGH guide to psychiatry in primary care.* New York, NY: McGraw-Hill.

Pavlov, I. P. (1927). *Conditioned reflexes: An investigation of the physiological activity of the cerebral cortex* (translated by G.V. Anrep). London: Oxford University Press.

Pi, E. H., & Simpson, G. M., (2005). Cross-cultural psychopharmacology: A current clinical perspective. *Psychiatric Services, 56*, 31–33.

Reimherr, F. W., Amsterdam, J. D., Quitkin, F. M., Rosenbaum, J. F., Fava, M., Zajecka, J., . . . & Sundell, K. (1998). Optimal length of continuation therapy in depression: A prospective assessment during long-term fluoxetine treatment. *The American Journal of Psychiatry, 155*(9), 1247–1253.

Renner, J. A., & Bierer, M. F. (1998). Approach to the alcohol-abusing patient. In T. A. Stern, J. B. Herman, & P. L. Slavin (Eds.). *The MGH guide to psychiatry in primary care.* New York, New York: McGraw-Hill.

Riss, J., Cloyd, J., Gates, J., & Collins, S. (2008). Benzodiazepines in epilepsy: Pharmacology and pharmacokinetics. *Acta Neurologica Scandinavica, 118*, 69–86.

Royner, B. W., Edelman, B. A., Cox, M. P., & Schmuely, R. (1992). The impact of antipsychotic drugs regulations on psychotropic prescribing practices in nursing homes. *American Journal of Psychiatry, 149*, 1390–1392.

Salzman, C. (1998). *Treatment of anxiety and anxiety-related disorders.* In C. Salzman (Ed.), *Clinical geriatric psychopharmacology.* Baltimore, MD: Williams & Wilkins.

Sheehan, D., et al. (1982). *The treatment of panic attacks with agoraphobia with alprazolam and ibuprofen: A controlled study.* Presentation to the annual meeting of the American Psychiatric Association in Toronto, Canada.

Stern, T. A., Herman, J. B., & Slavin, P. L (1998). *The MGH guide to psychiatry in primary care.* New York, NY: McGraw-Hill.

Sundaram, V. (2009). Immigrants gain right to medical interpreters. *New America Media,* January 26.

Taylor, J., & Jentch, D. (2000). Stimulant effects on striatal and cortical dopamine systems involved in reward-related behavior and impulsivity. In M. Solanto, A. Arnsten, & F. Castellaos (Eds.), *Stimulant drugs and ADHD* (pp. 104–133). New York, NY: Oxford University Press.

Vasudev, K., Macritchie, K., Geddes, J., Watson, S., & Young, A. (2011). Topiramate for acute affective episodes in bipolar disorder. *The Cochrane Database of Systematic Reviews,* Issue 8.

Wassner, S. J., Malekzadeh, M. H., Pennisi, A. J., Ettenger, R. B., Uilttenbogaart, C. H., & Fine, R. N. (1977). Allograft survival in patients receiving anticonvulsant medications. *Clinical Nephrology, 8*, 293–297.

Wells, B. G., Pieper, J. A., Self, T. H., Stewart, C. F., Waldon, S. L., Bobo, L., & Warner, C. (1986). The effect of ranitidine and cimetideine on imipramine disposition. *European Journal of Clinical Pharmacology, 31*(3), 285–290.

Wilkaitis, J., Mulvihill, T., & Nasrllah, H. (2009). Classical antipsychotic medications. In A. F. Schatzberg & C. B. Nemeroff (Eds.), *The American Psychiatric Publishing textbook of psychopharmacology*. Washington, DC: American Psychiatric Publishing.

Zweber, A. (2002). Cultural competence in pharmacy practice. *American Journal of Pharmaceutical Education, 66*(2), 172–176.

Chapter 10

RESEARCH IN CLINICAL PSYCHOPHARMACOLOGY

Robert E. McGrath

Of all the mental-health professions, psychologists receive the most extensive and intensive training as clinical researchers. Unfortunately, for many full-time clinicians, the opportunity to apply those skills declines after graduate school and the adage, "If you don't use it you lose it," applies. That pattern is likely to change as entities responsible for the reimbursement of health-care services increasingly expect clinical practices to be empirically defensible. Nowhere is the importance of maintaining and even enhancing research skills learned in graduate school as important as it is for the pharmacologically informed psychologist, for several reasons. First, practice standards for pharmacological treatment are rapidly updated in light of new research, a phenomenon that so far has no real parallel in psychosocial interventions. Some of the leading reference texts on psychotropic medications undergo significant revision every two to three years (Bezchlibnyk-Butler & Jeffries, 2007; Julien, 2007; Julien, Advocat, & Comaty, 2010; Virani, Bezchlibnyk-Butler, & Jeffries, 2009).

Second, the pharmaceutical industry regularly uses its tremendous resources to present its products in the most positive light possible. In recent years, comparisons between complete data reported to the Food and Drug Administration (FDA) and corresponding published articles have consistently demonstrated that the latter exaggerate medication efficacy through selective reporting of results (Turner, Matthews, Linardatos, Tell, & Rosenthal, 2008; Vedula, Bero, Scherer, & Dickersin, 2009). A comparison of seven meta-analyses published with pharmaceutical industry support versus parallel meta-analyses published under the auspices of the independent Cochrane Collaboration similarly found every one of the former recommended the medication without reservations, whereas none of the latter did, even though the mean effect sizes reported were similar (Jørgensen, Hilden, & Gøtzsche, 2006). Summaries of drug efficacy and safety provided in industry advertisements have also been found to be misleading (Villanueva, Peiró, Librero, & Pereiró, 2003; Wilkes, Doblin, & Shapiro, 1992). Finally, the prescribing psychologist must be prepared to deal with patients requesting medication based on direct-to-consumer advertising (Mintzes et al., 2003). The best defense against a distorted sense of a medication's efficacy and safety is a willingness to look at original literature and alternate sources of information, which requires a certain level of comfort with reading original research.

This chapter has several goals. First, it provides a review of basic concepts in research design and analysis that are particularly relevant to drug research. Second, it summarizes the drug approval process and some current findings concerning the relationship between pharmacotherapy and psychotherapy. Finally, I will talk about electronic resources relevant to maintaining currency in pharmacology. In doing so,

I will address the various research content domains identified for inclusion in the Psychopharmacology Examination for Psychologists (PEP).

RESEARCH METHODS

Research Validity

The *validity* of a research study refers to the extent to which inferences derived from that research must be considered conditional, that is, the extent to which those inferences are compromised by limitations of the study itself. Traditionally, the discussion of research validity focuses on four topics, though these should not be considered exhaustive (Wampold, Davis, & Good, 1990). *Internal validity* refers to the degree to which the inferred causes of a relationship are justified by the results. For example, Hokanson, Rubert, Welker, Hollander, and Hedeen (1989) found that social problems at the beginning of college were associated with whether a student becomes depressed over the ensuing months. If they had concluded from their findings that social problems were a cause of depression in college students, that would have compromised the internal validity of the study, because they did not have evidence of a causal relationship. Internal validity is compromised by the extent to which *confounds* or *nuisance variables*, variables that could cause *spurious relationships* between variables in the study, are not controlled. For example, preexisting differences between groups in a drug trial in level of motivation or hopefulness could create a spurious relationship between treatment condition and outcome. *Allegiance effects* can occur when one or more sites are particularly associated with one of the treatments, resulting in a heightened level of expectation for the efficacy of that treatment and unusually large treatment effects. The impact of allegiance on outcomes has been more thoroughly studied in relation to psychotherapy effects. For example, Gaffan, Tsaousis, and Kemp-Wheeler (1995) reanalyzed data from an early review of cognitive-behavioral therapy (CBT) that had found it superior to other treatments, and they concluded through the reanalysis that half of the difference was attributable to allegiance effects.

External validity has to do with the degree to which inferences are likely to generalize across populations and contexts. Hokanson et al. (1989) conducted their study on the relationship between social problems and depression at a large state university in Florida. The same results may be less likely at a school with a very different student population.

Though it is not the case in all research, the design of drug research often requires accepting a trade-off between internal and external validity. Specifically, *efficacy studies* are ones in which internal validity is emphasized, to the detriment of external validity. This is usually accomplished by selecting a fairly heterogeneous sample so that effects cannot be attributable to confounds such as other diagnoses. *Effectiveness studies* are those in which external validity is emphasized, to the detriment of internal validity. For example, the Treatment for Adolescents with Depression Study (TADS) is the largest study conducted to date of psychotherapy, pharmacotherapy, and their combination as treatments of depression. TADS was designed as an efficacy study. The protocol was intended to maximize the internal validity of the study, so that any differences between groups were likely to represent differential impact of the treatments on depression. Although the *inclusionary criteria* were reasonable—for example, participants were 12–17 years old and met criteria for major depressive disorder (MDD) at two measurement points—the protocol included 12 *exclusionary criteria*, including bipolar disorder, severe conduct disorder, and a history of treatment failure (The Treatment for Adolescents with Depression Study [TADS] Team, 2005). Out of 2,804 initial contacts, only 439 met criteria for participation, and 19 of those did not meet all criteria. Of the 2,365 who were rejected, 79.2% demonstrated stable depression during the screening. That means that, of approximately 2,312 adolescents who were stably depressed, only 439 (18%) met all the criteria. In carefully selecting a homogeneous sample, so that treatment effects are not likely to reflect changes in any other condition than depression,[1] the researchers generated results that can only be assumed applicable to a very specific population of depressed adolescents. Once efficacy studies demonstrate that a drug has an effect on the disorder, effectiveness studies with less tightly controlled conditions are used to evaluate whether they work in the real world. It is not unusual to find that compliance with medication regimens declines substantially in less tightly controlled circumstances, or that improvement over the control condition is not as great with more heterogeneous samples.

Construct validity has to do with the relationship between the operations performed in the process of conducting the study (the administration of questionnaires, standardized observations of participants, and treatment conditions) and the latent constructs they are intended to represent. For example, anxiety is a construct with physiological, experiential, and behavioral implications. Simply administering a self-report measure to gauge changes in anxiety resulting from drug treatment may not provide a sufficiently valid representation of the treatment's effect. Standardized observations require that raters are trained to assure consistency. This may involve some combination of formal training, observation of others collecting data, completion of pilot administrations, and continued training until some standard of acceptable performance is achieved. Both questionnaires and ratings should also meet standard psychometric expectations for reliability, which will be discussed further on. A treatment administered in an inadequate manner (medication given in insufficient dosage, or psychotherapy administered poorly) also represents a failure of construct validity. When the first major efficacy study on depression, the National Institute of Mental Health Treatment of Depression Collaborative Research Program, generated evidence that CBT was not as effective as medication, Jacobson and Hollon (1996) hypothesized that differences in outcomes for CBT when compared to previous studies suggested the treatment may not have been administered competently at some sites, a hypothesis to which the study authors responded (Elkin, Gibbons, Shea, & Shaw, 1996). Developing a construct-valid treatment protocol for a medication involves determining its *therapeutic window*, that is, the range of dosages in which the medication's effects are desirable. It also requires establishing a fixed set of steps for *titrating*, or adjusting, the dosage when appropriate.

Finally, *statistical conclusion validity* has to do with activities that compromise the validity of the conclusions derived from the quantitative data. Examples of threats to statistical conclusion validity include *fishing expeditions* (conducting numerous analyses and only reporting those that are significant), violation of statistical *assumptions*, and insufficient *power* (a topic discussed further, later in this chapter).

---

[1]Homogeneous samples are also more likely to produce significant results, all other factors being equal, because of less error variance or variability within groups.

Study Design

The most important factor contributing to the internal validity of a research study is the type of study conducted, whether it represents a true experiment, quasi-experiment, or observational study. A study represents a *true experiment* if (1) the researcher randomly assigns participants to treatment condition, and (2) the impact of differences in treatment condition (the *independent variable*) on some outcome (the *dependent variable*) is evaluated. A study represents a *quasi-experiment* if there are treatment conditions to which participants are not randomly assigned. *Observational research* (sometimes called correlational research) occurs when there is no assignment and no manipulation by the researcher as there is in treatment conditions. Each plays an important role in drug research.

True experiments always involve a *between-group design*, a comparison of two or more groups. True experiments conducted to test the efficacy of a treatment are often called *randomized controlled trials (RCT)*, also known as randomized clinical trials. By randomly assigning participants to an active treatment or a control group, the RCT offers control over potential confounds. Consider a study in which participants are assigned to an antidepressant or a placebo. If one group is more optimistic than the other, or less depressed to start with, or more socially involved, then these variables may account for better outcomes in that group rather than differences in the treatments assigned to the two groups. A word of caution is in order, however. Randomization is not a magic bullet; a certain minimum sample size is necessary. Just as a sample of two coin flips is much more likely to consist of 100% heads than a sample of 300 coin flips, groups are more likely to be equalized by randomization across all possible confounds as group size increases. In the only study conducted to date on this topic, Hsu (1989) examined the relationship between sample size and the likelihood of successful random assignment. He concluded that random assignment is likely to be effective when the number of participants in each of two groups is ≥40. Smaller group sizes (20–40) are generally acceptable. When the group size is 15 or less, random assignment is likely to fail 10% of the time or more.

Reports of RCTs are so important to the medical literature that guidelines for reporting results from RCTs have been developed. The *CONSORT statement* (CONsolidated Standards of Reporting Trials; www.consort-statement.org) consists of 25 recommendations covering every aspect of a research article for an RCT from the choice of title to the contents of the author footnotes. If you are involved in RCT research, the CONSORT statement can help you improve the quality of your manuscript. The CONSORT statement can also help you identify gaps in articles summarizing RCTs. When I find an article omits important elements covered in the CONSORT statement, I wonder why the authors chose to do so, and it helps me to be a more critical consumer of research.

Though the RCT is often touted as the methodological gold standard, several quasi-experimental designs appear with some regularity in the medication research. The first is the between-group study with nonrandom assignment, sometimes called the *preexisting groups design*. Nonrandom assignment usually occurs in clinical research for practical reasons; for example, the researcher may need to administer active treatment to the group that meets Thursday night and placebo to the group that meets Tuesday night. The absence of randomization to treatment increases the likelihood of preexisting group differences (though it may be reasonable to assume there is no basis for a systematic difference between participants who volunteered to attend on Tuesday versus Thursday night). Though analytic strategies will be described later that are intended to mitigate such differences, it is best to employ randomization if at all possible.[2]

A second quasi-experimental option sometimes found in the drug literature is the *repeated measures design* or *within-group design*. The most basic of these is the simple *pretest-posttest design*. This involves a single group that receives the active treatment, and the analysis focuses on aggregate change from pretest to posttest. This design has some obvious advantages in terms of the number of participants needed. However, the absence of a comparison to individuals who did not receive the active treatment clearly compromises its usefulness. Specifically, it is impossible to partition that portion of change attributable to the active treatment versus various potential confounds such as expectation of change or maturation, so that the treatment effects may overestimate the effect that would be found in a more controlled between-group study. In a large-scale analysis of the efficacy of psychosocial interventions, Lipsey and Wilson (1993) found effect sizes from one-group pretest-posttest designs were on average 61% larger than those resulting from between-group designs. Even so, the pretest-posttest design can be a reasonable option when (1) failure to provide an active treatment can have serious consequences for the participant, and/or (2) the dependent variable is unlikely to be responsive to confounding variables. The study of antiretrovirals as a treatment of the human immunodeficiency virus represents a good example of a situation in which the design is particularly useful. Preliminary animal trials of medications are similarly often conducted as one-group studies.

Some studies intended to demonstrate the effectiveness of psychotropic medication in humans are conducted using the pretest-posttest design. When a new treatment intervention is evaluated, researchers will often conduct a *pilot study*, a small-sample study that is often weak in terms of both internal and external validity. However, demonstration that a pilot study provided some evidence suggestive that the treatment is useful, combined with a reasonable rationale for that treatment, often provides the basis for a successful grant proposal. Results from the pilot study are also often used in the process of estimating the sample size for a more comprehensive study. Some pilot studies are designed as an *open trial* or *open-label trial*, in which all participants receive the targeted treatment and no one is *blind* to (unaware of) condition.

A more rigorous repeated measures design is the *crossover study*, in which each participant receives all the treatments. For example, one could conduct a study of aripiprazole in which schizophrenics sequentially receive the active treatment and a placebo. This design offers an alternative means of controlling between-group systematic differences in potential confounds by using the same participants in both conditions. It also cuts the number of participants needed in half. However, there are certain problems that the sequential design introduces, referred to generally as *order effects*. If participants can be expected to improve over the course of any treatment (generically called a *practice effect*) then the treatment administered second will tend to look better on average, all other factors being equal. If, instead, participants can be expected to deteriorate over the time frame of the study (a *fatigue effect*), then the opposite will occur. A third possibility is a *carryover effect*, a lingering effect from one treatment that interferes with assessing the true impact of the next treatment.

[2]Wilkinson and APA Task Force on Statistical Inference (1999) recommended calling the participants receiving the alternative to the focal treatment the *control group* if random assignment has occurred, the *comparison group* if it has not. This recommendation has never really caught on but I consider it a very good one.

Some control over these potential confounds is offered by two methodological tools specific to the crossover study. The first is the *washout period*, an interval between treatments that allows return to baseline. In some studies, the washout period is a fixed interval in which return to baseline is likely to occur, but the better option is to monitor the dependent variable during the washout period and delay implementation of the next treatment until the participant has returned to baseline level. Unfortunately, some conditions are unlikely to return to the baseline level once treatment has been implemented. This is especially true for certain mental disorders that are particularly sensitive to contextual circumstances such as depression.

The second tool is *counterbalancing*, alternating the order in which treatments are administered across participants. The best option is *full counterbalancing*, in which all possible orders of the treatments are employed. Full counterbalancing can be problematic when the number of treatments is large, because the number of orders is equal to the factorial of the number of treatments. If there are five treatments A–E, there are $5! = 5(4)(3)(2)(1) = 120$ possible orders, for example, ABCDE, DCEAB, CAEBD, AECDB, EDABC, and so forth. Although full counterbalancing provides the most complete protection against order effects in this situation, it would require at least 120 participants, and even then only one person would be exposed to each order. With a large number of treatments, *partial counterbalancing* is often the more practical option, which uses as many orders as there are treatments by simply moving the first treatment in one order to the end of the next order: ABCDE, BCDEA, CDEAB, DEABC, EABCD. Notice that each treatment appears in each serial position (A is first in one order, second in another order, etc.). Crossover studies tend to involve very few treatments, usually no more than three, so that full counterbalancing is possible (I will leave it to you to compute how many orders that would be). Whichever counterbalancing strategy is used, participants should be randomly assigned to order to avoid any systematic differences.

The crossover design is most likely to be useful when (a) the disorder is chronic and likely to remain consistent across the treatment period, (b) effects of the treatment are temporary so that return to baseline between treatments is feasible, and (c) the number of treatments is relatively small. Becausee the second condition is particularly unlikely in mental disorders, the crossover design is not nearly as common as the RCT.

The third quasi-experimental design that merits discussion in the context of drug research is the *single-subject design*, a study involving a single participant or a small group of participants administered treatment individually. Single-subject designs are potentially plagued by problems with both internal and external validity. The external validity problems are the more serious, though in reality perhaps not much more of an issue than in small-sample studies where participants are not randomly sampled from the population.

Various methodological tools are available for enhancing the internal validity of single-subject studies. One that is relevant in the context of drug research is the *ABAB design*, in which the treatment is alternately administered and removed. This strategy is similar to the within-group design. The second most popular single-subject design is the *multiple baseline design*. In the context of drug research, the multiple baseline design usually involves a small group of participants who begin baseline observation at the same time. After some period of baseline observation of all participants, in which the target condition is demonstrated to be stable, the first participant is administered the treatment. The rest of the sample remains in baseline observation. After some period determined by the researcher, treatment is extended to a second participant, and the process continues until treatment has been administered to all. The stepwise introduction of treatment allows a much stronger case for concluding that change reflected the treatment rather than other factors. It is this systematic approach to enhancing internal validity that distinguishes single-subject designs from *case studies*, which involve observation of a single individual without systematic manipulation of the treatment.

The case study is an example of an observational study. Research into the population of individuals receiving some medication without actual manipulation of the drug regimen by the researcher represents a particularly popular observational design. Observational studies can be *cross-sectional*, involving measurement at one point in time. For example, evaluating the rate of tardive dyskinesia among individuals taking atypical antipsychotics would represent a cross-sectional study. Cross-sectional studies can also be *retrospective*, in which participants are asked about events in the past. Individuals hospitalized for suicide attempts might be asked what antidepressants they took in the past. Alternatively, individuals using a certain antidepressant might be followed to observe changes in suicidal gestures over time. This would represent a *longitudinal design*, which is always *prospective*.

OTHER METHODOLOGICAL CONCEPTS

Controlling Expectations

Beyond the overall design of the study, there are a number of methodological concepts that are important to understand in the context of drug research. The first two have to do with controlling expectations and beliefs as contributors to treatment outcome. This is particularly important in the context of psychotropic medications, where changes in affect are often a key component of anticipated treatment effects and such changes are very sensitive to expectations. For this reason, a *waitlist control* is considered weak in internal validity, because the group receiving active treatment has greater expectations of improvement. A better alternative is a *comparator* condition. The most common comparator condition involves a *placebo*, some overtly similar intervention that should not demonstrate ameliorative physiological effects but should activate similar expectations of improvement. Although it is often difficult to identify a compelling placebo alternative to psychotherapy, since any reasonable psychosocial intervention may well meet the definition for psychotherapy, the sugar pill offers a reasonable placebo alternative to medication. In fact, an inert pill sufficiently activates beliefs about medication that researchers often notice *nocebo* effects, deterioration or side effects in response to the placebo (although the term *nocebo* is also sometimes used in relation to anticipated adverse events associated with a medication). The safety profile for a medication reflects the total number of adverse reactions experienced, but for obvious reasons the FDA is particularly concerned about differences between negative responses to the active drug and the placebo. It has also been suggested that, as exposure to drug advertising increases, placebo effects have been increasing, making it more difficult for drug companies to meet FDA criteria for drug approval (Silberman, 2009).

Even so, critics have argued that completely inert pills offer an insufficient alternative to drugs with activating effects on the central nervous system, because the experience of those effects can heighten expectations of change. In a classic review of studies in which antidepressants were compared to a placebo with activating effects,

Moncrieff, Wessely, and Hardy (1998) concluded that as much as half the effectiveness of antidepressants may be due to this activating effect.

The second methodological concept used to reduce effects due to expectations is blinding. It was mentioned previously that open trials typically do not involve any blinding. In the *single-blind study* participants are unaware of the treatment they are receiving. In a *double-blind study* both participants and care providers (psychologists, physicians, nurses, etc.) are unaware of treatment condition. In a *triple-blind study*, participants, care providers, and data gatherers (including trained raters) are unaware of treatment.[3] Though blinding is an important tool, it is important to recognize that information can still be transferred. As an interviewer in one study who was technically unaware of treatment condition once told me, "I may be blind, but I'm not deaf."

Third Variables

In addition to confounds, other variables can be important to consider in evaluating the relationship between a treatment variable (active versus control condition) and outcome variables. *Moderators* refer to third variables that influence the strength of the relationship between the treatment variable (active treatment versus placebo) and outcomes. Psychologists often equate moderation with the analysis of *interactions*, but a number of statistical methods are available for detecting moderators.

An important example of a moderator is provided in the *dose-response curve*, variation in the relationship between treatment and outcome across medication dosage. The dose-response curve is often represented by a graph in which dosage of the medication is plotted on the X axis, and mean or percent improvement is plotted on the Y axis. Evidence that improvement increases with dosage in the active treatment but not in the placebo condition provides powerful evidence for an efficacious medication. When designing studies, it is important to remember that the dose-response curve is never an infinitely increasing relationship. Most medications have a therapeutic window outside of which the medication is ineffective, or nocebo effects suppress treatment effects. A second important moderator is symptom severity. For example, Fournier et al. (2010) described a severity-response curve for antidepressants, where improvement over placebo is greatest for those with more severe depression, whereas treatment effects approach zero for those with mild-moderate depression.

A less common phenomenon involves the *nested design*. If treatment A is only administered by providers 1 and 2, whereas treatment B is only administered by providers 3 and 4, then provider is "nested within" treatment. Similarly, if treatment involves group meetings so that members of the group can influence each other, or if each hospital only administers a single treatment, then nesting has occurred. This nesting introduces potential error variance into the design. Baldwin, Murray, and Shadish (2005) demonstrate that when the statistical design ignores nesting in the research design, spurious significant findings can result.

---

[3]Devereaux et al. (2001) found the use of blinding terminology is not as standard as the text would suggest. Instead of assuming terms such as *triple blinding* are interpreted consistently, the CONSORT statement recommends that reports of drug trials should simply indicate which groups involved in the study were blinded.

STATISTICAL CONCEPTS

Inferential Strategies

Traditionally, the most popular statistical strategy for drawing inferences about populations from samples in psychology has been significance testing. Psychologists' inferential practices have been gradually changing over the years, and a quiet revolution is currently underway in statistical methods. More detailed discussions of this revolution are available (McGrath, in press; Rodgers, 2010); this section will provide brief summaries of the issues involved.

Significance testing refers to an inferential strategy first described by Sir Ronald Fisher that focuses on the rejection or retention of *null hypotheses* that usually— although not necessarily—hypothesized the absence of an *effect*, usually a relationship between two or more variables, in a population. If the null hypothesis is true, there are two possible outcomes: Retaining the null hypothesis, which represents a correct decision; or rejecting the null hypothesis, which would be an error. Although Fisher did not use this terminology, the latter has come to be referred to as a *Type I error*. Though a Type I error is always possible, the probability of a Type I error for circumstances in which the null hypothesis is true is easily set to whatever value is desired. This desired level has since come to be called the *alpha level*, and is usually set to 0.05 and sometimes to 0.01. This means that if the null hypothesis is true, the results of a study should only lead to rejection of the null hypothesis 5% (or 1% if alpha is set to 0.01) of the time.

Neyman and Pearson (1933) subsequently criticized Fisher for failing to consider the implications of rejecting or retaining the null hypothesis under conditions in which the null hypothesis is false. They introduced a complementary hypothesis, the *alternative hypothesis*, that suggested the existence of an effect. If the alternative hypothesis is true, then retention of the null hypothesis would represent a *Type II error*, and they referred to the desired probability of such an error (if the null hypothesis is false) as the *beta level*. They referred to the probability of a correct rejection of the null hypothesis as the power of the study. Where alpha is set easily, by selecting a *critical value* for the significance test that is associated with the desired probability if the null hypothesis is true, setting power is more difficult and requires a *power analysis*.

To summarize, there are four possible outcomes to the decision to reject or retain the null hypothesis:

		Fact	
		Null hypothesis (H_0) is true	Alternative hypothesis (H_1) is true
Statistical decision	Reject	Incorrect rejection (Type I error) $p(incorrect\ rejection) = \alpha$	Correct rejection $p(correct\ rejection) = 1 - \beta$ (power)
	Retain	Correct retention $p(correct\ retention) = 1 - \alpha$	Incorrect retention (Type II error) $p(incorrect\ retention) = \beta$

There are three factors that universally affect power (though there are others that are specific to certain statistical analyses). The larger alpha is, the greater the power is. However, you do not want to increase alpha beyond 0.05 because it will result in an excessive Type I error rate should the null hypothesis be true. Second, the larger the size of the effect in the population, the greater the power in the sample. Various *effect size statistics* have been developed in recent years to estimate population effects.

However, since the effect size is a *parameter*, a population value, the researcher does not have much control over its size. Finally, the larger the sample size, the greater the power of the study. This is the factor most directly under the control of the researcher. Therefore, power analysis involves identifying the sample size necessary to achieve a desired level of power given the desired alpha level and the estimated size of the effect in the population. Though once considered almost an intractable task because of its computational complexity, Cohen (1988) did a great deal to popularize and simplify power analysis, and the free GPower program (Erdfelder, Faul, & Buchner, 1996) is now used widely to conduct power analyses.

More recently, significance testing itself has been roundly criticized. There are various reasons for this criticism (see Kline, 2004), but several stand out. First, the idea of focusing completely on evaluating whether an effect exists, without ever trying to estimate that effect, represents a very odd strategy. To draw a parallel, imagine that all research on gravity tested the hypothesis "things drop" and never tried to estimate how fast they drop. Second, many psychological studies are underpowered: It has been suggested that the typical analysis in psychological research is associated with power of about 0.50, meaning that the null hypothesis is retained for half of the nonzero effects (e.g., Cashen & Geiger, 2004). This failure to reject null hypotheses even when they are not true has had all sorts of negative consequences for the accumulation of knowledge in psychology (Schmidt, 1996). As a result, psychological researchers increasingly rely on sample-based effect size estimates and *confidence intervals*, a range of values in which the true value is likely to fall. The most recent edition of the American Psychological Association (2010) *Publication Manual* stops just short of mandating their use, and it is likely the next edition will actively discourage the use of significance tests.

To understand the value of confidence intervals, consider this example. Two researchers studying different topics both find a sample correlation of 0.30 and reject the null hypothesis of no effect in the population. These results provide us with evidence of positive correlations in the population, but technically do not tell us much about how large those population correlations are. Both researchers also compute 95% confidence intervals for their correlations. Researcher A's confidence interval stretches from 0.03 to 0.45, whereas Researcher B's is bounded by 0.27 and 0.33. Clearly, 0.30 is a more trustworthy estimate of the population correlation in Research B's study than in Researcher A's. Confidence intervals and effect size estimates, computed using exactly the same data used to compute significance testing statistics, are much more informative about the population, and increasingly are considered mandatory elements of a research report.

Significance Testing Statistics

The most popular statistics in psychology developed specifically for significance testing are the t, F, and χ^2. These statistics are applicable to a wide variety of research settings and effect sizes. The t-test is used to evaluate simple differences between two groups, whether they are within-group or between-group, and to evaluate null hypotheses about correlations.

The F-test is used extensively in conjunction with the *analysis of variance* (ANOVA), which is a general strategy for evaluating the impact of categorical independent variables on dimensional dependent variables. Particularly useful variants in the context of drug research include the *mixed-factors ANOVA* (in which treatment condition represents a between-group factor and time of measurement such as baseline, posttreatment, and follow-up represent a within-group factor), and the *analysis of covariance* (ANCOVA). ANCOVA allows you to equalize participants on some potential confound, which is now called the *covariate*. The most common covariate is baseline level. That means that the results of the ANOVA are adjusted as if all participants had the same level of depression or psychotic symptoms at baseline. As a result, baseline no longer needs to be treated as a level of the within-group factor.

The χ^2 statistic is relevant when the independent and dependent variables are both categorical; for example, when the independent variable is treatment condition and the dependent variable is improved–not improved. This statistic is also increasingly used in conjunction with sophisticated statistical techniques that have become popular in recent years such as logistic regression, structural equation modeling, and survival analysis (described later). This flexibility reflects the statistic's usefulness as a general indicator of whether sample statistics support a particular model of how the elements in a set of variables relate to each other in the population.

Effect Size Statistics

Probably the best-known effect-size statistics among psychologists are the *standardized mean difference* and the *correlation coefficient*. The former is usually symbolized d, although variants are also symbolized by g and Δ (capital delta). This issue of variants is important, because I know many studies in which (a) it is hard to tell which formula is being used for the standardized mean difference, or (b) the wrong formula is used. In particular, there is a variant of d appropriate for within-group designs yet the between-group formula is very often used instead (Dunlap, Cortina, Vaslow, & Burke, 1996). The standardized mean difference computes the difference between two groups' means relative to the within-group standard deviations. A d value of 0.50 means the difference between the means is one-half the standard deviation, for example. In contrast, the correlation is a standardized measure of the degree to which one variable can be predicted from the other on a scale from –1.0 to +1.0, with 0 meaning no predictive value. The correlation and d represent two different approaches to understanding how strongly two variables are related.

A variety of effect-size statistics have also been developed specifically for circumstances in which the independent and dependent variables are both dichotomous. Table 10.1 provides data for a study in which two treatments are compared in terms of the number of individuals who improved/did not improve.

The correlation could be computed here (sometimes called the *phi coefficient* when both variables are dichotomous), and the value would be .20. However, at least three statistics specifically intended for two dichotomous variables might also be used:

1. The *relative risk ratio* (*RR*) compares the proportion of patients improving with medication versus the proportion improving with placebo:

Table 10.1   Example of Dichotomous Independent and Dependent Variables

	Improved	Not Improved
Medication	$n_{11} = 14$	$n_{12} = 36$
Placebo	$n_{21} = 6$	$n_{22} = 44$

$$RR = \frac{n_{11}/(n_{11} + n_{12})}{n_{21}/(n_{21} + n_{22})} = \frac{14/(14 + 36)}{6/(6 + 44)} = 2.33$$

If there is no effect, then $RR = 1.0$, for effective treatments $RR > 1.0$, and for ineffective treatment, RR is between 0 and 1.0. A value of 2.33 means that a person taking the medication is 2.33 times as likely to improve as the person taking placebo.

2. The *odds ratio* (OR) represents the odds of improving with medication versus the odds of improving with placebo:

$$OR = \frac{n_{11}/n_{12}}{n_{21}/n_{22}} = \frac{14/36}{6/44} = 2.85$$

If there is no effect, then $OR = 1.0$, for effective treatments $OR > 1.0$, and for ineffective treatment OR is between 0 and 1.0. Because a no-effect point of 1.0 is potentially confusing, researchers often report the natural log of the odds ratio instead, so that the no-effect value is shifted to 0 as is the case for d and r.[4]

A number of articles have been published critical of the odds ratio (e.g., Sackett, Deeks, & Altman, 1996). Perhaps the most serious problem with this statistic is that people do not appreciate the difference between odds and the proportions used to compute *relative risk*. If 75 out of 100 people improve on the medication, the proportion improving is 75/100 = 0.75 but the odds of improving are 75 to 25 = 75/25 = 3. Notice that a proportion is always limited to the range 0–1; there is no limit to the range of odds. I have seen published articles in which the authors confused the odds ratio with the risk ratio, for example, suggesting an odds ratio of 2.85 means those taking the medication are 2.85 times as likely to improve, but what it really means is that the *odds* of improvement are 2.85 times as large. I suspect this mistake occurs because people have a better intuitive grasp of proportions than odds. Unfortunately, certain more complicated statistical procedures, such as logistic regression, rely heavily on the odds ratio, so it will remain a popular statistic. Be careful how you interpret this statistic!

3. The *number needed to treat* (NNT) represents the number of cases needed to receive the active treatment to generate one more positive outcome than the comparison treatment:

$$NNT = \frac{1}{n_{11}/(n_{11} + n_{12}) - n_{21}/(n_{21} + n_{22})} = \frac{1}{14/(14 + 36) - 6/(6 + 44)} = 6.25$$

This value means that if you treat 6.25 people with the medication, you will get one more positive outcome than you would from treating those 6.25 people with placebo. NNT differs from the two previous statistics in that smaller NNT values are better. One problem with NNT is that it is scaled oddly, though the scaling makes sense in the context of the information that the statistic is trying to provide. When there is no effect, so the proportion improving from medication is the same as that improving from placebo, then the denominator is 0 and NNT is infinitely large.

---

[4]Standard mean difference and correlation coefficient, respectively.

If everyone taking medication improves and no one on placebo improves then NNT is 1.0. Therefore, values closer to 1.0 are more desirable for positive outcomes.

These statistics are also often used to compare the safety of the active treatment with placebo. When the NNT is used to evaluate the number of cases needed to receive the active treatment to generate one more adverse event than the comparison treatment, it is often referred to as the *number needed to harm*.

The example provided in Table 10.1 demonstrates one of the important lessons to learn about commonly used effect size statistics. These statistics estimate the efficacy of medication's relative risk, the probability of improvement in the active treatment relative to the control condition. Compared to this placebo, the medication tested in Table 10.1 was relatively more efficacious. This is a very different issue than the medication's *absolute risk*, the probability of improvement in the active treatment. Improvement occurred for substantially less than half of those who took the medication. This is not a criticism of the medication or the statistics: Finding the medication is better than placebo is a worthwhile finding. However, consumers of research often ignore the difference between absolute and relative efficacy, a lapse that can tend to encourage overestimating the likelihood of improvement in response to the medication.

It was noted earlier that the confidence interval is an increasingly important inferential tool in individual studies. In fact, the computation of confidence intervals has probably become the standard in medical research. Across studies, the most important inferential tool in use today is the *meta-analysis*. Meta-analysis is a complex topic. There are competing approaches available, numerous (at times inconsistent) sources available on how best to conduct a meta-analysis (e.g., Borenstein, Hedges, Higgins, & Rothstein, 2009; Hunter & Schmidt, 2004), various statistical concepts and formulas to master, and a variety of decisions to be made during the process that can change the outcome of the analysis dramatically. At heart, though, the concept of a meta-analysis is quite simple, which is the averaging of effect size estimates across studies so the resulting mean can be considered as a best estimate of the population effect size. Given the limitations of significance testing noted earlier, it is not surprising that meta-analysis has revolutionized the integration of findings across studies. The *PRISMA statement* (Preferred Reporting Items for Systematic Reviews and Meta-Analyses; http://www.prisma-statement.org), formerly called QUOROM (QUality Of Reporting Of Meta-analyses) does for meta-analyses what the CONSORT statement does for RCTs. PRISMA consists of 27 recommendations for the conduct and reporting of meta-analyses. Again, failure of a meta-analytic study to comply with PRISMA recommendations should be considered a red flag.[5]

Attrition

All drug studies suffer from attrition, some more than others, and various statistical strategies have been developed to address issues of attrition. One approach to attrition is simply to ignore those individuals who left the trial early, the *observed cases* approach. In an antidepressant versus placebo drug trial in which 100 people

---

[5]It is not really relevant to the present topic, but for the sake of completeness I will note there is a third statement called STARD (STAndards for the Reporting of Diagnostic accuracy studies; www.stard-statement.org) that consists of 25 recommendations for studies that attempt to classify participants into groups.

are assigned to each treatment, if only 35 participants in the active treatment condition and 63 in the placebo condition complete the 12-week trial, then analysis is based on 98 cases.

It is often suggested that this approach inevitably provides a skewed perspective on the efficacy of the medication, because one would expect withdrawal is not a random phenomenon. The alternative is some form of *intent to treat* analysis, in which all participants are included in the analysis regardless of whether they completed the trial. The most common variant is the *last observation carried forward* approach. In the antidepressant study mentioned in the previous paragraph, if participant 132 completed three weeks of the trial before withdrawing, that participant's Week-3 data is entered into the final analysis. Including all participants enhances the power of the analysis, since the sample size is 200 rather than 98. However, it means mixing data from various points in the trial into a single analysis. Intuitively, one would expect observed cases and last observation carried forward analyses to result in very different results, but this does not always prove to be the case (e.g., Kirsch, Moore, Scoboria, & Nicholls, 2002).

The methods described so far focus on how to deal with attrition as a problem in drug research. *Survival analysis* differs in that it is used specifically to study the attrition process. Survival analysis is actually a suite of statistical tools used to estimate the length of time until some event occurs. The word *survival* has a broad meaning here. In industry it has to do with how long it will be before some part fails, and in medical-research settings, survival analysis is often used to estimate how long it will be before a patient dies. Of course, mortality can be a focus of interest even in drug research, but in the context of psychotropic medications, survival analysis is most commonly used to study the topic of attrition: how many people are likely to drop out of each treatment, and what variables predict attrition and time to attrition.

Construct Validity

The final set of statistical concepts to be discussed here has to do with ensuring the construct validity of the questionnaires and ratings used in drug trials. *Classical test theory* represents the dominant approach to evaluating measurement devices in psychology, though this approach has significant limitations (McGrath, in press). At the heart of classical test theory is the demonstration of *reliability*, a term that has been defined mathematically in terms of the proportion of variance in a set of scores that is not error variance. Reliability is usually estimated in one of three ways. For a multi-item questionnaire, *internal reliability* can be estimated. Internal or test reliability has to do with consistency in responding across the items. The most common statistic used for this purpose is *coefficient alpha*, alternatively called Cronbach's alpha. External or *test-retest reliability* is estimated by administering the same instrument twice under conditions in which responding should be consistent. The most common statistic used to evaluate consistency across retests is some form of the *intraclass correlation coefficient*, a statistic closely related to the traditional correlation coefficient. For cases in which trained observers make ratings, reliability across multiple raters can be evaluated. This *inter-rater reliability* is also usually evaluated using the intraclass correlation coefficient.

Note that the computation of reliability always requires multiple observations: multiple items in the case of internal reliability, multiple administrations of the same scale over time for test-retest reliability, and observation by multiple raters in the case of inter-rater reliability. Reliability in the population is always on a scale from

0 to 1.0, 0 meaning all the variance in scores is due to error (no consistency in the multiple observations for any one person) and 1.0 meaning none of the variance is due to error (no inconsistency in the multiple observations for any one person). When correlations of 0.30 are common in psychology between measures of different variables, the multiple observations that comprise a measurement should match closely. Reliability values for measures used in research should be at least 0.60, and values of 0.80 or higher are desirable (Shrout, 1998).

BEST PRACTICES IN DRUG RESEARCH

The Drug Approval Process

The process of drug approval research in the United States is regulated by the FDA.[6] Prior to initiating this process, the sponsoring organization typically has conducted a series of preliminary studies attempting to gauge the *pharmacodynamics* (the drug's effect on the body), *pharmacokinetics* (the body's effect on the drug), and toxicity of the drug when administered to humans. The drug is not administered to humans at this point, but it may be studied *in vitro* (test tubes) or *in vivo* (in animals or in culture). Based on findings from previous studies without human participants, the organization has the option of conducting a small-sample study involving administration of a single, subtherapeutic dose of the medication to humans to verify that the medication acts in humans as expected (*Phase 0*).

If preliminary studies produce encouraging results, clinical trials can begin. These trials consist of four phases. *Phase I: Human Pharmacology* trials also involve small samples. Phase I investigations tend to focus on three issues: (1) by far the most important issue is safety and toxicity; (2) evaluation of pharmacodynamics and pharmacokinetics in humans; and (3) *dose ranging*, identifying the range of dosages that is likely to define the therapeutic window. Phase I trials generally involve healthy volunteers except when medications are being tested for serious conditions for which alternative treatment options are unavailable. *Phase II: Therapeutic Exploratory* trials expand the study of safety (and sometimes dose-ranging) to a larger sample. They also represent the first large-scale evaluation of efficacy in patients. *Phase III: Therapeutic Confirmatory* trials represent large-scale multisite investigations. Organizations are hesitant to fund such large trials unless they have good reason to believe the medication will survive greater scrutiny, so most drugs that fail the process are terminated at the end of Phase II. Often, the organization will sponsor several Phase III trials with the recognition that there will be some variability in outcomes. The strongest results from these trials will be highlighted in the marketing of the medication, including selective reporting of results in manuscripts submitted for publication. Once the Phase III trials are completed, the entire body of evidence collected to date is submitted for FDA approval of the medication for distribution and sale. *Phase IV: Therapeutic Use* trials represent the expectation of ongoing monitoring. From a public health perspective, Phase IV is very important for the detection of very low-base, high-impact side effects such as liver damage or suicidality that can lead to additional *black box warnings* (warnings of serious side effects) and even withdrawal of the medication from the market. Though a few such withdrawals have

---

[6]See Chapter 8, Figure 8.8.

garnered a great deal of attention, such as that for Vioxx, FDA approval is withdrawn for about 3% of medications (Lasser et al., 2002). Phase IV is also important for evaluating the medication's efficacy and safety in populations not included in the prior trials, such as pregnant women. From the company's perspective, this can also be a period to gather information about whether the drug can have unanticipated benefits for other conditions comorbid with the approved condition. Increasingly, drug manufacturers continue to pursue additional uses for their medications once an initial use has been approved.

Special Populations

The evaluation of medications in special populations based on age, pregnancy, or cultural status is an issue involving practical, ethical, and public health implications. Even in Phase III trials with thousands of participants, the number of participants of minority background is often minuscule (U.S. Department of Health and Human Services, 2001). This disparity can reflect difficulties recruiting individuals representing cultural minorities into research and/or difficulties finding members of such minorities who meet the stringent criteria for an efficacy study. To some extent, difficulties recruiting individuals of minority background can be addressed through involving community leaders in the research through churches, schools, or a community advisory board.

There is a similar lack of efficacy evidence for the use of medications with children, so that many of the medications used with children represent off-label use. The Best Pharmaceuticals for Children Act of 2002 was intended to address this shortfall. In return for conducting pediatric efficacy research, the FDA can extend a drug maker's *market exclusivity* (prohibition of generic alternatives) for up to six months. It also permitted the FDA to request the National Institutes of Health to fund research into specified topics in pediatric pharmacology. The Pediatric Research Equity Act of 2003 went further, allowing the FDA to mandate manufacturer-sponsored pediatric drug trials if such research is deemed necessary for the public health and other mechanisms have failed to generate action.

Ethical Conduct of Research

Any organization receiving federal funding that conducts research with humans is expected to maintain an *Institutional Review Board* (IRB) charged with reviewing and approving all research conducted under the auspices of that organization. IRB procedures are defined by the U.S. Department of Health and Human Services. Canada has established a parallel system of Research Ethics Boards, and the International Conference on Harmonisation has attempted to establish universal standards for research review. Among the issues IRBs evaluate when approving research are the use of *informed consent*, confidentiality, and weighing of the potential benefits against the potential risks and costs of participating.

Informed consent is often the most problematic of these factors. Informed consent should include at least the following: (a) a statement that this is a consent for research; (b) a description of the research and what is expected of the participant, including duration of expected involvement; (c) the risks/costs of participating, and any procedures used to mitigate those risks and costs; (d) the potential benefits of participating; (e) any consequences resulting from not participating or withdrawing;

and (f) issues of confidentiality and privacy.[7] Pediatric research typically requires consent from both the child and a guardian.

One final issue of growing concern in drug research is *conflict of interest*. Most journals now expect authors to report any conflict of interest that would potentially compromise their objectivity as researchers. Unfortunately, it is often the case that the individuals most qualified to conduct and evaluate drug research are the individuals who are most beholden to the pharmaceutical industry for support of their research.

STAYING CURRENT

The final topic I address is the various tools that are available to help pharmacologically trained psychologists remain current in their knowledge of best practices. As a practical matter of accessing information during the course of a patient consult, various tools have been developed for computers and personal digital assistants. The best known of these are Lexi-Comp and ePocrates. The latter is available for free download with reduced functionality. For purposes of evaluating the current state of knowledge about medications, there are several useful sources. The clinicaltrials.gov website provides information about current clinical trials in progress, and guidelines.gov is a clearinghouse of treatment guidelines. These guidelines are often problematic because they are often formulated by the same individuals who are receiving pharmaceutical industry funding. A more independent source of information is provided by the Cochrane reviews (www.cochrane.org/cochrane-reviews), because industry funding of the reviews is prohibited. Finally, MedWatch (www.fda.gov/Safety/MedWatch/default.htm) is the FDA's program for gathering adverse event information. Psychologists committed to remaining current in their understanding of medications will maintain a subscription to ePocrates or Lexi-Comp, receive regular e-mail alerts from MedWatch, review guidelines relevant to the patients they treat at guidelines.gov, and establish a critical stance toward medications through Cochrane reviews. Involvement in pharmacotherapy requires a level of commitment to currency and research consumption that is unusual for the psychologist but will become increasingly important for our profession.

CHAPTER 10 KEY TERMS

ABAB design: A single-subject design that involves sequential administration and removal of the active treatment.

Absolute risk: The probability of improvement in the active treatment.

Allegiance effects: A confound involving differences due to sites that are particularly associated with one of the treatments, resulting in a heightened level of expectation for the efficacy of that treatment and unusually large treatment effects.

Alpha level: The acceptable (researcher-defined) probability of a Type I error.

Alternative hypothesis: The proposition that some effect exists in a population.

---

[7]See www.hhs.gov/ohrp/humansubjects/assurance/consentckls.htm for a more complete description of informed consent elements.

Analysis of covariance: An analysis similar to analysis of variance that allows for equalization of participants on some potential confound.

Analysis of variance: A statistical method developed by Sir Ronald Fisher that involves one or more categorical independent variables of two or more groups and one dimensional dependent variable.

Assumptions: Statistical requirements underlying the use of a statistical method.

Beta level: The acceptable (researcher-defined) probability of a Type I error.

Between-group design: A comparison of two or more separate groups.

Black box warning: A warning of serious side effects associated with a medication.

Blind: Unaware of a condition or independent variable.

Carryover effect: A confound in repeated measures studies in which one treatment influences response to the next.

Case studies: Relatively unsystematic observation of single individuals; contrasted with single-subject designs.

Classical test theory: A dominant approach to evaluating measurement devices in psychology that focuses on the estimation of reliability.

Coefficient alpha: The most popular statistic for the estimation of internal reliability.

Comparator: A treatment alternative to the original treatment.

Confidence intervals: A range of values derived from a sample in which a parameter is likely to fall.

Conflict of interest: Economic or other factors that could compromise a researcher's objectivity in a research study.

Confounds: Variables that could cause spurious relationships between variables in a study.

CONSORT statement: A set of recommendations for the conduct of randomized controlled trials.

Construct validity: Having to do with the relationship between the operations performed in the process of conducting the study and the latent constructs they are intended to represent.

Correlation coefficient: A standardized measure of the degree to which one variable can be predicted from the other.

Counterbalancing: Systematic changes in the order of administration of treatments in a repeated measures study to minimize order effects.

Covariate: A confound controlled through an analysis of covariance.

Critical value: The value for some test statistic at which the null hypothesis is rejected given a predefined alpha level.

Crossover study: A repeated measures study in which the same participants receive all treatments.

Cross-sectional study: An observational study that involves measurement at one point in time.

Dependent variable: The outcome variable in a true or quasi-experiment.

Dose ranging: Identifying the range of dosages likely to define the therapeutic window.

Dose-response curve: Variation in the relationship between treatment and outcome across medication dosage.

Double-blind study: A study in which participants and care providers are unaware of participants' treatment conditions.

Effect size statistics: Statistics that are designed to estimate the size of an effect in a sample or population.

Effect: Some hypothesized relationship or pattern.

Effectiveness studies: Studies in which external validity is emphasized, to the detriment of internal validity.

Efficacy studies: Studies in which internal validity is emphasized, to the detriment of external validity.

Exclusionary criteria: Criteria of excluding a participant from a study.

External validity: The degree to which inferences are likely to generalize across populations and contexts.

Fatigue effect: An order effect involving deterioration over time.

Fishing expedition: A study in which numerous analyses are conducted but only those that are significant are reported.

Full counterbalancing: Counterbalancing using all possible orders of treatments.

In vitro research: Research conducted in test tubes.

In vivo research: Research conducted with humans or in culture.

Inclusionary criteria: Criteria for including a participant in a study.

Independent variable: The manipulated variable in a true or quasi-experiment.

Informed consent: Agreement to participate in research under conditions of full disclosure.

Institutional Review Board: A committee that must approve any research conducted by an organization hoping to receive federal funding for research.

Intent to treat: An analysis involving all individuals for whom there was an intention of treatment, regardless of their level of participation.

Interaction: A statistical product of a moderator relationship in analysis of variance.

Internal reliability: A method of estimating reliability based on responses across multiple items of a test.

Internal validity: The degree to which the inferred causes of a relationship are justified by the results.

Inter-rater reliability: A method of estimating reliability based on responses across multiple raters using the same test.

Intraclass correlation coefficient: A statistic used to estimate reliability.

Last observation carried forward: An intent to treat comparison using the final observation for all participants in the study.

Longitudinal design: A study that involves observation over an extended period of time.

Market exclusivity: The period during which FDA approval permits a company to market a medication exclusively.

Meta-analysis: A variety of methods used to estimate outcomes across a series of studies (usually effect size statistics) to provide a summative analysis of some body of literature.

Mixed-factors ANOVA: An analysis of variance involving at least one between-group and at least one within-group independent variable.

Moderators: Third variables that influence the strength of the relationship between the treatment variable and outcomes.

Multiple baseline design: A single-subject design that involves introducing intervention at different times across participants or settings.

Nested design: An experimental design in which the variables are arranged in an explicit hierarchy.

Nocebo: Deterioration or side effects in response to a placebo; or, any adverse event associated with a treatment.

Nuisance variables: See *confounds*.

Null hypothesis: The proposition that a given effect is absent in a population.

Number needed to harm: An effect size statistic in circumstances where both variables are dichotomous estimating the number of additional patients who would need to receive the active treatment to achieve one more negative outcome (e.g., some side effect).

Number needed to treat: An effect size statistic in circumstances where both variables are dichotomous estimating the number of additional patients who would need to receive the active treatment to achieve one more positive outcomes.

Observational research: A study in which there is no assignment or manipulation by the researcher.

Observed cases: A comparison of treatments based only on participants who completed the study.

Odds ratio: An effect size statistic in circumstances where both variables are dichotomous based on the relative odds of improvement in two treatments.

Open-label trial: See open trial.

Open trial: A study in which all participants receive the targeted treatment and are aware of the treatment.

Order effects: Confounds in repeated measures studies having to do with the order in which treatments are received.

Parameter: A population statistic.

Partial counterbalancing: Counterbalancing using some possible orders of treatments.

Pharmacodynamics: A drug's effect on the body.

Pharmacokinetics: The body's effect on a drug.

Phase 0: A term used in the FDA approval process to refer to a small-sample study involving administration of a single, subtherapeutic dose of the medication to humans to verify that the medication acts in humans as expected.

Phase I (Human Pharmacology): A term used in the FDA approval process to refer to a small-sample study that focuses on safety, pharmacodynamics, pharmacokinetics, and dose ranging in humans.

Phase II (Therapeutic Exploratory): A term used in the FDA approval process to refer to the first large-sample studies conducted to evaluate safety, dose-ranging, and efficacy in humans.

Phase III (Therapeutic Confirmatory): A term used in the FDA approval process to refer to large, multisite studies focusing on efficacy.

Phase IV (Therapeutic Use): A term used in the FDA approval process to refer to research after approval, focusing on safety and new uses.

Phi coefficient: The correlation coefficient in circumstances where both variables are dichotomous.

Pilot study: A preliminary small-sample study that is often weak in terms of both internal and external validity.

Placebo: An alternative overtly similar to the active treatment that should not demonstrate ameliorative physiological effects but should activate similar expectations of improvement.

Power: The probability of rejecting the null hypothesis when the null hypothesis is false; the complement of beta.

Power analysis: A procedure for estimating the appropriate sample size to achieve a desired level of power.

Practice effect: An order effect involving improvement over time.

Preexisting groups design: A between-group study with non-random assignment.

Pretest-posttest design: A study involving a single group that receives the active treatment.

PRISMA statement: A set of recommendations for the conduct of meta-analyses.

Prospective study: A study in which events are used to predict events at later periods.

Quasi-experiment: A study that involves conditions to which participants are not randomly assigned.

Randomized controlled trials: A true experiment in which individuals are assigned to treatment conditions.

Relative risk: The probability of improvement in the active treatment relative to the control condition.

Relative risk ratio: An effect size statistic in circumstances where both variables are dichotomous based on the relative probability of improvement in two treatments.

Reliability: The degree to which variability within a set of scores is attributable to true variation rather than random error.

Repeated measures design: A comparison of matched groups, because of a dependency between groups or a within-group design.

Retrospective study: A cross-sectional study in which information about past events is gathered.

Significance testing: An inferential strategy developed to evaluate whether null hypotheses are true in a population.

Single-blind study: A study in which participants are unaware of their treatment condition.

Single-subject design: A study in which treatment is systematically manipulated in one participant at a time.

Spurious relationships: Relationships between variables that are attributable to a third variable.

Standardized mean difference: Several effect size statistics (e.g., *d*) that present the difference between two groups relative to the size of the standard deviation within groups.

Statistical conclusion validity: Activities that compromise the validity of the conclusions derived from the quantitative data.

Survival analysis: A set of statistics used to study the attrition process itself.

Test-retest reliability: A method of estimating reliability based on responses across multiple administrations of some test.

Therapeutic window: The range of dosages in which the medication is efficacious.

Titrating: A method for determining the endpoint of a reaction, and therefore the precise quantity of a drug needed to achieve the reaction.

Triple-blind study: A study in which participants, care providers, and data gatherers are unaware of participants' treatment conditions.

True experiment: A study in which the researcher randomly assigns participants to condition and differences in condition on some outcome that is evaluated.

Type I error: An error that involves rejecting the null hypothesis when the null hypothesis is true.

Type II error: An error that involves retaining the null hypothesis when the null hypothesis is false.

Validity: The extent to which inferences derived from a research study must be considered conditional or compromised by limitations of the study itself.

Waitlist control: An alternative to the active treatment involving no treatment.

Washout period: An interval between administration of repeated measures treatments to allow return to baseline.

Within-group design: A study in which the same participants are exposed to all conditions.

Chapter 10 Questions

1. A new medication proves to be more effective when evaluated by its developers than by any other researchers. This is an example of a(n):
   a. Allegiance effect.
   b. Interaction.
   c. Moderator.
   d. All of the above.

2. Legislation enacted intended to enhance the availability of medications for children includes which of the following?

   a. Permitting NIH to request that the FDA fund research into certain topics

   b. Allowing the FDA to fund research in pediatric pharmacology

   c. Allowing the FDA to extend market exclusivity to companies for conducting research in pediatric pharmacology

   d. Allowing NIH to mandate companies conduct research in pediatric pharmacology when other mechanisms have failed

3. Three out of every four people in the active treatment improve, whereas one out of every four in the placebo treatment improves. The odds ratio equals:

   a. 3

   b. 9

   c. 0.75

   d. None of the above.

4. Three out of every four people in the active treatment improve, whereas one out of every four in the placebo treatment improves. 0.75 represents the:

   a. Relative risk ratio.

   b. Absolute risk.

   c. Relative risk.

   d. Odds ratio.

5. A double-blind study would mean which of the following are unaware of treatment condition?

   a. Participants

   b. Data analysts

   c. Data gatherers

   d. Two of the above.

6. Which of the following is NOT an effect size statistic?

   a. d

   b. r

   c. odds ratio

   d. t

7. Whether pregnant women metabolize a medication more slowly than nonpregnant women represents a question in:

   a. Pharmacokinetics.

   b. Pharmacodynamics.

   c. Carryover effects.

   d. None of the above.

8. A study conducted to evaluate whether pregnant women metabolize a medication more slowly than nonpregnant women would involve all the following EXCEPT:

   a. A between-group design.

   b. Informed consent.

   c. A comparator.

   d. A quasi-experimental design.

9. At which phase are medications most likely to be pulled from the approval process?

   a. Before Phase I
   b. Before Phase II
   c. Before Phase III
   d. Before Phase IV

10. Recommendations for the conduct and reporting of meta-analyses may be found in the:

    a. CONSORT statement.
    b. PRISMA statement.
    c. STARD statement.
    d. None of the above.

11. The failure to use an activating placebo represents a threat to:

    a. Statistical conclusion validity.
    b. External validity.
    c. Construct validity.
    d. Internal validity.

12. A study finds no difference between a medication and a placebo as a measure of depression, so the researchers conclude the medication is inefficacious. It turns out the measure of depression used is very unreliable. This represents a problem for:

    a. External validity.
    b. Construct validity.
    c. Internal validity.
    d. All the above.

   Answers: (1) d, (2) c, (3) b, (4) b, (5) a, (6) d, (7) a, (8) c, (9) c, (10) b, (11) d, and (12) d

REFERENCES

American Psychological Association. (2010). *Publication manual of the American Psychological Association* (6th ed). Washington, DC: Author.

Baldwin, S. A., Murray, D. M., & Shadish, W. R. (2005). Empirically supported treatments or type I errors? Problems with the analysis of data from group-administered treatments. *Journal of Consulting and Clinical Psychology, 73*, 924–935.

Bezchlibnyk-Butler, K., & Jeffries, J. J. (2007). *Clinical handbook of psychotropic drugs* (17th ed.). Cambridge, MA: Hogrefe & Huber.

Borenstein, M., Hedges, L. V., Higgins, J. P. T., & Rothstein, H. R. (2009). *Introduction to meta-analysis*. Hoboken, NJ: Wiley.

Cashen, L. H., & Geiger, S. W. (2004). Statistical power and the testing of null hypotheses: A review of contemporary management research and recommendations for future studies. *Organizational Research Methods, 7*, 151–167.

Cohen, J. (1988). *Statistical power analysis for the behavioral sciences* (2nd ed.). Hillsdale, NJ: Erlbaum.

Devereaux, P. J., Manns, B. J., Ghali, W. A., Quan, H., Lacchetti, C., Montori, V. M., . . . Guyatt, G. H. (2001). Physician interpretations and textbook definitions of blinding terminology in randomized controlled trials. *JAMA: Journal of the American Medical Association, 285,* 2000–2003.

Dunlap, W. P., Cortina, J. M., Vaslow, J. B., & Burke, M. J. (1996). Meta-analysis of experiments with matched groups or repeated measures designs. *Psychological Methods, 1,* 170–177.

Elkin, I., Gibbons, R. D., Shea, M. T., & Shaw, B. F. (1996). Science is not a trial (but it can sometimes be a tribulation). *Journal of Consulting and Clinical Psychology, 64,* 92–103.

Erdfelder, E., Faul, F., & Buchner, A. (1996). GPOWER: A general power analysis program. *Behavior Research Methods, Instruments, & Computers, 28,* 1–11.

Fournier, J. C., DeRubeis, R. J., Hollon, S. D., Dimidjian, S., Amsterdam, J. D., Shelton, R. C., & Fawcett, J. (2010). Antidepressant drug effects and depression severity: A patient-level meta-analysis. *JAMA: Journal of the American Medical Association, 303,* 47–53.

Gaffan, E. A., Tsaousis, J., & Kemp-Wheeler, S. M. (1995). Researcher allegiance and meta-analysis: The case of cognitive therapy for depression. *Journal of Consulting and Clinical Psychology, 63,* 966–980.

Hokanson, J. E., Rubert, M. P., Welker, R. A., Hollander, G. R., & Hedeen, C. (1989). Interpersonal concomitants and antecedents of depression among college students. *Journal of Abnormal Psychology, 98,* 209–217.

Hsu, L. (1989). Random sampling, randomization, and equivalence of contrasted groups in psychotherapy outcome research. *Journal of Consulting and Clinical Psychology, 57,* 131–137.

Hunter, J. E., & Schmidt, F. L. (2004). *Methods of meta-analysis: Correcting error and bias in research findings* (2nd ed.). Thousand Oaks, CA: Sage.

Jacobson, N. S., & Hollon, S. D. (1996). Cognitive–behavior therapy versus pharmacotherapy: Now that the jury's returned its verdict, it's time to present the rest of the evidence. *Journal of Consulting and Clinical Psychology, 64,* 74–80.

Jørgensen, A. W., Hilden, J., & Gøtzsche, P. C. (2006). Cochrane reviews compared with industry supported meta-analyses and other meta-analyses of the same drugs: Systematic review. *BMJ, 333* (October 14), 782, doi: 10.1136/bmj.38973.444699.0B.

Julien, R. M. (2007). *A primer of drug action* (11th ed.). New York, NY: Worth.

Julien, R. M., Advokat, C. D., & Comaty, J. E. (2010). *A primer of drug action* (12th ed.). New York, NY: Worth.

Kirsch, I., Moore, T. J., Scoboria, A., & Nicholls, S. S. (2002). The emperor's new drugs: An analysis of antidepressant medication data submitted to the U.S. Food and Drug Administration. *Prevention & Treatment, 5,* Article 23.

Kline, R. B. (2004). *Beyond significance testing: Reforming data analysis methods in behavioral research.* Washington, DC: APA Books.

Lasser, K. E., Allen, P. D., Woolhandler, S. J., Himmelstein, D. U., Wolfe, S. M., & Bor, D. H. (2002). Timing of new black box warnings and withdrawals for prescription medications. *JAMA: Journal of the American Medical Association, 287,* 2215–2220.

Lipsey, M. W., & Wilson, D. B. (1993). The efficacy of psychological, educational, and behavioral treatment: Confirmation from meta-analysis. *American Psychologist, 48,* 1181–1209.

McGrath, R. E. (2011). *Quantitative models in psychology.* Washington, DC: APA Books.

Mintzes, B., Barer, M. L., Kravitz, R. L., Bassett, K., Lexchin, J., Kazanjian, A., . . . & Marion, S. A. (2003). How does direct-to-consumer advertising (DTCA) affect prescribing? A survey in primary care environments with and without legal DTCA? *Canadian Medical Association Journal, 169,* 405-412.

Moncrieff, J., Wessely, S., & Hardy, R. (1998). Meta-analysis of trials comparing antidepressants with active placebos. *British Journal of Psychiatry, 172,* 227–231.

Neyman, J., & Pearson, E. S. (1933). On the problem of the most efficient tests of statistical hypotheses. *Philosophical Transactions of the Royal Society of London, 231A*, 289–337.

Rodgers, J. L. (2010). The epistemology of mathematical and statistical modeling: A quiet methodological revolution. *American Psychologist, 65*, 1–12.

Sackett, D. L., Deeks, J. J., & Altman, D. G. (1996). Down with odds ratios! *Evidence-Based Medicine, 1*, 164–166.

Schmidt, F. L. (1996). Statistical significance testing and cumulative knowledge in psychology: Implications for training of researchers. *Psychological Methods, 1*, 115–129.

Shrout, P. E. (1998). Measurement reliability and agreement in psychiatry. *Statistical Methods in Medical Research, 7*, 301–317.

Silberman, S. (2009, August 24). Placebos are getting more effective. Drugmakers are desperate to know why. *Wired Magazine*. Downloaded August 22, 2010, from www.wired.com/medtech/drugs/magazine/17-09/ff_placebo_effect

The Treatment for Adolescents with Depression Study (TADS) Team. (2005). The Treatment for Adolescents with Depression Study (TADS): Demographic and clinical characteristics. *Journal of the American Academy of Child and Adolescent Psychiatry, 44*, 28–40.

Turner, E., Matthews, A., Linardatos, E., Tell, R., & Rosenthal, R. (2008). Selective publication of antidepressant trials and its influence on apparent efficacy. *The New England Journal of Medicine, 358*, 252–260.

U.S. Department of Health and Human Services. (2001). *Mental health: Culture, race, and ethnicity—A supplement to mental health: A report of the Surgeon General*. Rockville, MD: U.S. Department of Health and Human Services, Substance Abuse and Mental Health Services Administration, Center for Mental Health Services.

Vedula, S. S., Bero, L., Scherer, R. W., & Dickersin, K. (2009). Outcome reporting in industry-sponsored trials of gabapentin for off-label use. *New England Journal of Medicine, 361*, 1963–1971.

Villanueva, P., Peiró, S., Librero, J., & Pereiró, I. (2003). Accuracy of pharmaceutical advertisements in medical journals. *Lancet, 361*, 27–32.

Virani, A. S., Bezchlibnyk-Butler, K., & Jeffries, J. J. (2009). *Clinical handbook of psychotropic drugs* (18th ed.). Cambridge, MA: Hogrefe & Huber.

Wampold, B. E., Davis, B., & Good, R. H., III. (1990). Hypothesis validity of clinical research. *Journal of Consulting and Clinical Psychology, 58*, 360–367.

Wilkes, M. S., Doblin, B. H., & Shapiro, M. F. (1992). Pharmaceutical advertisements in leading medical journals: Experts' assessments. *Annals of Internal Medicine, 116*, 912–919.

Wilkinson, L., & APA Task Force on Statistical Inference. (1999). Statistical methods in psychology journals: Guidelines and explanations. *American Psychologist, 54*, 594–604.

Chapter 11

PROFESSIONAL, LEGAL, ETHICAL, AND INTERPROFESSIONAL ISSUES IN CLINICAL PSYCHOPHARMACOLOGY

Lisa Cosgrove

Bret A. Moore

Every profession is faced with a unique set of professional, legal, ethical, and collaborative challenges and guidelines. If absent, the profession lacking in structure would cease to exist. Therefore, in order to thrive, directions and methods for engaging in ethical, legal, and effective interprofessional collaboration must be established at the outset.

Psychologists' prescribing is a somewhat different animal. Caught between the well-established profession of psychology and the practice of psychopharmacology—which has traditionally been the purview of medicine—prescribing psychology has struggled with its identity. Does it follow the ethical and practice guidelines of the American Psychological Association (APA) or adopt those of the American Psychiatric Association? How does it handle collaborative issues with psychiatrists, physicians, and nonprescribing psychologists? Will the pharmaceutical industry exert the same influences and pressure on psychologists as it has on psychiatrists?

In this chapter we address several prominent professional issues most relevant to psychologists' prescribing. First, we discuss the ethical codes and standards as they pertain to pharmacological practice and the most pertinent issues surrounding current practice guidelines and standards of care regarding prescribing psychotropic medications. Second, we offer critical information about federal and state laws and statutes for psychologists' prescribing psychotropic medications. Third, we discuss the ethical and professional implications of pharmaceutical influences on prescribing psychologists. And last, we cover the issue of patient's rights.

ETHICAL CODES, STANDARDS, AND PRACTICE GUIDELINES RELATED TO PHARMACOLOGICAL PRACTICE

As McGrath and Rom-Rymer (2010) aptly point out, a discussion about the various professional issues surrounding psychologists' prescribing is premature without an understanding of the different levels of practice.

Resulting from an APA Board of Directors ad hoc task force on factors related to pursuing prescriptive authority, Smyer et al. (1993) recommended three levels of training in psychopharmacology for psychologists: (1) basic psychopharmacology education resulting from a graduate-level course; (2) collaborative practice, which would allow psychologists to incorporate collaboration on medication management into psychosocial treatments; and (3) prescription privileges allowing independent practice.

The ethical and practice issues that the pharmacologically trained psychologist will encounter will undoubtedly be influenced by the level at which he or she practices. For example, a psychologist with Level I training may be faced with the dilemma of to what degree he or she should discuss the side effects, limitations, and benefits of a psychotropic medication prescribed by a medical provider. This will be of less concern for the Level II trained psychologist and of little or no concern for the Level III independent practitioner. Although this example is a limited, yet basic, dilemma that occurs in everyday practice, it serves to prompt the larger question of "What is the status of ethical and practice guidelines for prescribing medical psychologists?"

A PROGRESSION TOWARD PRACTICE GUIDELINES

In the recent book *Pharmacotherapy for Psychologists: Prescribing and Collaborative Roles*, in their chapter, titled "Ethical Considerations in Pharmacotherapy for Psychologists," McGrath and Rom-Rymer (2010) present a clear and informative progression of practice standards for psychologists engaged in pharmacotherapy. In brief, the chapter describes a three-stage evolution initiated by a 1996 paper by Buelow and Chafetz, which provided a number of generic recommendations regarding ethical standards for psychologists involved in pharmacotherapy, such as: "Prescribing psychologists should exercise special care when treating medically ill patients."

In 2004, McGrath and colleagues put forth a second series of recommended practice standards, which dealt with several prominent issues for prescribing psychologists. An example, and probably the most notable and contentious between opponents and proponents of prescriptive authority for psychologists, is the need for prescribing psychologists to maintain their professional identity as psychologists. Other examples of issues broached included continuing education requirements and interacting with pharmaceutical companies (see latter part of this chapter).

In 2009, a task force from the APA Division 55 (American Society for the Advancement of Pharmacotherapy) developed the most comprehensive list of practice guidelines for psychologists involved in pharmacotherapy to date. Totaling 17 specific guidelines broken down into five themes (general, education, assessment, intervention and consultation, and relationships), *Practice Guidelines Regarding Psychologists' Involvement in Pharmacological Issues* was the first comprehensive source document for psychologists engaged in pharmacotherapy at all three levels of training in psychopharmacology. Although considered aspirational in nature and not intended as mandates, the guidelines do provide practical guidance via recommendations, which have their foundation in the APA Ethics Code. See Table 11.1 for an outline of the content areas of the guidelines.[1]

---

[1]Also, see Chapter 1, Table 1.1, for a fuller description of APA's *Practice Guidelines Regarding Psychologists' Involvement in Pharmacological Issues*.

Table 11.1   Content Areas of the *Practice Guidelines Regarding Psychologists' Involvement in Pharmacological Issues*

Guideline 1. Psychologists are encouraged to consider objectively the scope of their competence in pharmacotherapy and to seek consultation as appropriate before offering recommendations about psychotropic medications.

Guideline 2. Psychologists are urged to evaluate their own feelings and attitudes about the role of medication in the treatment of psychological disorders, as these feelings and attitudes can potentially affect communications with patients.

Guideline 3. Psychologists involved in prescribing or collaborating are sensitive to the developmental, age and aging, educational, sex and gender, language, health status, and cultural/ethnicity factors that can moderate the interpersonal and biological aspects of pharmacotherapy relevant to the populations they serve.

Guideline 4. Psychologists are urged to identify a level of knowledge concerning pharmacotherapy for the treatment of psychological disorders that is appropriate to the populations they serve and the type of practice they wish to establish, and to engage in educational experiences as appropriate to achieve and maintain that level of knowledge.

Guideline 5. Psychologists strive to be sensitive to the potential for adverse effects associated with the psychotropic medications used by their patients.

Guideline 6. Psychologists involved in prescribing or collaborating are encouraged to familiarize themselves with the technological resources that can enhance decision-making during the course of treatment.

Guideline 7. Psychologists with prescriptive authority strive to familiarize themselves with key procedures for monitoring the physical and psychological sequelae of the medications used to treat psychological disorders, including laboratory examinations and overt signs of adverse or unintended effects.

Guideline 8. Psychologists with prescriptive authority regularly strive to monitor the physiological status of the patients they treat with medication, particularly when there is a physical condition that might complicate the response to psychotropic medication or predispose a patient to experience an adverse reaction.

Guideline 9. Psychologists are encouraged to explore issues surrounding patient adherence and feelings about medication.

Guideline 10. Psychologists are urged to develop a relationship that will allow the populations they serve to feel comfortable exploring issues surrounding medication use.

Guideline 11. To the extent deemed appropriate, psychologists involved in prescribing or collaboration adopt a biopsychosocial approach to case formulation that considers both psychosocial and biological factors.

Guideline 12. The psychologist with prescriptive authority is encouraged to use an expanded informed consent process to incorporate additional issues specific to prescribing.

Guideline 13. When making decisions about the use of psychological treatments, pharmacotherapy, or their combination, the psychologist with prescriptive authority considers the best interests of the patient, current research, and, when appropriate, the needs of the community.

Guideline 14. Psychologists involved in prescribing or collaborating strive to be sensitive to the subtle influences of effective marketing on professional behavior and the potential for bias in information in their clinical decisions about the use of medications.

Guideline 15. Psychologists with prescriptive authority are encouraged to use interactions with the patient surrounding the act of prescribing to learn more about the patient's characteristic patterns of interpersonal behavior.

(continued)

Table 11.1   (Continued)

Guideline 16. Psychologists with prescriptive authority are sensitive to maintaining appropriate relationships with other providers of psychological services.

Guideline 17. Psychologists are urged to maintain appropriate relationships with providers of biological interventions.

Note: Adapted from APA (2009). *Practice guidelines regarding psychologists' involvement in pharmacological issues.* Washington, DC: Author. Available at www.apa.org/practice/guidelines/pharmacological-issues.pdf
Also see Table 1.1 of Chapter 1.

CLINICAL STANDARDS OF CARE AND PRACTICE

As correctly pointed out by Ally (2010), writing a prescription is not as simple as pulling out a pen from the drawer and signing your name. There are countless steps and procedures that must be followed leading up to this point, as well as critical issues to be subsequently managed.

What's In a Name?

Utilizing the correct title and representing oneself in an ethical and legal manner is imperative as a prescriber. Although the terms *prescribing psychologist* and *medical psychologist* are often used interchangeably, they are not the same. The term *prescribing psychologist* first appeared during the *Department of Defense Psychology Demonstration Project* (*PDP*) (see Sammons, 2010 for a thorough review) as the label used to distinguish those psychologists who participated in the PDP and subsequently prescribed in the military. More recently, the term was adopted by the New Mexico Board of Psychologist Examiners as the official term for psychologists engaged in pharmacotherapy licensed in that state. In Louisiana, the legal term approved by the representative licensing board is *medical psychologist* (*MP*). However, as noted in the introductory chapter, use of the latter term by psychologists engaged in pharmacotherapy is not without controversy.

Knowing how to represent oneself to patients is not a trivial matter—it's both a legal and an ethical issue. For example, legally, in New Mexico where psychologist prescribers are initially granted a *conditional prescribing certificate*, state regulation requires disclosure of this title and practice level to the patient. Specifically, disclosure that the psychologist is under the supervision of a licensed physician is required. Moreover, ethically, it is poor form not to provide the patient with the psychologist's limitations regarding scope of practice, education, training, and expertise. Without this information up front, it can be argued that the patient is not making a fully informed choice, as some patients may prefer to see a physician or other medical provider for medication management services.

Documentation

There are two primary issues related to documentation, which are unique to psychologists practicing pharmacotherapy: (1) enhanced clinical notes and (2) the prescription. Unlike standard psychological evaluations, clinical documentation by prescribers needs to include a more thorough medical history. Although a standard review of medical history is commonplace in psychological practice, documentation of specific factors such as physical and neurological exams, past response to medications by immediate family members, history of *adverse drug reactions*, current and anticipated pregnancy status, and the pharmacodynamic and pharmacokinetic properties of current medications are not commonplace. Other critical points concerning documentation for prescribers include vital signs (blood pressure, pulse); physical exam (height and weight at a minimum); potential *drug–drug* and *drug–food interactions*; risks, benefits, and limitations of the medication(s); recommended laboratory tests and relevant past laboratory values; and a description of the patient information about the medication provided.

Furthermore, there are several important pieces of information required on the prescription itself (see Figure 11.1). These are:

- Patient's name, address, and phone number
- Patient's age and/or date of birth
- Date of the prescription
- Name of the medication
- Whether the brand-name medication is medically required or generic is acceptable
- Medication dosage
- How many doses to be taken (e.g., two pills)
- How the medicine will be taken (e.g., oral, intramuscular [IM], rectal)
- How many times during the day the medicine will be taken and what time of the day
- Number of refills
- Drug Enforcement Administration (DEA) number and signature

Each piece of information on the prescription serves a critical role in ensuring that the patient receives appropriate pharmacotherapy and minimizes risks associated with human error. If the prescription is not completed correctly, the chance of injury and even death from an adverse drug reaction increases.

In addition to written orders, the prescriber should also be aware of the risks associated with *verbal orders*. In some situations, the psychologist will be required to provide a verbal order for a medication via telephone or in person. Oftentimes, this is associated with more emergent cases (e.g., patient presenting to emergency room with psychosis). Although this is an expeditious way to handle crisis situations, the chance of miscommunication resulting in a medication error is a real possibility. One way to minimize this risk is to have the person receiving the verbal order via telephone (i.e., nurse, emergency room physician) repeat back the medication instructions. The health care provider receiving the oral medication order can reduce risk of miscommunication by immediately writing the order down on paper.

Patient Education

Helping patients make informed decisions about pharmacotherapy begins during the initial encounter; however, it is cemented during the *patient education* phase of treatment. One of the biggest contributors to medication noncompliance is poor patient

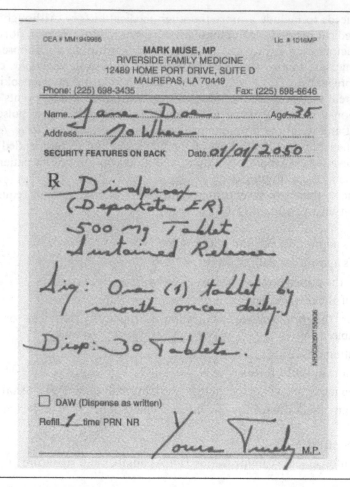

Figure 11.1   Sample Prescription

education. Whether it is related to the prescriber's discomfort, lack of attention, or lack of information, neglecting to inform the patient of potential side effects, both serious and mild, sets the stage for incomplete treatment.

It is important to keep in mind that pharmacy handouts and online patient education resources are not a substitute for talking with the patient about potential side effects and the proper way to take the medication. Most patients will not review the literature once they have left the office. On the flip side, for those who do read the literature, appropriate education up front can minimize any fear or anxiety that will arise once the patient digests the laundry list of potential side effects noted in the package insert.

Restrictions on Prescribing

The ethical and competent prescriber must be aware of various restrictions associated with his or her practice. The most obvious, and the one the prescriber will encounter first, is institutional *medication formulary* restrictions. In almost all health care settings, limitations on which drugs can be dispensed are in place. In most cases this is due to financial reasons. For example, some pharmacies will not dispense a name-brand medication if the generic equivalent is available; this is especially true in HMO-based pharmacies. Along the same lines, if a drug similar to the more expensive prescribed drug is available, then the less expensive drug will be dispensed. A prime example is when patients are switched by institutional protocol from escitalopram to citalopram. However, this is not necessarily absolute. When the prescriber can make a compelling case as to why the more expensive medication is warranted, some pharmacies may make concessions; also, the prescribing medical psychologist has the option of specifying "*Dispense as written (DAW)*" on the prescription, which alerts the dispenser not to make substitutes without first conferring with the prescriber.

Psychologists engaged in psychopharmacology will also encounter state, federal, and organizational restrictions associated with controlled substances. For example, in New Mexico and Louisiana, psychologists cannot prescribe Schedule I or Schedule II and III narcotic drugs (prescribing medical psychologists can prescribe Schedule II and III nonnarcotic medications in the two states). Also, phone or electronic orders for Schedule II medications are not accepted unless in clear emergency situations, and require a *hard copy script*. Nevertheless, the psychologist is unlikely to be in an emergency situation in which a Schedule II medication is required.

A *chemical restraint* is a form of medical restraint in which a drug is used to restrict the freedom or movement of a patient. This intervention is used in emergency and psychiatric settings to minimize risk of harm to the patient or those near the patient. Chemical restraint should be a last resort. Furthermore, it should never be utilized out of convenience or as a disciplinary measure. For medical psychologists engaged in prescribing, the most common drugs used for chemical restraint are benzodiazepine and antipsychotic medications. It is important to know your organization's policies regarding this practice as well as pertinent state law.

STATE AND FEDERAL STATUTES

In 2002, New Mexico became the first state to grant appropriately trained psychologists the authority to prescribe. Louisiana followed in 2004. Even though both laws were passed around the same time and succeeded in accomplishing the same goal of providing psychologists the opportunity to prescribe, the two states differ in their laws and allowable practices. One glaring difference is the regulatory body that governs psychologists' prescribing. In New Mexico the New Mexico Board of Psychologist Examiners[2] regulates the practice of prescribing psychologists whereas the Louisiana State Board of Medical Examiners[3] regulates the practice of medical psychologists.

Understanding the rights and limitations associated with the legal statutes of the state in which the psychologist practices is crucial. For example, Louisiana requires of the initial medical psychologist consultation, collaboration, and concurrence with the patient's primary care physician when prescribing or changing a medication treatment protocol. However, with three years of experience as a medical psychologist,

---

[2]See http://www.rld.state.nm.us/psychology/index.html
[3]See http://www.lsbme.louisiana.gov

treatment of 100 patients with psychotropic medications, and the recommendation of two collaborating physicians of collaborative practice a "Certificate of Advanced Practice" can be obtained, which encourages collaboration with the patient's primary care physician as a best practice standard, but does not mandate it. In contrast, New Mexico requires collaboration, but not necessarily concurrence. Other examples include differences in continuing education, documentation, and residency requirements.

At the time of this writing, prescribing in a federal agency is not connected to state licensing. In other words, the psychologist's prescribing practices are regulated by the governmental organization in which he or she practices. The two most prominent examples are the United States military and the Indian Health Services. The former has separate credentialing requirements for the Army, Navy, and Air Force. At present, credentialing of the latter is handled at the individual hospital or service unit level. In such cases, a federal DEA number is issued, which is extraterritorial.

One requirement consistent with practice in both states and within federal agencies is the requirement to obtain a DEA number through the U.S. Department of Justice's Drug Enforcement Administration.[4] In a relatively straightforward process, the psychologist is allowed to apply for the DEA number after obtaining state licensure and registering with the representative state board of pharmacy. Once this process is completed, the psychologist is listed under the unfortunate rubric of "midlevel practitioner." This is unfortunate because there is nothing midlevel about psychologists' training and practice as doctoral-level independent practitioners. Medical terminology, however, is slow to revise out-of-date nomenclature.

RELATIONSHIPS WITH PHARMACEUTICAL COMPANIES: FINDING A BALANCE IN RESEARCH AND PRACTICE

Over the past 10 years, government spending on biomedical research has significantly decreased. In 1985 the ratio of government spending to industry spending was over 2:1 (Center for the Health Care Professions, 2005), but now only 58% of all *biomedical research* is federally funded (Dorsey et al., 2010). During this time period, revenues of the pharmaceutical industry have substantially grown; in 2008 the pharmaceutical industry was the third most profitable business in the United States (Fortune, 2009) with sales of psychotropic medications reaching $24.2 billion (IMS Health, 2009). Moreover, as industry profits have grown, so too have concerns about the ways in which financial *conflicts of interest* (FCOIs) may compromise biomedical research. Although industry-academic relationships can result in unethical behavior that is clearly intentional, FCOIs do not always translate into scientific misconduct. Industry financial relationships can also affect researchers' and clinicians' behavior in subtle ways that may result in implicit bias. Because of the close partnership between industry and academe, clinicians must work harder than ever to make sure that they are fully educated about the risk/benefit ratio of psychotropic medications, and they need to critically evaluate the diagnostic and treatment information that is being produced and disseminated. Critical thinking should not be conflated with an antimedication approach, for it is in patients' and clinicians' best interest to carefully review any data on the efficacy and safety of psychotropic medications, however prestigious the

---

[4]See http://www.deadiversion.usdoj.gov

source. This section identifies some of the ethical challenges that arise for clinicians in today's industry-dominated climate. It first describes the problems that are incurred by FCOIs, and then makes some specific suggestions for ensuring that *evidence-based pharmacological practice* is distinct from *pharmaceutical marketing practice*.

Why should clinicians be concerned that industry-academic relationships may result in imbalanced or even biased results and pharmacotherapy recommendations? Psychologists are rightly skeptical about the practice of *pharmaceutical detailing* (i.e., when industry representatives provide information about their company's products to individual health care providers and, in return for the provider's time, the reps give gifts, such as trips or expensive dinners). Medical psychologists are skeptical because they wonder if they are receiving fully accurate and balanced information—it comes, after all, from a pharmaceutical company representative who is being paid (usually on commission) to sell the company's drugs. However, many medical providers do not use their critical thinking skills when assessing the information disseminated in a *clinical practice guideline* (*CPG*) or published in a prestigious medical journal. Most people assume that if a study is published in a highly respected medical journal or cited in a CPG that is produced by a professional medical organization they can trust the information. This assumption rests on other assumptions—that the vast majority of researchers adhere to the norms of science and that the peer-review process protects against the dissemination of scientifically flawed studies, invalid results, or questionable conclusions. We want to believe that clinical trial designs, disclosure policies, and conflicts of interest policies are all robust enough to provide adequate safeguards. Unfortunately, meta-analyses, qualitative reviews, and medical journal editors have documented the ways in which industry funding of Phase III randomized clinical trials (RCTs) results in the publication of pro-industry results, overestimation of efficacy, and underreporting of harms (see, e.g., Angell, 2004; Bekelman, Li, & Gross, 2003; Bodenheimer, 2000; Djulbegovic et al., 2000; Perlis et al., 2005; and Pitrou, Boutron, Ahmad, & Ravaud, 2009). In turn, publication and trial design bias result in the proliferation of *me-too drugs*—medications that are neither more effective nor safer than first-generation drugs.

What are some industry practices that clinicians should be aware of? Over four decades' worth of research from social psychology clearly demonstrates that gifts— even small ones—create obligations to reciprocate (Katz, Caplan, & Merz, 2003; Mather, 2005; Mauss, 1967). Thus, when researchers or authors of psychiatric taxonomy or CPGs serve on speakers bureaus, receive honoraria, are given research funding, or hold equity in a company, these relationships may engender the same sort of obligations or dispositions that are inherent when gifts are given to individual providers. Moreover, researchers and guideline authors may be unaware of the ways in which these ongoing relationships create a demand for reciprocity (Sismondo, 2008) that can result in implicit bias (e.g., choices of what results to emphasize or conclusions to be drawn from RCTs; decisions about revisions to the *Diagnostic and Statistical Manual of Mental Disorders*). In light of the fact that there are no biological markers for mental illness, psychiatry is particularly vulnerable to industry influence and thus to subtle, implicit biases when developing diagnostic criteria or when prioritizing treatment recommendations. For example, the fact that 90% of the authors of three major CPGs produced by the American Psychiatric Association for major depressive disorder, bipolar disorder, and schizophrenia had ties to the companies that manufactured the medications recommended as treatments for these disorders raises questions about undue industry influence (Cosgrove, Bursztajn, Krimsky, Anaya, & Walker, 2009).

The *DSM*'s Relationship to Big Pharma: Three Examples of Industry's Capture of Controversial Disorders

Although some *DSM* disorders may have questionable validity and have been the subject of intense scrutiny, they may nonetheless be used by industry to support applications for medications. This is because the Food and Drug Administration (FDA) does not simply grant approval of new medications—it grants approval based on a particular use or condition (Angell, 2004). In this way, current psychiatric taxonomy can play a subtle but critical role in the FDA's decision to approve a new psychotropic drug. Hence, it is important for the clinician to be cognizant of what some have referred to as the "unholy alliance" among the FDA, the *DSM*, and the American Psychiatric Association. When the FDA considers a new indication for a drug, there must be empirical support or well-accepted diagnostic criteria for the indication. Thus, when Eli Lilly requested approval for the use of its drug Sarafem (fluoxetine hydrochloride; previously marketed as Prozac) for the treatment of premenstrual dysphonic disorder (PMDD), Lilly had to provide evidence that PMDD was "distinct from other disorders that are characterized by affective symptoms such as . . . major depressive disorder" (Food and Drug Administration, 1999). The Sarafem/Prozac story is an example of a company essentially looking for a *patent extender* (Angell, 2004), and an important lesson can be learned from this story. The wise clinician should look carefully at the empirical evidence that supports the validity of new, or controversial, *DSM* diagnoses—especially when these disorders are being used to support patent-extending drugs or new drugs.

As can be seen in Eli Lilly's use of PMDD, the *DSM* can too frequently play handmaiden to industry (see, e.g., Lewis et al., 2001). Hypoactive sexual desire disorder (HSD) is another example of a diagnosis with questionable validity that was used to support a company's drug application to the FDA. HSD is defined as "a deficiency or absence of sexual fantasies and desire for sexual activity (American Psychiatric Association, 2000, p. 539) and a prevalence rate of 33% for women is given. (No prevalence rates are given for men.) Supporters of the diagnosis use the *DSM*'s nosology to claim it is a legitimate condition. However, this disorder has been the subject of much controversy because it is based on the assumption that there is a universal, staged, and biologically based sexual response pattern, the human sexual response cycle model (HSRCM). Questions have been raised about the validity and generalizability of the HSRCM as a universal norm (Tiefer, 2004; Wood, Koch, & Mansfield, 2006). The assumption that sexual problems are biologically driven undermines an appreciation for women's lived experiences and for the gendered power dynamics in which sexual problems are inevitably embedded. For example, the HSRCM, as a universal model, does not address the needs and experiences of women who have been sexually molested or who are currently in abusive relationships. The *DSM* clearly states that there are no "normative age- or gender-related data on frequency or degree of sexual desire [and] the diagnosis must rely on clinical judgment" (American Psychiatric Association, 2000, p. 539). Nonetheless, a prevalence rate of 33% is given for women with HSD. The *DSM*'s own acknowledgment of the lack of normative data renders the reliability and validity of HSD suspect, even before the more far-reaching criticisms just noted are considered.

Despite these concerns about the validity of HSD, in June 2010 the pharmaceutical company Boehringer-Ingelheim submitted an application to the FDA for approval of Flibanserin (a serotonergic drug) for the treatment of HSD. An especially important issue in terms of the request for FDA approval of Flibanserin is *iatrogenic harm*; paradoxically, one of the best-known side effects of serotonergic agents is sexual dysfunction. Recent reviews suggest that the prevalence of sexual side effects (e.g., loss of libido, difficulty achieving orgasm) can be anywhere from 30% to 70% with SSRIs (Gregorian et al., 2002; Montejo, Llorca, Izquierdo, & Rico-Villademoros, 2001). There also is increasing evidence that serotonergic agents have a host of adverse side effects, ranging from increased risk of upper gastrointestinal tract bleeding (Dalton et al., 2003; de Abajo & García-Rodríguez, 2008) to documented adverse neonatal outcomes in relation to maternal exposure to SSRIs and other newer serotonergic/noradrenergic antidepressants (see Tuccori et al., 2009, for review). In addition, serotonergic drugs have been shown to have deleterious effects on the metabolism and therapeutic efficacy of tamoxifen and other antineoplastic agents (Spina, Santoro, & D'Arrigo, 2008). Because of the lack of evidence that Flibanserin increased sexual desire, and because of concern over side effects, the FDA rejected Boehringer-Ingelheim's application, although "the company was encouraged to continue its research" (Wilson, 2010, June 19).

A third example of the connections among industry, the FDA, and the *DSM* can be found in a newly proposed disorder, "attenuated psychotic symptoms syndrome," which is being considered for inclusion in the *DSM-5* (www.dsm5.org). This syndrome describes symptoms of psychosis that are theorized to appear in individuals at risk for developing schizophrenia before they are actually diagnosed with the disease. Supporters of this new diagnosis use prophylactic treatment as their rationale; if clinicians can diagnose and treat soft psychotic symptoms early enough, they can prevent at-risk individuals from developing schizophrenia. However, the data do not bear out this reasoning (Gopal, Cosgrove, & Bursztajn, 2010). Various studies have demonstrated that only 16% to 30% of people with symptoms of psychosis end up developing schizophrenia later in life (McGorry et al., 2009; Yung, Nelson, Thompson, & Wood, 2010). Serious questions also remain about whether treatment with antipsychotic medications reduces their risk for developing schizophrenia any more than treatment with a placebo (McGlashan et al., 2006), and some researchers warn that the risk/benefit ratio does not justify treating those at risk for psychosis with these medications (de Koning et al., 2009; McGorry et al., 2009). However, industry-sponsored publications maintain that "attenuated psychotic symptoms syndrome" is a valid diagnostic category despite concerns over the validity of this syndrome (Woods et al., 2009) and industry publications advocate the use of antipsychotic medications as one of the main treatment interventions (McGlashan et al., 2006; see also Gopal et al., 2010). As Moncrieff and Leo (2010) note, a recent non-industry-funded study found that risperidone impaired working memory in individuals who presented with a first episode of psychosis (Reilley, 2006). Indeed, there are significant discrepancies between industry and non-industry-funded research on the validity and treatment of "attenuated psychotic symptoms syndrome." Inclusion of this disorder in the *DSM* may open the door for more aggressive antipsychotic treatment to ever younger patients, raising the issue of iatrogenic harm; adverse side effects of antipsychotic medications also include, but are not limited to, movement disorders, weight gain, and diabetes.

Inappropriate use of exclusion criteria may produce results that are favorable to industry. A subtle (and seldom discussed) industry practice that may have an impact on the results of RCTs is the use of exclusion criteria that allow for favorable drug outcomes but also make it hard to generalize the results to clinical practice (Geddes, 2003; Healy, 2009; Seeman, 2001). For example, excluding patients from RCTs for antidepressants or antipsychotics who have coexisting Axis II disorders, anxiety, medical conditions, or more severe depression limits the generalizability of the study. It has been predicted that the common practice of excluding patients with Hamilton Rating Scale for Depression (HRSD) scores above 18 in most RCTs may exclude almost half of all patients with depression (Zimmerman, Posternak, & Chelminski, 2002). In addition, as Dubovsky and Dubovosky (2007) astutely point out, while dropout rates are typically reported, most industry-supported studies do not report on the number of participants who were "screened in" to get an adequately powered study: "[This number] tells us how much the deck was stacked in favor of the study drug by enriching the sample and what percent of the actual clinical population is represented by the subjects" (p. 71). As industry increasingly relies on for-profit entities such as *contract research organizations* (*CROs*) rather than on academic medical centers, the potential for bias increases because of inappropriate screening in and inappropriate exclusion criteria. This shift to CROs has been dramatic; whereas in 1993 CROs received $1.6 billion of research funding from pharmaceutical companies, by 2003 they netted $7.6 billion in funding according to *CenterWatch* (as cited in Lenzer, 2008, p. a1332). The lack of peer review of research design and research management engendered by this shift opens the door for undue industry influence (see, e.g., Dubovsky & Dubovosky, 2007).

Disease-oriented rather than patient-oriented outcome measures: efficacy versus effectiveness. "Often an *'efficacy-effectiveness' gap* exists between the results achieved in efficacy trials and those observed by usual practitioners treating real patients in common settings" (Lagomasino, Dwight-Johnson, & Simpson, 2005, p. 649).

The reason that RCTs have become the gold standard in evidence-based medicine is that they require randomization of participants, which in turn allows for a true intent-to-treat analysis (researchers are thus able to conclude that differences in outcome reflect real differences—they are not due to confounding variables). However, without proper allocation concealment, blinding, and statistical methods to control for attrition (described in more detail later), the RCT is not randomized and the results may get distorted. Moreover, perhaps one of the most potentially biasing factors in favor of the study drug is the use of conceptually flawed outcome measures and, concomitantly, the use of disease-oriented rather than patient-oriented outcome measures (Shaughnessy, 2009; Shaughnessy & Slawson, 2004). For example, although the Hamilton Depression Rating Scale (HDRS) is one of the most frequently used outcome measures in RCTs for antidepressant medications, its conceptual flaws have been well documented (Bagby, Ryder, Schuller, & Marshall, 2004). The HDRS was developed by an industry researcher looking for ways to document the study drug's effect (Bech, 2009). It is a remarkably brief survey instrument that is heavily focused on neurovegetative symptoms and has few questions on the subjective experience of depression, mood, or affect. The National Institute for Health and Clinical Excellence (NICE) requires an effect size of 0.50 as criteria of clinical significance, defined as a 50% reduction in depression rating scale scores (National Institute for Health and Clinical Excellence, 2009). This requirement translates into a 3-point difference on the HDRS, because remission is rarely selected as the goal of treatment for RCTs. It is therefore possible that participants in RCTs for depression can show statistically significant improvement on the HDRS (e.g., by slight improvements in sleeping and eating habits and/or energy level) but still have the subjective experience of depression. This is an example of how an accepted outcome measure can generate a statistically significant result that is not clinically meaningful. Clearly, there is a need to develop and incorporate meaningful patient-oriented outcome measures in order to ensure that favorable drug study results have relevance to clinical practice. It is important to emphasize that the issue is not that industry-sponsored researchers, or government sponsored researchers for that matter, intentionally look for inappropriate outcome measures.[5] As noted here, in RCTs for antidepressants, the standard acceptable practice is to use an industry-friendly disease-oriented outcome measure. Under our current regulatory system, industry is not incentivized—and one could argue that it is deincentivized—to develop patient-centered measures.

Also, the relatively short duration of RCTs makes it very difficult to determine if the drug is truly effective and not simply efficacious on a disease-oriented outcome measure. Many clinicians reading study results are not aware of this important distinction: The World Health Organization defines effectiveness as "the likelihood and extent of desired **clinically relevant effects** [emphasis added] in patients with a specified condition" (as cited in Bero & Rennie, 1996, p. 209). In contrast, efficacy refers to "any arbitrarily chosen effect which **may or may not be clinically relevant** [emphasis added]." In 2007 the FDA mandated that all RCTs identify both primary and secondary outcome measures within 21 days of the enrollment of the first patient (Food and Drug Administration, 2007), which will mitigate the opportunity for industry to choose *surrogate outcome measures* to produce favorable efficacy results. Nonetheless, this requirement will only provide a safeguard and will require great vigilance on the part of editors and reviewers to prevent misuse of secondary measures. Also, the fact that most RCTs last only 6 to 8 weeks (Klantel, 2010) makes it difficult to determine whether the drug is truly effective in the long term. The short duration of RCTs makes it challenging to document side effects and thus address the issue of iatrogenic harm. In addition, it has been argued that Phase IV trials (the vast majority of which have corporate sponsorship) frequently use suboptimal trial designs. These designs are not flawed per se, but they are developed to provide data that will be favorable to industry rather than to maximize medical information (Falit, 2007). In so doing, such designs may reinforce the false superiority of me-too drugs.

Controlling for attrition. One of the most intractable problems in developing a sufficiently powered study is making sure that there is a sufficient number of participants who complete the study. Although attrition is an issue for all RCTs, it is a particular problem for psychotropic drug studies. In fact, average dropout rates of 50% to 64% have been reported in antipsychotic studies and 37% in antidepressant studies (Leon et al., 2006). The last observation carried forward (LOCF) is an intent-to-treat model that is accepted by the FDA as a statistical method to control for attrition even though other techniques might better control for bias (Wooley et al., 2009). Specifically, when a participant drops out of an RCT, his or her last result (e.g., score on the HDRS) is carried forward and considered and computed as the final value. This model assumes a randomization of dropouts that is not supported by any theory or any data (Kenward & Molenberghs, 2009; Leon et al., 2006), and it is also a model that fails to assess outcomes in patients who keep taking the drug:

> In randomized trials SSRIs appeared to be at least as effective as tricyclic antidepressants such as imipramine, because imipramine is not as well tolerated

---

[5]Yet, examples of intentional manipulation and/or fabrication of research results exist. Witness the findings of the Office of Research Integrity, U.S. Department of Health and Human Services, that "Eighty-nine percent of the 133 research misconduct findings made over the entire period (1994–2003) were based on falsification or fabrication singularly or in combination" (Rhoades, 2004).

and is more likely to be discontinued early, but for more severely depressed patients who are more motivated to continue it until it works, imipramine may be more helpful. [Use of LOCF] misses the impact of **adherence** [emphasis added] to treatment. (Dubovsky & Dubovosky, 2007, p. 51)

Thus, insofar as LOCF misses the impact of adherence to treatment, as can be seen in the example, it may fail to provide information about real patients' eventual outcomes. This technique may introduce bias such that the study drug may appear to be more efficacious than it actually is (Molnar, Man-Son-Hing, Hutton, & Fergusson, 2009), although the direction or extent of the bias incurred by the uncritical use of LOCF is not able to be predicted (Wooley et al., 2009). Clinicians should thus pay close attention to the rationale for use of LOCF when reading RCT results, and editors and reviewers should consider carefully the question, "Would other techniques have controlled for attrition while introducing less bias?"

PATIENT'S RIGHTS

Given the ethical dilemmas one faces practicing in today's industry-dominated climate, what does the psychologist, especially the prescribing medical psychologist, need to know? Ethical pharmacological practice requires collaborative decision making, which can be achieved only if there is transparency and *informed consent*. Informed consent, defined by the Nuremberg Code, updated in 2000 by the World Medical Association Declaration of Helsinki (World Medical Association, 2004), and articulated by professional organizations, requires (among other considerations) the ability to assess the risks and benefits of the proposed treatment, alternatives to the proposed treatment, and disclosure of important information. Certainly, protecting patient autonomy and improving informed consent practices in an industry-dominated climate are arduous tasks. It is thus helpful to understand informed consent as a relational, dialogical process. It is an exercise (Bluhm, 2009), not something that can be achieved once and for all by disclosing currently known risks, benefits, alternatives to treatment, and FCOIs. Ethical practice is enhanced because informed consent is conceptualized as a partnership and conversation that occurs over time (Bluhm, 2009) and not as a static event. Hopefully, patients who believe that their prescribing psychologist has their best interests at heart are better able to engage in shared decision making. A therapeutic alliance grounded in trust is essential to bringing strength and hope to the lives of individuals who struggle with emotional distress and behavioral difficulties. Thus, when a medication proves ineffective or has adverse side effects, a patient who has been meaningfully informed of those possibilities has a better chance to maintain trust in the clinician, and thereby stay in treatment long enough to try another medication or another form of therapy, than a patient for whom the bad outcome is a devastating surprise (Cosgrove & Bursztajn, 2010).

In order to improve informed consent practices, we offer the following suggestions.

1. Pharmaceutical companies are for-profit entities whose fiduciary responsibility to their shareholders inevitably creates conflicted sponsors—that is, corporate sponsors that are financially incentivized to make money rather than optimize public health (Falit, 2007). Hence, psychologists should not rely on pharmaceutical manufacturers

to voluntarily disseminate complete and balanced information regarding efficacy and risks. It is thus important for prescribing medical psychologists to educate themselves about the various pharmaceutical manufacturers' track records with respect to disclosing adverse efficacy and safety data, as some companies' records are better than others. The FDA's website is a useful resource for assessing a company's disclosure history (http://www.fda.gov/Drugs/default.htm).

2. As noted before, manufacturers of psychotropic medications are profit-minded companies and rely on marketing strategies to sell their products—especially second- (or third-) generation medications, often referred to as me-too drugs. Although psychologists might tend to think they will not succumb to marketing techniques, these techniques are subtle, powerful, and effective, so it is imperative to educate yourself about pharmaceutical marketing strategies (Carlat, 2010), as well as about *semantic decision-making biases* (Bursztajn, Chanowitz, Gutheil, & Hamm, 1992; Hamm, 2009). Industry has a vested interest in framing the kind of questions companies would like prescribing providers to ask about new medications. For example, the more advertising frames the salient question as "Which among this new class of drugs is better than the others?" the easier it is to fail to ask "How are these new, usually more expensive, drugs any better than the old ones, or better than alternative treatments?"

3. The peer-review process is absolutely essential in terms of ensuring adherence to the norms of science. In today's industry-dominated climate, peer review is necessary but insufficient in protecting the integrity of the scientific process and the public's health. It should not be assumed that high-impact, prestigious medical journals[6] are immune from publishing studies with design flaws, inappropriate statistical analyses, or questionable conclusions regarding the study drug. It is especially important to read the methods and results section carefully—never relying solely on the abstract and conclusion to provide one with accurate information. For example, the FDA requires that new drug applications be compared against a placebo rather than a comparator drug (i.e., head-to-head comparisons are not required). Therefore, when reading results that favor the study drug, be sure to consider its relevance to real-world prescribing decisions. It is critical to ask whether there is enough information to suggest that this new drug is more effective over the long term than current drugs on the market. Don't be fooled by the use of intermediate or surrogate outcomes. Clinicians should be wary when reading an article where "researchers replace their pre-specified outcome measure with a new one" (Pigott, Leventhal, Alter, & Boren, 2010, p. 269). It is important to ask the following questions: "Does the article/study address the issue of effectiveness (not just short-term efficacy) on a measure that is meaningful to patients?" "What outcome measures were used and are they patient-oriented and clinically relevant?" "Is there enough information on *both* efficacy *and* safety to justify a higher-cost medication?"

4. When reading an industry-sponsored study/article, pay close attention to the financial disclosure statement and, concomitantly, to what role, if any, the funding source played in the design, analysis, or drafting of the study/article. Most medical journals now require authors to precisely identify their individual contributions at the end of the article, which can provide the reader with helpful information about potential conflicts of interest. It has now become more common to see reviewing

---

[6]Witness *The Lancet*'s retraction of previously published research conducted on the causes of autism by Andrew Wakefield (*The Lancet, 375*, issue 9713, February 6, 2010, p. 445).

bodies or editors make statements that they found no evidence of influence because of these financial ties. Unfortunately, it is far less common for there to be transparency about this review process, for typically no information is provided about how this determination was made. In light of this lack of transparency, it is important to look for studies that are not sponsored by industry and compare these results with industry-sponsored ones. The *Cochrane Central Register of Controlled Trials*[7] is part of an international effort to "create an unbiased source of data for systematic reviews" and is an informative and impartial resource.

5. Because continuing medical education (CME) events are often industry sponsored, it is suggested that prescribing psychologists seek out educational events that do not have corporate sponsorship. For example, PharmedOut is an excellent source of CME events that are web-based and aim to provide unbiased information about medications. This nonprofit organization is a Georgetown University Medical Center project "run by physicians for physicians and other providers in order to document and disseminate information about how pharmaceutical companies influence prescribing" (http://www.pharmedout.org/aboutus.htm).

6. Medical subspecialty organizations that are themselves conflicted—because they rely heavily on various forms of pharmaceutical funding—will produce practice guidelines that are equally conflicted. Shaneyfelt and Centor (2009) sum this point up well: "Too many current guidelines have become marketing and opinion-based pieces . . . only when likely biases of industry and specialty societies have been either removed or overcome by countervailing interests can impartial recommendations be achieved" (pp. 868–869). Although the American Psychiatric Association has taken many important steps to restore public trust and increase transparency, concerns remain as to whether these policy changes have resulted in the development of objective, balanced, and cogent treatment recommendations.

For example, in 2008 and in 2010, two meta-analyses on the efficacy of antidepressants were published in *Public Library of Science* (*PLoS*) and *Journal of the American Medical Association* (*JAMA*), respectively. The *JAMA* study found that "the magnitude of benefit of AD medication compared with placebo increases with severity of depression symptoms and may be minimal or non-existent, on average, in patients with mild or moderate symptoms" (Fournier et al., 2010). The research team who previously conducted a meta-analysis drew an even stronger conclusion: "[T]he relationship between initial severity and antidepressant efficacy is attributable to **decreased responsiveness to placebo among very depressed patients rather than increased responsiveness to medication** [emphasis added]" (Kirsch et al., 2008). In October 2010, the American Psychiatric Association published a new CPG on major depressive disorder in which the authors reference these important meta-analytic studies. However, the major depressive disorder guideline produced by the Association makes the following recommendation: "An antidepressant medication is recommended as an initial treatment choice for patients with mild to moderate depression" (American Psychiatric Association, 2010, p. 17). Although to the Association's credit, the authors suggest that patient preference and other clinical features should be taken into account when developing a treatment plan and that use of psychotherapy alone may also be a choice for mildly depressed individuals, there

---

[7]See http://uscc.cochrane.org/en/newPage3.html

is far more coverage devoted to pharmacological interventions than to psychothera-peutic or lifestyle changes even for mild depression.

It is not surprising that these guidelines are promoting its members' interests. "[T]he guild of healthcare professionals—including their specialty societies—has a primary responsibility to promote its members' interests. . . . It is only in healthcare that the same group that provides a service tells us how valuable that service is and how much of it we need" (Quanstrum & Hayward, 2010, p. 1078). Until the development of practice guidelines is centralized under a government agency (see, e.g., Shaneyfelt & Centor, 2009), it will not be possible to eliminate undue industry influence and achieve balanced, concise, and impartial recommendations. Therefore, medical psychologists should adopt the same critical and reflective comportment toward practice guidelines as they do toward peer-reviewed journal articles.

Finally, it should be clear that a researcher's mere association with industry does not imply that any particular researcher will inevitably engage in scientific misconduct or will make unintentional design or data choices that favored industry. In fact, some have argued that framing the problem as conflict of interest is itself problematic for that very reason—it focuses attention only on individuals and makes it seem like industry ties "are a purely individual problem—that an individual has a conflict and we need to manage it" (Elliott, 2010, p. 161). Financial ties between industry and academic researchers point out the generic risk (Thompson, 2009) that the research process may be compromised or that public trust could be eroded; "the point is to minimize or eliminate circumstances that would cause reasonable persons to sus-pect that professional judgment has been improperly influenced, **whether or not it has** [emphasis added]" (Thompson, 2009, p. 137). In order to enhance public trust in the biomedical field, particularly patient trust in psychopharmacological treatments, we need to develop mechanisms and policies that restore integrity to the scientific process (e.g., by creating firewalls between industry and academic researchers) and thus elimi-nate practices that allow for bias and corruption.

CHAPTER 11 KEY TERMS

Adverse drug reaction: Response to a drug that is noxious and unintended and that occurs at doses normally used for prophylaxis, diagnosis, or therapy of disease.

Biomedical research: Basic research, applied research, or translational research con-ducted to aid and support the body of knowledge in the field of medicine.

CenterWatch: Largest online database of global clinical trials involving new drugs and devices regulated by the FDA and the Department of Health and Human Services.

Chemical restraint: Form of medical restraint in which a drug is used to restrict the freedom or movement of a patient or in some cases to sedate a patient.

Clinical practice guidelines: A document with the aim of guiding decisions and crite-ria regarding diagnosis, management, and treatment in specific areas of health care.

Cochrane Central Register of Controlled Trials: Bibliographic database of definitive controlled trials.

Conditional prescribing certificate: Certificate provided by the New Mexico Board of Psychologist Examiners to qualified prescribing psychologists, which requires them to practice under the supervision of a licensed physician for two years. Subsequently, the prescribing psychologist can apply for an unrestricted certificate.

Conflict of interest: Occurs when an individual or organization is involved in multiple interests, one of which could possibly corrupt the motivation for an act in the other.

Contract research organization (CRO): Also called a clinical research organization, a CRO is a service organization that provides support to the pharmaceutical and biotechnology industries in the form of outsourced pharmaceutical research services.

Department of Defense Psychology Demonstration Project (PDP): The 1991 Department of Defense (DoD) initiated program designed to train doctoral-level psychologists to prescribe psychotropic medications. The program was housed in the psychology department at Walter Reed Army Medical Center and trained 10 psychologists.

Dispense as written (DAW): Indication on a prescription that the prescribed medication should not be substituted for a different or generic medication.

Drug–drug interaction: An alteration of the effect of a drug when administered with another drug.

Drug–food interaction: An alteration of the effect of a drug when administered with a particular food.

Efficacy-effectiveness gap: Difference between results achieved in efficacy trials and those observed by practitioners treating real patients in common settings.

Evidence-based pharmacological practice: Pharmacology practice based on available evidence supporting use of particular medications with particular disorders, diseases, or conditions.

Hard copy script: Medication or medical procedure order written out by hand or printed on paper.

Iatrogenic harm: Harm caused to the patient due to the medical intervention.

Informed consent: A legal procedure to ensure that a patient understands all of the risks and costs involved in a treatment. The elements of informed consent include informing the client of the nature of the treatment, possible alternative treatments, and the potential risks and benefits of the treatment.

Medication formulary: A list of generic and brand-name medications that a pharmacy or clinic has available to dispense.

Me-too drug: A drug that is structurally very similar to already known drugs, with only minor differences. The term is generally used in a negative manner to describe the pharmaceutical industry's desire to make money instead of adding a novel therapy.

Patent extender: Making a minor change in the molecular structure of a new drug in order to extend the exclusive rights to market a previously successful medication.

Patient education: Process by which health professionals impart information to patients that will alter their health behaviors or improve their health status.

Pharmaceutical detailing: The practice of pharmaceutical representatives to provide information about their company's products to individual health care providers and, in return for the provider's time, give gifts, such as trips or expensive dinners.

Pharmaceutical marketing practice: Pharmaceutical companies' practice of influencing health care providers and patients regarding choices of medical therapy.

Practice Guidelines Regarding Psychologists' Involvement in Pharmacological Issues: First comprehensive practice guidelines for psychologists engaged in pharmacotherapy at all three levels of training in pharmacotherapy. Consists of 17 specific guidelines broken down into five themes (general, education, assessment, intervention and consultation, and relationships).

Semantic decision-making bias: Phenomenon in which fine shades of the meaning of words bias decisions.

Surrogate outcome measures: Substitutes for real clinical outcome measures, or measured in parallel to such measures. They are often chosen as they can be quantified to produce statistical significance by studying a smaller population than would be needed to study the real clinical outcomes of actual overall morbidity or mortality on an intention-to-treat basis.

Verbal order: An order for a medication or medical procedure either in person, via phone, or via some form of electronic media. It is a substitute, often in emergency situations, for a written order.

Chapter 11 Questions

1. Surrogate decision making
   a. Is for patients who have lost the ability to make rational and logical decisions.
   b. May require that a surrogate be designated by a court.
   c. Is usually performed by the next of kin.
   d. All of the above.
2. The general elements that must be addressed in the process of obtaining informed consent for treatment are
   a. Information and consent.
   b. Age and intelligence.
   c. Intelligence and psychopathology.
   d. Comprehension and coercion.
3. What is the primary business objective of pharmaceutical companies?
   a. To generate profits for stockholders
   b. To promote the welfare of all people
   c. To advance scientific knowledge
   d. To educate prescribers
4. Involuntary drug treatment could be the basis of a civil suit based on all of the following *except*
   a. A malpractice claim of battery.
   b. Negligent failure to provide informed consent.
   c. A violation of constitutional right to privacy.
   d. The insanity defense.

5. The biomedical ethical principle of *autonomy* is concerned with
   a. The right of the government to assert its parens patriae authority over individuals in need.
   b. The right of the individual to govern his or her affairs without external restraint.
   c. The right of parents to direct the behavior of their children.
   d. The right of health care providers to determine the proper course of treatment.

6. When a patient is seeing two providers concurrently and they appear to disagree on approaches to treatment, what is the best course for the first provider to pursue?
   a. Obtain a release and tell the patient to have the other provider contact him or her.
   b. Ask the patient to decide which approach he or she thinks is best.
   c. Explain fully why one's own approach is preferable.
   d. Obtain a release, discuss the matter with the other provider, and review the issues later with the patient.

7. According to many state laws and court rulings, competent mentally ill prisoners may refuse medication
   a. Under all circumstances.
   b. Only if they obtain a court injunction.
   c. Unless they are judged dangerous to themselves or others.
   d. Only for bona fide religious reasons.

8. In deciding what information to provide to a patient in obtaining informed consent, the courts have generally endorsed
   a. The prevailing cultural standard.
   b. The reasonable person standard.
   c. The professional practice standard.
   d. The *de minimis* standard.

9. How long can psychotropic medication be administered during a psychiatric emergency?
   a. According to delineated state laws
   b. For 24 hours
   c. For as long as the emergency exists
   d. Until the patient refuses

10. In a semistructured environment such as the military, one factor that may potentially impact voluntary health care decision making by individuals is
    a. Learned helplessness.
    b. Coercion by those in authority.
    c. Perceived power and control of the organization over the individual's privileges.
    d. Antiauthoritarian personality traits.

    Answers: (1) d, (2) a, (3) a, (4) d, (5) b, (6) d, (7) c, (8) b, (9) c, and (10) c.

REFERENCES

Ally, G. A. (2010). Nuts and bolts of prescriptive practice. In R. E. McGrath, B. A. Moore, R. E. McGrath, & B. A. Moore (Eds.), *Pharmacotherapy for psychologists: Prescribing and collaborative roles* (pp. 71–87). Washington, DC: American Psychological Association.

American Psychiatric Association. (2000). *Diagnostic and statistical manual of mental disorders: DSM-IV-TR* (4th ed., text rev.). Washington, DC: Author.

American Psychiatric Association. (2010). *Practice guideline for the treatment of patients with major depressive disorder* (3rd ed.). Washington, DC: Author.

American Psychological Association Council of Representatives. (2009). *Practice guidelines regarding psychologists' involvement in pharmacological issues*. Washington, DC: Author. Available at www.apa.org/practice/guidelines/pharmacological-issues.pdf

Angell, M. (2004). *The truth about drug companies: How they deceive us and what to do about it*. New York, NY: Random House.

Bagby, R., Ryder, A., Schuller, D., & Marshall, M. (2004). The Hamilton Depression Rating Scale: Has the gold standard become a lead weight? *American Journal of Psychiatry, 161*(12), 2163–2177.

Bech, P. (2009). Fifty years with the Hamilton scales for anxiety and depression: A tribute to Max Hamilton. *Psychotherapy and Psychosomatics, 78*(4), 202–211.

Bekelman, J. E., Li, Y., & Gross, C. P. (2003). Scope and impact of financial conflicts of interest in biomedical research: A systematic review. *JAMA: Journal of the American Medical Association, 289*, 454–465.

Bero, L., & Rennie, D. (1996). Influences on the quality of published drug studies. *International Journal of Technology Assessment in Health Care, 12*(2), 209–237.

Bluhm, R. (2009). Evidence-based medicine and patient autonomy. *International Journal of Feminist Approaches to Bioethics, 2*(2), 134–151.

Bodenheimer, T. (2000). Uneasy alliance: Clinical investigators and the pharmaceutical industry. *New England Journal of Medicine, 342*(20), 1539–1544.

Buelow, G., & Chafetz, M. (1996). Ethical practice guidelines for clinical pharmacopsychology: Sharpening a new focus in psychology. *Professional Psychology: Research and Practice, 27*(1), 53–58.

Bursztajn, H. J., Chanowitz, B., Gutheil, T. G., & Hamm, R. M. (1992). Micro-effects of language on risk perception in drug prescribing behavior. *Bulletin of the American Academy of Psychiatry & the Law, 20*, 59–66.

Carlat, D. (2010). *Unhinged—The trouble with psychiatry: A doctor's revelation about a profession in crisis*. New York, NY: Free Press.

Center for the Health Care Professions, University of California, San Francisco. (2005). *Trends in US funding for biomedical research*. Retrieved from University of California, San Francisco, Center for the Health Care Professions website: http://www.futurehealth.ucsf.edu/summaries/trends_summary.html

Cosgrove, L., & Bursztajn, H. (2010). Strengthening conflict-of-interest policies in medicine. *Journal of Evaluation in Clinical Practice, 16*(1), 21–24.

Cosgrove, L., Bursztajn, H., Krimsky, S., Anaya, M., & Walker, J. (2009). Conflicts of interest and disclosure in the American Psychiatric Association's clinical practice guidelines. *Psychotherapy and Psychosomatics, 78*(4), 228–232.

Dalton, S., Johansen, C., Mellemkjaer, L., Nørgård, B., Sørensen, H., & Olsen, J. (2003). Use of selective serotonin reuptake inhibitors and risk of upper gastrointestinal tract bleeding: A population-based cohort study. *Archives of Internal Medicine, 163*(1), 59–64.

de Abajo, F., & García-Rodríguez, L. (2008). Risk of upper gastrointestinal tract bleeding associated with selective serotonin reuptake inhibitors and venlafaxine therapy: Interaction with nonsteroidal anti-inflammatory drugs and effect of acid-suppressing agents. *Archives of General Psychiatry, 65*(7), 795–803.

de Koning, M., Bloemen, O., van Amelsvoort, T., Becker, H., Nieman, D., van der Gaag, M., & Linszen, D. (2009). Early intervention in patients at ultra high risk of psychosis: Benefits and risks. *Acta Psychiatrica Scandinavica, 119*(6), 426–442.

Djulbegovic, B., Lacevic, M., Cantor, A., Fields, K. K., Bennett, C. L., Adams, J. R., . . . Lyman, G. H. (2000). The uncertainty principle and industry-sponsored research. *Lancet, 356*(9230), 635–638.

Dorsey, E. R., de Roulet, J., Thompson, J. P., Reminick, J. I., Thai, A., White-Stellato, Z., . . . & Moses, H., III. (2010). Funding of US Biomedical Research, 2003–2008. *Journal of the American Medical Association, 303*(2), 137–143.

Dubovsky, S. L., & Dubovsky, A. N. (2007). *Psychotropic drug prescriber's survival guide: Ethical mental health treatment in the age of Big Pharma.* New York, NY: W. W. Norton.

Elliott, C. (2010). *White coat, black hat: Adventures on the dark side of medicine.* Boston, MA: Beacon.

Falit, B. P. (2007). Curbing industry sponsors' incentive to design post-approval trials that are suboptimal for informing prescribers but more likely than optimal designs to yield favorable results. *Seton Hall Law Review, 37*, 969–1049.

Food and Drug Administration. (2007). *Public Law 110–85—Sept. 27, 2007* (H.R. 3580). Washington, DC: U.S. Government Printing Office.

Food and Drug Administration, Center for Drug Evaluation and Research, Psychopharmacological Drugs Advisory Committee. (1999). *Consideration of NDA 18-936 (S), Prozac® (fluoxetine hydrochloride) Eli Lilly & Co.* (Minutes ID No. 3542m1). Retrieved from http://www.fda.gov/ohrms/dockets/ac/99/minutes/3543m1.pdf

Fortune. (2009). Fortune 500: Our annual ranking of America's largest corporations. *Fortune, 159*(9), F1–F60.

Fournier, J., DeRubeis, R., Hollon, S., Dimidjian, S., Amsterdam, J., Shelton, R., & Fawcett, J. (2010). Antidepressant drug effects and depression severity: A patient-level meta-analysis. *JAMA: Journal of the American Medical Association, 303*(1), 47–53.

Geddes, J. (2003). Generating evidence to inform policy and practice: The example of the second generation "atypical" antipsychotics. *Schizophrenia Bulletin, 29*(1), 105–114.

Gopal, A., Cosgrove, L., & Bursztajn, H. (2010). Commentary: The public health consequences of an industry-influenced psychiatric taxonomy: "Attenuated psychotic symptoms syndrome" as a case example. *Accountability in Research, 17*(5), 264–269.

Gregorian, R., Golden, K., Bahce, A., Goodman, C., Kwong, W., & Khan, Z. (2002). Antidepressant-induced sexual dysfunction. *Annals of Pharmacotherapy, 36*(10), 1577–1589.

Hamm, R. M. (2009). Automatic thinking. In M. W. Kattan (Ed.), *Encyclopedia of medical decision making* (pp. 45–49). Thousand Oaks, CA: Sage Publications.

Healy, D. (2009). Trussed in evidence?: Ambiguities at the interface between clinical evidence and clinical practice. *Transcultural Psychiatry, 16*(1), 16–37.

IMS. (2009). *IMS Health lowers 2009 global pharmaceutical market forecast to 2.5–3.5 percent growth.* Danbury, CT: Author.

Katz, D., Caplan, A. L., & Merz, J. F. (2003). All gifts large and small: Toward an understanding of the ethics of pharmaceutical industry gift-giving. *American Journal of Bioethics, 3*(3), 39–46.

Kenward, M., & Molenberghs, G. (2009). Last observation carried forward: A crystal ball? *Journal of Biopharmaceutical Statistics, 19*(5), 872–888.

Kirsch, I., Deacon, B., Huedo-Medina, T., Scoboria, A., Moore, T., & Johnson, B. (2008). Initial severity and antidepressant benefits: A meta-analysis of data submitted to the Food and Drug Administration. *PLoS Medicine, 5*(2), e45.

Lagomasino, I., Dwight-Johnson, M., & Simpson, G. (2005). Psychopharmacology: The need for effectiveness trials to inform evidence-based psychiatric practice. *Psychiatric Services, 56*(6), 649–651.

Lenzer, J. (2008). Contract research organizations: Truly independent research? *British Journal of Medicine, 337*(211), a1332.

Leon, A., Mallinckrodt, C., Chuang-Stein, C., Archibald, D., Archer, G., & Chartier, K. (2006). Attrition in randomized controlled clinical trials: Methodological issues in psychopharmacology. *Biological Psychiatry, 59*(11), 1001–1005.

Lewis, S., Baird, P., Evans, R. G., Ghali, W. A., Wright, C. J., Gibson, E., & Baylis, F. (2001). Dancing with the porcupine: Rules for governing the university-industry relationship. *Canadian Medical Association Journal, 165*(6), 783–785.

Mather, C. (2005). The pipeline and the porcupine: Alternate metaphors of the physician-industry relationship. *Social Science & Medicine, 60*(6), 1323–1334.

Mauss, M. (1967). *The gift: Forms and functions of exchange in archaic societies* (I. Cunnison, Trans.) New York, NY: W.W. Norton.

McGlashan, T., Zipursky, R., Perkins, D., Addington, J., Miller, T., Woods, S., . . . Breier, A. (2006). Randomized, double-blind trial of olanzapine versus placebo in patients prodromally symptomatic for psychosis. *American Journal of Psychiatry, 163*(5), 790–799.

McGorry, P., Nelson, B., Amminger, G., Bechdolf, A., Francey, S., Berger, G., . . . Yung, A. (2009). Intervention in individuals at ultra-high risk for psychosis: A review and future directions. *Journal of Clinical Psychiatry, 70*(9), 1206–1212.

McGrath, R. E. (2004). Saving our psychosocial souls. *American Psychologist, 59*(7), 644–645.

McGrath, R. E., & Rom-Rymer, B. N. (2010). Ethical considerations in pharmacotherapy for psychologists. In R. E. McGrath, B. A. Moore, R. E. McGrath, & B. A. Moore (Eds.), *Pharmacotherapy for psychologists: Prescribing and collaborative roles* (pp. 89–104). Washington, DC: American Psychological Association.

McGrath, R. E., Wiggins, J. G., Sammons, M. T., Levant, R. F., Brown, A., & Stock, W. (2004). Professional issues in pharmacotherapy for psychologists. *Professional Psychology: Research and Practice, 35*(2), 158–163.

Molnar, F., Man-Son-Hing, M., Hutton, B., & Fergusson, D. (2009). Have last-observation-carried-forward analyses caused us to favour more toxic dementia therapies over less toxic alternatives? A systematic review. *Open Medicine, 3*(2), e31–e50.

Moncrieff, J., & Leo, J. (2010). A systematic review of the effects of antipsychotic drugs on brain volume. *Psychological Medicine, 40*(9), 1409–1422.

Montejo, A., Llorca, G., Izquierdo, J., & Rico-Villademoros, F. (2001). Incidence of sexual dysfunction associated with antidepressant agents: A prospective multicenter study of 1022 outpatients. Spanish Working Group for the Study of Psychotropic-Related Sexual Dysfunction. *Journal of Clinical Psychiatry, 62*(Suppl), 310–321.

National Institute for Health and Clinical Excellence. (2009). *Depression: The NICE guideline on the treatment and management of depression in adults* (updated ed.). London, UK: Author.

Perlis, R. H., Perlis, C. S., Wu, Y., Hwang, C., Joseph, M., & Nierenberg, A. A. (2005). Industry sponsorship and financial conflict of interest in the reporting of clinical trials in psychiatry. *American Journal of Psychiatry, 162*, 1957–1960.

Pigott, H., Leventhal, A., Alter, G., & Boren, J. (2010). Efficacy and effectiveness of antidepressants: Current status of research. *Psychotherapy and Psychosomatics, 79*(5), 267–279.

Pitrou, I., Boutron, I., Ahmad, N., & Ravaud, P. (2009). Reporting of safety results in published reports of randomized controlled trials. *Archives of Internal Medicine, 169,* 1756–1761.

Quanstrum, K., & Hayward, R. (2010). Lessons from the mammography wars. *New England Journal of Medicine, 363*(11), 1076–1079.

Rhoades, L. (2004). *ORI closed investigations into misconduct allegations involving research supported by the Public Health Service: 1994–2003.* Washington, DC: Office of Research Integrity.

Sammons, M. T. (2010). The Psychopharmacology Demonstration Project: What did it teach us, and where are we now? In R. E. McGrath, B. A. Moore, R. E. McGrath, & B. A. Moore (Eds.), *Pharmacotherapy for psychologists: Prescribing and collaborative roles* (pp. 49–67). Washington, DC: American Psychological Association.

Seeman, S. V. (2001). Clinical trials in psychiatry: Do results apply to practice? *Canadian Journal of Psychiatry, 46,* 352–355.

Shaneyfelt, T., & Centor, R. (2009). Reassessment of clinical practice guidelines: Go gently into that good night. *JAMA: Journal of the American Medical Association, 301*(8), 868–869.

Shaughnessy, A. (2009). Evaluating and understanding articles about treatment. *American Family Physician, 79*(8), 668–670.

Shaughnessy, A., & Slawson, D. (2004). Blowing the whistle on review articles. *British Medical Journal, 328*(7440), E280–E282.

Sismondo, S. (2008). How pharmaceutical industry funding affects trial outcomes: Causal structures and responses. *Social Science & Medicine, 66*(9), 1909–1914.

Smyer, M. A., Balster, R. L., Egli, D., Johnson, D. L., Kilbey, M., Leith, N. J., & Puente, A. E. (1993). Summary of the report of the Ad Hoc Task Force on Psychopharmacology of the American Psychological Association. *Professional Psychology: Research and Practice, 24*(4), 394–403.

Spina, E., Santoro, V., & D'Arrigo, C. (2008). Clinically relevant pharmacokinetic drug interactions with second-generation antidepressants: An update. *Clinical Therapeutics, 30,* 1206–1227.

Thompson, D. (2009). The challenge of conflict of interest in medicine. *Zeitschrift für Evidenz, Fortbildung und Qualität im Gesundheitswesen, 103*(3), 136–140.

Tiefer, L. (2004). *Sex is not a natural act & other essays* (2nd ed.). Boulder, CO: Westview.

Tuccori, M., Testi, A., Antonioli, L., Fornai, M., Montagnani, S., Ghisu, N., & Del Tacca, M. (2009). Safety concerns associated with the use of serotonin reuptake inhibitors and other serotonergic/noradrenergic antidepressants during pregnancy: A review. *Clinical Therapeutics, 31*(11), 1426–1453.

Wilson, D. (2010, June 19). Drug for sexual desire disorder opposed by panel. *New York Times,* B3.

Wood, J. M., Koch, P. B., & Mansfield, P. K. (2006). Women's sexual desire: A feminist critique. *Journal of Sex Research, 43*(3), 236–244.

Woods, S., Addington, J., Cadenhead, K., Cannon, T., Cornblatt, B., Heinssen, R., . . . McGlashan, T. (2009). Validity of the prodromal risk syndrome for first psychosis: Findings from the North American Prodrome Longitudinal Study. *Schizophrenia Bulletin, 35*(5), 894–908.

Woolley, S. B., Cardoni, A. A., & Goethe, J. W. (2009) Last-observation-carried-forward imputation method in clinical efficacy trials: Review of 352 antidepressant studies. *Pharmacotherapy, 29,* 1408–1416.

World Medical Association. (2004). Declaration of Helsinki: Ethical principles for medical research involving human subjects. Retrieved from http://web.archive.org/web/20071027224123/www .wma.net/e/policy/pdf/17c.pdf

Yung, A., Nelson, B., Thompson, A., & Wood, S. (2010). The psychosis threshold in ultra high risk (prodromal) research: Is it valid? *Schizophrenia Research, 120*(1–3), 1–6.

Zimmerman, M., Posternak, M., & Chelminski, I. (2002). Symptom severity and exclusion from antidepressant efficacy trials. *Journal of Clinical Psychopharmacology, 22*(6), 610–614.

Subject/Author* Index

ABAB design, 436, 447
Abilify (aripiprazole), 119, 145–146, 151, 204, 207, 255, 331, 363, 371, 389, 417–418, 435
Absence seizures, 139, 163, 173
Absolute risk, 443, 447, 453
Absorption, 98, 196, 198, 200, 208, 218, 221–224, 236, 261, 263, 276, 321, 327–328, 331, 335, 337, 340–341, 343, 374, 394, 402, 423, 425
Abstinence-violation effect, 422
Academy of Medical Psychology, 2, 6, 11
Accuracy, 250, 251, 273
Acetylation, 330, 343
Acetylcholine, 57, 59, 62–63, 82, 85, 90, 92, 101, 110, 144, 152, 165, 177, 215, 222, 225, 270, 273, 410
Acetylcholinesterase inhibitors, 270, 273
Action potential, 48, 53–56, 72, 90–91, 93, 97–98, 101, 141, 159, 214, 217, 399
Activated microglia, 108, 110, 163
Activation ratio, 118, 163
Active transport, 51, 197, 220, 223, 230
Activities of Daily Living (ADL), 245, 269, 273, 307
Acute pain, 158–159, 163, 387
Adderall (amphetamine), 38, 144, 147, 156, 204, 227, 260, 269, 288, 292–293, 295, 322, 343, 366–367, 370, 377, 394–395, 407, 410–411, 420–421, 427
Addiction medicine, 290, 296, 311
Addison disease, 260
Adenosine, 57, 61, 70, 71, 196, 206, 226
Adenosine triphosphate (ATP), 59, 164, 166, 195, 211, 230
Adiocytes, 227, 230
Adipose, 197, 207, 230, 254

Adverse drug event, 265, 273
Adverse drug reaction (ADR), 265–267, 273, 373, 395–399, 422, 461, 473
Afferent, 48, 84, 86, 90, 93, 94, 96
After-depolarization, 56, 93
After-hyperpolarization, 56, 93
Agonist, 47, 59, 93, 118, 144, 146, 154, 156, 157, 173, 304, 312, 405, 411, 418, 419, 421, 423
Akathisia, 151, 153, 157, 163, 308, 309, 310, 312
Akathisia (iatrogenic neuroleptic), 309, 311
Akinesia, 148, 149, 151, 152, 163, 167
Albumin, 206, 210, 225, 254, 258, 273, 274
Albuterol, 303, 311
Alcohol-related neurodevelopmental disorders, 123, 163
Algorithms, 20, 23, 25, 30–32, 33, 35
Allegiance effects, 432, 447
Ally, Glenn, x–xi
ALP (alkaline phosphatase), 225, 258, 273
Alpha level, 439, 440, 447, 448
Alpha synuclein, 115, 116, 163
Alpha-1 glycoprotein, 405
Alprazolam (Xanax), 219, 360, 361, 383, 415, 416
ALT (alanine amino transferase), 258, 273
Alternative hypothesis, 439, 447
Ambien (zolpidem), 361, 405, 416
American Society for the Advancement of Pharmacotherapy, x, 2, 11, 241, 458
Amphetamine, 144, 147, 204, 227, 269, 370, 394, 395, 407, 410, 420
Amitriptyline, 116, 263, 266, 355, 369, 377, 413
Amyloid beta, 108, 163, 168

---

* Authors are indexed in italics.

485

Poor metabolizer (PM), 313
Portal circulation, 373, 374
Potency, 22, 146, 361, 415
Postconcussive Syndrome, 134, 135, 173
Postganglionic fibers, 92
Postictal sleep, 139, 173
Power, 10, 143, 433, 439, 440, 444, 451, 466
Power analysis, 439, 440, 451
Practice effect, 435, 451
Practice guidelines, 6, 7, 8, 12, 242, 276,
    457, 458, 459, 460, 472, 473, 475
Prader-Willi syndrome, 124, 173
Preexisting groups design, 434, 451
Preganglionic fibers, 92, 98
Premorbid personality, 291
Prescriptive authority for psychologists,
    5, 12, 154, 458
Presenting complaint, 244, 276, 299
Preston, John, 266
Presumptive clues, 286, 313
Pretest-posttest design, 436, 451
Primary brain injury, 136, 174
Primary care psychology, 1, 3, 12, 272
Prion protein, 116, 174
PRISMA statement, 443, 451
Prodrug, 399, 421
Prolactin, 65, 145, 174, 203, 205, 263, 264,
    364, 388, 389, 390
Prolonged QT Interval, 217, 235,
    276, 388, 418
Prominence, 225, 235
Prophylaxis, 292, 399, 400, 419, 424
Prospective study, 451
Protein kinase, 61, 98
Proteolytic enzymes, 136, 174
Prozac (fluoxetine), 376, 404, 414, 466
Psychobiosocial, 1, 3, 4, 5, 6, 17, 19, 24, 34,
    47, 111, 157, 246, 270, 294, 421
Psychopharmacology, 1, 2, 3, 4, 6, 9, 10,
    17, 23, 25, 32, 33, 61, 63, 64, 152, 161,
    193, 203, 210, 212, 217, 241, 244, 247,
    248, 249, 256, 260, 267, 269, 271, 291,
    295, 311, 353, 354, 373, 413, 431, 457,
    458, 463
Psychopharmacology Examination for
    Psychologist (PEP), 247, 276
Psychosocial interventions, 19, 21, 22, 25,
    28, 35, 296, 431, 435
Psychosomatic medicine, 287, 289, 313
Reduplicative paramnesia, 284, 313

Review of systems (ROS), 244, 246, 276,
    289, 301, 313
Purkinje cell, 50, 88, 98
Putamen, 83, 98, 115, 126, 149, 174
Pyramidal cell, 79, 80, 83, 98, 143
Pyramidal neurons, 67, 80, 143, 174
Pyrimidine, 47, 98
Pyrogens, 199, 235

Quadrants, 250, 276
Quantal dose response curve, xxiii
Quasi-experiment, 434, 435, 436, 451
Quetiapine (Seroquel), 145, 418
Quillin, James, 242

Rabbit syndrome, 151, 152, 153, 174
Racemic mix, 420
Randomized controlled trials, 25,
    434, 451
Rapamycin, 126, 174
Raphe nuclei, 65, 66, 86, 88, 98
Reality distortion syndrome, 142, 174
Receptor potential, 53, 98
Reduction, 25, 27, 75, 118, 122, 143,
    146, 162, 173, 264, 308, 376, 380, 381,
    382, 383, 384, 385, 397, 401, 410, 411,
    416, 468
Rehabilitation psychology, 1, 12, 244
Reinforcer, 146, 147, 174
Relapse prevention, 399, 400, 408, 424
Relative risk, 142, 201, 202, 442, 443, 451
Relative risk ratio, 441, 451
Reliability, 250, 299, 403, 433, 444, 445,
    451, 466
Remeron (mirtazapine), 358
Renin, 208, 235
Repeated measures design, 435, 451
Resorption, 209, 225, 235
Restless leg, 148, 149, 157, 174
Retinohypothalamic fibers, 87, 98
Retrograde messenger, 69, 70, 98
Retrograde neuronal transport, 76, 98
Retrospective study, 451
Retrosplenial cortex, 82, 98
Reuptake, 51, 57, 62, 63, 64, 66, 67, 68, 69,
    92, 98, 116, 144, 147, 175, 204, 263, 270,
    305, 359, 368, 380, 381, 403, 413, 414,
    419, 420, 421
Review of systems (ROS), 244, 246, 276,
    289, 301, 313